Infectious Disease:
Pathogenesis, Prevention, and Case Studies

N. Shetty
Department of Clinical Microbiology,
University College London Hospitals

J.W. Tang
Division of Microbiology/Molecular Diagnostic Centre,
Department of Laboratory Medicine,
National University Hospital,
Singapore

J. Andrews
Department of Clinical Microbiology,
University College London

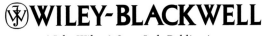

WILEY-BLACKWELL

A John Wiley & Sons, Ltd., Publication

This edition first published 2009, © 2009 by N. Shetty, J.W. Tang and J. Andrews

Blackwell Publishing was acquired by John Wiley & Sons in February 2007. Blackwell's publishing program has been merged with Wiley's global Scientific, Technical and Medical business to form Wiley-Blackwell.

Registered office: John Wiley & Sons Ltd, The Atrium, Southern Gate, Chichester, West Sussex, PO19 8SQ, UK

Editorial offices: 9600 Garsington Road, Oxford, OX4 2DQ, UK
      The Atrium, Southern Gate, Chichester, West Sussex, PO19 8SQ, UK
      111 River Street, Hoboken, NJ 07030-5774, USA

For details of our global editorial offices, for customer services and for information about how to apply for permission to reuse the copyright material in this book please see our website at www.wiley.com/wiley-blackwell

Library of Congress Cataloguing-in-Publication Data
Shetty, N. (Nandini)
   Infectious disease : pathogenesis, prevention, and case studies / N. Shetty, J.W. Tang, J. Andrews.
     p. ; cm.
   Includes bibliographical references and index.
   ISBN 978-1-4051-3543-6 (hardcover : alk. paper) 1. Communicable diseases. I. Tang, J.W. (Julian W.)
II. Andrews, J. (Julie) III. Title.
   [DNLM: 1. Communicable Diseases–etiology. 2. Communicable Disease Control–methods.
WC 100 S554i 2009]
   RC111.S458 2009
   616.9–dc22

                       2008042548

ISBN: 9781405135436

A catalogue record for this book is available from the British Library.

Set in 11/13pt Bembo by Graphicraft Limited, Hong Kong
Printed and bound in Malaysia by Vivar Printing Sdn Bhd

1 2009

Contents

Editors and Contributors, iv
Preface, v
Glossary of abbreviated terms, vii

PART 1 GENERAL PRINCIPLES OF INFECTIOUS DISEASES, 1

1 Microbial etiology of disease N. Shetty, E. Aarons, J. Andrews, 3
2 Structure and function of microbes N. Shetty, E. Aarons, J. Andrews, 15
3 Host defence versus microbial pathogenesis and the mechanisms of microbial escape N. Shetty, E. Aarons, J. Andrews, 41
4 Diagnosis of microbial infection N. Shetty, M. Wren, E. Aarons, J. Andrews, 85
5 General principles of antimicrobial chemotherapy N. Shetty, E. Aarons, J. Andrews, 124
6 Basic concepts of the epidemiology of infectious diseases N. Shetty, 157

PART 2 A SYSTEMS BASED APPROACH TO INFECTIOUS DISEASES, 177

7 Infections of the skin, soft tissue, bone, and joint N. Shetty, J.W. Tang, 179
8 Gastroenteritis N. Shetty, J.W. Tang, 212
9 Cardiac and respiratory tract infections N. Shetty, J.W. Tang, J. Andrews, 238
10 Infections of the central nervous system N. Shetty, J.W. Tang, 271
11 Infections of the genitourinary system N. Shetty, R. Smith, 294

PART 3 INFECTIONS IN SPECIAL GROUPS, 333

12 Obstetric, congenital and neonatal infections N. Shetty, J.W. Tang, J. Andrews, 335
13 Infections in the immunocompromised host D. Mack, N. Shetty, 363
14 Healthcare associated infections N. Shetty, 393
15 The fever and rash conundrum: rashes of childhood J.W. Tang, 414

PART 4 INFECTIONS OF GLOBAL IMPACT, 435

16 Tuberculosis S. Srivastava, N. Shetty, 437
17 Malaria D. Mack, 458
18 Human immunodeficiency virus (HIV) and acquired immunodeficiency syndrome (AIDS) J.W. Tang, 476
19 Viral hepatitis J.W. Tang, 491
20 Influenza J.W. Tang, P.K.S. Chan, 506
21 Infections in the returning traveler N. Shetty, 521

PART 5 EMERGING AND RESURGENT INFECTIONS, 551

22 Viral hemorrhagic fevers J.W. Tang, 553
23 Emerging infections I (human monkeypox, hantaviruses, Nipah virus, Japanese encephalitis, chikungunya) J.W. Tang, 567
24 Emerging infections II (West Nile virus, dengue, severe acute respiratory syndrome-associated coronavirus) J.W. Tang, P.K.S. Chan, 583
25 Diphtheria N. Shetty, 599
26 Agents of bioterrorism J.W. Tang, 607

Answers to test yourself questions, 627
Index, 647

Editors and Contributors

N. Shetty
Consultant Microbiologist and Honorary Senior Lecturer, Department of Clinical Microbiology, University College London Hospitals

J.W. Tang
Consultant Virologist, Division of Microbiology/Molecular Diagnostic Centre, Department of Laboratory Medicine, National University Hospital, Singapore

J. Andrews
Consultant Microbiologist, Department of Clinical Microbiology, University College London

E. Aarons
Consultant Virologist, University College London, UK

P.K.S. Chan
Professor, Department of Microbiology, The Chinese University of Hong Kong, Prince of Wales Hospital, Hong Kong

D. Mack
Consultant Microbiologist, Barnet & Chase Farm Hospitals, London, UK

R. Smith
Consultant Microbiologist, The Royal Free Hospital, London, UK

S. Srivastava
Specialist Registrar in Microbiology, Royal Devon and Exeter Hospitals, Exeter, Devon, UK

M. Wren
Consultant Biomedical Scientist, University College London Hospitals, UK

Preface

Infectious Disease: Pathogenesis, Prevention, and Case Studies is a new textbook written in the modern era of widespread and ready access to internet resources. The book is aimed at university students with interest in infectious diseases. The level of the text is at an intermediate to senior undergraduate college level and will give the student a sense of the many areas of infectious disease in which he/she may want to specialize further, e.g. an infectious disease clinician, a public health physician, a basic science researcher, or perhaps even a medical journalist specializing in infectious diseases.

Topics covered include hospital-acquired infections, emerging and re-emerging infections, infections in the immunocompromised, in pregnancy and in children. The multidisciplinary text makes it suitable for clinical (and perhaps some more basic) microbiology, public health and infectious disease epidemiology courses. A special feature is the extensive use of illustrative clinical cases (many of them based on real cases seen by the authors), which have been included to reinforce some of the concepts touched upon in that chapter.

The text is organized into chapters on infections of specific organ systems as well as chapters on specific organisms. This has been done to allow the text to be used on a wide variety of different courses, as well as by different student learning strategies. The style as well as the detail of the text varies from chapter to chapter, reflecting the specialties of the individual authors, but also includes standard items, i.e. sections on epidemiology, pathogenesis, clinical features, diagnosis and treatment, as well as Q&A sections (with answers in the back) and boxes describing specific areas of interest and relevance in each chapter theme. Other boxes are designed to encourage students to think about certain issues, and here, answers are not provided and the student is encouraged to read further.

The textbook is sufficient for a complete course in infectious diseases, covering all the major pathogen groups (i.e. bacteria, fungi, parasites, and viruses). It can also be used in specialist modules that may last only one or two semesters, e.g. on hospital-acquired infections, emerging infections, infections of childhood, pregnancy, returning travelers, or the immunocompromised. Teaching can be organized at an organ system level, with specialist modules on specific organisms, e.g. respiratory infections with further detail in a chapter on influenza or infections of the immunocompromised with a specialist chapter on HIV. Although there is extensive cross-referencing between the chapters, each chapter has been written to also stand alone, and the book does not necessarily need to be read in the order in which the chapters are presented.

Since the worldwide severe acute respiratory syndrome (SARS) outbreaks of 2003, the ongoing HIV/AIDS pandemic, and the more recent preparedness for a possibly approaching influenza pandemic, internet resources for infectious diseases have become invaluable for tracking and updating information on infectious diseases worldwide. These include comprehensive, easily navigated websites at the Center for Disease Control and Prevention (CDC: http://www.cdc.gov/), the World Health Organization (WHO: http://www.who.int/), and email alert systems like ProMED (http://www.promedmail.org/). In addition, there are now excellent online medical resources, such as eMedicine (www.emedicine.com/) and Medscape (www.medscape.com/).

This text incorporates some of these online resources as part of the recommended 'Further Reading' in many of the chapters, as it is understood by the authors that the reference journal articles and textbooks, which are also listed, may be less accessible to many readers.

In addition, many of the images used in the book are from freely available online resources, particularly the CDC Public Health Image Library (http://phil.cdc.gov/phil/home.asp), which allows students to download such images (after having been directed to them by the main text) for their own use, either as revision and aidé-memoirs, or for their own presentations. A CD is also included containing other images created specially for this book for similar purposes.

This text has been reviewed by teaching staff at many universities. The authors have taken the feedback/comments seriously and made appropriate amendments to the text to enhance its quality for both accuracy and student teaching.

Nandini Shetty, Julie Andrews (University College London)
Julian Tang (National University Hospital, Singapore)

Glossary of abbreviated terms

AAC	*N*-acetyltransferases
AAD	antibiotic associated diarrhea
Ab	antibody
ADCC	antibody-dependent cellular cytotoxicity
ADE	antibody-dependent enhancement
ADEM	acute disseminated encephalomyelitis
ADPR	adenine diphosphate ribose
AIDS	acquired immune deficiency syndrome
ALT	alanine amino transferase
ANT	*O*-adenyltransferases
APC	antigen presenting cell
APH	*O*-phosphotransferases
ARDS	acute respiratory distress syndrome
ART	antiretroviral therapy
ASP	amnesic shellfish poisoning
ATP	adenosine triphosphate
ATS	American Thoracic Society
AZT	azidothymidine
BAL	bronchoalveolar lavage
BBB	blood–brain barrier
BCG	Bacille Calmette Guerin
BCYE	buffered charcoal yeast extract
BL	Biosafety Level
BOOP	bronchiolitis obliterans organizing pneumonia
BSAC	British Society for Antimicrobial Chemotherapy
BSE	bovine spongiform encephalopathy
BSI	bloodstream infections
BTWC	Biological and Toxin Weapons Convention
BV	bacterial vaginosis
CAP	community acquired pneumonia
CCHF	Crimean-Congo hemorrhagic fever
CDC	Centers for Disease Control and Prevention
CF	cystic fibrosis
CFA	colonizing factor antigen
CGD	chronic granulomatous disease
CLSI	Clinical and Laboratory Standards Institute
CMV	cytomegalovirus
CNS	central nervous system
CoNS	coagulase negative staphylococci
COPD	chronic obstructive pulmonary disease
CoV	coronaviruses
CPE	cytopathic effect
CRC	congenital rubella syndrome
CRF	circulating recombinant forms
CRP	C reactive protein

CSF	cerebrospinal fluid
CSF	colony-stimulating factor
CT	computed tomography
CTL	cytotoxic T lymphocytes
CVS	congenital varicella syndrome
CWD	chronic wasting disease
d4T	stavudine
DAP	diaminopimelic acid
DDC	zalcitabine
DDI	didanosine
DDT	dichloro-diphenyl-trichloroethane
DFA	direct fluorescent assay
DHF	dengue hemorrhagic fever
DHF	dihydrofolate
DIC	disseminated intravascular coagulation
DIN	Deutsches Institut für Normung (English: the German Institute for Standardization)
DNA	deoxyribonucleic acid
DSP	diarrheic shellfish poisoning
dsRNA	double-stranded ribonucleic acid
DSS	dengue shock syndrome
DTH	delayed-type hypersensitivity
EAEC	entero-aggregative *E. coli*
EB	elementary body
EBV	Epstein–Barr virus
ECL	electrochemiluminescence
EEG	electroencephalography
EF	elongation factor
EGD	esophagogastroduodenoscopy
EHEC	enterohemorrhagic *E. coli*
EIA	enzyme-linked immunoassay
EIEC	enteroinvasive *E. coli*
EKG	electrocardiogram
ELISA	enzyme-linked immunosorbent assay
ELONA	enzyme-linked oligonucleotide assay
EM	electron microscopy
EPEC	entero-pathogenic *E. coli*
EPP	exposure-prone procedures
ER	emergency room
ESBL	extended spectrum beta-lactamase
ET	exfoliatin toxin
ETEC	entero-toxigenic *E. coli*
EV	enterovirus
FDA	Food and Drug Administration
FPA	fluorescence polarization assay
FRET	fluorescence (or Forster) resonance energy transfer
G6PD	glucose-6-phosphate dehydrogenase deficiency
GABHS	group A beta-hemolytic streptococci
GBS	group B beta-hemolytic streptococci
G-CSF	granulocyte-colony stimulating factor
GE	gastroenteritis

GI	gastrointestinal
GISA	glycopeptide intermediate *Staphylococcus aureus*
GLC	gas–liquid chromatography
GM-CSF	granulocyte/monocyte colony stimulating factor
GMS	Gomori methenamine silver
GRE	glycopeptide-resistant enterococci
GTP	guanosine triphosphate
GTPase	guanosine triphosphatase
GVHD	graft versus host disease
HAART	highly active antiretroviral therapy
HACEK	*Haemophilus, Actinobacillus, Cardiobacterium, Eikenella, Kingella*
HAI	healthcare associated infections
HAV	hepatitis A
HBeAg	HBe antigen
HBIG	HBV immunoglobulin
HBoV	human bocavirus
HBsAg	hepatitis B surface antigen
HBV	hepatitis B virus
HCMV	human cytomegalovirus
HCV	hepatitis C virus
HCW	healthcare workers
HDsAg	hepatitis D surface antigen
HDV	hepatitis D virus
HEL	human embryonic lung
HERV	human endogenous retrovirus
HEV	hepatitis E virus
HFMD	hand-foot-and-mouth disease
HFRS	hemorrhagic fever with renal syndrome
HHV	human herpes virus
HI	herd immunity
Hib	*Haemophilus influenzae* type b
HIG	human immune globulin
HIT	herd immunity threshold
HIV	human immunodeficiency virus
hMPV	human metapneumovirus
HPS	hantavirus pulmonary syndrome
HPV	human papilloma virus
HRP-2	histidine-rich protein 2
HSCT	hematopoietic stem cell transplantation
HSV	herpes simplex virus
HTLV	human T cell leukemia/lymphoma virus
HUS	hemolytic uremic syndrome
ICP	intracranial pressure
ICU	intensive care unit
IDDM	insulin-dependent diabetes mellitus
IDSA	Infectious Disease Society of America
IDU	injecting drug users
IE	infective endocarditis
IF	immunofluorescence
IFA	immunofluorescence assay

IFN	interferon
Ig	immunoglobulin
IL	interleukin
IM	intramuscular
IPT	intermittent preventive treatment
ITN	insecticide-treated net
IUGR	intrauterine growth retardation
IV	intravenous
IVDU	intravenous drug user
IVIg	intravenous immunoglobulin
JCV-PML	JC virus progressive multifocal leukoencephalopathy
JE	Japanese encephalitis
KSHV	Kaposi's sarcoma associated herpes virus
LAM	lipoarabinomannan
LDH	lactate dehydrogenase
LGV	lymphogranuloma venereum
LLO	listeriolysin O
LPS	lipopolysaccharide
LRT	lower respiratory tract
LT	labile toxin
LTA	lipoteichoic acids
LTBI	latent TB infection
M	macrophage
MAC	*Mycobacterium avium* complex
MALT	mucosal associated lymphoid tissue
MAT	microagglutination test
MBL	mannose binding lectin
MBP	major basic protein
MCP	monocyte chemoattractant protein
MCV	meningococcal conjugate vaccine
MDCK	Madin-Darby canine kidney
MDR-TB	multi-drug resistant tuberculosis
MHC	major histocompatibility complex
MIC	minimum inhibitory concentration
MIP	macrophage inflammatory protein
MMR	measles-mumps-rubella
MMWR	*Morbidity and Mortality Weekly Report*
MR	mannose receptors
MRI	magnetic resonance imaging
MRSA	methicillin resistant *Staphylococcus aureus*
MS	multiple sclerosis
MSM	men who have sex with men
MTB	*M. tuberculosis*
MTCT	mother-to-child-transmission
MVA	Modified Vaccinia Virus Ankara
NAD	nicotinamide adenine dinucleotide
NAG	*N*-acteylglucosamine
NAI	neuraminidase inhibitors
NAM	*N*-acetylmuramic acid
NASBA	nucleic acid sequence-based amplification

NGU	nongonococcal urethritis
NICU	neonatal intensive care unit
NK	natural killer
NPA	nasopharyngeal aspirate
NPV	negative predictive value
NRTI	nucleoside reverse transcriptase inhibitor
NSAIDs	non-steroidal anti-inflammatory drugs
NSP	neurotoxic shellfish poisoning
NTM	nontuberculous mycobacteria
OAS	oligonucleotide synthetase
PABA	para-amino benzoic acid
PAF	platelet activation factor
PAM	primary amebic meningitis/meningoencephalitis
PAMPS	pathogen associated molecular patterns
PBP	penicillin binding protein
PCR	polymerase chain reaction
PEP	postexposure prophylaxis
*Pf*EMP	*Plasmodium falciparum* erythrocyte membrane protein
PG	prostaglandins
PHI	primary HIV infection
PI	protease inhibitor
PID	pelvic inflammatory disease
PIF	parainfluenza
PIM	phosphatidylinositol mannosides
PK	protein kinase
PLDH	*Plasmodium* lactate dehydrogenase
PMN	polymorphonuclear neutrophil
POCT	point of care test
PPD	purified protein derivative
PPV	positive predictive value
PRR	pattern-recognition receptor
PSP	paralytic shellfish poisoning
PSS	postsplenectomy sepsis
PT	prothrombin time
PTLD	post-transplant lymphoproliferative disease
PTT	partial thromboplastin time
PVB19	parvovirus B19
QA	quality assurance
QC	quality control
R	effective net reproductive rate
R_0	basic reproductive rate
RB	reticulate body
RBCs	red blood cells
RDT	rapid diagnostic tests
RFLP	restriction fragment length polymorphisms
RIA	radioimmunoassay
RIBA	recombinant immunoblot assay
RMSF	Rocky Mountain spotted fever
RNA	ribonucleic acid
rRNA	ribosomal RNA

RSV	respiratory syncytial virus
RT-PCR	reverse transcription polymerase chain reaction
RVF	Rift Valley fever
SAR	secondary attack rate
SARA	sexually acquired reactive arthritis
SARS	severe acute respiratory syndrome
SARS-CoV	severe acute respiratory syndrome-associated coronavirus
SCF	stem cell factor
SCID	severe combined immunodeficiency
SDS–PAGE	sodium dodecylsulfate polyacrylamide gel electrophoresis
SE	staphylococcal enterotoxins
SIRS	systemic inflammatory response syndrome
SIV	simian immunodeficiency virus
SLE	systemic lupus erythematosus
SLT	shiga like toxins
SN	Sin Nombre
SPE	streptococcal pyrogenic exotoxins
SSI	surgical site infection
SSPE	subsclerosing panencephalitis
SSSS	staphylococcal scalded skin syndrome
STD	sexually transmitted disease
STI	sexually transmitted infection
T-20	enfuvirtide
TB	tuberculosis
3TC	lamivudine
TCR	T cell receptor
THF	tetrahydrofolate
TK	thymidine kinase
TLR	toll like receptor
TMA	transcription mediated amplification
TME	transmissible mink encephalopathy
TMP-SMX	trimethoprim-sulfamethoxaole
TNF	tumor necrosis factor
TRFA	time resolved fluorescence assay
TSS	toxic shock syndrome
TSST-1	toxic shock syndrome toxin-1
TST	tuberculin skin test
TTP	thrombotic thrombocytopenic purpura
TTV	transfusion-transmitted virus
TU	tuberculin units
UNSCOM	United Nations Special Commission
URT	upper respiratory tract
URTI	upper respiratory tract infection
USAMRIID	US Army Medical Research Institute for Infectious Diseases
UTI	urinary tract infection
VAP	ventilator associated pneumonia
VHF	viral hemorrhagic fever
VIG	vaccinia immunoglobulin
VISA	vancomycin intermediate *S. aureus*
VL	visceral leishmaniasis

vmRNA	viral messenger RNA
VRE	vancomycin-resistant enterococci
VRSA	vancomycin resistant *Staphylococcus aureus*
VT	verotoxin
VTM	viral transport medium
VZIG	VZV immunoglobulin
VZV	varicella zoster virus
WBCs	white blood cells
WHO	World Health Organization
WNV	West Nile virus
YEL-AVD	yellow fever vaccine-associated viscerotropic disease

Part 1

General principles of infectious diseases

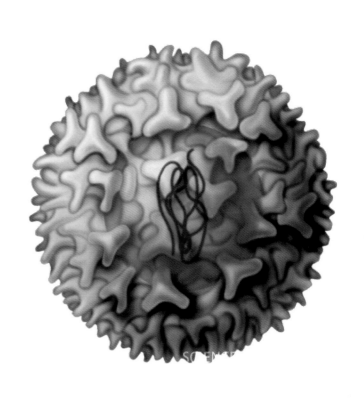

Chapter 1
Microbial etiology of disease

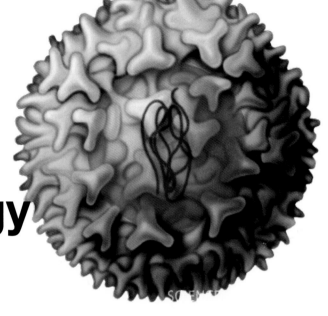

N. Shetty, E. Aarons, J. Andrews

Prokaryotic and eukaryotic cells
Bacteria
Sizes, shapes and arrangement of bacteria
Phases of bacterial growth
Viruses
General properties
Viral transmission

Fungi
Fungi of medical importance
Protozoa
Classification
Helminths

Microbes and their habitats have held a peculiar fascination for mankind ever since **Antony van Leeuwenhoek** (1632–1723) recorded some of the most important discoveries in the history of biology. Once Leeuwenhoek succeeded in creating the simple microscope, he described bacteria, free-living and parasitic creatures, sperm cells, blood cells, microscopic nematodes and much more. His publications opened up an entire world of microscopic life for scientific study. Microbes continue to excite intense research because of their virulence; their ability to cause tissue damage and death. They have been responsible for the great plagues and epidemics and have often changed the course of human history. The HIV pandemic has emerged as the single most defining occurrence in the history of infectious diseases of the late 20th and early 21st centuries. Microbes continue to baffle human ingenuity; they defy attempts at control by chemotherapeutic agents, vaccines, and the human immune system. The threat of a future pestilence is never far away.

In order to study the microbial etiology of infectious disease, an understanding of the basic principles of microbiology and their interaction with the human host are essential. There are four basic groups of microbes:

- Bacteria
- Viruses
- Fungi: yeasts and molds
- Protozoa.

Multicellular organisms such as helminths also need to be included in the broad description of infectious disease agents.

Table 1.1 Differences between prokaryotic and eukaryotic cells

Cell structure	Prokaryotic	Eukaryotic
Cell wall	Complex cell wall containing peptidoglycan/lipopolysaccaride Some cells have a capsule	Animal cells lack cell walls; plants, algae and fungi do have cell walls, but they differ in composition from those of bacteria
Cytoplasmic membrane	Cytoplasmic membrane without carbohydrates and usually lacking sterols. Incapable of endocytosis and exocytosis	Cytoplasmic membrane contains sterols and carbohydrates and is capable of endocytosis (phagocytosis and pinocytosis) and exocytosis
Nuclear body	Not bounded by a nuclear membrane Usually contains one circular chromosome composed of deoxyribonucleic acid (DNA). No nucleolus. May contain extrachromosomal DNA – the plasmid	Nucleus is bounded by a nuclear membrane, connecting it with the endoplasmic reticulum. Contains one or more paired, linear chromosomes composed of DNA. Nucleolus present
Cytoplasmic structures	70S ribosomes composed of a 50S and a 30S subunit. Mitochondria, endoplasmic reticulum, Golgi apparatus, vacuoles, and lysosomes are absent. No microtubules. Contains only actin-like protein that contribute to cell shape. Spore formation may occur	Ribosomes composed of a 60S and a 40S subunit; mitochondria, endoplasmic reticulum, Golgi apparatus, vacuoles, and lysosomes present. Mitotic spindle involved in mitosis. Cytoskeleton with microtubules, actin, and intermediate filaments
Respiratory enzymes and electron transport chains	Located in the cell membrane	Located in the mitochondria
Cell division	Usually by binary fission. No mitosis or meiosis	By mitosis; sex cells in diploid organisms are produced through meiosis
Organelles of locomotion	Some have hair-like flagellae, fimbriae or pili may also be present. No cilia	May have flagella or cilia: organelles involved in locomotion; consist of a distinct arrangement of sliding microtubules surrounded by a membrane

Prokaryotic and eukaryotic cells

The cell is the basic unit of life, whether it is of human or bacterial origin. Differences in bacterial (prokaryotic cells) and human (eukaryotic cells) have been exploited for diagnostic and treatment purposes. It is important to understand what these differences are and how they contribute to disease pathogenesis (Table 1.1).

Bacteria

Sizes, shapes and arrangement of bacteria

Bacteria are unicellular organisms, ranging from 0.4 μm to 2.0 μm in size. They exist broadly in one of three morphological forms, spheres (cocci), rods (bacilli), or spirals. All of these forms are subject to variation depending on existing growth conditions. The morphology of a bacterium is maintained by a unique cell wall structure and it is the chemical nature of this cell wall that is exploited by the Gram staining

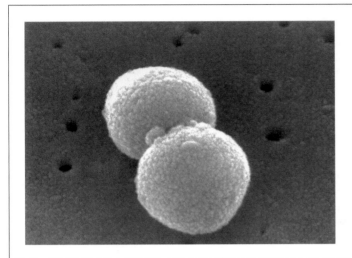

Figure 1.1 Scanning electron micrograph of a diplococcus. Image provided by Dr Richard Facklam. Courtesy of the Centers for Disease Control and Prevention; from CDC website: http://phil.cdc.gov/phil/details.asp

technique (see Chapter 4). The Gram stain remains the single most important diagnostic test in the study of infection – dividing bacteria into two basic groups: **Gram positive** bacteria and **Gram negative** bacteria – thereby influencing the all too important decision: which antibiotic does the clinician use immediately and empirically before full microbiological results are available.

With the help of the Gram stain and a microscope it is possible to visualize the size (relative to a human red or white cell), the shape, the arrangement (if distinctive), and the Gram reaction of the bacterial cell. All the above features are important clues that help identify the infectious agent from a patient's clinical specimen.

Cocci are spherical or oval bacteria having one of several distinct arrangements based on their planes of division:

1 Division in **one plane** produces either a **diplococcus** (paired; Figure 1.1) or **streptococcus** (chain) arrangement.
If you were to Gram stain a smear of the specimen containing a putative diplococcus you would be able to see a Gram positive (purple) or -negative (pink) coccus in pairs; note the size relative to a polymorphonuclear leukocyte (Figure 1.2a and b). Streptococci, including medically important ones such as *Streptococcus pyogenes*, are Gram positive (Figure 1.3). The streptococci can be arranged in pairs (e.g. *Streptococcus pneumoniae*, Figure 1.2a) or in chains (e.g. *S. pyogenes*, Figure 1.3).
2 Division in **random planes** produces a **staphylococcus** arrangement. Note the Gram stained smear of a pus sample showing numerous polymorphs 'pus cells' and staphylococci: cocci in irregular, grape-like clusters (Figure 1.4). Ordered division in two or three planes can result in sarcinial arrangements (tetrads) respectively.

Bacilli are rod-shaped bacteria (Figure 1.5). Bacilli divide in one plane and are arranged singly or in chains as in *Bacillus anthracis*. For many clinically important bacilli the arrangement is not distinctive; some bacilli may be rounded off looking more coccoid; they are often called cocco-bacillary forms. Bacilli, like cocci, can be Gram positive or -negative (Figure 1.6)

Other common shapes of bacteria are: curved bacteria as in *Campylobacter* (Figure 1.7) and *Vibrio* species; *Spirillum* species have thick rigid spirals; and spirochaete forms such as *Leptospira* species have flexible spirals (Figure 1.8). Spirals range in size from 1 μm to over 100 μm in length.

It is worth remembering that not all bacteria stain with the Gram stain. In Chapter 2 we will discuss organisms that do not take up the Gram stain readily, those that do not have typical bacterial cell wall structures or arrangements, and those that are obligate intracellular microorganisms.

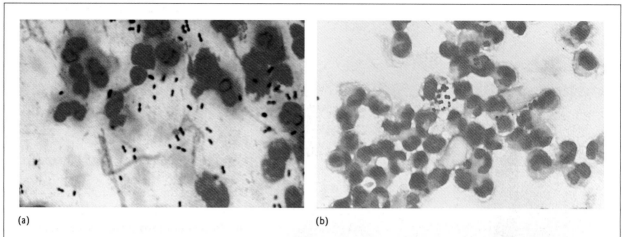

(a)　　　　　　　　　　　　　　(b)

Figure 1.2 (a) Gram stain of sputum (1000×) showing numerous polymorphs and Gram positive cocci in pairs (e.g. *Streptococcus pneumoniae* or pneumococci). (b) Gram stain of CSF (1000×) showing numerous polymorphs and Gram negative cocci in pairs (e.g. *Neisseria meningitidis* or meningococci). © Bayer

Figure 1.3 Gram positive cocci in chains: the streptococci

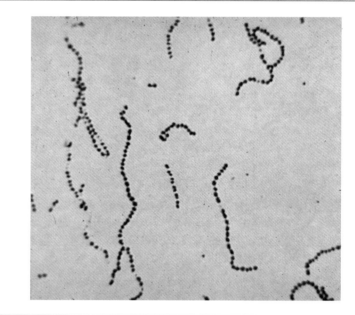

Figure 1.4 Gram stain of a smear (1000×) from pus showing numerous polymorphs and Gram positive cocci in clusters (e.g. *Staphylococcus aureus*)

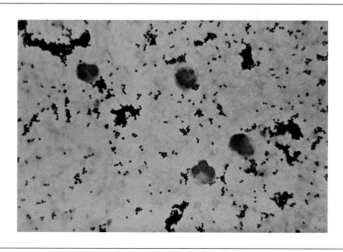

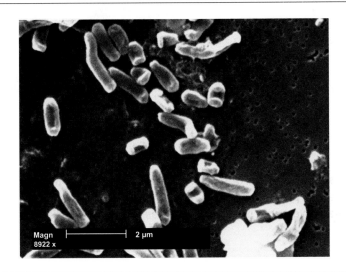

Figure 1.5 Scanning electron image of a bacillus (rod). Image provided by Ray Butler and Janice Carr. Courtesy of the Centers for Disease Control and Prevention; from CDC website: http://phil.cdc.gov/phil/details.asp

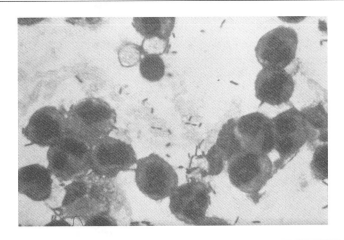

Figure 1.6 Gram stained smear of urine (1000×) showing polymorphs and Gram negative rods (e.g. *Escherichia coli*)

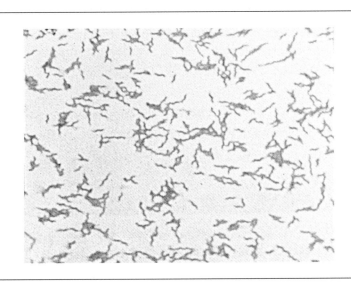

Figure 1.7 Gram stain image (1000×) of *Campylobacter* species, showing curved Gram negative rods

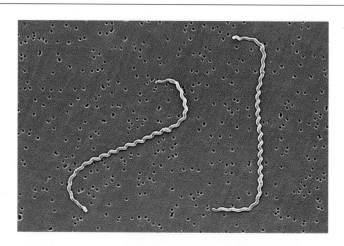

Figure 1.8 Scanning electron micrograph of *Leptospira* species. Image provided by Rob Weyant. Courtesy of the Center for Disease Control and Prevention; from CDC website: http://phil.cdc.gov/phil/details.asp

Phases of bacterial growth

When an organism is inoculated into suitable media such as a liquid culture medium in the laboratory or if it were to encounter a susceptible human/animal host it will exhibit a growth curve (Figure 1.9).

In the **lag phase** the microorganism adapts to a new and often more favourable environment. During this phase, there is a marked increase in enzymes and intermediates, in preparation for active growth. The lag phase is a period of adjustment necessary for the accumulation of metabolites until they are present in concentrations that permit cell division to resume.

In the exponential or **logarithmic phase**, cells are in a state of balanced growth. The cells increase in number and there is a logarithmic expansion of mass and volume. In other words imagine a single cell dividing into two, each further divides in a binary manner and two becomes four, four to eight, eight to sixteen, and so on. A steady state is reached where one of many factors come into play; either essential nutrients become exhausted, there is accumulation of waste products, change in pH, induction of host immune mechanisms and other obscure factors exert a deleterious effect on the culture, and growth is progressively slowed.

During the **stationary phase**, accumulation of toxic products or exhaustion of nutrients causes net growth to cease. The viable cell count remains constant. The formation of new organisms equals the death of organisms in the system. The stationary phase is important to the clinical microbiologist as microbial toxins, antimicrobial substances and other proteins such as bacteriocins and lysins accumulate to significant levels at the end of the stationary phase. Thus, they affect not only growth in the laboratory but also pathogenesis of disease in the host.

As factors detrimental to the bacteria accumulate, more bacteria are killed than are formed. During the **phase of decline** there is a negative exponential phase, which results in a decrease in the numbers of viable bacteria within the system.

Figure 1.9 The bacterial growth curve showing the four phases of growth. (a) The lag phase; (b) the exponential phase; (c) the stationary phase; (d) the phase of decline

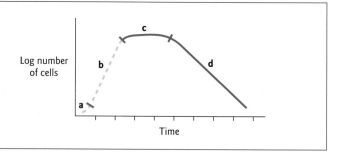

Viruses

General properties

Of all the agents infectious to man, and indeed to other living things, viruses are the smallest. (See Box 1.1 for a description of prions.) An individual infectious unit, comprising a nucleic acid genome, packaged inside a protein coat with or without a surrounding lipid-containing envelope membrane, is known as a viral particle or **virion** (Figure 1.10).

Only the very largest of these, the poxviruses measuring up to 400 nm in their longest dimension and the even larger mimivirus, can be visualized with a light microscope. Cell-free, intact virions are entirely

---

Box 1.1 Prions

Even smaller infectious agents have been identified that, amazingly, lack a nucleic acid genome. It would appear that the protein alone is the infectious agent. This infectious agent has been called a **prion**, short for **pro**teinaceous **in**fectious particle. They are unique structures as they lack DNA or RNA (the very code for life in a living microorganism) and they resist all conventional attempts at inactivation. The discovery that proteins alone can transmit an infectious disease has led to much debate and controversy in the scientific community.

Prion diseases target the brain and are often called **spongiform encephalopathies**. The post

mortem appearance of the brain is characteristic, with large vacuoles in the cortex and cerebellum. Many mammalian species develop these diseases. Specific examples include:

- **Scrapie** in sheep
- **TME** (transmissible mink encephalopathy) in mink
- **CWD** (chronic wasting disease) in muledeer and elk
- **BSE** (bovine spongiform encephalopathy) in cows; this led to banning of British beef worldwide (commonly known as mad cow disease).

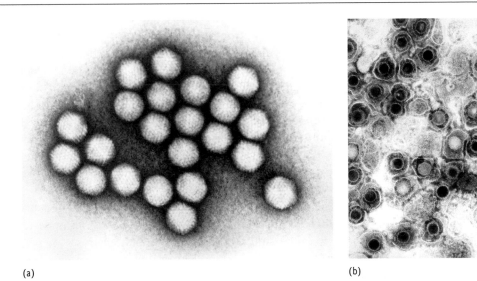

(a)   (b)

Figure 1.10 Electron photomicrograph of: (a) a nonenveloped virus, the adenovirus; (b) an enveloped virus, the herpes virus. Courtesy of: (a) Dr G. William Gray Jr; (b) Dr Fred Murphy; from CDC website: http://phil.cdc.gov/phil/details.asp

metabolically inert: they cannot be said to be "alive" at all. Yet, on entering an appropriate cell (which is anything but a matter of chance proximity), the cellular machinery is hijacked and diverted towards production of new viral particles. Normal cellular function may be disrupted to a greater or lesser extent and the consequences of this may be manifest as disease.

As viruses can replicate themselves only inside living prokaryotic or eukaryotic cells, they have evolved alongside cellular organisms and specific viral infections are known in mycoplasma and other bacteria, algae, fungi, plants, and animals. In that certain viruses depend on co-infection of their cellular targets with other viruses, viruses might be said to even parasitize each other (e.g. hepatitis D virus cannot replicate in the absence of hepatitis B virus (HBV) because it requires the HBV protein coat for the packaging of its own nucleic acid).

The **host range** for a given virus may be relatively broad (e.g. influenza A, which can infect ducks, chickens, pigs and horses as well as humans), or extremely narrow (e.g. measles, which infects only humans). This is known as **host-specificity**. Within a multicellular host, a particular virus may be able to infect many types of cell (e.g. Ebola virus) or be restricted to the cells of only certain tissues. This phenomenon is known as **tissue tropism**. Both host-specificity and tissue tropism are determined largely by the molecular properties of the viral surface (the viral envelope proteins or in the absence of an envelope, the viral coat proteins) precisely interacting with specific cell surface molecules. In the absence of the cell surface molecule(s) required, the virus cannot enter the cell. This will be discussed further later in this chapter.

The "purpose" of a virus, then, is to find a susceptible cell, enter it and replicate in such a way as to facilitate its progeny finding susceptible cells in new hosts, i.e. transmission. The strategies used to achieve this end are hugely diverse, and accomplished with the most extraordinary economy of material. A virion may carry an enzyme or two, necessary for the initiation of the replication cycle, but is essentially just a sophisticatedly addressed package bearing an auto-start program: a blueprint for making more of itself. Compared with the genomes of cellular organisms, viral genomes are minute. For comparison, the human genome comprises 3×10^6 kilobases (kb), that of *Haemophilus influenzae* 1.8×10^3 kb, that of a pox virus around 200 kb, and that of hepatitis B virus (HBV) only 3.2 kb. The numbers of genes encoded by viral genomes are commensurately small. HBV encodes just four. Moreover, there is almost no redundancy in viral genomes and, not infrequently, genes overlap, with different proteins being transcribed from different open reading frames (see Chapter 19). The possession of relatively so few genes does not however imply that viruses are easily understood and hence eliminated by human intervention. It should be noted that while the 9.7-kb genome of the human immunodeficiency virus (HIV) was first fully sequenced in 1985 by Ratner and his co-workers, over 20 years later, we do not entirely understand its pathogenesis, have no cure, and no preventative vaccine.

Viral transmission

Many viral diseases that occur in humans are **zoonoses**, i.e. they are communicable from animals to humans under natural conditions. Unlike most other human pathogens, viruses have no free-living form outside their host(s). In the environment, a virus particle can do no more than passively survive intact and any damage is liable to render it noninfectious. In this respect it is important to note that the lipid bilayer of enveloped viruses is very vulnerable to disruption by desiccation, detergents, and solvents. Because infectivity depends on the integrity of the envelope bearing its viral attachment (glyco)proteins, these viruses do not survive long in the environment and are readily susceptible to decontamination methods (e.g. even simple soap and water). Conversely, nonenveloped viruses tend to be considerably more durable. Caliciviruses are particularly resilient and the difficulty of adequately decontaminating **fomites** (contaminated inanimate objects) in the context of norovirus outbreaks has no doubt contributed to outbreak persistence on many occasions.

Despite their passivity in the environment, viruses have evolved so as to maximize their chances of transmitting from host to host. Some viruses, **ar**thropod **bo**rne or **arboviruses**, multiply to high viral loads in the bloodstream and are transferred to new hosts by arthropods that feed on human blood. Transmission is also assured if viruses shed in vast numbers into human body fluids – respiratory secretions, saliva, genital secretions, urine, and stool. Human behavior takes care of the rest: face to face conversation, sexual activity, use of the hands for eating as well as for toileting facilitates transmission and continued survival. Certain viruses, influenza and rotavirus for example, go even further by causing the volume of the infectious fluid to be considerably increased and literally sprayed into the environment by sneezing or explosive, watery diarrhea respectively. Mother-to-child transmission (also known as **vertical transmission**) is usually an incidental means of transmission rather than the predominant one. The transmission of **blood-borne viruses** through parenteral exposure (blood transfusion, contaminated surgical implements, tattooing, sharing of equipment for IV drug use, etc.) is of course an artifact of very recent (in evolutionary terms) human behavior, where the major means of transmission is mucosal or skin lesion contact with blood or genital secretions. In the absence of universal immunization, knowledge of the route by which a viral disease is transmitted is essential to the control of that infection in human populations.

Fungi

Fungi are an extremely diverse group of organisms, ubiquitous in the environment. They are found as two main forms, **yeasts** and **molds**. They are nonphotosynthetic organisms with the ability to absorb soluble nutrients by diffusion from living or dead organic matter. Molds consist of branching filaments (**hyphae**), which interlace to form a mycelium. The hyphae of the more primitive molds remain aseptate (without walls) whereas those of the more developed groups are septate with a central pore in each cross wall. Yeasts are unicellular organisms consisting of separate round or oval cells. They do not form a mycelium, although the intermediate yeast-like fungi form a pseudomycelium consisting of chains of elongated cells.

Many fungi, including some of clinical importance, can exist in both forms dependent on temperature and other environmental conditions. These are known as **dimorphic** fungi.

Like mammalian cells, fungi are **eukaryotes** (Table 1.1) with DNA organized into chromosomes within the cell nucleus. Fungi also have distinct cytoplasmic organelles including Golgi apparatus, mitochrondria, and storage vacuoles. Homology with mammalian cells also extends to biosynthesis, where fungi share similar pathways for both protein synthesis and DNA replication.

A formal classification scheme of fungi has little medical relevance so a simplified clinical classification for **pathogenic** fungi, based on initial site of infection, is more commonly used (Table 1.2).

Cutaneous superficial fungal infections are very common. The majority are caused by three groups of fungi: mold dermatophytes such as *Microsporium* spp. and *Trichophyton* spp., *Candida albicans*, and *Malassezia* spp. Keratin-containing structures such as hair shafts, nails, and skin are affected. Dermatophyte skin infection (sometimes called ringworm) is commonly named after the area affected, for example tinea capitis (head) or tinea corporis (body).

The **systemic** fungi include *Coccidioides immitis*, *Paracoccidioides braziliensis*, and *Histoplasma capsulatum*. These are thermally dimorphic fungi, meaning they have both yeast-like and filamentous forms. They are environmental organisms, which enter the body usually via inhalation. Infection is geographically

Table 1.2 Classification of fungi associated with human infection (mycoses)

Classification	Examples (and form)
Cutaneous and mucocutaneous infection	*Microsporium* spp. (mold) *Trichophyton* spp. (mold) Candida vaginal infection (vaginal thrush) Candida mouth infection in babies (oral thrush)
Systemic infection	*Coccidioides immitis* (dimorphic) *Histoplasma capsulatum* (dimorphic)
Infections of the immunocompromised host	*Candida* spp. (yeast) *Aspergillus* spp. (mold)

circumscribed and often clinically mild. Severe disseminated disease can occur, however, particularly in immunocompromised patients.

The main fungi that cause disease in immunocompromised patients are the yeasts **C. albicans** and related species such as *Candida krusei*. **Aspergillus** species are important environmental filamentous fungi, which may cause pulmonary or disseminated infection. The yeast-like fungi **Cryptococcus neoformans** can cause chronic meningitis in patients with HIV infection.

Fungi of medical importance

Over 200 000 species of fungi have been described although only about 200 have been associated with human disease. With a few exceptions, fungal infections of humans originate from an exogenous source in the environment and are acquired through inhalation, ingestion, or traumatic implantation.

A few species of fungi are capable of causing significant disease in otherwise normal individuals. Many more are only able to produce disease when the host has some aspect of impaired immunity e.g. HIV seropositivity, or during treatment for malignancy. With the increasing number of **immunocompromised** patients, fungi previously considered to be nonpathogenic are being recognized as the cause of sporadic infections. Any fungus capable of growing at the temperature of the human host (37°C) must now be regarded as a potential human pathogen.

Recent DNA sequencing work has shown that **Pneumocystis jiroveci**, long believed to be a protozoon, is in fact also a fungus. This organism is an important pathogen in immunocompromised patients, especially those with AIDS.

Protozoa

Protozoa are unicellular microorganisms, which are found in almost every type of environment. Almost two-thirds of the world population live in conditions in which infection with protozoa or **helminths** (see later) are thought to be unavoidable. Protozoan lifecycles are extremely diverse and can be complex and thus they display a much wider range of morphology than bacteria or viruses. Many species are parasites of higher plants and animals but this chapter will deal only with those that cause disease in humans.

Protozoans such as *Plasmodium* spp., *Leishmania* spp., and *Entamoeba histolytica* are important causes of morbidity and mortality in the tropics but can be seen in the developed world in the returning traveler. Pathogens such as *Cryptosporidium parvum* and *Giardia lamblia* are important causes of morbidity in both the developed and developing world. Protozoan organisms including *Toxoplasma gondii*, *Leishmania* spp., and *C. parvum* have been shown to cause particularly severe disease in patients with AIDS. With increased levels of international travel and the immunosuppressive effects of infection with HIV, one needs to have a raised awareness of diseases caused by protozoa.

Classification

The classification of protozoa that are medically important can be simplified by subdivision into four main groups, which in part relate to the method of locomotion (Table 1.3). These distinctions are by no means absolute, for example some organisms may be flagellate or amoeboid at different stages of their lifecycle. Flagellates are often divided into organisms causing intestinal or urogenital infection such as *Giardia lamblia* or *Trichomonas vaginalis*, and flagellates found in the blood or tissues (hemoflagellates) such as *Leishmania* spp. or *Trypansoma* spp.

Helminths

For completeness a short section on helminths has been included here. Helminths are multicellular organisms that range from less than 1 cm to more than 10 m in length. The helminths that infect man include the

Table 1.3 A simplified classification scheme for the medically important Protozoa and example(s) in each group

Classification	Most important examples
Sporozoa	*Plasmodium* spp. *Toxoplasma gondii* *Cryptosporidium parvum* *Isospora belli* *Cyclospora cayetanensis*

Flagellates
  Intestinal/urogenital
  Blood/tissue
	Giardia lamblia, Trichomonas vaginalis
	Leishmania spp., *Trypanosoma brucei, Trypanosoma cruzi*

Ameboid	*Entamoeba histolytica*
Ciliates	*Balantidium coli*

Table 1.4 Some medically important helminths and the associated infections

Species name	Infection caused
Roundworms (nematodes)	
Ascaris lumbricoides	Intestinal roundworm
Trichuris trichiura	Whipworm
Ancylostoma duodenale/Necator americanus	Hookworm
Strongyloides stercoralis	Strongyloidiasis
Enterobius vermicularis	Thread worm or pin worm
Trichinella spiralis	Trichinellosis
Wuchereria bancrofti	Filariasis
Loa loa	Loiasis
Onchocerca volvulus	River blindness
Toxocara canis	Visceral larva migrans
Tapeworms (cestodes)	
Taenia solium	Cysticercosis
Taenia saginata	Beef tapeworm
Hymenolepis nana	Dwarf tapeworm
Diphyllobothrium latum	Fish tapeworm
Echinococcus granulosus	Hydatid disease
Flukes (trematodes)	
Schistosoma spp.	Schistosomiasis
Fasciola hepatica	Liver fluke
Paragonimus westermani	Lung fluke
Clonorchis sinensis	Chinese liver fluke

nematodes (roundworms) and platyhelminths (flatworms), the latter group consisting of **cestodes** (tapeworms) and **trematodes** (flukes). Worms are covered by a cuticle that protects them from environmental stresses. The lifecycle of all worms includes an egg, one or more larval stages, and the adult. The prevalence of helminthic infection is greatest in developing countries where poverty leads to increased exposure because of lack of clean water, poor sanitation, and inadequate housing. Table 1.4 demonstrates some of the most important helminths known to infect humans.

Further reading

Chiodini PL, Moody A, Manser DW. *Atlas of Medical Helminthology and Protozoology*, 4th edition. London: Churchill Livingstone, 2001

Winn WC, Koneman EW, Allen SD, et al. *Koneman's Color Atlas and Textbook of Diagnostic Microbiology*, 6th edition. Baltimore, MD: Lippincott Williams and Wilkins, 2006

Chapter 2
Structure and function of microbes

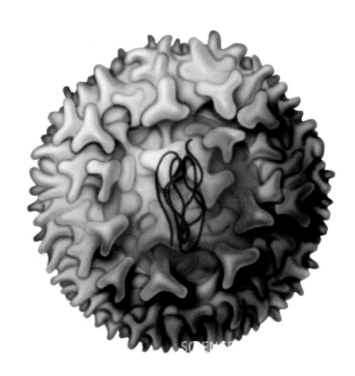

N. Shetty, E. Aarons, J. Andrews

Bacterial cell structure and function
  Nuclear equivalent
  Cell membrane
  Cell wall
  Flagella
  Fimbriae
  Capsule and slime production
Obligate intracellular microorganisms
  Rickettsiae
  Chlamydiae

Viral structure and component function
  The viral lifecycle
  Virus classification
  Viruses as parasites
Fungi: structure and function
  Fungal cell membrane
  Fungal cell walls
  Reproduction
Protozoa: structure and function
  Structure
  Lifecycles

Open your newspaper, log on to your current news website or switch on the television and before long you will come across a news story that relates to an infectious agent. Microbes, their victims, and their hunters are locked in an age old battle that is still relevant today. To understand what makes the microbe so successful and how we create the "magic bullet" that will selectively destroy a microbial cell leaving the host cell intact we need to delve a little deeper into the cellular structure and function of microorganisms: bacteria, viruses, fungi, and protozoa.

Bacterial cell structure and function
Within the single cell, bacteria pack a number of complex structures that ensure their survival and propagation.

Nuclear equivalent

The bacterial chromosome is a single circular double-stranded, helical, supercoiled DNA molecule. The chromosome is several hundred to a thousand times longer than the length of the cell and frequently contains as many as 3500 genes.

To enable a circular structure this large to fit within the bacterium, histone-like proteins bind to the DNA, segregating the DNA molecule into around 50 chromosomal domains and making it more compact. In addition, an enzyme called DNA gyrase supercoils each domain around itself forming a compact, supercoiled mass of DNA approximately 0.2 μm in diameter. A group of unique bacterial enzymes called DNA topoisomerases are essential in the unwinding, replication, and rewinding of the circular, supercoiled bacterial DNA. **DNA gyrase and the topoisomerses are important targets for antimicrobial killing action on bacteria**.

Unlike the eukaryotic nucleus, the bacterial chromosome is not contained within a membrane-bound nucleus.

Bacteria often contain extrachromosomal DNA material called **plasmids**. Plasmids exist as circular double-stranded DNA. Plasmids are not essential for normal bacterial growth and bacteria may lose or gain them without harm. They can, however, provide an advantage under certain environmental conditions. **Many plasmids code for resistance or "R" factors, which render the organism resistant to one or more antimicrobial agents. Plasmids also code for toxins and other virulence factors produced by bacteria**.

All bacteria possess **ribosomes** and ribosomal RNA (rRNA). Ribosomes are composed of two subunits with densities of 50S and 30S. ("S" is the Svedberg unit of density). The two subunits combine during protein synthesis to form a complete 70S ribosome. A typical bacterium may have as many as 15 000 ribosomes. Many antibacterial agents target ribosomes, achieving bacterial cell death by switching off bacterial protein biosynthesis.

Bacterial cells may contain one or other type of inclusion granule. **Inclusions** are distinct granules that may occupy a substantial part of the cytoplasm. Inclusion granules are usually reserve materials of some sort. For example, *Corynebacterium diphtheriae*, the organism that causes diphtheria, may contain inclusion bodies, known as metachromatic granules, which are composed of inorganic polyphosphates (volutin) that serve as energy reserves. Other bacteria may contain glycogen or fat granules that are also thought to function as carbon and energy reserves.

Two clinically important genera of bacteria produce **endospores**: the genus *Bacillus* (e.g. *Bacillus anthracis*) and the genus *Clostridium* (e.g. *Clostridium tetani*). Endospores are resistant, dormant forms of the organism and are produced during unfavorable environmental conditions. Many endospores are resistant to heat, disinfectants, and drying. In the presence of unfavorable conditions the bacterium transforms itself into a spore form by a process called sporulation.

Sporulation generally takes around 15 hours. Spores pose an important threat of transmission of infection to humans and animals (they can also whip up a mass frenzy). Spores finding their way into susceptible host tissue will germinate in the presence of favorable conditions of moisture, nutrition and temperature and cause disease (Box 2.1).

Box 2.1 White powder scare on jet airplane

Passengers on a west bound flight have been forced to wait three hours during a white powder scare.

The jet airplane on its way from New York to Los Angeles had touched down at St Louis when the substance was found in the overhead baggage locker.

Police and antiterrorist squads attended and isolated the plane before a team of scientists including a microbiologist was brought in to test the white powder.

The microbiologist did a smear analysis on the substance and deemed that it was not an immediate bacterial risk as he could see no evidence of spore structures of the anthrax or other bacterial groups. He said further tests were needed to confirm this. Passengers were reassured of the low risk and alternative arrangements were made for their onward travel.

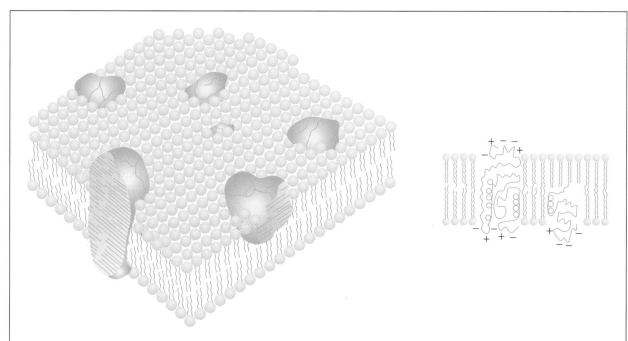

Figure 2.1 Fluid mosaic model of the cell membrane. Membrane phospholipids arrange themselves to form a fluid bilayer. Some membrane proteins span the bilayer and may form transport channels through the membrane

Cell membrane

The cell membrane lies internal to the cell wall. Like all biological membranes it is a phospholipid bilayer complexed with proteins. Dispersed within the bilayer are various structural and enzymatic proteins, which carry out most membrane functions. Most proteins are partly inserted into the membrane, or possibly even traverse the membrane as channels from the outside to the inside. The arrangement of proteins and lipids to form a membrane is called the **fluid mosaic model**, and is illustrated in Figure 2.1.

Bacterial cell membranes differ from eukaryotic cell membranes in that they lack sterols, except for the mycoplasmas which incorporate sterols when grown in sterol rich media.

Major functions of the cell membrane are in: (i) selective permeability and transport of solutes; (ii) electron transport and oxidative phosphorylation; (iii) removal of waste; (iv) carriage of enzymes and other proteins required for cellular bio-synthesis; (v) the bearing of receptors; and (vi) coordination of DNA replication and segregation with septum formation and cell division.

The cell memberane functions mainly as a selective **permeability barrier** that regulates the passage of substances into and out of the cell. Selective permeability of water and solutes occurs by passive diffusion and active transport. Water, dissolved gases such as carbon dioxide and oxygen, and lipid-soluble molecules diffuse across the phospholipid bilayer. Water-soluble ions generally pass through small pores – less than 0.8 nm in diameter – in the membrane . All other molecules require carrier molecules to transport them through the membrane. For further information on bacterial transport mechanisms see *Medical Microbiology* by Jawetz et al. (Further reading).

Mesosomes appear as infoldings of the bacterial cytoplasmic membrane and are often seen in electron micrographs. Mesosomes may also represent specialized membrane regions involved in DNA replication and segregation, cell wall synthesis, or increased enzymatic activity.

Some antibiotics such as polymyxins and many disinfectants and antiseptics, such as chlorhexidine, hexachlorophene, and alcohol, **alter the bacterial cell membrane** causing **leakage of cellular contents**.

Cell wall

Most bacteria have a rigid **cell wall**. The cell wall is an essential structure that helps the bacterium retain its shape while protecting it from mechanical damage and from osmotic rupture or **lysis**. The bacterial cell wall is unique in that it:

- is composed of unique components found nowhere else in nature
- is one of the most important sites for attack by antibiotics such as penicillin
- provides ligands for adherence and receptor sites for drugs or viruses
- elicits specific immunological responses in the host
- is the basis for immunological distinction and immunological variation among strains of bacteria.

The cell wall is made of a network of repeating, cross-linked monomer units composed of polymers of peptidoglycan, a component of all bacterial cell walls. A **peptidoglycan monomer** consists of alternating units of amino sugars, *N*-acetylglucosamine (NAG) and *N*-acetylmuramic acid (NAM), with a tetra or pentapeptide chain attached to the NAM. The types and the order of amino acids in the side chain show some slight variation between Gram positive and Gram negative bacteria (Figure 2.2a and b).

The Gram positive cell wall

In **Gram positive bacteria such as *Staphylococcus aureus*** (those that retain the purple crystal violet dye when subjected to the Gram staining procedure) the cell wall is thick (15–80 nm), consisting of up to 40 layers of peptidoglycan much like the layers of an onion. While the tetra or pentapeptide unit attached to the NAM may vary within the species, the invariant feature of this component is the presence of D-alanine, which is always the linkage unit between peptidoglycan chains. A peptidoglycan monomer of *S. aureus* consists of two joined amino sugars, *N*-acetylglucosamine (NAG) and *N*-acetylmuramic acid (NAM), with a pentapeptide attached to the NAM. In *S. aureus*, the pentapeptide consists of the amino acids L-alanine, D-glutamine, L-lysine, and one or two D-alanines (Figure 2.2a).

Each layer of peptidoglycan is attached to the next by an **interpeptide bridge** of amino acids that connects a free amino group on lysine to a free carboxy group on D-alanine of a nearby side chain. In

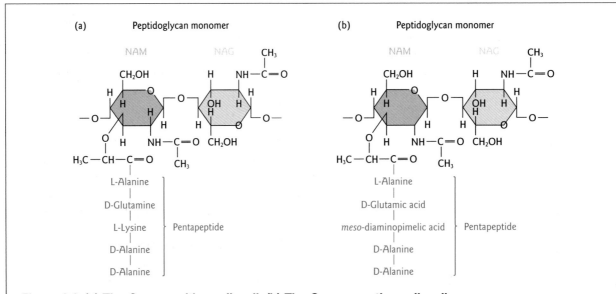

Figure 2.2 (a) The Gram positive cell wall. (b) The Gram negative cell wall

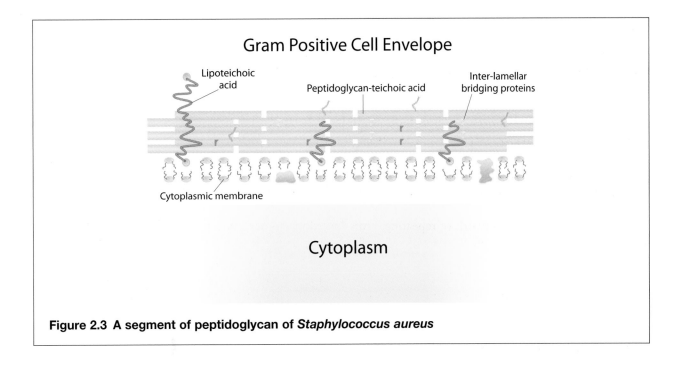

Gram Positive Cell Envelope

Lipoteichoic acid

Peptidoglycan-teichoic acid

Inter-lamellar bridging proteins

Cytoplasmic membrane

Cytoplasm

Figure 2.3 A segment of peptidoglycan of *Staphylococcus aureus*

S. aureus, this interlamellar bridge (Figure 2.3) is a peptide consisting of five glycine molecules (called a **pentaglycine bridge**).

Assembly of the pentaglycine bridge in Gram positive cell walls is mediated by a group of enzymes called transglycosylases, transpeptidases, and carboxypeptidases, and is inhibited by the action of beta-lactam antibiotics. These enzymes are also referred to as penicillin binding proteins (PBPs). Hence, beta-lactam antibiotics are said to act by "inhibition of cell wall synthesis" in bacteria. Gram positive bacteria are more sensitive to beta-lactam antibiotics than Gram negative bacteria because the peptidoglycan is a more abundant and exposed molecule. In Gram positive bacteria, peptidoglycans may vary in their amino acid side chains, and in the exact composition of the interpeptide bridge. At least eight different types of peptidoglycan exist in Gram positive bacteria.

Attached to the rigid peptidoglycan framework of the cell wall are various polysaccharides which are covalently linked to the peptidoglycan; their function remains uncertain.

In some cases the cell wall of Gram positive bacteria may contain proteins of special significance. Examples of these are the M, T and R proteins of Group A streptococcus and protein A of *S. aureus*.

The Gram negative cell wall

In **Gram negative bacteria** (stain pink with the counterstain after decolorisation) the cell wall is relatively thin (10 nm) and is composed of a single layer of peptidoglycan surrounded by a membranous outer coat called the **outer membrane**. The outer membrane of Gram negative bacteria invariably contains a unique component, **lipopolysaccharide** (**LPS**), also called **endotoxin**. Endotoxin is present in bacteria not normally considered to be pathogens. When released by lysis of the bacterial cell, they may be toxic to humans and animals.

Peptidoglycan structure and arrangement in *Escherichia coli* is representative of many Gram negative bacteria (Figure 2.4). A peptidoglycan monomer as in all bacteria consists of two joined amino sugars, *N*-acetylglucosamine (NAG) and *N*-acetylmuramic acid (NAM), with a pentapeptide attached to the NAM. In *E. coli*, the pentapeptide consists of the amino acids L-alanine, D-glutamic acid, *meso* diaminopimelic acid (DAP), and two D-alanines (Figure 2.2b).

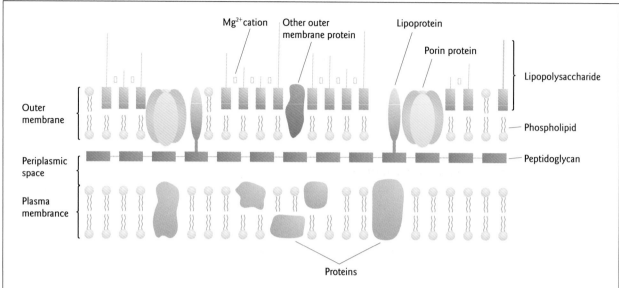

Figure 2.4 Schematic illustration of the outer membrane, peptidoglycan cell wall, and plasma membrane (inner membrane) of a Gram negative bacterium

Gram negative bacteria may contain a single monolayer of peptidoglycan in their cell walls, unlike Gram positive bacteria which are thought to have several layers, similar to an "onion skin," of peptidoglycan. **Strands of peptidoglycan** are assembled in the periplasm and are connected to form a continuous glycan molecule that encompasses the cell. Wherever their proximity allows it, the tetrapeptide chains that project from the NAM part of the glycan backbone can be cross-linked by an **interpeptide bond** between a free amino group on DAP and a free carboxy group on a nearby D-alanine. The assembly of peptidoglycan on the outside of the plasma membrane is mediated by the same group of enzymes, i.e. transglycosylases, transpeptidases, and carboxypeptidases, as in Gram positive bacteria. The mechanism of action of penicillin and related beta-lactam antibiotics to **block transpeptidase and carboxypeptidase enzymes** during assembly of the peptidoglycan cell wall is also similar to Gram positive bacteria.

The glycan backbone of the peptidoglycan molecule can be cleaved by an enzyme called **lysozyme** that is present in tissues and secretions, such as tears and saliva, and in the phagocyte. This function constitutes an innate mechanism of defence against infectious agents. Some Gram positive bacteria are very sensitive to lysozyme. Gram negative bacteria are less vulnerable to attack by lysozyme because their peptidoglycan is shielded by the outer membrane.

The outer membrane of Gram negative bacteria

The **outer membrane of Gram negative bacteria** is a discrete bilayered structure on the outside of the peptidoglycan sheet (Figure 2.4). It functions mainly as a permeability barrier, but because of its lipopolysaccharide content, it is responsible for the many interesting and important characteristics of Gram negative bacteria. The outer membrane is a lipid bilayer intercalated with proteins, superficially resembling the plasma membrane. The inner face of the outer membrane is composed of phospholipids similar to the plasma membrane. The outer face of the outer membrane may contain some phospholipid, but it is largely composed of lipopolysaccharide (LPS) or endotoxin. Outer membrane proteins usually traverse the membrane and some act to anchor the outer membrane to the underlying peptidoglycan sheet.

The LPS molecule (Figure 2.5) that forms part of the outer face of the outer membrane is composed of a hydrophobic region, called **Lipid A**, that is attached to a hydrophilic linear polysaccharide region, consisting of the **core polysaccharide** and the **O-specific polysaccharide**.

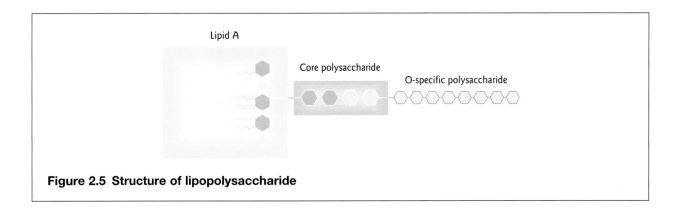

Figure 2.5 Structure of lipopolysaccharide

The Lipid A head of the molecule inserts into the interior of the membrane, and the polysaccharide tail of the molecule faces the aqueous environment. Bacterial lipopolysaccharides are toxic to humans and animals. When injected in small amounts LPS or **endotoxin** activates macrophages to produce pyrogens, activates the complement cascade causing inflammation, and collectively activates the systemic inflammatory response syndrome (SIRS). Endotoxins thus play a major role in infection by Gram negative bacteria. The toxic component of endotoxin (LPS) is Lipid A. The O-specific polysaccharide may provide ligands for bacterial attachment and confer some resistance to phagocytosis. Variation in the exact sugar content of the O polysaccharide (also referred to as the O antigen) accounts for multiple antigenic types (serotypes) among Gram negative bacterial pathogens.

The proteins in the outer membrane of *E. coli* are well characterized. A group of trimeric proteins called **porins** form pores of a fixed diameter through the lipid bilayer of the membrane. The **omp C** and **omp F** porins of *E. coli* are designed to allow passage of hydrophilic molecules up to a molecular weight of about 750 daltons. Larger molecules or harmful hydrophobic compounds (such as bile salts in the intestinal tract) are excluded from entry.

Porins in Gram negative bacteria allow passage of useful molecules (nutrients) through the barrier of the outer membrane, but they exclude the passage of harmful substances from the environment. The ubiquitous **omp A** protein in the outer membrane of *E. coli* has a porin-like structure, and may function in uptake of specific ions; it is also a receptor for the F pilus and an attachment site for bacterial viruses. As a result of genetic mutation, alteration in porin protein size and shape is one way Gram negative bacteria exclude antibiotics from entering the periplasmic space, acting as a permeability barrier and conferring resistance to antimicrobial agents.

Cell wall-less forms

A few bacteria are able to live or exist without a cell wall. The mycoplasmas are a group of bacteria that lack a cell wall. Mycoplasmas have sterol-like molecules incorporated into their membranes and they are usually inhabitants of osmotically protected environments. *Mycoplasma pneumoniae* is the cause of atypical bacterial pneumonia. For obvious reasons, beta-lactam antibiotics which target cell wall biosynthesis are ineffective in the treatment of this type of pneumonia. Sometimes, under the pressure of antibiotic therapy, pathogenic streptococci can revert to cell wall-less forms (called **spheroplasts**) and persist or survive in osmotically protected tissues. When the antibiotic is withdrawn from therapy the organisms may regrow their cell walls and reinfect unprotected tissues.

The acid-fast cell wall

Some bacteria are described as being acid-fast because they resist decolorization with an acid–alcohol mixture during the acid-fast stain procedure. They retain the initial dye carbol fuchsin and appear red (Figure 2.6).

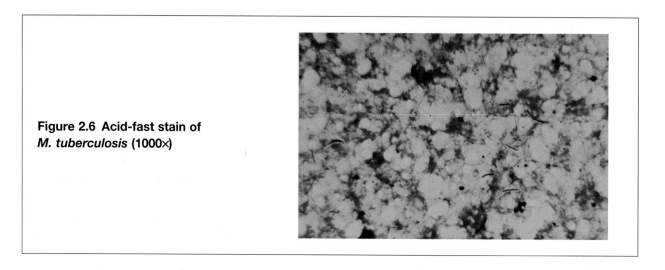

**Figure 2.6 Acid-fast stain of
M. tuberculosis (1000×)**

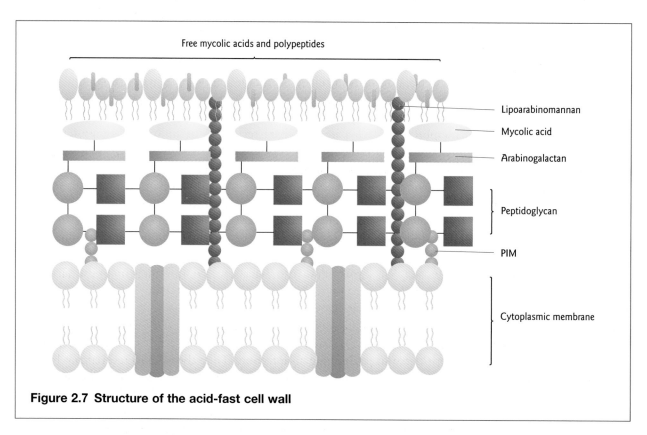

Figure 2.7 Structure of the acid-fast cell wall

Common acid-fast bacteria of medical importance include *Mycobacterium tuberculosis*, *Mycobacterium leprae*, and *Mycobacterium avium-intracellulare* complex. The unique cell wall structure (Figure 2.7) of these bacteria is the reason for their acid-fastness, and also why they do not stain well by the Gram stain.

In addition to peptidoglycan, the acid-fast cell wall of *Mycobacterium* species is characterized by unique **glycolipids, called the mycolic acids**, that make up approximately 60% of the acid-fast cell wall. The peptidoglycan layer is linked to arabinogalactan (D-arabinose and D-galactose), which in turn is linked to the mycolic acid sheet. The arabinogalactan/mycolic acid layer is overlaid with a layer of polypeptides and mycolic acids consisting of free lipids, glycolipids, and peptidoglycolipids. Other glycolipids include lipoarabinomannan and phosphatidylinositol mannosides (PIM) as shown in Figure 2.7.

The complex acid-fast cell wall performs many functions: the peptidoglycan prevents osmotic lysis as in all bacteria. The mycolic acids and other glycolipids make these organisms more resistant to chemical agents and lysosomal digestion by phagocytes than most bacteria.

Flagella

Flagella are filamentous protein structures that protrude external to the cell wall; they provide bacteria with motility. The flagellar filament is rotated by a motor apparatus in the plasma membrane, driven by proton motive force; it allows the cell to swim in fluid environments. Many pathogenic bacillary forms of bacteria and all of the spiral and curved bacteria are motile by means of flagella. By contrast, very few cocci are motile, which reflects their adaptation to dry environments.

Flagellar protein is a potent antigen. Often called the "H" antigen in some bacterial species such as *E. coli* and salmonellae, the H antigen helps to immunologically characterize and differentiate within the genus and species.

Flagella are arranged on the surface of bacteria in one of several distinct patterns. They may be **polar** (one or more flagella arising from one or both poles of the cell) or **peritrichous** (lateral flagella distributed over the entire cell surface) (Figure 2.8). Flagellar distribution is a genetically distinct trait that is occasionally used to characterize or distinguish bacteria. For example, among Gram negative rods, the polar flagella of pseudomonads distinguish them from enteric bacteria, which have peritrichous flagella.

Spirochetes (see Figure 1.8) move by using **axial filaments** that are similar to bacterial flagella in structure. These filaments run along the outside of the protoplasm, but within the periplasmic space; they give the bacterium a characteristic cork screw motility.

Flagella endow the organism with the ability to move or swim in response to environmental stimuli. During chemotaxis a bacterium can sense (using chemoreceptors in the cytoplasmic membrane) certain chemicals in its environment and swim towards them (if they are useful nutrients) or away from them (if they are harmful substances). Motility and chemotaxis probably help some intestinal pathogens to move through the mucous layer so they can attach to the epithelial cells of the mucous membranes.

Fimbriae

Fimbriae and **pili** are interchangeable terms used to designate short, hair-like structures on the surfaces of bacterial cells. Like flagella, they are protein in nature, and protrude from the cytoplasmic membrane lying external to the cell wall.

They perform the important functions of colonization and attachment of bacterial cells to host cells. In human infections, they are major determinants of bacterial virulence because they facilitate adherence of bacterial cells to host cells, the first step to establishing an infection. They also help to resist attack by phagocytic neutrophils and macrophages. For example, pathogenic *Neisseria gonorrhoeae* adheres specifically to the human cervical or urethral epithelium by means of its fimbriae; enterotoxigenic strains of *E. coli* adhere to the mucosal epithelium of the intestine by means of specific fimbriae; the M-protein and associated fimbriae of *Streptococcus pyogenes* are involved in adherence to upper respiratory tract epithelium.

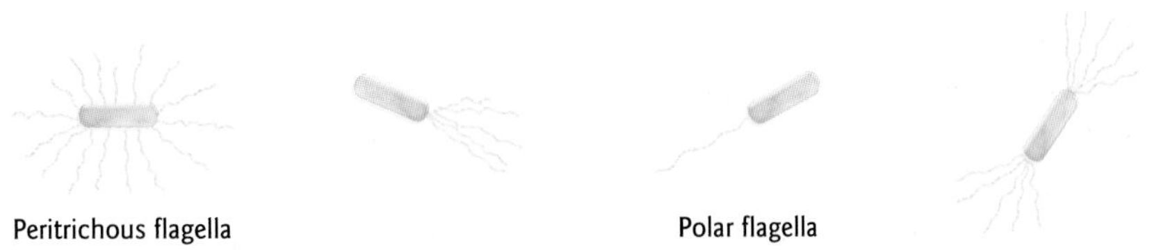

Peritrichous flagella   Polar flagella

Figure 2.8 Peritrichous and various polar arrangements of bacterial flagella

In *E. coli* and other organisms, a specialized type of pilus, the **F or sex pilus**, mediates the transfer of DNA between mating bacteria during the process of **conjugation**.

Capsule and slime production

All bacteria secrete an outer glycocalyx or viscous covering of fibers extending from the cell wall. If it forms an organized outer layer of gelatinous material adhering to the cell wall, it is called a capsule. If the glycocalyx appears unorganized and loosely attached, it is referred to as a slime layer.

The capsule is usually polysaccharide or polypeptide in nature. The capsule is a major virulence determinant of some bacterial species, it enables certain bacteria to resist phagocytic engulfment by human neutrophils or macrophages. Examples of bacteria that use their capsule to resist phagocytic engulfment include *Streptococcus pneumoniae*, *Haemophilus influenzae* type b, *Neisseria meningitides*, *Bacillus anthracis*, and *Bordetella pertussis*.

The slime layer produced by some bacteria enables them to adhere to environmental and tissue surfaces (intravascular catheters and other prostheses, root hairs, teeth, etc.) and hence to colonize and resist flushing. Some bacteria that reside as normal skin flora (e.g. coagulase negative staphylococcus species) produce slime or glycocalyx to form a "biofilm" on intravascular catheters and prostheses. A "**biofilm**" consists of layers of bacterial populations adhering to host cells and embedded in a common capsular mass. Bacteria embedded in biofilm can cause serious systemic infections and are difficult to treat, as most antibiotics are unable to penetrate or eradicate "biofilms."

Streptococcus mutans, a bacterium partially responsible for dental caries, breaks down sucrose into glucose and fructose. It produces a slime layer rich in a sticky polysaccharide called dextran and allows the *S. mutans* and other bacteria to adhere to tooth enamel and form a plaque.

Obligate intracellular microorganisms

Rickettsiae

Rickettsiae are small organisms compared to the conventional bacteria that we have studied so far. They are typically 0.3–1.0 μm in size, and morphologically they appear as pleomorphic bacillary or coccobacillary forms. Most are obligate intracellular parasites, dependent on the host cell for all their energy requirements. After the bacterium adheres to the surface of the host cell, it is engulfed into the host cell by endocytosis (phagocytosis) and lives within an endocytic vacuole.

Rickettsia rickettsii causes Rocky Mountain Spotted Fever and is transmitted to humans by infected wood ticks in the Western United States and by dog ticks in the East. *Rickettsia prowazekii* causes epidemic typhus fever and is transmitted by body lice. *Rickettsia typhi*, the causative agent of endemic typhus fever, is transmitted by infected fleas, and the vector for *Ehrlichia*, the rickettsia causing human granulocytic erlichiosis, is the deer tick.

Chlamydiae

The chlamydiae are small coccoid bacteria, 0.2–0.7 μm in size. They are also obligate intracellular parasites dependent on the host cell for energy and essential metabolism. They have a unique intracellular cycle of replication. The infectious form is the elementary body, it enters the host cell by phagocytosis where it develops into a larger reticulate body within a cytoplasmic vacuole. The reticulate body then divides by binary fission and condenses to form more elementary bodies that are then released from the host cell to infect other cells. *Chlamydia trachomatis* is one of the most important causes of sexually transmitted infections in women worldwide; it also causes trachoma, a leading cause of blindness in resource-poor countries. In the United States, it is the primary cause of nongonococcal urethritis (NGU); it is also commonly implicated as a cause of epididymitis, pelvic inflammatory disease (PID), and neonatal respiratory and eye infections. *Chlamydia pneumoniae* is loosely described as one of the causes of "atypical" pneumonia in the community.

Viral structure and component function

Functionally, a virus particle comprises a payload and delivery system (Figure 2.9). The payload is the viral genome, which is *either* RNA *or* DNA, not both, and which can be single or double-stranded, linear or circular, and segmented (analogous to having chromosomes) or unsegmented. The genome may code for regulatory proteins as well as structural proteins that ultimately make up part of the mature virion. In some virus families, the payload includes some enzymes that are required to initiate the first, pre-transcription steps of viral replication. Retroviruses, for example, carry reverse transcriptase.

The delivery system invariably involves a protein shell surrounding, stabilizing and protecting the payload. This shell is also known as the **capsid** and is made up of multiple virus-encoded protein subunits, usually symmetric, that tend to self-assemble into a hollow structure with either helical or icosahedral symmetry (Figure 2.10). Some viruses such as the pox viruses have complex capsid symmetry. The morphological subunits seen on electron microscopy are called **capsomeres**. The protein–nucleic acid complex representing the packaged form of the viral genome is referred to as the **nucleocapsid**.

For some viruses, such as human papilloma and polio viruses, the nucleocapsid is the complete virion. For others, however, such as herpes simplex and influenza viruses, the delivery system also includes an outer lipid-bilayer membrane: the **envelope** (Figure 2.9). This is acquired during viral maturation when the virus buds through a cellular membrane. Therefore it is mainly host derived but incorporates virus-encoded glycoproteins. Whether the outer surface of the mature virion is capsid or envelope, it is the virus-encoded

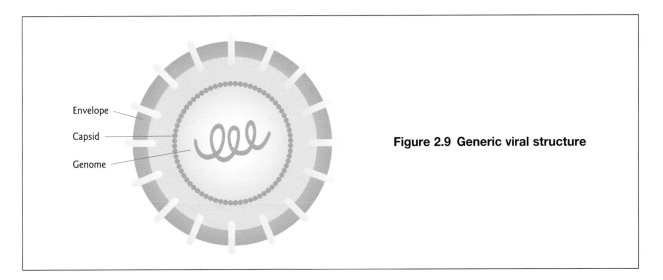

Envelope
Capsid
Genome

Figure 2.9 Generic viral structure

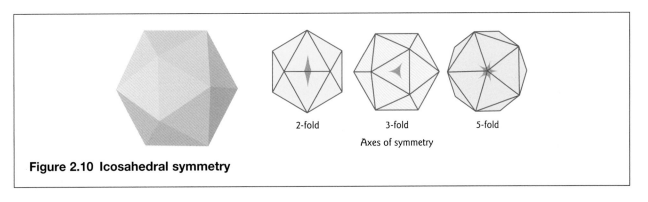

2-fold   3-fold   5-fold

Axes of symmetry

Figure 2.10 Icosahedral symmetry

(glyco)protein *here* that determines that virus's host specificity and tissue tropism. Since lipid bilayers are disrupted by detergents, it follows that enveloped viruses are susceptible to detergent inactivation of infectivity, even though the nucleocapsid remains intact.

The viral lifecycle

The same basic series of events occurs in all animal virus lifecycles (Figure 2.11). For any given virus, a detailed understanding of the processes involved is vital for the design of drugs that selectively inhibit viral replication without interfering with host cell function.

Attachment

This initial interaction between the surface of a virus particle and a particular cell surface protein is a prerequisite for entry of the virus into that cell. Viruses have evolved to use all sorts of different cell surface

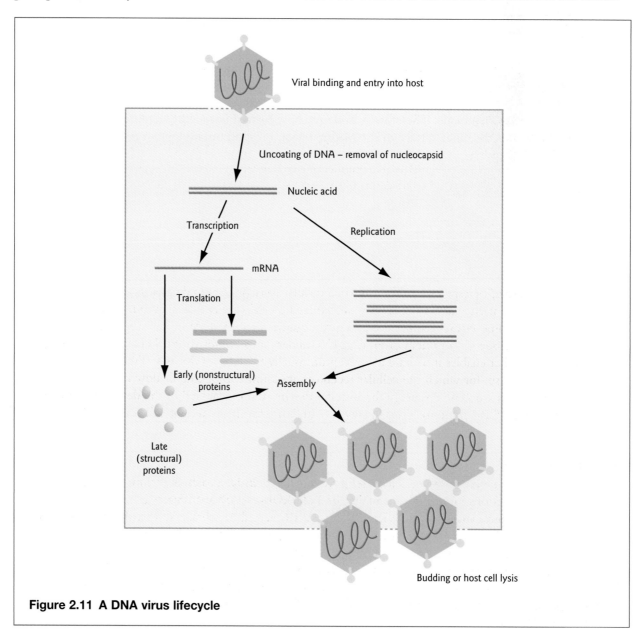

Figure 2.11 A DNA virus lifecycle

Table 2.1 Some cellular receptors for selected animal viruses (reproduced from Wagner EK, Hewlett MJ, *Basic Virology*, 2nd edition. Oxford: Blackwell Science Ltd, 2004, table 6.1, p. 63, with permission from Blackwell Science Ltd)

Name	Cellular function	Virus receptor for
ICAM-1	Intracellular adhesion	Poliovirus
CD-4	T-lymphocyte functional marker	HIV
MHC-I	Antigen presentation	Togavirus, SV40
MHC-II	Antigen presentation/stimulation of B-cell differentiation	Visnavirus (lentivirus)
Fibronection	Integrin	Echovirus (picornavirus)
Cationic amino acid transporter	Amino acid transport	Murine leukemia virus (oncornavirus)
LDL receptor	Intracellular signaling molecule	Subgroup A avian leukosis virus (oncornavirus)
Acetylcholine receptor	Neuronal impulse transducer	Rabies virus
EGF	Growth factor	Vaccinia virus
CR2/CD21	Complement receptor	Epstein–Barr virus
HVEM	Tumor necrosis factor receptor family	Herpes simplex virus
Sialic acid	Ubiquitous component of extracellular glycosylated proteins	Influenza virus, reovirus, coronavirus

molecules as "receptors," irrespective of their normal cellular role. As already discussed, the host range and tissue tropism of a particular virus is largely determined by the type and distribution of receptor molecule it utilizes. Some viruses require the presence of more than one kind of cell surface receptor. For instance, the envelope glycoprotein of HIV, gp120, undergoes a conformational change on binding to its receptor CD4 that enables it to bind a coreceptor, usually CCR5 or CXCR4. Table 2.1 shows some examples of viruses for which the cellular receptors are known. Blockade or downregulation of cell surface receptors is a potential strategy for antiviral therapy and this has led to the development and licensing of the first CCR5 inhibitor drug (maraviroc) in 2007, for the treatment of HIV.

Penetration (entry)

A nonenveloped virus enters its target cell by receptor-mediated **endocytosis** after numerous co-localizing virion–receptor interactions initiate the formation of a **clathrin–coated pit** (Figure 2.12). Entry of enveloped viruses requires **fusion** of the viral envelope with the cell membrane so that the nucleocapsid is emptied into the cell cytoplasm. In some cases, the fusion process occurs *after* receptor-mediated endocytosis and the cell membrane involved is therefore that of the endocytotic vesicle. For influenza A and HIV viruses in particular, the series of conformational changes exhibited by the envelope glycoproteins that results in the fusion of the two lipid bilayers into one has been characterized in detail. Drugs that interfere with the function of the HIV fusion protein, gp41, are now part of the armory of anti-HIV therapy.

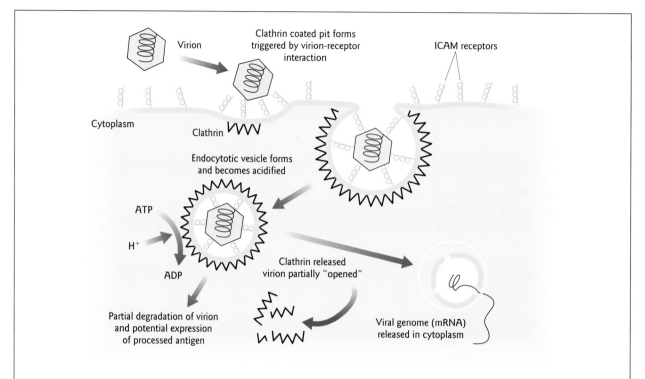

Figure 2.12 Schematic of receptor-mediated endocytosis utilized by poliovirus for entry into the host cell. The endocytotic vesicle forms as a consequence of close association between the poliovirus–receptor complex and the plasma membrane. Reproduced from Wagner EK, Hewlett MJ, *Basic Virology*, 2nd edition. Oxford: Blackwell Science Ltd, 2004, figure 6.2, with permission from Blackwell Publishing Ltd

Disassembly (uncoating)

In order that the viral genome can gain access to the synthetic machinery of the cell, it must be released from its protective capsid coat. In some cases, receptor binding of nonenveloped viruses may directly initiate the necessary conformational changes in the capsid proteins. For viruses that enter cells by endocytosis, the acidic environment that develops within the endocytotic vesicle may cause specific changes to the capsid proteins. Pleconaril and amantadine are drugs that specifically interfere with the uncoating of enteroviruses and of influenza A virus respectively. Further interactions between viral and cellular proteins may be required for the trafficking of the viral genome to the appropriate part of the cell for transcription.

Transcription

Differences between groups of viruses in their methods of transcription provide the basis for the Baltimore classification of viruses (see Further reading). Positive-sense RNA virus genomes serve directly as mRNA for the synthesis of viral proteins. However, negative-sense RNA genomes require *either* an RNA-dependent RNA polymerase to generate positive mRNA transcripts *or* a reverse transcriptase to generate DNA provirus that in turn serves as the transcription template for mRNA. As such enzymes are not provided by the host cell, they must be brought into the cell contained within the virus particle.

For the most part, DNA viruses use their host cells' DNA-dependent RNA polymerase and viral transcription must therefore take place in the nucleus. Pox virus particles carry their own DNA-dependent RNA polymerase and transcription takes place in the cytoplasm.

Because they are irrelevant to host cell function, viral transcription enzymes make excellent drug targets. Reverse transcriptase inhibitors are the mainstay of combination drug therapies against HIV.

Translation

Some viral mRNAs are translated only after splicing. Viruses use cellular machinery for the translation of viral proteins from mRNA transcripts. For this reason, the translation of virus-specific proteins is not a particularly good target for drug intervention. Viral polypeptides may undergo extensive post-translational modification including cleavage and glycosylation. The former process is often mediated by viral protease and such enzymes are major targets for antiviral chemotherapy: HIV protease inhibitors are an important class of antiretroviral drugs.

Replication

Synthesis of new viral genomes is usually under the control of regulatory viral proteins synthesized earlier in the viral lifecycle. As far as DNA viruses are concerned, the larger ones, such as herpes and pox viruses, encode their own DNA-dependent DNA polymerase, whereas the smaller viruses like adenovirus, parvovirus, and papillomavirus, use the host cell enzyme. The DNA genomes of hepatitis B virions are produced by reverse transcription from large RNA transcripts! RNA viruses mostly depend on viral polymerases for their replication. Once again, virus-specific enzymes make good drug targets: a major mechanism of action of aciclovir against herpes simplex virus is the differential inhibition of the viral DNA polymerase as compared with the host cell DNA-polymerase. Similarly, reverse transcriptase inhibitors are effective against hepatitis B.

Assembly

Following synthesis of the various structural elements, new virus particles are assembled. In tissue culture, the accumulations of viral components may be visible within infected cells as **inclusion bodies**. The process of assembly in small icosahedral viruses is facilitated by the tendency of major capsid proteins to polymerize and so self-assemble into hollow capsid-like structures. With large icosahedral viruses, the process of capsid assembly is complex, with scaffolding proteins providing internal supports for the immature capsid prior to insertion of the viral genome. Virus-specific proteases are often involved in the maturation of infectious viral particles (before or after cellular release), again serving as potential drug targets. For enveloped viruses, the nascent nucleocapsids must accumulate in the vicinity of the appropriate cell membrane into which envelope glycoproteins have been inserted.

Release

Release of new viral particles from an infected cell requires that either the cell must undergo lysis, as is the case for most nonenveloped viruses, or that the virions must bud from the cell surface, like HIV and influenza virus, or that they must be exocytosed like HSV. In influenza A and B virus infections, the final separation of new virions from the host cell surface requires the action of a virus encoded neuraminidase. Inhibition of this enzyme keeps the virus trapped on the infected cells and is the mechanism of action of a new class of drugs, the neuraminidase inhibitors (NAIs, e.g. zanamivir and oseltamivir), which are effective against both influenza A and B (amantadine and its sister drug, rimantidine, are both only active against influenza A).

Virus classification

Viruses can be classified in a great many different ways: by host type, symptomatology, particle morphology or genomic properties to name a few. A universal system of virus taxonomy has been established to separate viruses into major groupings – **families** – on the basis of virion morphology and strategies of replication. Families are subdivided into **genera** on the basis of physicochemical or serologic differences. Virus family names carry the suffix – **viridae** and virus genus names carry the suffix – **virus**. Conventionally virus families are grouped together according to genome type and physical virion characteristics (Table 2.2). Other classifications based on genome type and transcription strategy (Baltimore classification) exist. (See Further reading.)

Table 2.2 Classification of families of animal viruses that contain members able to infect humans

Genome type	Genome structure	Virion structure	Virus family and example
DNA	Double-stranded (ds)	Enveloped	Herpesviridae, e.g. HSV
			Poxviridae, e.g. vaccinia virus
		Nonenveloped	Adenoviridae, e.g. adenovirus
			Papovaviridae, e.g. papillomavirus
	Single-stranded (ss)	Nonenveloped	Parvoviridae, e.g. parvovirus B19
	ds/ss	Enveloped	Hepadnaviridae, e.g. HBV
RNA	ds, positive-sense, segmented	Nonenveloped	Reoviridae, e.g. rotavirus
	ss, positive-sense, nonsegmented	Enveloped	Flaviviridae, e.g. HCV Coronaviridae, e.g. SARS virus Togaviridae, e.g. rubella virus
			Retroviridae, e.g. HIV
		Nonenveloped	Astroviridae, e.g. astrovirus Caliciviridae, e.g. norovirus Picornaviridae, e.g. poliovirus
	ss, negative-sense, segmented	Enveloped	Orthomyxoviridae, e.g. influenza A virus
	ss, negative-sense and ambisense, segmented		Arenaviridae, e.g. Lassa virus Bunyaviridae, e.g. Hantaan virus
	ss, negative-sense, nonsegmented		Filoviridae, e.g. Ebola virus Paramyxoviridae, e.g. mumps virus Rhabdoviridae, e.g. rabies virus

Viruses as parasites

Viruses are truly parasitological: they have an absolute requirement for their host merely in order to replicate, and their presence is almost invariably to the detriment of the host. The concepts of **normal flora**, **colonization** and **mutualistic symbiosis** really do not apply! Viruses can only replicate intracellularly and, hence, aside from contamination, the presence of viable virions at any site in/on the human body necessarily implies that there is ongoing viral replication, although this may be localized (e.g. human papilloma virus infection of the uterine cervix) rather than disseminated. Having said that, there are some common viruses which, despite replicating extensively and successfully, transmitting themselves from person to person, seem to cause little if any recognizable pathology (e.g. SEN virus, TTV, GBV-C) and there are others, notably all the members of the herpes family, that are never cleared from the human body but remain in a harmless **latent** state in certain cells from which, however, they may later reactivate.

Despite the fundamentally parasitological nature of viruses, there is nevertheless a group of human viruses that might reasonably be considered to have a somewhat mutualistic relationship with their host. These are the human **endogenous retroviruses** (HERVs), the legacy of ancient germ cell infections by exogenous retroviruses (not to be confused with retroviruses such as HIV that cause disease) over the last 60 million years. It is thought that endogenous retroviruses are present, integrated in the genome of every cell, in every species of vertebrate. Here they replicate in Mendelian fashion, as an integral part of the sexual reproduction of the host, without the necessity for formation of infectious virus particles. Remarkably, 8% of the human genome consists of complete HERV genomes and, if HERV fragments are also counted, then the roughly half our DNA is retroviral in origin! The presence of HERV DNA in human cells may well be responsible for a variety of human genetic diseases, cancers, and autoimmune diseases. However, there is much evidence that expression of ERV-encoded proteins makes a critical contribution to mammalian placental function: the formation of the synctial layer that provides the physiological barrier between the maternal and fetal circulations. HERVs have also been found to contribute physiologically in other human tissues.

Fungi: structure and function

Fungal cell membrane

Fungal cells like mammalian cells contain a **cell membrane** that serves an important role in cell structure and metabolism (Figure 2.13). Complex lipid particles, called **sterols**, account for about 25% of the weight of the fungal cell membrane. The principal sterol in many fungal species is **ergosterol**, which differs from the principle sterol found in mammalian cell membranes, cholesterol.

Fungal cell walls

Not all species of fungi have cell walls but in those that do, the semi-rigid **cell walls** are composed of a complex network of carbohydrates and proteins (Figure 2.13). These molecules vary in composition depending on the fungal species. Carbohydrates present in the fungal cell wall may include **glucan polymers** such as beta (1,6)-glucan, beta (1,3)-glucan, and **chitin**, the same carbohydrate that gives strength to the exoskeleton of insects. The fungal cell wall gives shape and form, protects against mechanical injury and osmotic lysis, and also limits the entry of molecules that may be toxic to the fungus, like plant-produced

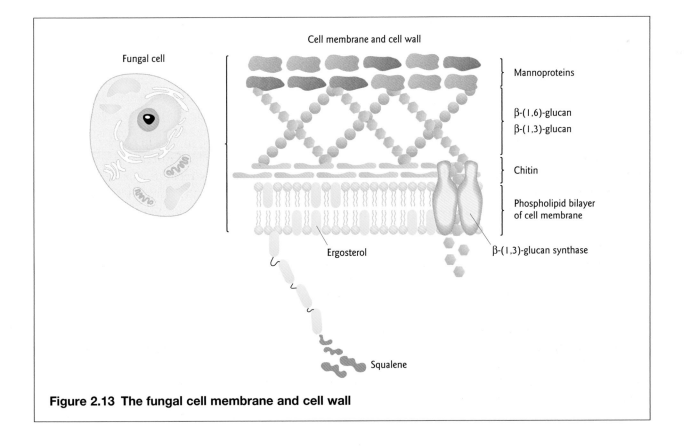

Figure 2.13 The fungal cell membrane and cell wall

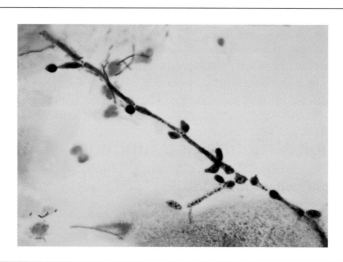

Figure 2.14 Gram stain of *Candida albicans* showing pseudohyphae and budding cells. Provided by Dr Stuart Brown. Courtesy of the Centers for Disease Control and Prevention; from CDC website: http://phil.cdc.gov/phil/details.asp

fungicides. The fungal cell wall is also an important site for filtration of ions and proteins, as well as metabolism of more complex nutrients. Cell wall surface molecules are responsible for attachment of fungi to several types of surfaces, including host cells in the case of pathogenic fungi.

Reproduction

During their evolution most fungi have relied upon a combination of both sexual and asexual reproduction to aid survival. Sexual spores and the structures that develop around them may aid fungal classification. However, the asexual stage in many fungi has proved so successful as a means of rapid dispersal in the environment that the sexual stage has ceased. In these fungi the shape of the asexual spores and the arrangement of associated structures are of more importance in identification.

Molds reproduce by the formation of several kinds of sexual and asexual spores that develop from the vegetative mycelium, or from aerial mycelium that aids air-borne dissemination. Yeasts reproduce sexually with the formation of spores or asexually by budding. The bud may become detached from the parent cell (true yeast) or it may remain attached and itself produce another bud (pseudoyeast). *Candida* species are examples of yeast like fungi. *Candida albicans* is the commonest candida causing human infection. It has a dimorphic lifecycle with yeast and hyphal stages. The yeast produces hyphae (strands) and pseudohyphae. The pseudohyphae are so called because they can give rise to yeast cells by apical or lateral budding (Figure 2.14). Conversion to hyphal form occurs if there is tissue invasion.

Protozoa: structure and function

Structure

Protozoa are unicellular **eukaryotes**, whose DNA exists as chromosomes within a nucleus. The nucleus is surrounded by a nuclear membrane, which has multiple channels connecting the nucleoplasm with the endoplasm. Some organisms have a single nucleus, and others may be binucleate (e.g. *Giardia lamblia*) or have multinucleate cysts (e.g. *Entamoeba histolytica*). The nucleus may contain single or multiple linear chromosomes.

The **endoplasm** is the inner portion of the cytoplasm immediately surrounding the nucleus. It contains chromatoid bodies, endoplasmic reticulum, Golgi bodies, mitochrondria, food vacuoles, and microsomes. The **ectoplasm** is the metabolically active portion of the cell, and is involved in respiration, locomotion, and phagocytosis. The cell is limited by the plasma membrane, which controls the intake and output of nutrition and waste products. It may vary in shape and form pseudopodia for locomotion (e.g. in *E. histolytica*).

Protozoa may have a number of structures external to the plasma membrane. These include an external glycocalyx (as in *Leishmania donovani*), or an outer shell that allows it to survive outside the body for long periods and makes it resistant to chlorine disinfection (as in *C. parvum*), or a tough cyst wall to enable the organism to survive in the external environment (as in *E. histolytica*). Production of a cyst or **encystation** is triggered by alteration in nutrition or oxygen supply, pH, or dessication.

Some protozoa have specialized organelles; for example *Leishmania* spp. possess flagella which arise from a specialized kinetoplast containing its own DNA. Others, such as *Balantidium coli*, express cilia, which beat in formation to propel the organism.

Due to factors such as their complex lifecycles and differentiation of the single cell into organelles that perform particular functions (e.g. cilia), the microscopic morphology of protozoa is often diagnostic, particularly after staining. This differs from bacteria, which often require culture and biochemical testing for diagnosis. In fact as protozoa have complex nutritional requirements, laboratory culture is possible only in rare cases.

Lifecycles

Protozoa have more complex reproductive cycles compared to bacteria and these lifecycles may involve a number of different hosts and environments. Unlike bacteria which have only limited sexual function, based on transfer of genome fragments by various means, protozoa have well-developed sexual reproduction.

Amoebae have the simplest lifecycle of all the protozoa. Only one species, *E. histolytica*, is recognized as a true pathogen in human disease. The motile feeding **trophozoite** form (Figure 2.15a) causes invasive infection, presenting most often with dysentery or liver abscesses, but the disease is transmitted by non-motile resistant **cysts** via contaminated food or water (Figure 2.15b). Excystation occurs in the intestinal tract and organisms multiply by binary fission; trophozoites then colonize the caecal area. Definitive diagnosis is by recognition of motile trophozoites containing red blood cells in the patient's stool or biopsy material. Microscopic detection of cysts of the correct size and appearance in fecal specimens is suggestive but not conclusive as these must be differentiated from the cysts of the nonpathogenic *Entamoeba coli*.

The intestinal and urogenital flagellates also have a lifecycle that is relatively simple, resembling that of the amoebae. Most simple flagellates have both a cyst and trophozoite stage, but *Trichomonas vaginalis* lacks a cyst stage and the trophozoite of these organisms serves as the infective stage.

Giardia lamblia is one of the most common intestinal parasites worldwide infecting up to 20% of the world's population. It is a common cause of diarrhoea and is transmitted in the cyst form, mainly by infected

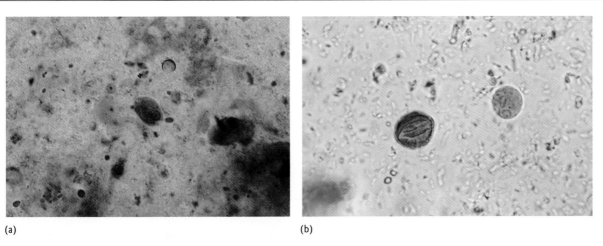

(a) (b)

Figure 2.15 (a) Trophozoites of *Entamoeba histolytica*. (b) Cysts of *Entamoeba histolytica*. From CDC website: http://www.dpd.cdc.gov/dpdx/HTML/

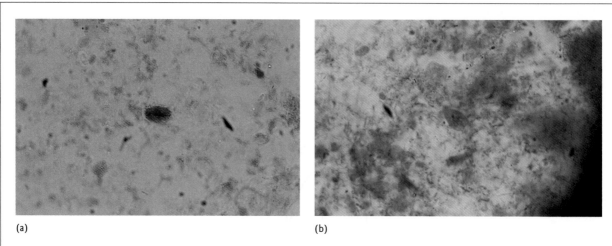

(a)   (b)

Figure 2.16 *Giardia lamblia.* **(a) Cyst form (Trichrome stained). (b) Trophozoite form (Trichrome stained).**

water. Cysts of *G. lamblia* are oval with up to four nuclei (Figure 2.16a) and trophozoites are pear shaped, bilaterally symmetrical with two nuclei and four pairs of flagella (Figure 2.16b).

Trichomonas vaginalis is the most common pathogenic protozoan of humans in industrialized countries (Figure 2.17). This organism resides in the female lower genital tract and the male urethra and prostate, where it replicates by binary fission. It is transmitted through close sexual contact, in the trophozoite form, and is a common cause of vaginitis in women and urethritis in males.

The medically important hemoflagellates have more complex lifecycles and are transmitted by **vectors**. A **vector-borne** disease is one in which the pathogenic microorganism is transmitted from an infected individual to another individual by an arthropod or other agent, sometimes with other animals serving as intermediary hosts. The transmission depends upon the attributes and requirements of at least three different living organisms: the pathologic agent (either a virus, protozoa, bacteria, or helminth); the vector (commonly arthropods such as ticks or mosquitoes); and the human host. In addition, intermediary hosts such as domesticated and/or wild animals often serve as a reservoir for the pathogen until susceptible human populations are exposed. The distribution of vector-associated diseases is restricted to the geographical area where the vector is found.

Figure 2.17 Trophozoites of
***Trichomonas vaginalis.* From**
CDC website: http://www.dpd.cdc.gov/
dpdx/HTML/

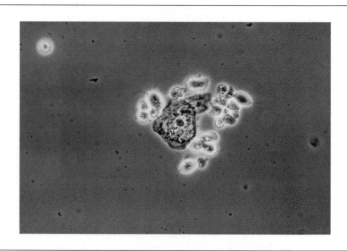

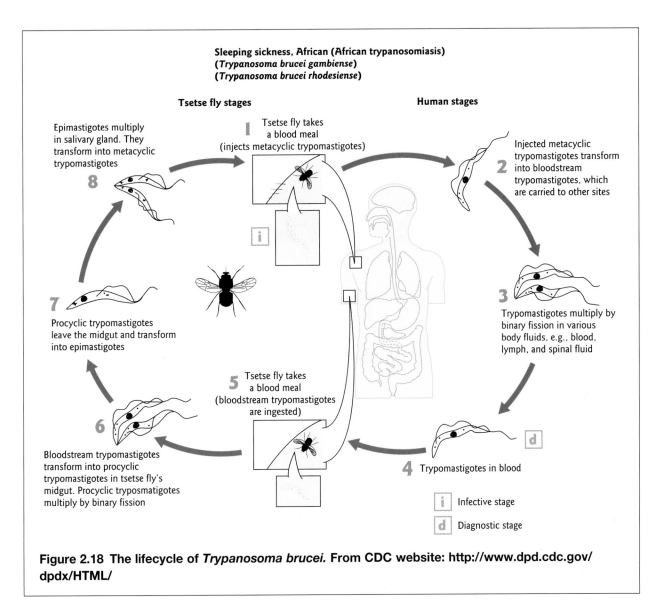

Sleeping sickness, African (African trypanosomiasis)
(*Trypanosoma brucei gambiense*)
(*Trypanosoma brucei rhodesiense*)

Tsetse fly stages

Human stages

8 Epimastigotes multiply in salivary gland. They transform into metacyclic trypomastigotes

1 Tsetse fly takes a blood meal (injects metacyclic trypomastigotes)

2 Injected metacyclic trypomastigotes transform into bloodstream trypomastigotes, which are carried to other sites

7 Procyclic trypomastigotes leave the midgut and transform into epimastigotes

3 Trypomastigotes multiply by binary fission in various body fluids, e.g., blood, lymph, and spinal fluid

5 Tsetse fly takes a blood meal (bloodstream trypomastigotes are ingested)

6 Bloodstream trypomastigotes transform into procyclic trypomastigotes in tsetse fly's midgut. Procyclic tryposmatigotes multiply by binary fission

4 Trypomastigotes in blood

i Infective stage

d Diagnostic stage

Figure 2.18 The lifecycle of *Trypanosoma brucei*. From CDC website: http://www.dpd.cdc.gov/ dpdx/HTML/

Trypanosoma brucei is the cause of African sleeping sickness and is transmitted by infected *Glossina* spp. flies (also known as tsetse flies). There are two main infecting species, *T. brucei gambiense* which causes West African sleeping sickness and *T. brucei rhodesiense* which causes the less acute East African sleeping sickness. Figure 2.18 demonstrates the lifecycle of *T. brucei*; note that trypomastigotes (Figure 2.19) multiply by binary fission and the role of the tsetse fly as the vector in the lifecycle.

Another flagellate, *Trypanosoma cruzi*, is the cause of Chagas disease (American trypanosomiasis), a disease geographically restricted to South and Central America. *T. cruzi* is transmitted by another vector, the "kissing" or reduviid bug (*Triatoma infestans*) (Figure 2.20).

Leishmania spp. promastigotes are transmitted to man by the bite of a sandfly (*Phlebotomus* spp.). There are many species of *Leishmania* parasites causing two main diseases syndromes, cutaneous and the more serious, visceral leishmaniasis. The lifecycle of *Leishmania* parasites is shown in Figure 2.21, again note the role of the sandfly vector. **Amastigotes** are the stage of the lifecycle seen in humans multiplying in various types of cells including macrophages (Figure 2.22).

Plasmodium species are the causative agent of malaria, which is the most common and globally important protozoal illness. There are four main species of medical importance: *Plasmodium falciparum*, *P. vivax*, *P. ovale*, and *P. malariae*. Malaria is another vector-borne illness, *Plasmodium* spp. sporozoites are transmitted to man by

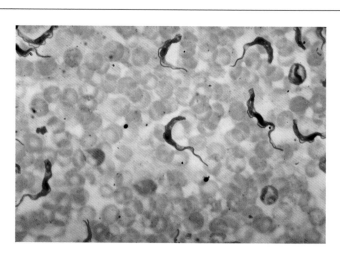

Figure 2.19 *Trypanosoma brucei* trypomastigotes in a peripheral blood smear (stained with Giemsa). From CDC website: http://www.dpd.cdc.gov/ dpdx/HTML/

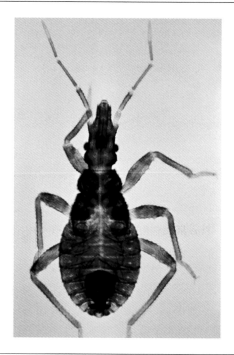

Figure 2.20 *Triatoma infestans.* From CDC website: http://www.dpd.cdc.gov/ dpdx/HTML/

the bite from a female *Anopheles* mosquito. It is important to fully understand the lifecycle of *Plasmodium* species in order to comprehend the pathogenesis of malaria and to appreciate the medications that can be used to combat this important disease. The lifecycle is therefore fully outlined in Chapter 17, which is devoted to malaria, and not covered here any further.

Other medically important sporozoan parasites whose lifecycle warrants coverage include *Toxoplasma gondii*, *Cryptosporidium parvum*, *Isopora belli* and *Cyclospora cayetenensis*.

Cats are the definitive hosts for the sexual stages of *T. gondii* and thus are the main reservoirs of infection. After **tissue cysts** or **oocysts** are ingested by the cat, viable organisms are released and invade epithelial cells of the small intestine. Here they undergo an asexual followed by a sexual cycle and then form oocysts,

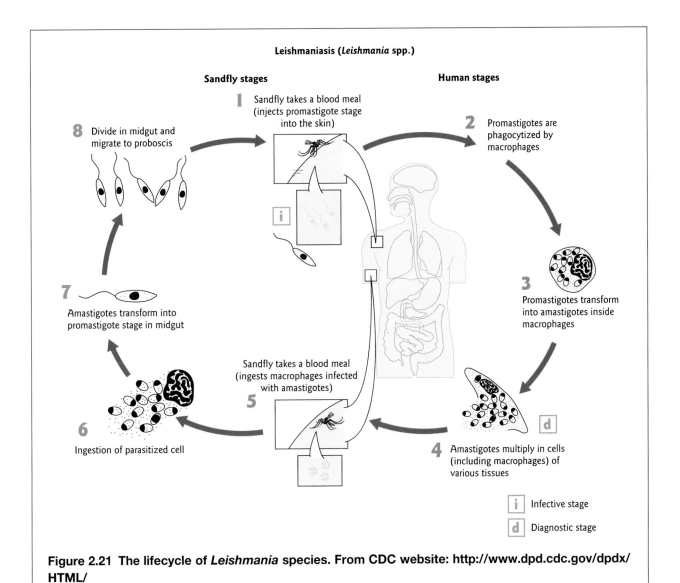

Leishmaniasis (*Leishmania* spp.)

Sandfly stages

Human stages

1 Sandfly takes a blood meal (injects promastigote stage into the skin)

2 Promastigotes are phagocytized by macrophages

8 Divide in midgut and migrate to proboscis

3 Promastigotes transform into amastigotes inside macrophages

7 Amastigotes transform into promastigote stage in midgut

Sandfly takes a blood meal (ingests macrophages infected with amastigotes)

5

6 Ingestion of parasitized cell

4 Amastigotes multiply in cells (including macrophages) of various tissues

i Infective stage

d Diagnostic stage

Figure 2.21 The lifecycle of *Leishmania* species. From CDC website: http://www.dpd.cdc.gov/dpdx/ HTML/

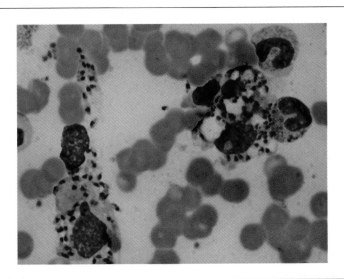

Figure 2.22 Amastigotes of *Leishmania tropica* seen within a macrophage from a patient with cutaneous leishmaniasis. Courtesy: Department of Parasitology, University College London Hospitals

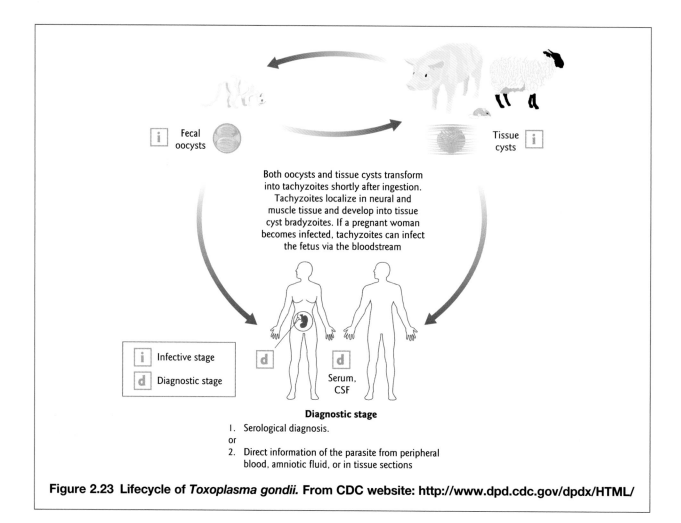

Both oocysts and tissue cysts transform into tachyzoites shortly after ingestion. Tachyzoites localize in neural and muscle tissue and develop into tissue cyst bradyzoites. If a pregnant woman becomes infected, tachyzoites can infect the fetus via the bloodstream

Fecal oocysts

Tissue cysts

| i | Infective stage |
| d | Diagnostic stage |

Serum, CSF

Diagnostic stage

I. Serological diagnosis.

or

2. Direct information of the parasite from peripheral blood, amniotic fluid, or in tissue sections

Figure 2.23 Lifecycle of *Toxoplasma gondii*. From CDC website: http://www.dpd.cdc.gov/dpdx/HTML/

which are excreted (Figure 2.23). The unsporulated oocyst takes 1–5 days after excretion to **sporulate** (become infective). Oocysts can survive in the environment for several months and are remarkably resistant to disinfectants, freezing, and drying.

Human toxoplasmosis infection may be acquired in several ways including consumption of undercooked infected meat containing sporulated oocysts, ingestion of the oocyst from fecally contaminated hands or food, organ transplantation, blood transfusion, or transplacental transmission. The parasites form tissue cysts, most commonly in skeletal muscle, myocardium, and brain.

Cryptosporidium parvum is another common intestinal parasite, which is transmitted by water, milk, and direct contact with farm animals. Person-to-person contact can also occur. Symptomatic infection, presenting as cramps and watery diarrhea, is more common in children under 5 and those with HIV infection.

The sexual and asexual lifecycles of *C. parvum* occur in the same host. Ingestion of the infective oocyst (Figure 2.24) initiates the asexual cycle with the release of **sporozoites**. These penetrate the intestinal mucosal border and mature into trophozoites, which when mature rupture to release **merozoites**. Merozoites penetrate other cells, either to continue asexual reproduction or to transform into gametes of the sexual reproductive cycle to produce more oocysts.

Infection with *I. belli* is seen less often than *C. parvum* but the symptoms are clinically indistinguishable. Like *C. parvum*, infection in most is self-limiting, whereas immunocompromised patients may have protracted symptoms. The lifecycle of *I. belli* is very similar to that of *C. parvum* but the oocyst requires 48 hours of existence outside the body before it becomes infective.

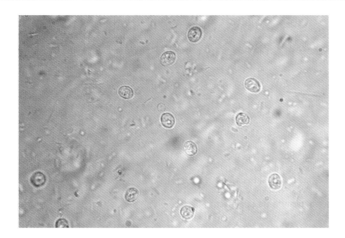

Figure 2.24 Wet preparation demonstrating *Cryptosporidium parvum* oocysts. From CDC website: http://www.dpd.cdc.gov/dpdx/HTML/

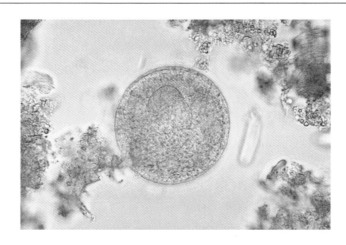

Figure 2.25 *Balantidium coli* cyst. From CDC website: http://www.dpd.cdc.gov/dpdx/HTML/

Cyclospora cayetanensis is primarily seen in immunocompetent patients returning from areas in which the organism is endemic, such as Central America and East Asia. *C. cayetanensis* may cause prolonged but self-limiting diarrhea. The lifecycle has not been fully elucidated in humans as yet but is likely to be similar to *C. parvum* and *I. belli*. However unlike these pathogens, person-to-person transmission is unusual as the oocysts have been shown to require a week outside the body to become infective.

Only one ciliate, *Balantidium coli*, is considered a pathogen for humans. Most people with infection are asymptomatic, but the organism may cause a self-limiting diarrhea. The lifecycle is similar to that of the amoebae, with the cyst (Figure 2.25) being the infective stage for the human host. The round thick walled cyst is large, averaging 45–75 μm and is covered with short cilia.

For a detailed description of helminthic (worm infestations) diseases of humans, see CDC website (http://www.dpd.cdc.gov/dpdx).

Further reading

Brooks GF, Butel JS, Morse SA. *Jawetz, Melnick, & Adelberg's Medical Microbiology*, 24th edition. New York: McGraw-Hill Medical, 2007

Chiodini PL, Moody A, Manser DW. *Atlas of Medical Helminthology and Protozoology*, 4th edition. London: Churchill Livingstone, 2001

Koonin EV. Virology: Gulliver among the Lilliputians. *Curr Biol* 2005;15(5):R167–R169

Morag C, Timbury A, McCartney, Thakker B, Ward K. *Notes on Medical Microbiology*. London: Churchill Livingstone, 2004

Ratner L, Doran EL, Rafalski JA, et al. Complete nucleotide sequence of the AIDS virus, HTLV-III. *Nature* 1985;313(6000):277–284

Ryan FP. Human endogenous retroviruses in health and disease: a symbiotic perspective. *J R Soc Med* 2004;97(12):560–565

Winn WC, Koneman EW, Allen SD, et al. *Koneman's Color Atlas and Textbook of Diagnostic Microbiology*, 6th edition. Baltimore, MD: Lippincott Williams and Wilkins, 2006

Chapter 3
Host defence versus microbial pathogenesis and the mechanisms of microbial escape

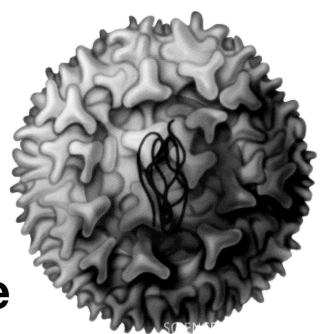

N. Shetty, E. Aarons, J. Andrews

Host defence
  Innate immunity
  Adaptive immunity
  The immunization success story

Microbial pathogenesis and escape mechanisms
  Bacterial and fungal pathogens
  Viruses
  Protozoa and helminths

In this chapter we will attempt to understand the interplay between host defence, microbial pathogenesis, and mechanisms of microbial escape. The chapter will present this theme in two broad sections:

1 Host defence mechanisms:
  – innate and adaptive immunity
  – immunization: passive and active.
2 Microbial pathogenesis and mechanisms of escape in:
  – bacterial and fungal pathogens
  – viruses
  – protozoa and helminths.

Host defence

A formidable range of infectious agents use the human body as a sanctuary to raise their offspring. **Host defence against microbial invasion** comes in the form of a mighty triad (innate immunity, antibody, and cellular immunity). To this we can add the protection offered by **immunization** which, in a sense, is a manipulation of the adaptive immune process. However, it merits discussion as a separate subject.

This chapter will deal with host defence by these well-recognized entities:

Table 3.1 Cell types involved in the defence against microbes

Phagocytic cells	**Polymorphonuclear neutrophils** **Mononuclear phagocytes** (include monocytes in blood and macrophages in tissues) **Eosinophils**
Lymphocytes: functionally lymphocytes are divided into: **B cells**	become antibody producing **plasma cells**
T cells	are involved in cell-mediated immune response and provide B cell help to produce antibody
Large granular lymphocytes	also called **null cells or natural killer (NK) cells** – kill other rogue cells in a nonspecific manner

- Innate immunity:
  - constitutional factors
  - natural barriers and normal flora
  - phagocytosis
  - complement.
- Adaptive immunity:
  - antibody
  - cell-mediated immunity (including cytokines).
- Immunization:
  - passive
  - active.

Before we commence our discussions on innate and adaptive specific immunity, let us review the tissues and cell types involved in defence. These are summarized in Table 3.1.

Innate immunity

Among the nonspecific or innate defence mechanisms there are those that form a set of ill understood and perhaps grossly under-emphasized **constitutional factors** that make one species innately susceptible and another resistant to certain infections.

These constitutional factors are listed below.

1. Genetic – between species
For example:

- *Mycobacterium leprae* seems to infect humans and armadillos only.
- *Bacillus anthracis* is an infection of humans though not of chickens.
- Gonorrhoea is a disease of man and chimpanzees and not of any other species.

Some species seem to be able to harbor organisms within their body tissues while the same organism may cause another species to succumb to such an infection. Within man, there are certain well known **racial differences** in disease susceptibility:

- Dark skinned individuals have an increased susceptibility to coccidioidomycosis.
- Certain dark skinned people lack the red cell Duffy antigen and are not susceptible to vivax malaria.
- Genetic control of disease has been shown to be strongly associated with the major histocompatibility complex (see Further reading).

2. Age

The very young are more susceptible to many infections, such as *Escherichia coli* meningitis; this may be because bactericidal IgM does not cross the placenta. At the other end of the spectrum rickettsial infections and certain viral infections of children are more severe with age.

3. Metabolic factors

Hypoadrenal and hypothyroid states decrease resistance to infection. In diseases such as diabetes mellitus where altered metabolism causes increase in blood glucose, decrease in pH, and a reduced influx of phagocytes – infection can be a severe complication. Steroid hormones are known to affect many modalities of the immune response.

4. Neuroendocrine factors

There is a growing body of evidence that supports the hypothesis that immune processes can be influenced by neuroendocrine factors. Immunologic cells have receptors for a whole range of hormones. Corticosteroids, androgens, estrogens, and progesterone depress immune responses, whereas growth hormone, insulin, and thyroxine do the opposite. Immunologic organs are innervated by autonomic and primary sensorial neurons; hormone secretion is balanced by neural control. It therefore seems reasonable to say that immune responses are finely tuned by neuroendocrine circuits. At a more physiologic level, stress and circadian rhythms modify the functioning of the immune system.

5. Environment

Poor living conditions, overcrowding, and malnutrition also increase susceptibility to infection.

Natural barriers to infectious agents are simple yet effective means of innate defence (Figure 3.1). A major form of defence in this context is the **intact skin** which is impermeable to most infectious agents. Many fungal infections appear to require some breach in skin before infection can be established. Bloodstream infections caused by *Candida* species are often associated with breaches of the skin by intravascular catheters. Dermatophytic fungi cause a variety of skin infections without a breach in the skin but do not cause more

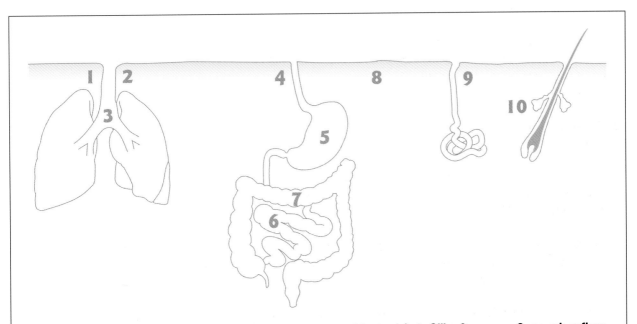

Figure 3.1 Natural barriers to infection (structures are not to scale). 1, Cilia; 2, mucus; 3, cough reflex; 4, mucus; 5, acid in gastric reflux; 6, intestinal enzymes; 7, colonic flora; 8, intact skin; 9, sweat; 10, sebum

invasive disease because they prefer temperatures below body temperature of 37°C. **Sweat glands** and **sebaceous glands** are potential points of entry for the infectious agent, however, most bacteria fail to enter due to the low pH and direct inhibitory effects of **lysozymes**, **lactic acid** and other **fatty acids** of sweat and sebaceous secretions. An exception is *Staphylococcus aureus* which commonly infects the hair follicle and glands.

Mucus secretions of the tracts that connect internal organs to external surfaces form an important form of defence. They entrap and immobilize bacteria and hence, prevent adherence and colonization of epithelial surfaces. **Hairs at the external nares**, the **cough reflex**, and the **ciliated mucus membrane** of the respiratory tract help drive entrapped organisms upwards and outwards.

Mechanical factors which help protect mucosal tracts are the **washing action of tears, saliva, and urine.** Many secretions contain bactericidal components such as **acid in gastric juice**; **lysozyme** in tears, nasal secretions and saliva; **proteolytic enzymes** in intestinal secretions; **spermine and zinc in semen**, and **lactoperoxidase in breast milk**.

Normal microbial flora

Normal flora is essential to well-being, playing a vital part in promoting health: preventing disease, protecting against invasive pathogenic microorganisms, and maintaining equilibrium within the host. Our bodies are like hosts that carry an aura of living microbes about them. Rich in biodiversity we are home to vast numbers of bacterial cells. This normal bacterial flora lives on the external body surfaces, along mucosal surfaces, and in the gut.

The composition of the normal flora varies somewhat from individual to individual. Some bacterial species may be carried only transiently. Most, however, are fairly permanent. It is extremely difficult to alter the composition of or eradicate the normal flora of, say, the skin in a healthy individual. Hand washing removes transient bacterial flora but skin gets rapidly re-colonized after washing. Some members of the normal flora can become pathogenic if they acquire additional virulence factors (e.g. *E. coli*) or are introduced into normally sterile sites (e. g. coagulase negative staphylococci in blood).

Normal flora may prevent pathogenic microorganisms from getting a foothold on body surfaces (a phenomenon known as colonization resistance). Administration of broad-spectrum antibiotics has a profound effect on the normal flora and can result in colonization with antibiotic-resistant organisms. Antibiotic-mediated disruption of the normal flora can lead to fungal infections, such as superficial or, in the critically ill, invasive candidiasis, or to antibiotic-associated colitis caused by *Clostridium difficile*.

Even though most bacteria that constitute normal microbial flora of the human skin, nails, eyes, oropharynx, genitalia, and gastrointestinal tract are harmless in healthy individuals, these organisms may cause disease in compromised hosts. Here they are said to act as opportunists exploiting the susceptibility of the host to cause infection. Viruses and eukaryotic parasites are not considered members of the normal microbial flora.

There are multiple viruses (endogenous, latent or nonpathogenic, e.g. hepatitis G virus) that coexist with humans harmlessly. They may contribute actively to our well-being but are still not normal microbial flora, which conventionally just refers to bacteria and some fungi.

Colonization versus infection

Colonization and infection are commonly confused terms and may lead to unnecessary anxiety for patients and their families. Colonization occurs when microorganisms inhabit a specific body site (such as the skin, bowel, or chronic ulcers) but do not cause signs and symptoms of infection. For the most part colonizing bacteria live in an ecological niche on the human host and pose no threat to the individual.

However, colonized pathogens do have the potential to cause infection if they enter a different site on the same patient (e.g. from skin into wound or from skin into the bloodstream through an intravenous catheter); or if they spread to another more susceptible person through the environment or via hands of healthcare staff. Often colonization may precede infection: a typical example is *Neisseria meningitidis*, an organism that is known to colonize the upper respiratory tract before infecting the central nervous system of susceptible patients, causing meningitis.

Common colonizing bacteria that cause particular concern in hospital environments are methicillin-resistant *Staphylococcus aureus* (MRSA), *C. difficile*, and vancomycin- or glycopeptide-resistant enterococci (VRE/GRE). Besides healthcare staff working in hospital environments, individuals at risk for colonization are generally those who may have had prolonged hospitalizations, chronic wounds, or who have received treatment with multiple antibiotics.

These potential pathogens can be transmitted within healthcare facilities from reservoirs of unrecognized colonized patients or healthcare staff and from contaminated environments. Certain individuals are heavy shedders of colonizing bacteria, typically such individuals have eczema or dermatitis and shed large amounts of skin scales each of which acts like a magic carpet carrying thousands of microorganisms.

Should infection occur, it is usually evidenced by the onset of fever, a rise in the white blood cell count or inflammation and purulent drainage from a wound or body cavity. The distinction between colonization and infection is a clinical one. Such a distinction should be determined by the clinician and not by culture results alone.

Why is normal flora critical to the host?

Most of our understanding of the beneficial effects of normal microbial flora comes from studies on germ free animals (animals which lack any bacterial flora). Bacterial flora of the gastrointestinal tract, perhaps because of their sheer weight in numbers and species diversity, seem to have the greatest overall impact on their host.

Normal bacterial flora prevents colonization by pathogens (also called colonization resistance) by competing for attachment sites and for essential nutrients. This is thought to be their most important beneficial effect, and has been demonstrated in the oral cavity, the intestine, the skin, and the vaginal epithelium. Figure 3.2 illustrates some of the factors that are important in the competition between the normal flora and bacterial pathogens.

Other putative beneficial effects of normal flora are less well studied:

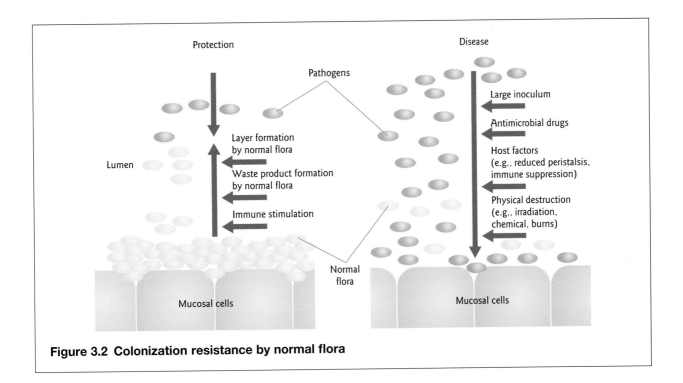

Figure 3.2 Colonization resistance by normal flora

- **Normal flora may offer protection to the host by antagonizing other bacteria** through the production of substances which inhibit or kill nonindigenous species. The intestinal bacteria produce a variety of substances ranging from relatively nonspecific fatty acids and peroxides to highly specific bacteriocins, which inhibit or kill other bacteria. Lactobacilli in the vagina create an acidic environment which protects against infection with *Neisseria gonorrhoeae*.

- **Resident bacteria may stimulate the production of cross-reactive antibodies.** Antigenic components of resident bacteria may induce an immunological response. Low levels of antibodies produced against these components are known to cross-react with certain related pathogens, preventing infection or invasion.

- **Normal flora may play an important role in the development of certain tissues.** There is evidence that the cecum of germ-free animals is enlarged, thin-walled, and fluid-filled, compared to that of conventional animals. Intestinal lymphatic tissues such as Peyer's patches of germ-free animals are poorly developed compared to conventional animals and are less able to respond to immunologic stimulation.

- **Components of normal bowel flora synthesize and excrete vitamins** in excess of their own needs; these are absorbed as nutrients by the host. For example, enteric bacteria secrete vitamin K and vitamin B_{12}.

Constituents of normal microbial flora in the human host

The composition of normal flora in humans is related to factors such as age, sex, diet, and nutrition. Some bacteria are found resident at particular anatomical sites; others are transient. Developmental changes in humans such as weaning, eruption of teeth, puberty, menstruation, and menopause, invariably affect the composition of the normal flora in the skin, the oral cavity, and the vagina. Despite the limits posed by these variations, bacterial flora at different sites of the human host is relatively predictable.

It has been calculated that the human body is home to more bacterial cells (there are more than 10^{14} in the gut alone) than the total number of human eukaryotic cells in all the organs in the body.

Skin

It is said that healthy, clean and dry skin stains "Gram positive." If areas become sweaty, unwashed or broken the spectrum changes with Gram negative organisms moving in to take residence. Skin thus provides a good example of biodiversity in different microenvironments. The adult human is covered with approximately 2 square meters of skin. The density and composition of the normal flora of the skin varies with the anatomical site. Bacteria on the skin near any body orifice may be similar to those in the orifice.

The majority of skin microorganisms consist of Gram positive organisms: coagulase negative staphylococci, for example, *Staphylococcus epidermidis*, *Micrococcus* sp., and diptheroids such as corynebacteria. These are generally nonpathogenic and constitute normal flora, although they can be opportunistic pathogens in patients with intravascular catheters, prostheses, and postoperative sternal wound infections. Sometimes the potentially pathogenic *S. aureus* is found in warm moist and sweaty areas of the body such as the hairline, axilla, perineum, and anterior nares: appropriate screening sites to detect carriage.

Oral and upper respiratory tract flora

A large number of bacterial species colonize the mouth and the upper respiratory tract. The predominant species are nonhemolytic and alpha-hemolytic streptococci and *Neisseria*.

All mucosal surfaces, and the oral cavity is no exception, by virtue of mucosal folds such as deep gingival crevices are home to a variety of aerobic and anaerobic bacteria. The presence of food debris, nutrients, and other secretions makes the mouth a rich ecological niche. Oral bacteria include streptococci, lactobacilli, staphylococci and spirochaetes, and a variety of anaerobes, especially fusobacteria and bacteroides.

The pathogenic potential of oral and upper airway microflora is well known. Dental caries and periodontal disease, which affects nearly 80% of the population in the western world, is due to *Streptococcus mutans*, an organism normally resident in the mouth. Oral streptococci, particularly *S. milleri* in association with anaerobes in the oral flora, are implicated in purulent sinusitis, and in brain and lung abscesses. Mouth streptococci that translocate into the bloodstream, as a result of periodontal infection, are the commonest organisms causing native valve infective endocarditis, particularly those with pre-existing valvular damage.

Pathogens such as *Streptococcus pneumoniae*, *Streptococcus pyogenes*, *Haemophilus influenzae*, and *Neisseria meningitidis* can also be found colonizing the pharynx in some individuals. If the respiratory tract epithelium becomes damaged, as in smokers, patients with chronic bronchitis or viral pneumonia, individuals who are colonized become susceptible to infection by pathogens residing in the damaged mucosa of the nasopharynx (e.g. *H. influenzae* or *S. pneumoniae*). The lower respiratory tract (trachea, bronchi, and pulmonary tissues) is otherwise free of microorganisms, mainly because of the efficient cleansing action of the ciliated epithelium which lines the tract.

Gastrointestinal (GI) flora

The bacterial flora of the GI tract of humans and animals has been the subject of intense study. In humans, GI flora differs with age, diet, cultural conditions, and the use of antibiotics. Administration of broad spectrum antibiotics is the single most important factor associated with alteration of normal GI flora and its consequences.

At birth the entire intestinal tract is sterile; soon after, the neonatal gut is colonized with the first feed. Initial colonizing bacteria vary with the type of feed. In breast-fed infants bifidobacteria account for more than 90% of the total intestinal bacteria; they play an important role in preventing colonization of the infant intestinal tract by diarrhea-causing pathogenic bacteria.

In the upper GI tract of adult humans, the esophagus contains transient swallowed bacteria from saliva and food. High acidity of the gastric juice precludes the long-term survival of many bacteria. In achlorhydria (where the acidity of gastric juice is not maintained) and malabsorption syndrome bacterial counts increase in the upper GI tract. However, at least half the population in the USA is colonized by *Helicobacter pylori*, an organism that not only survives but flourishes in the acid environment of the stomach. This organism has been implicated in gastric ulcers and is strongly associated with gastric cancer. Rapid peristalsis and the presence of bile also inhibit organisms in the upper GI tract.

Further along the jejunum and into the ileum, bacterial populations begin to increase, and at the ileocecal junction they reach levels of 10^6 to 10^8 organisms/ml, with streptococci, lactobacilli, anaerobes, and bifidobacteria predominating. Fecal flora contains concentrations of 10^9 to 10^{11} bacteria/g and includes a bewildering array of more than 400 bacterial species. Almost 95–99% belong to the anaerobic genera of *Bacteroides*, *Bifidobacterium*, *Eubacterium*, *Peptostreptococcus*, and *Fusobacterium*. In a highly anaerobic environment these bacteria grow and metabolize to produce characteristic metabolic waste products such as acetic, butyric, and lactic acids. These metabolic end products are responsible for inhibiting the growth of other bacteria in the large bowel; they are also used as means of identifying anaerobes in clinical samples. The remaining 1–5% of the flora is made up of *E. coli* and other enteric Gram negative bacilli.

The pathogenic potential of gut flora is manifold. Anaerobes in the intestinal tract are the primary agents of intra-abdominal infections and peritonitis. Bowel perforations as a result of conditions such as diverticulitis and appendicitis; cancer, infarction, surgery, or trauma can cause severe and life-threatening fecal peritonitis. Mucositis in patients undergoing cancer chemotherapy is a predisposing factor for severe Gram negative sepsis in neutropenic (abnormally low or absent white blood cells) and immunosuppressed patients.

Treatment with broad spectrum antibiotics is the single most important risk factor for hospital acquired antibiotic associated colitis. Certain anaerobic species, notably *C. difficile*, remain viable and overgrow in a patient undergoing antimicrobial therapy, and is the cause of intractable and distressing diarrhea.

Urogenital flora

The vagina becomes colonized soon after birth with corynebacteria, coagulase negative staphylococci, streptococci, and lactobacilli. During the reproductive years, from puberty to menopause, circulating estrogens cause vaginal epithelium to secrete glycogen. Lactobacilli predominate in the healthy vagina being able to metabolize the glycogen to lactic acid. The resultant acid pH of the adult vagina, attributed

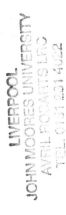

to lactobacilli colonizing the healthy vagina, protects against infection with *N. gonorrhoeae* and *Candida* species. In bacterial vaginosis, a syndrome affecting many sexually active women, the ecological balance of the healthy vagina is disturbed. Gram positive lactobacilli and streptococci are overgrown by mixed anaerobic flora and *Gardnerella* species accounting for the thin watery and foul smelling discharge in bacterial vaginosis. Group B beta hemolytic streptococci (GBS) are carried as normal flora in 20–40% of women and is the commonest cause of neonatal sepsis. Some women may also experience maternal infections and urinary tract infection with GBS. After menopause, the pH again rises, less glycogen is secreted, and the flora returns to that found in prepubescent females.

The distal urethra of males and females is colonized with coagulase negative staphylococci, streptococci, nonpathogenic neisseria, and diphtheroids. This is the reason that patients are advised to collect mid-stream specimens of urine (allowing for the initial voiding of urine to wash away the distal urethral flora) for microbiological examination. Contamination of a urine sample with distal urethral flora can lead to misleading and uninterpretable urine culture results. To preclude this, routine urine microbiology is one of the few specimens where bacterial growth is quantified and a significant culture result is reported as $>10^5$ colony forming units/ml of urine.

Conjunctival flora

The conjunctiva is only sparsely colonized, usually with coagulase negative staphylococci and certain coryneforms. *Staphylococcus aureus*, some streptococci, *Haemophilus* sp., and *Neisseria* sp. are occasionally found. The mechanical action of blinking, tears, and enzymatic action of lysozyme in lachrymal secretions protect the conjunctiva against bacterial infection.

If microorganisms do penetrate the body, two main defensive operations come into play – **phagocytosis** and the bactericidal effect of **soluble chemical factors** (molecules such as complement proteins, acute phase proteins, and cytokines constitute an innate defence mechanism; some play a part in the adaptive defence strategy). Cells other than the polymorphonuclear neutrophil (PMN) may be involved: these cells (basophils, mast cells, and eosinophils) also release inflammatory mediators.

Phagocytosis

The engulfment and digestion of infectious agents is assigned to two major cell populations: the polymorphonuclear neutrophil (PMN) and the macrophage (M). Phagocytosis is a multiphasic act (Figure 3.3), requiring recognition, movement of PMNs out of blood vessels towards the irritant, attachment to microorganisms, ingestion and intracellular killing.

Pattern recognition and ingestion

Phagocytic cells are among the most important defence cells, endowed with a variety of receptors capable of recognizing molecular patterns expressed on the surface of pathogens or pathogen associated molecular patterns (PAMPS); these are shared by a large group of infectious agents and are clearly differentiated from "self" patterns. For example bacterial flagellar protein, flagellin, is potent PAMP. Most body defence cells (neutrophils and macrophages particularly) have **pattern–recognition receptors** (PRRs) for common pathogen-associated molecular patterns (Figure 3.4) and so there is an immediate response against the invading microorganism. Pathogen-associated molecular patterns can also be recognized by a series of soluble pattern-recognition receptors in the blood that function as **opsonins** (Box 3.1) and initiate the complement pathways. In all, the innate immune system is thought to recognize approximately 10^3 molecular patterns.

Most of these PRRs are lectin-like and bind to externally displayed microbial sugars. They are glycoprotein in nature and are also known as **toll-like receptors** and are found on the surface of various body defence cells. They are so named because they recognize and bind to pathogen-associated molecular patterns – molecular components associated with microorganisms but not found as a part of eukaryotic cells. These include bacterial molecules such as peptidoglycan, teichoic acids, lipopolysaccharide, mannans, flagellin, pilin, and bacterial DNA. There are also pattern-recognition molecules for viral double-stranded

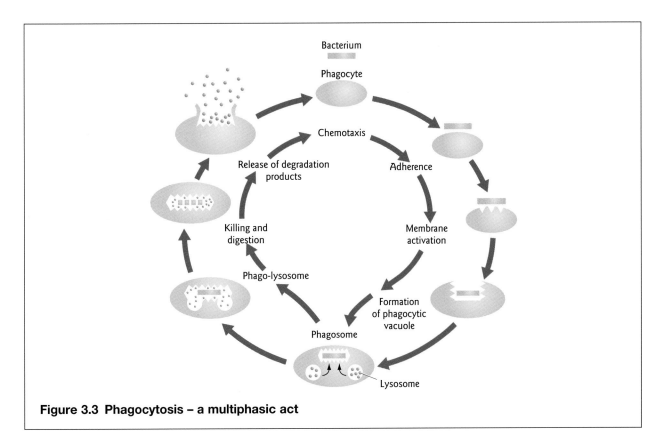

Figure 3.3 Phagocytosis – a multiphasic act

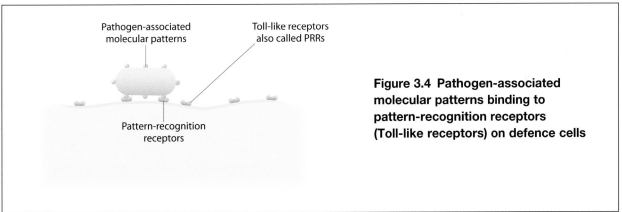

Figure 3.4 Pathogen-associated molecular patterns binding to pattern-recognition receptors (Toll-like receptors) on defence cells

Box 3.1 What is an opsonin?

The term opsonin is derived from the Greek word "opsons" meaning to prepare food for: (phagocytes). A classic description of opsonin was given in 1906, by George Bernard Shaw, in his play *The Doctor's Dilemma*. The lead character Sir Colenso Ridgeon was closely patterned after the British scientist Almroth Wright. "The phagocytes," Ridgeon says in the play, "won't eat the microbes unless the microbes are nicely buttered for them. Well the patient manufactures the butter for himself alright, that butter, I call opsonin." There are two principal classes of opsonin: specific serum antibody and complement component fragments. Other proteins such as C reactive protein (CRP) also act as opsonins.

RNA (dsRNA) and fungal cell wall components such as lipoteichoic acids, glycolipids, mannans, and zymosan. Binding of the microbial molecule to the toll-like receptor sends a signal through the cytoplasm to the nucleus of the cell where it activates genes coding for the synthesis and secretion of cytokines.

There is evidence that an adherent particle may initiate ingestion by activating an actin-myosin contractile system which extends pseudopods around the particle. The particle is eventually enclosed completely in a vacuole – the phagosome. Lysosomal granules come into contact and finally fuse with the phagosome forming a phagolysosome. Several hydrolytic enzymes are now released into the phagolysosome which act optimally at a low pH.

Intracellular killing

Intracellular killing utilizes two mechanisms: (i) oxygen dependent mechanisms and (ii) oxygen independent mechanisms (Table 3.2).

Table 3.2 Oxygen dependent and independent mechanisms

Oxygen dependent mechanisms			
$Glucose + NADP^+$	Hexose monophosphate shunt $\longrightarrow$	Pentose phosphate + NADPH	O_2 burst + generation of superoxide anion
$NADPH + O_2$	Cytochrome b-245	$NADP^+ + O_2$	
$2O_2 + 2H^+$	Spontaneous dismutation $\longrightarrow$	$H_2O_2 + {}^1O_2$	
$O_2 + H_2O_2$	$\longrightarrow$	$OH + OH^- + {}^1O_2$	Spontaneous formation of further microbicidal agents
$H_2O_2 + Cl^-$	Myeloperoxidase $\longrightarrow$	$OCl^- + H_2O_2$	
$OCl^- + H_2O_2$	$\longrightarrow$	${}^1O_2 + Cl^- + H_2O_2$	Myeloperoxidase and generation of microbicidal molecules
$2O_2 + 2H^+$	Superoxide dismutase $\longrightarrow$	$O_2 + H_2O_2$	Protective mechanism used by host and many microbes
$2H_2O_2$	Catalase $\longrightarrow$	$2H_2O + O_2$	
Oxygen independent mechanisms			
Cationic proteins (incl. cathepsin G), α-defensins, cationic proteins		Damage to microbial membranes	
Lysozyme		Splits mucopeptide in bacterial cell wall	
Lactoferrin		Deprives proliferating bacteria of iron	
Proteolytic enzymes and a variety of other hydrolytic enzymes		Digestion of killed organisms	

Oxygen dependent mechanisms

With the formation of the phagolysosome, there is a dramatic increase in activity of the hexose monophosphate shunt, increased glycolysis and increased oxygen consumption with an exaggerated formation of hydrogen peroxide, lactic acid and a subsequent fall in pH – a prerequisite for optimal functioning of hydrolytic enzymes. Collectively the stimulation of all these pathways is called a "respiratory burst." The hexose monophosphate shunt generates NADPH, which is ultimately utilized to reduce molecular oxygen bound to cytochrome, causing a burst of oxygen consumption. As a result oxygen is converted to superoxide anion (O_2), hydrogen peroxide, singlet O_2 ($^1O_2$), and hydroxyl radicals (OH) – all of which are powerful microbicidal agents. Furthermore the combination of peroxide, myeloperoxidase, and halide (Cl^-) ions constitutes a potent halogenating system capable of killing both bacteria and viruses.

Killing by nitric oxide

Nitric oxide is known to be a physiologic mediator similar to factors that relax the endothelium. It is formed within most cells, particularly neutrophils and macrophages, and generates a powerful antimicrobial effect. It is thought to be particularly effective against *Salmonella* and *Leishmania*, pathogens known to live comfortably within the cell and yet escape phagocytic killing.

Oxygen independent mechanisms

As a result of the oxygen dependent mechanisms the pH of the vacuole rises so as to allow several cationic proteins which are microbicidal to act optimally. These molecules are known as α-defensins and act selectively on microbial lipid components. Other substances such as the neutral proteinase (cathepsin G) are also powerful microbicidal agents. Lysozyme and lactoferrin also constitute bactericidal or bacteriostatic factors which are oxygen independent and can function under anaerobic conditions. Finally the killed organisms are digested by hydrolytic enzymes and the degraded products released to the exterior.

Extracellular killing

Natural killer cells (NK cells) are large granular lympocytes. Their main role is to kill virus infected cells, this they do by secreting a cytolysin called perforin that attacks the membrane of the infected cell. Large parasites such as helminths cannot be physically phagocytosed. Extracellular killing by **eosinophils** (using the complement pathway, see below) has evolved as a way of defence against these parasites. Remember eosinophilia can sometimes be an indirect clue that the patient has a parasitic infestation.

Soluble (humoral) bactericidal factors

Of the soluble bactericidal substances elaborated by the body, perhaps the most abundant and widespread is the enzyme **lysozyme**, a muramidase which splits the peptidoglycan of the bacterial cell wall.

Human β-defensins are proteins that play an important role in defending against microbial invaders along mucosal tracts.

There are also a number of plasma proteins collectively called the "**acute phase proteins**" which show a dramatic increase during infection. These include **C-reactive protein (CRP), serum amyloid A, α_1 antitrypsin, mannose-binding protein, fibrinogen**, and **caeruloplasmin**.

During infection, microbial substances such as endotoxins stimulate the release of a cytokine called **interleukin 1** (IL-1) – an endogenous pyrogen (a substance that induces a fever). IL-1 in turn induces the liver to release more CRP. The prime function of CRP is to bind to a number of microorganisms (in a calcium dependent fashion) which contain phosphorylcholine. This then enhances activation of complement and thereby induces the acute inflammatory response. CRP therefore acts as an opsonin, coating organisms and triggering complement-mediated lysis. **Interferons** (also cytokines) are antiviral agents synthesized by cells that are infected by viruses. They are secreted into the extracellular fluid where they bind to receptors on uninfected cells, the bound interferon exerts an antiviral effect and prevents the uninfected cell from becoming infected. (See later section for a more detailed description of the cytokines.)

However, many of these remarkable defence mechanisms are powerless in the face of overwhelming infection. Experience with chronically ill or debilitated patients indicates that many of these patients become "secondarily" infected – a reflection of the waning innate or natural defence mechanism in the host. Should innate immunity fail for some reason, other strategies of defence, far more powerful and exquisitely precise, are brought into play, in the form of **adaptive specific immunity**. The following section is an overview of adaptive immunity in relation to infectious diseases, it is not meant to be exhaustive.

Complement

The complement system is the primary humoral mediator or facilitator of the host's attack against foreign antigen. The system consists of at least 26 chemically and immunologically distinct plasma proteins, capable of interacting with each other, with antibody, and with cell membranes. Following activation of this system, these interactions lead to the generation of a wide range of biological activity from lysis of different kinds of cells, bacteria and viruses to direct mediation of the inflammatory process. In addition, complement is able to recruit and enlist the participation of other cellular effector systems: to induce histamine release from mast cells, migration of leukocytes, phagocytosis, and release of lysosomes from phagocytes.

There are two parallel but entirely independent pathways leading to the terminal most active part of the complement system. The two pathways are called the **classical** and the **alternative** pathways. Each pathway is triggered by different substances (Table 3.3). The end result of complement activation is **cytolysis** or **cytotoxicity**.

Biological significance of the complement system

The sum total effect of the integrated complement system is that it is able to produce inflammation and facilitate the localization of an infective agent. Phagocytes bear receptors on their surface for antibody and for complement components. Foreign antigenic substances induce antibody and complement formation. These foreign antigenic particles are coated with opsonins, these are antibody and complement components or complement alone. This coating attracts the phagocyte bearing receptors for both antibody and complement and facilitates phagocytosis. This process is called opsonization (Figure 3.5).

Other biological effects such as smooth muscle contraction, vascular permeability, and chemotaxis of leukocytes further facilitate the acute inflammatory process. Evidence for the biological importance of this system can be obtained from human and animal complement deficiency states: marked increase in susceptibility to infection is a dominant feature.

Table 3.3 Activators of the complement system

	Classical	Alternative
Immunologic	Antigen–antibody complexes, where antigen may be a bacterial substance	IgA, IgG (types of antibodies)
Nonimmunologic	Trypsin-like enzymes DNA C-reactive protein Staphylococcal protein A	Lipopolysaccharide Plant and bacterial polysaccharides Cobra venom Trypsin-like enzymes

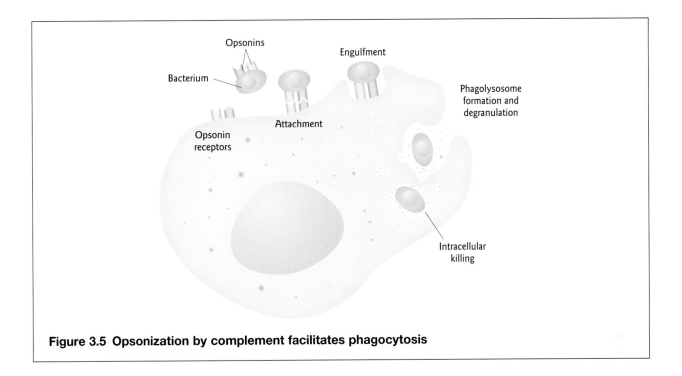

Figure 3.5 Opsonization by complement facilitates phagocytosis

Adaptive immunity

Specific adaptive immunity is a mighty tool that comprises:

- antibody
- cell-mediated immunity (including cytokines).

Before we embark on a discussion of adaptive immunity in the defence of microbes, let us review the different subsets of lymphocytes that play a vital role in this process.

When cells of the immune system encounter an antigen, a humoral (antibody-mediated) immune response or cellular (cell-mediated) immune response, or both may occur.

Humoral immunity is mediated by B cells, which after stimulation proliferate and differentiate into antibody producing plasma cells. T cell subsets of the T-helper lineage, the **Th2 cells**, enhance and supplement the activity of B cells (Table 3.4).

Cellular immunity is mediated by T cells, which become activated to secrete a number of substances important in the immune response: the **cytokines**; they also kill virus infected cells directly, fulfilling the role of cytotoxic T lymphocyte (CTL or Tc cell) or killer T cells. Killer T cell activity is helped along by the other subset of the T helper cell, **Th1 cells** (Table 3.4). It is therefore obvious that T cells and B cells need to communicate and interact with each other and with other antigen presenting cells. This they do through receptors, soluble factors, and various cell adhesion molecules.

The antigen presenting cell

Antigen presenting cells (APCs) are key players in immune defence. To illustrate the role of the APC we will restrict our discussion to the macrophage as the main cell involved in antigen presentation.

Broadly, the macrophage serves two major functions: to ingest and destroy particulate matter – a function greatly enhanced when the foreign matter is coated by complement or antibody. The term opsonin is used

Table 3.4 T cell subsets and how they function in the defence against microbes

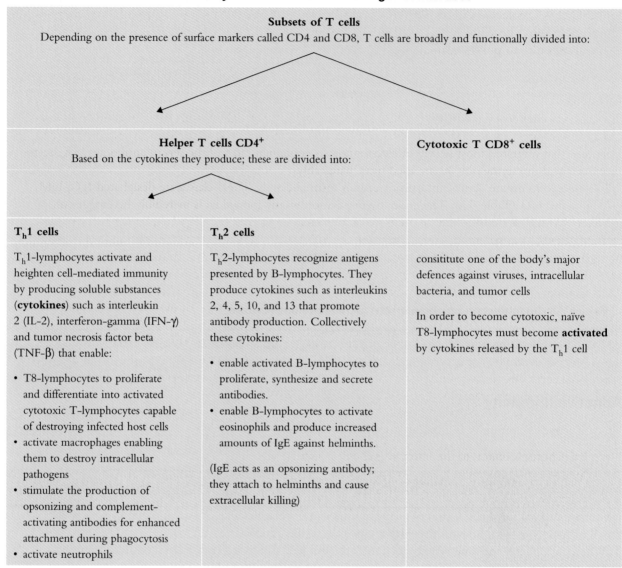

Subsets of T cells Depending on the presence of surface markers called CD4 and CD8, T cells are broadly and functionally divided into:		
Helper T cells CD4$^+$ Based on the cytokines they produce; these are divided into:		**Cytotoxic T CD8$^+$ cells**
T$_h$1 cells	**T$_h$2 cells**	
T$_h$1-lymphocytes activate and heighten cell-mediated immunity by producing soluble substances (**cytokines**) such as interleukin 2 (IL-2), interferon-gamma (IFN-γ) and tumor necrosis factor beta (TNF-β) that enable: • T8-lymphocytes to proliferate and differentiate into activated cytotoxic T-lymphocytes capable of destroying infected host cells • activate macrophages enabling them to destroy intracellular pathogens • stimulate the production of opsonizing and complement-activating antibodies for enhanced attachment during phagocytosis • activate neutrophils	T$_h$2-lymphocytes recognize antigens presented by B-lymphocytes. They produce cytokines such as interleukins 2, 4, 5, 10, and 13 that promote antibody production. Collectively these cytokines: • enable activated B-lymphocytes to proliferate, synthesize and secrete antibodies. • enable B-lymphocytes to activate eosinophils and produce increased amounts of IgE against helminths. (IgE acts as an opsonizing antibody; they attach to helminths and cause extracellular killing)	consititute one of the body's major defences against viruses, intracellular bacteria, and tumor cells In order to become cytotoxic, naïve T8-lymphocytes must become **activated** by cytokines released by the T$_h$1 cell

to describe this coating with both antibody and complement to facilitate phagocytosis (Box 3.1). The other function involves the initial recognition, processing and presentation of antigen to the T-cell to elicit the specific immune response.

Role of major histocompatibility (MHC) antigen

Virtually every human cell bears a surface antigen called the major histocompatibility (MHC) antigen. These antigens play an important role in the defence against foreign antigens. They are classed into two broad groups: the class I and class II MHC antigens.

The true physiologic role of the MHC class I antigens lies in the cell-mediated lysis of virus infected cells. T cells do not recognize viral antigen; antigen must first be **processed** by an antigen presenting cell such as the macrophage and then **presented** in association with MHC class I. In other words, T cells are blind to native antigen and will "see" antigen only when processed and presented together with an MHC molecule.

To reiterate a general rule of thumb: the CD8$^+$ T (cytotoxic T) cell recognizes antigen in association with an MHC class I molecule (Figure 3.6) and a CD4$^+$ T cell recognizes antigen in conjunction with an MHC class II molecule. The CD4$^+$ T cell (helper T cell)–MHC class II molecule interaction provides T cell help to B cells in order to produce antibody.

Antibody

The first real chemical information regarding the structure of antibodies was provided by **Tiselius and Kabat** in the early 1940s. These workers demonstrated that the fraction of serum proteins (the gamma globulins) that migrated most slowly in electrophoresis contained most of the serum antibodies. The terms antibodies and immunoglobulins are used interchangeably.

Immunoglobulins are classed into major groups termed classes. These classes are designated IgG, IgM, IgA, IgE, and IgD (Table 3.5). The antibody population in any individual is incredibly heterogenous. In effect, this means that the normal immune system can generate an immunoglobulin for every possible immunogen that the system may encounter during its life time. This antibody diversity is possible as a result of a process called **somatic recombination**. The DNA in the germ cells (in the male sperm and the female egg) or in the early embryo contains several bits and pieces of the gene that eventually dictates antibody formation. These bits and pieces are shuffled and spliced together (yielding an enormous number of permutations and combinations) in the DNA of the B-lymphocyte to yield the required antibody.

The classes of antibody differ from each other in their ability to carry out certain secondary biological functions. For example, the IgG and IgM fix complement most efficiently; IgG also binds to receptors on phagocytic cells, NK (natural killer) cells, and placental syncytiotrophoblasts; also to staphylococcal protein A. IgE binds to specific receptors on mast cells and basophils.

Table 3.5 Characteristics of the immunoglobulin classes

Characteristics	IgG	IgM	IgA	IgE	IgD
Sedimentation coefficient	7S	19S	11S	8S	7S
Molecular weight	150 000	900 000	160 000	200 000	185 000
Functions	Most abundant in extravascular spaces; combats microorganisms and their toxins	Early in immune response. Effective in agglutination; first line defence in bacteraemia	Major Ig in seromucus secretions, defends external body surfaces	Protects external body surface, responsible for symptoms of allergy. Raised in parasitic infections	Mostly present on surface of B lymphocytes
Complement fixation:					
Classical	++	+++	–	–	–
Alternative	–	–	+	–	–
Cross placenta	+	–	–	–	–
Fix to homologous mast cells/basophils	–	–	–	+	–
Bind to macrophages and polymorphs	+	–	+	–	–

Cell-mediated immunity

It soon became evident that antibody and complement-mediated defence was woefully inadequate when it came to mounting an attack on intracellular bacteria and viruses and complex structures such as parasites. In all of these instances, antigen is not overt but is either too complex or masked within the body's own cell systems. The host relies on cellular defence mechanisms against such infectious agents. A summary of these defence strategies is presented here.

Cell-mediated immunity involves three major defence strategies:

1 Activating antigen-specific cytotoxic T-lymphocytes (CTLs) that are able to lyse body cells displaying foreign antigen on their surface.
2 Activating macrophage and natural killer (NK) cells and antibody dependent cell cytotoxicity.
3 Stimulating cells to secrete a variety of cytokines that influence the function of other cells involved in adaptive immune responses and innate immune responses.

Activating antigen-specific cytotoxic T-lymphocytes

Cytotoxic T cells kill target cells by direct cell lysis or by apoptosis (a deliberate and programmed cell death). The T cytotoxic cells recognize antigen in conjunction with MHC class I molecules, are stimulated by Th1 helper cells, and then turn cytotoxic (Figure 3.6). T cytotoxic cells are the major effector pathway of cell-mediated immunity to certain viruses.

Activating macrophage and natural killer cells and antibody dependent cell cytotoxicity

Activated macrophages are the effector cells in the cell-mediated immune response to various microorganisms. The ability of activated macrophages to kill microorganisms is enhanced by cytokines in a nonspecific fashion. For example, a macrophage that has been activated to kill intracellular *Listeria monocytogenes* would also kill *Salmonella* organisms more efficiently.

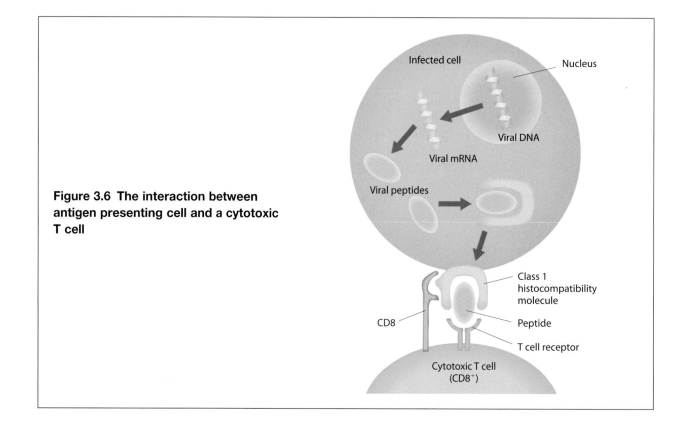

Figure 3.6 The interaction between antigen presenting cell and a cytotoxic T cell

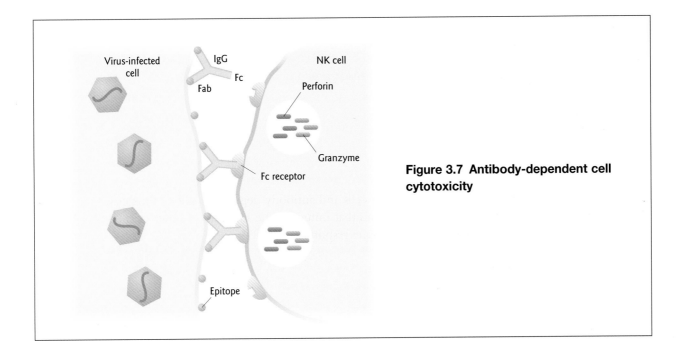

Figure 3.7 Antibody-dependent cell cytotoxicity

Natural killer cells are large granular lymphocytes that do not require prior exposure to antigen to become cytotoxic and their activity is not MHC restricted. Cytokines such as interleukin 2 (IL-2) and interferon-gamma (IFN-γ) produced by Th1 lymphocytes activate NK cells. NK cells also secrete the cytokine IL-1 and in response to IL-2, they become super killers.

NK cells are also capable of **antibody-dependent cellular cytotoxicity (ADCC)**. When NK cells are carrying out ADCC, they are sometimes also referred to as killer K cells (K cells). A specific antibody is generated against a target foreign antigen displayed on the cell surface; this acts like a bridge between the foreign antigen bearing target cell and the K cell (Figure 3.7). The K cell then releases pore-forming perforins, proteolytic enzymes called granzymes and cytokines that cause cell apoptosis and cell lysis similar to the mechanism of killing described for CTLs.

Monocytes, neutrophils, and eosinophils can also participate in ADCC. Eosinophils, for example, are effective killers of antibody coated schistosomulae, the larval forms of schistosomes. The mechanism of killing involves binding of the eosinophil to the larva via an antibody molecule. The eosinophil releases basic proteins and other molecules from its granules, leading to formation of pores in the target cell membrane. The organism dies because of the leaky membrane.

Stimulating cells to secrete a variety of cytokines

Cytokines are soluble substances produced by a variety of cell types that amplify and regulate a range of immune responses. Some cytokines are crucial in cell-mediated immune reactions, whereas others play a critical role in antibody responses. A variety of cytokines affect cellular immunity by:

- mediating the innate immune response
- regulating hematopoiesis (formation of the cellular components of blood)
- influencing cell-mediated immunity directly.

Cytokines that affect the inflammatory response generally **upregulate innate immunity**. These cytokines also play a role in mediating resistance to viral infections and causing the cardinal signs of inflammation (pain, redness, swelling, and heat). Included in this group are the Type I Interferons (IFN-α and IFN-β), tumor necrosis factor (TNF), interleukin 1, interleukin 6, and interleukin 8.

Type I IFNs

Type I IFNs include IFN-α and IFN-β. Type I IFN has several sources and several effects. For simplicity, Type I IFN inhibits viral replication in virus-infected cells. IFN-α has been used to treat HIV. IFN-α is made predominantly by neutrophils, and IFN-β is made predominantly by fibroblasts.

Tumor necrosis factor

Tumor necrosis factor (TNF-α and β) is made predominantly by monocytes and macrophages following stimulation with bacterial LPS (TNF-α) or by activated CD4$^+$ T-cells (TNF-β). TNF has many biological functions; it is probably most important in inducing the production of acute phase proteins by the liver. It also induces fever. This is one of the first cytokines to appear during an inflammatory response.

Interleukin 1

Interleukin 1 is also made by cells of the monocyte–macrophage cell lineage. It has many of the same functions as TNF, but it typically appears somewhat later in an inflammatory response. Like TNF, IL-1 is an endogenous pyrogen, so it induces fever. IL-1 is also a co-stimulator of CD4$^+$ T-helper cells.

Interleukin 6

Interleukin 6, like IL-1, has two major functions: to mediate inflammation, and to regulate the growth and differentiation of lymphocytes. IL-6 has a function similar to TNF in that it induces the synthesis of acute phase reactants by the liver. In addition, IL-6 also serves as a growth factor for plasma cells.

Interleukin 8

Interleukin 8 is produced by monocytes. IL-8 is a chemoattractant for neutrophils. It also induces adherence of neutrophils to vascular endothelial cells and aids their migration into tissue spaces.

Interleukin 11

Interleukin 11 is produced by bone marrow cells and shares the functional activity of IL-6. It is also produced by macrophages and might be anti-inflammatory.

Other chemokines

Other chemokines such as macrophage inflammatory protein (MIP-1a), MIP-1b, monocyte chemoattractant protein (MCP-1), MCP-2, and MCP-3 enable migration of these cells to the site of inflammation. They also induce certain morphologic, metabolic and functional changes in macrophages that enhance the cells' ability to kill microorganisms and tumor cells.

Several cytokines play a major role in hematopoiesis in the bone marrow. The best characterized of these are granulocyte/monocyte-colony stimulating factor (GM-CSF), granulocyte-colony stimulating factor (G-CSF), stem cell factor (SCF), interleukin 3, interleukin 7, and interleukin-9. Some of these cytokines are being used to treat patients that have deficiencies in hematopoiesis, such as cancer patients who are bone marrow suppressed due to anti-cancer therapy.

Specific cellular immune responses are mediated by T-lymphocytes. Activation of T cells requires the presence of antigen. Cytokines serve as "second signals" to drive the growth and differentiation of antigen-activated lymphocytes. Some cytokines act predominantly on T cells, others on both T and B cells.

Interleukin 2

Interleukin 2 is the primary growth and differentiation factor for T-cells. IL-2 causes antigen-primed cytotoxic T cells to proliferate and become aggressively cytotoxic. IL-2 is produced by CD4$^+$ T-helper cells.

Type II interferon or interferon γ

Type II interferon or interferon γ (IFN-γ) is produced by T-helper cells. It is an important cytokine for activating macrophages. An activated macrophage is more phagocytic, it processes and presents antigen more efficiently, it produces more cytokines, and becomes more bactericidal than resting macrophages. Activated macrophages are an important mediator of cellular immunity.

A summary of host defence mechanisms against viral infections is illustrated in Figure 3.8.

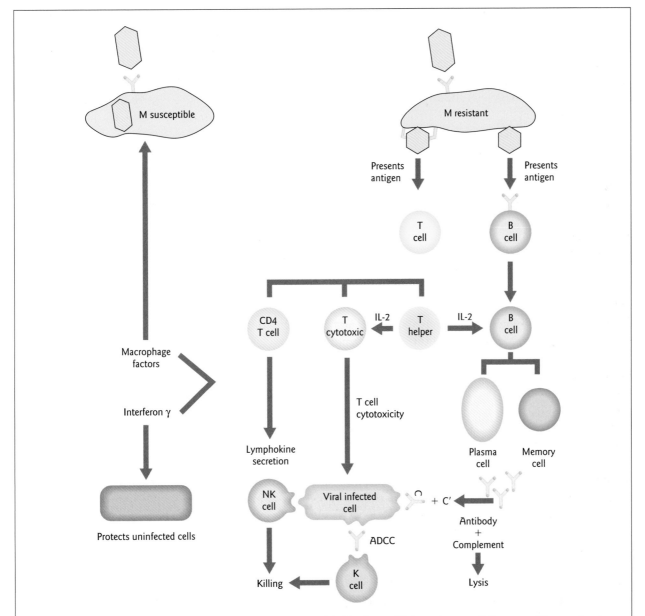

Figure 3.8 Host defence mechanisms against viral infections. Macrophages (M) may either enhance viral replication when susceptible or restrict viral growth when resistant. B cells after antigen presentation by macrophages differentiate into memory cells and plasma cells. T cells have a multifunctional role: they provide B cell help, cause cytotoxicity, and secrete lymphokines. The virally infected cell is hence subjected to complement-mediated lysis, T cell cytotoxicity, NK cell activity, and ADCC

Table 3.6 Milestones in immunization

Event	Year
Variolation	1721
Vaccination	1796
Rabies vaccine	1885
Diphtheria toxoid	1925
Tetanus toxoid	1925
Pertussis vaccine	1925
Viral culture in chick embryo	1931
Yellow fever vaccine	1937
Influenza vaccine	1943
Viral tissue culture	1949
Polio vaccine (Salk)	1954
Polio vaccine (Sabin)	1956
Measles vaccine	1960
Tetanus immune globulin (human)	1962
Rubella vaccine	1966
Mumps vaccine	1967
Hepatitis B vaccine	1975
Licensure of first recombinant vaccine (hepatitis B)	1986
Meningococcus C conjugated vaccine	1999
Live oral rotavirus vaccine	2006
Human papillomavirus vaccines	2007

The immunization success story

The greatest triumph of modern medicine has been the successful use of immunization procedures in the control of potentially fatal infectious diseases. The concept of immunization rose from the observation that individuals who recover from certain diseases are protected for life from recurrences. The introduction of small quantities of fluid from active smallpox pustules into uninfected persons (variolation) was an effort at mimicking natural infection. Jenner introduced vaccination in 1796 using cow pox to protect against smallpox. This was the first documented use of live attenuated vaccination and the beginning of modern immunization. Historical milestones in immunization are listed in Table 3.6.

Primary and secondary immune responses

The first exposure to an antigen evokes a **primary response**. Immediately after introduction of immunogen little or no antibody is detected. This is called the inductive or latent period (Figure 3.9). During this period, the immunogen is recognized as foreign and processed. The duration of this period is variable and depends on the type of antigen used, species of animal, and route of immunization. During the logarithmic

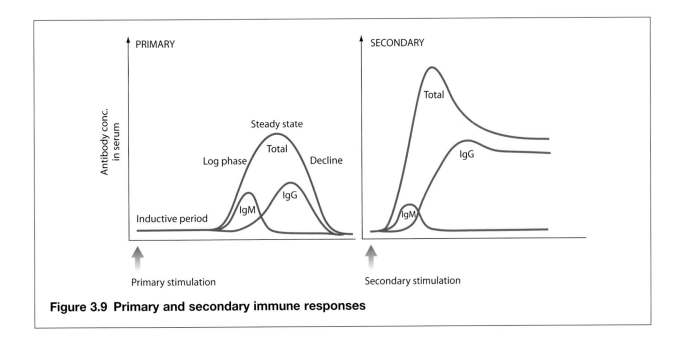

Figure 3.9 Primary and secondary immune responses

phase, antibody concentration increases logarithmically for 4–10 days, until it reaches a peak. This peak antibody level usually takes 4–5 days for erythrocytes, 8–12 days for soluble proteins, and 2–3 months for the toxoid of *Corynebacterium diphtheriae*.

The log phase is followed by a steady phase, where rates of antibody synthesis equal rates of antibody catabolism. The decline phase follows where antibody synthesis steadily falls, finally reaching pre-immunization levels. The early primary response is characterized by a predominance of IgM over IgG, IgM production is transient and within 2 weeks of initiation of the response IgG predominates.

The **secondary immune response** occurs upon second exposure to the same immunogen, weeks, months or even years later. The secondary immune response is accompanied by an accelerated response from already committed B lymphocytes in the memory pool. Rapid proliferation and differentiation into plasma cells yields a higher antibody output. The secondary response is characterized by an initial negative phase, which is due to the immediate reaction of pre-existing antibody with new immunogen. An enhanced response follows due to anamnestic recall of pre-committed memory cells. This enhanced response underlies the principle of administering booster doses after specific time intervals during immunization procedures. Immunologic memory can last for years, providing long lasting immunity to certain bacterial and viral infections. The evolution of immunologic memory is a function of T helper cells. T independent antigens therefore cannot elicit memory or for that matter a secondary IgG response.

Immunization can be a passive or an active process

Passively acquired immunity
Passive immunity is acquired: (i) by the newborn from the mother; (ii) by administering preformed immunoglobulins to an individual.

Maternal transfer of antibodies
The neonate is endowed with a relatively immature lymphoid system; the premature baby with a grossly ineffective immune mechanism. In early life, the newborn is thus protected by maternally derived antibodies (IgG) transferred passively via the placenta. Colostrum and breast milk also afford significant protection to the neonate. The major immunoglobulin in milk is the secretory IgA, which remains in the gut of the

newborn, protecting the intestinal mucosal surfaces from enteric pathogens. Interestingly, it has been found that the secretory IgA in the breast milk is specific for bacterial and viral antigens found in the mother's gut. It is presumed that IgA producing cells responding to gut antigens migrate from the gut mucosa to colonize breast tissue, now considered to be a part of the **mucosal associated lymphoid tissue (MALT)**. Here the IgA producing cells secrete specific antibodies which appear in milk. This circuit has also been termed the **entero-mammary axis**.

Administered gamma globulins

Antibody, either as whole serum or concentrated gamma globulins (immune globulin), is obtained from human volunteers who have recovered from a specific infectious disease or have received immunization. The globulin consists predominantly of IgG. Administration of such human immune globulin (HIG) offers immediate protection to individuals who are at risk, particularly where active immunization may take 7–10 days for effective antibody production. Passive immunization is also useful to those individuals who are unable to produce antibody for themselves. Hazards associated with administering human immune globulin (as pooled serum) include transmission of blood borne viruses – hepatitis B or C viruses and the human immunodeficiency virus (HIV). Purified IgG preparations are, however, free of these virus particles.

Antibodies may also be available from animal sera. However, such immunoglobulins are less desirable, as nonhuman proteins are cleared away by the host immune response against them. In addition, hazardous immune reactions against animal proteins may lead to the development of anaphylaxis or serum sickness. Neither human nor animal immune globulin should be administered intravenously for fear of anaphylactic reactions.

Human immune globulin against varicella, the varicella zoster immune globulin, is indicated in individuals who are at risk of severe varicella infection, pregnant women and those with defective immune systems such as premature infants, children with immunodeficiency diseases, and patients on steroid treatment who have no antibodies to varicella zoster virus. Rabies and hepatitis B immune globulin is administered to individuals who have been exposed and are at risk. Hepatitis B immune globulin is often used in association with hepatitis B vaccine for the prevention of infection in nonimmune individuals accidentally inoculated with hepatitis B virus and for the prevention of mother–child transmission (see Chapter 19). Diphtheria and botulism antitoxin is used as therapy in patients who have contracted the disease. The equine source of these latter two antibodies is still widely used. Tetanus antitoxin, now a human immune globulin, is given both prophylactically and therapeutically in appropriate cases.

Antibodies (equine) for noninfectious conditions are also available: antivenin against black widow spider and snake venoms. Human immune globulin to the Rh blood group is widely used to prevent hemolytic disease of the newborn.

Active immunity

Besides suffering the disease (and surviving it!), vaccination is the only other way of acquiring active immunity against an infectious agent. The advantages of active over passive immunization are due to the fact that the individual's immune system is stimulated to produce an immune response against a given antigen. Host participation ensures that both the humoral and cellular components of the immune system are activated. Consequently, T cell help is recruited and immunologic memory is available to boost the response after subsequent exposure to the antigen. Antibodies so formed are longer lasting and continuously replenished as compared to passively acquired immunoglobulin.

Active immunization may be performed with killed or live attenuated vaccines, toxoids, and polysaccharide conjugated vaccines.

Killed vaccines are obtained by inactivating the infectious agent using a chemical such as formaldehyde.

Live attenuated vaccines contain the live organisms but with their virulence factors removed, even so they must never be administered to the immunosuppressed individual or pregnant women as they can cause disseminated disease.

Toxoids are derived from protein **toxins** secreted by certain bacteria such as *C. diphtheriae* and *C. tetani* (see section on exotoxins on page 68). The toxin is extracted and treated by heat or chemicals so that its toxic, disease causing property is inactivated but its capacity to stimulate the formation of an immune response remains. The resultant antibody formed is able to neutralize the toxin if the patient happens to become infected.

Some bacterial antigens require to be **conjugated** to a protein molecule so as to elicit T cell help in making robust antibody responses. The bacteria for which conjugated vaccines are designed have an important structural feature in common. They are all surrounded by a polysaccharide (carbohydrate) capsule. The three most common causes of bacterial meningitis – the meningococcus, pneumococcus, and *H. influenzae* type B – are all capsulated. The immune system of children under 2 years of age, the age group at greatest risk from bacterial meningitis, does not respond to carbohydrate antigens. Older vaccines, produced from pure carbohydrate – polyvalent pneumococcal vaccines and Group A and Group C meningococcal vaccines – are of no use in young children. Even in older children and adults, these vaccines induce only short-term immunity. This is because B cells make antibodies to carbohydrate antigens without help from T cells. This has several consequences. This mechanism of antibody production does not develop reliably until children are around 2 years old. The range of antibody types produced is rather limited and no memory cells are formed so immunity is short-lived. Conjugate vaccines are so-called because their production involves the conjugation of the polysaccharide antigen with a protein. This conjugation converts the T cell independent carbohydrate antigen into a T cell dependent antigen, with all the associated benefits in terms of immunologic response.

The commonly used killed vaccines are:

- Bacterial vaccines for:
  - typhoid
  - cholera
  - pertussis
  - plague.
- Viral vaccines for:
  - rabies
  - poliomyelitis (the Salk vaccine)
  - hepatitis A
  - seasonal flu vaccines are purified subunit components from inactivated preparations.

Live attenuated vaccines include:

- Bacterial:
  - BCG – a live attenuated *Mycobacterium bovis* against tuberculosis
  - Ty21a – live oral attenuated mutant typhoid bacillus.
- Viral:
  - live vaccinia virus for smallpox, rubella, measles, mumps, polio (the Sabin vaccine), yellow fever virus, varicella zoster, rota virus
  - besides these, there are **toxoid vaccines** for diphtheria and tetanus.

There are polysaccharide conjugated vaccines for:

- *Haemophilus influenzae* type B (polyribosyl-ribitol-phosphate, conjugated to tetanus protein).
- *Neisseria meningitidis* (a combination vaccine against groups A,C,Y,W135 and the new meningococcus C conjugated vaccine).
- *Streptococcus pneumoniae* (a polyvalent 23 valent polysaccharide vaccine and the new 7-valent conjugated vaccine).

And recombinant vaccine for:

- Hepatitis B virus.

Live attenuated vaccines have many **advantages**. Attenuation mimics the natural behaviour of the organism without causing disease. The immunity conferred with live attenuated vaccines is superior because actively multiplying organisms provide a sustained antigen supply. The immune response takes place largely at the site of natural infection as in the case of the live polio vaccine and the oral typhoid vaccine producing an obviously advantageous local secretory IgA response.

The **hazards of using attenuated vaccines**, though uncommon, must be documented as the risk of developing complications is a very real one. A very small number of individuals develop encephalitis following measles vaccine; however, the danger of developing encephalitis from natural infection is far greater. There is the possibility of the attenuated virus reverting to its virulent form; chances of this decrease if the attenuation incorporates several gene mutations instead of just one. Preserving adequate cold storage facilities, and maintaining the cold chain from the laboratory into the field, is a continuing problem especially in the tropics. Live attenuated vaccines are not advised in patients with an immunodeficiency disease, in patients on steroid and other immunosuppressive treatment, and for those undergoing radiotherapy. Malignancies such as lymphomas and leukemias and pregnancy are all contraindications to the administration of live attenuated vaccines. The oral polio vaccine is contraindicated for any member of a household where there is a patient with a lymphoma or leukemia, as the live virus is shed in the stool of a vaccinated individual and poses a transmission risk. There is also the potential that the live vaccine strain could revert to a wild type that can cause paralytic poliomyelitis. Table 3.7 lists the current experimental and restricted use vaccines.

Recent developments in vaccine preparation

Since the process of attenuation is cumbersome and time consuming, recent developments in vaccine production use other methods.

Table 3.7 Experimental and restricted use vaccines

Vaccine	Status
Adenovirus	Live attenuated, for military recruits
Anthrax	For those with occupational exposure; military
Arboviruses **Kyasanur Forest Disease** **Japanese encephalitis**	Experimental only 50–60% protection. Killed vaccines
AIDS	Experimental
Cholera	New oral vaccine restricted for travellers
Cytomegalovirus	Experimental
Malaria	Experimental *Plasmodium falciparum* malaria vaccine based on the circumsporozoite protein
Gram negative bacteria	Experimental and restricted
Leprosy	Heat-killed *Mycobacterium leprae* + BCG. Clinical trials are ongoing
Palivizumab – though not a vaccine, is included here as it is a novel method of producing antibody (see Further reading on monoclonal antibodies)	Is a humanized monoclonal antibody to respiratory syncitial virus (RSV). Indicated for the prevention of serious lower respiratory tract disease caused by RSV in pediatric patients at high risk of RSV disease

Subunit vaccines

Subunit vaccines are being designed, which use only the relevant immunogenic portions of the organism. This has been possible using monoclonal antibodies and radio labelling techniques. Surface projections of the influenza virus, the measles virus and the rabies virus elicit neutralizing antibody and can be exploited for this purpose. If the low immunogenicity of these subunits can be overcome, such vaccines are stable, free from extraneous proteins and nucleic acids, and precise in their composition.

Biosynthesis of immunogenic proteins

Specific immunogenic surface proteins need to be available in large quantities for vaccine preparation. The problem of isolating and characterizing antigenic protein moieties has been overcome by cloning the genes that code for these proteins in bacterial or eukaryotic (yeast) cells or in the vaccinia virus. In 1986, the first recombinant (cloned) viral vaccine was licensed for use. The hepatitis B surface antigen (HBsAg) is the immunogen that stimulates protective immunity. The gene that codes for HbsAg has been cloned most successfully in the yeast cell. The antigen prepared by growing the yeast cells containing the recombinant gene in mass culture is widely used as a safe and effective vaccine.

New approaches to immunization

Novel delivery

With a few exceptions, most vaccines are currently given by intramuscular (IM) injection, which is a rather primitive way of delivering drugs. The development of mucosally delivered vaccines, i.e. given orally or nasally, has several advantages. One significant benefit is that this technology will provide a more convenient method that is pain-free and therefore more acceptable to recipients, so increasing compliance. Not having to use needles for administration will avoid the risks of blood borne virus transmission associated with failure to use a sterile needle for each and every injection. In addition, mucosally delivered vaccines will stimulate immune responses at mucosal sites, the entry point for most pathogens, responses that are poorly stimulated by IM vaccines.

Novel adjuvants

Live attenuated vaccines are generally highly effective at generating an immune response but vaccines containing dead organisms (inactivated vaccines) or pieces of the infectious organisms or their toxins (subunit, recombinant or toxoid vaccines) generally need an "adjuvant" to boost their effectiveness. Currently, the most commonly used adjuvants are aluminum salts known as alum. However, more efficient adjuvants such as MF-59 are in development.

Novel content

New and powerful scientific methods have revolutionized the way in which microbial pathogenesis and vaccine design are studied. These include genome sequencing, *in silico* analysis (i.e. computer modeling), proteomics, DNA microarrays, and *in vivo* expression technology. These have given rise to novel vaccination strategies, such as the use of synthetic peptides, viral vectors, naked DNA, and anti-idiotype antibodies, which are discussed below.

Synthetic peptide vaccines – A limited number of sites on an organism are involved in evoking an immune response. If these sites, consisting mainly of peptide fragments, can be synthesized they provide a possible means of obtaining chemical polypeptides as vaccines.

Unfortunately, this task has been made harder by the finding that immunogenic peptides are not simple, linear sequences of amino acids and the final configuration of the protein cannot always be synthesized in the form that B cells recognize. Besides, amino acid sequences of these peptides are discontinuous and are brought together by folding of the molecule.

Vector vaccines – Poxviruses (including fowlpox and vaccinia) are the most common live vector vaccine candidates. Their large genomes are fairly readily modified to incorporate segments of foreign DNA encoding the proteins of the target pathogen: "transgenes." The recombinant viral vector is then used to carry the transgenes into the cells of the vaccinee, resulting in the *in vivo* expression of a large amount of foreign protein. This provokes both a humoral and cell-mediated immune response. Fowlpox is a good live-vector candidate because it is able to infect but not replicate itself in mammalian cells. Modified Vaccinia Virus Ankara (MVA) is a highly attenuated strain of vaccinia virus that was developed by extensive passage of vaccinia virus in chicken cells, towards the end of the campaign for the eradication of smallpox. MVA has lost about 10% of the vaccinia genome and with it the ability to replicate efficiently in primate cells. Despite its limited replication, MVA provides similar levels of recombinant gene expression to those of replication-competent vaccinia viruses in human cells.

Nonreplicating viral vector vaccines are made by deleting one or more genes from a virus normally capable of entering and replicating in human cells, and inserting transgenes (see above) in their place. Vaccines derived from adenovirus serotype 5 have been generated in this way but the efficacy of such vaccines could be compromised by pre-existing immunity to the adenovirus.

DNA vaccines are usually circular plasmids that include a gene, derived from a pathogenic organism, encoding the target antigen (or antigens). The gene for the target antigen is under the transcriptional control of a promoter region active in human cells. The plasmids, which are cheaper and easier to produce than protein or peptide vaccines and are more stable, are injected intramuscularly or intradermally, whereupon some are taken up by host cells. Transcription results in the expression of the target antigen and the induction of both a humoral and a cell-mediated immune response to it. While immune responses to DNA alone have been relatively weak in humans, combination with adjuvants or with recombinant viral vectors in "prime-boost" approaches has resulted in greater potency. Many such DNA prime, recombinant viral vector boost regimens are under investigation for immunization against malaria and HIV.

These and other strategies such as using **anti-idiotypes** as vaccines are still experimental, but animal and early human studies have been encouraging.

Microbial pathogenesis and escape mechanisms

Pathogenicity (the disease process) is directly related to a number of virulence factors that microbes possess in their armamentarium. The infectious dose of a pathogen, route of entry, and underlying compromising factors in the host are often the first precipitating factors for an infection. Infection, invasion, and disease are established despite the host defence strategies outlined above. Besides displaying virulence factors, microbes have evolved mechanisms of escape including antimicrobial drug resistance so as to survive within a susceptible host.

Interaction between host and pathogen is a complex and dynamic process. The pathogenesis of many bacterial infections may be related to a particularly vigorous host immune response. Immuno-pathological mechanisms of disease ascribe much of the tissue damage to host immune response rather than to microbial virulence. Classic examples of immune response-mediated pathogenesis are seen in diseases caused by certain hepatitis viruses, Gram negative bacterial sepsis, tuberculosis, and tuberculoid leprosy. These pathological mechanisms can vary from being immune complex- to cytokine-mediated; in reality patients often deteriorate after appropriate therapy before (and if) they make a recovery.

Bacterial and fungal pathogens

Attachment and colonization

Mucous membranes are constantly exposed to microorganisms from the environment. To colonize the mucous membranes bacteria must have the ability to adhere closely to membrane surfaces and multiply there. We know that *Streptococcus mutans* causes dental caries. The organism has a constitutive enzyme, glucosyl transferase, which is able to convert sucrose to dextran which is utilized by the organism for adhesion to the tooth surface. Attachment is most often mediated by surface receptors on both host and bacterial cells. Group A β hemolytic streptococci adhere by the M antigen, the protein component of surface fimbriae. In *Escherichia coli*, the adhesive factor is a protein filament on the bacterial surface, designated the K88 antigen. Gonococci adhere to epithelial cell surfaces by pili. Candida species are able to colonize mucosal surfaces once normal flora has been altered, for example by antibiotics. These are just a few examples of novel methods of attachment, some to specific receptors on human cells. Attachment ensures that the organism is not washed off by body secretions such as saliva, mucus, or urine, and the organism need no longer compete with normal flora for a place to "pitch its tent."

Since adherence to epithelial cells of the mucous membranes is so vital to establish infection, the host has devised several mechanisms to overcome this ploy. Specific targeted **secretory antibody**, IgA, affords protection in secreted body fluids such as tears, saliva, nasal and intestinal secretions. IgA prevents bacterial adherence to mucosal surfaces. If an infectious agent succeeds in dodging the IgA barrier, it is confronted with the immunoglobulin IgE, which is present in mucosal secretions. IgE-mediated release of mast cell contents helps enhance the inflammatory response.

Resistance to phagocytosis

The principal host defence mechanism is ingestion and destruction by phagocytosis. This is effectively overcome by the capsular material that some bacteria produce. Capsulated strains of *Streptococcus pneumoniae* and *Bacillus anthracis* are resistant to phagocytosis. The principal factor responsible for this resistance is the polysaccharide of the capsule of *S. pneumoniae* and the polypeptide in the capsule of *B. anthracis*. *Cryptococcus neoformans* also possesses an antiphagocytic polysaccharide capsule. In addition, the *C. neoformans* capsule depletes complement and dysregulates cytokine secretion. Other organisms such as coagulase negative staphylococci have the ability to cover themselves in a layer of slime, producing a biofilm that is impenetrable by phagocytes (and to antimicrobial agents).

The host defence mechanism operates to circumvent this problem by ensuring that **opsonization** by specific antibody or complement takes place. Opsonization greatly facilitates phagocytosis and is the basis of immunity to such infections. Opsonization with C3b attracts cells with the complement CR I receptor, such as primate red cells. Complexes with aggregates of red cells are then transported to the liver for phagocytosis. The lipopolysaccharide of Gram negative organisms activates complement via the alternative pathway leading to cell lysis. Biologically active substances such as C3a and C5a aid chemotaxis and enhance the inflammatory response.

Intracellular growth by bacteria

Some bacteria are resistant to intracellular killing. Tubercle and leprosy bacilli and the *Brucella* species are able to survive and multiply within phagocytes and are thereby easily disseminated within body tissues. These organisms defy the killing mechanism within phagocytes in a variety of ways. *Mycobacterium tuberculosis* and *Salmonella typhi* and chlamydiae inhibit fusion of lysosome with phagosome, *Mycobacterium leprae* has a resistant outer coat, some rickettsiae slip out of the phagosome to survive undisturbed in the cytosol. Other organisms are resistant to inhibition and killing by lysosomal constituents after the formation of the phago-lysosome. *B. anthracis*, *M. tuberculosis*, and *Staphylococcus aureus* all possess mechanisms to survive intracellular killing in macrophages.

Where antibody or complement have no access to intracellular organisms, the human immune mechanism reacts using **cellular immunity**. Both cytotoxic T cells and activated macrophages play an important part in cell-mediated killing of intracellular organisms. Chronic granulomatous reaction represents an attempt by the body to wall off persistent infection. The activated macrophage has an abundance of hydrolytic enzymes and densely packed macrophages are the prominent feature of chronic granulomas.

Competition for iron

Iron is essential for metabolism and growth. Although blood is a rich source of iron, most of the iron is bound either to hemoglobin in erythrocytes or to transferrin in plasma, making it unavailable to bacteria.

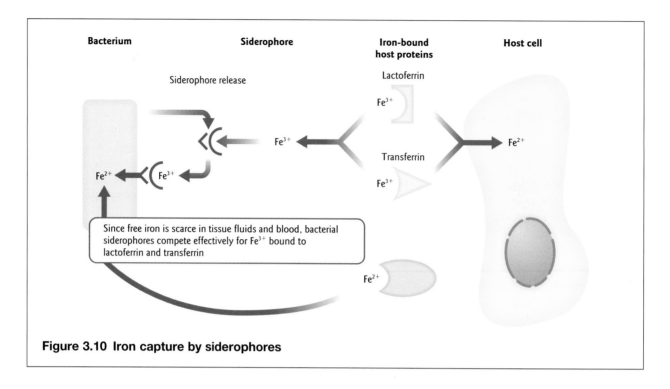

Figure 3.10 Iron capture by siderophores

Within the figure:

Bacterium   Siderophore   Iron-bound host proteins   Host cell

Siderophore release

Lactoferrin Fe^{3+}

Fe^{3+}

Fe^{2+} Fe^{3+} Fe^{2+}

Transferrin Fe^{3+}

Since free iron is scarce in tissue fluids and blood, bacterial siderophores compete effectively for Fe^{3+} bound to lactoferrin and transferrin

Fe^{2+}

Similarly, iron in milk and other secretions (e.g. tears, saliva, bronchial mucus, bile, and gastrointestinal fluid) is bound to lactoferrin.

Some bacteria express receptors for iron-binding proteins (e.g. transferrin-binding outer membrane proteins on the surface of *Neisseria* spp.). These specialized receptors are used to acquire bound iron, making it available for bacterial growth.

Other bacteria have evolved elaborate mechanisms to extract iron from host proteins. Siderophores are substances produced by many bacteria to capture iron from the host. The absence of iron triggers transcription of genes coding for enzymes that synthesize siderophores, as well as for a set of surface protein receptors that recognize siderophores carrying bound iron. Siderophore affinity for iron is so high that even iron bound to transferrin and lactoferrin is confiscated and taken up by bacterial cells (Figure 3.10). Both *Escherichia* and *Salmonella* species utilize siderophores to mobilize iron.

Microbial toxins and enzymes

A formidable array of toxins and enzymes are produced by microorganisms to promote their survival in the human host. These can be classed as exotoxins, enzymes, and bacterial endotoxin. Some fungi produce lytic enzymes but evidence for toxin production is limited. *Aspergillus* species, for example, produce aflatoxins but the precise role of these toxins as major virulence factors is unknown. The salient differences between bacterial exotoxins and endotoxin is described in Table 3.8.

Exotoxins

Exotoxins constitute a class of poisons that are among the most potent, per unit weight, of all toxic substances. Exotoxins are not essential for bacterial growth and metabolism and the genes for most can be deleted with no noticeable effect. In contrast to the extensive systemic and cytokine-mediated effects of endotoxin, the site of action of most exotoxins is localized to particular cell types or cell receptors. Exotoxins are potent immunogens: some elicit neutralizing antibodies (also known as antitoxins) that react with key enzymatic sites on the exotoxin, resulting in toxin inactivation. Antitoxins harvested from humans and animals are widely used for immediate therapy of acute life-threatening infectious diseases such as

Table 3.8 Exotoxins and endotoxins

Exotoxin	Endotoxin
Produced by Gram positive and Gram negative bacteria	Produced only by Gram negative bacteria
Protein; many antigenic types	Lipid A of lipopolysaccharide, single type
Secreted extracellularly	Integral part of the bacterial cell wall
Heat labile	Heat stable
Act on target cells via specific receptors; produce specific host effects, highly toxic and often fatal	Act on a wide range of host cells and tissues; producing abnormal physiological changes and systemic disease; weakly toxic and not directly fatal
Toxoid formation of the toxin used in protective immunization	Toxoid production not possible, no role in immunization
Intensely antigenic and elicit antibodies; also called antitoxin	Poorly immunogenic

---

Box 3.2 Identify the toxin (from Kansas Department of Health and Environment. National Immunization Program; Division of Field Epidemiology, Epidemiology Program Office, CDC)

On August 15, 1993 a 57-year-old man with noninsulin-dependent diabetes sought treatment at an emergency department for a puncture wound to his foot that occurred when he stepped on a rusty nail earlier that day. Treatment in the emergency department included wound cleaning and administration of the appropriate toxoid (0.5 cc).

On August 19, the man returned to the emergency department, reporting onset on August 18 of severe pain in the affected foot, fever, chills, and vomiting. He was hospitalized and treated for cellulitis. On August 20, he complained of pain and stiffness in his neck; he had had difficulty chewing and swallowing. Examination noted trismus ("lockjaw"); he subsequently had a cardiopulmonary arrest, was resuscitated, and was placed on mechanical ventilation. He remained on mechanical ventilation and died following a cardiac arrest on September 16.

1. Name the toxin responsible, list its key properties.
2. Why did the administration of a toxoid on first presentation not prevent the disease?

---

tetanus and diphtheria. Others induce lifelong protection of the host by inducing a systemic antibody response. Read on to identify the toxin in Box 3.2.

Based on their pathological profile exotoxins are best grouped into:

- Neurotoxins
- Cytotokins
- Enterotoxins.

Neurotoxins are best exemplified by the toxins produced by the *Clostridium* spp.: botulinum toxin formed by *C. botulinum* and the tetanus toxin produced by *C. tetani*. Botulinum toxin is a potent neurotoxin that acts on motor neurons by preventing the release of acetylcholine at neuromuscular junctions, preventing muscle excitation, and resulting in flaccid paralysis. The report in Box 3.3 is a typical example of the presentation seen in patients with botulism. (Note: wound botulism is emerging as an important public health problem in

Box 3.3 Wound botulism among black tar heroin users – Washington, 2003 (*MMWR* September 19, 2003/52(37);885–886)

During August 22–26, 2003, four injection-drug users (IDUs) in Yakima County, Washington, sought medical care at the same hospital with complaints of several days of weakness, drooping eyelids, blurred vision, and difficulty speaking and swallowing. All four were regular, nonintravenous injectors of black tar heroin, and one also snorted black tar heroin. This report summarizes the investigation of these cases, which implicated wound botulism as the cause of illness.

Two patients, both subcutaneous IDUs ("skin poppers"), progressed to respiratory failure despite antitoxin administration and required mechanical ventilation. The third and fourth patients, both intramuscular IDUs with milder presentations, were discharged with minimal residual weakness 17 and 9 days after admission, respectively.

At the Washington State Public Health Laboratories, botulinum toxin type A was detected by mouse bioassay in serum specimens obtained from the first two patients.

Box 3.4 What is BOTOX®?

BOTOX® is the commercial trade name for botulinum toxin type A. In the 1960s, the muscle-relaxing properties of botulinum toxin type A were used in realigning crossed eyes. These early studies paved the way for treating other conditions caused by overactive muscles with botulinum toxin type A.

When a small amount of highly diluted toxin is injected into muscles, botulinum toxin has a local effect. It blocks transmission between the nerve endings and muscle fibres around the injection site to cause weakness of the nearby muscle.

What is BOTOX® used for?

Cosmetic
BOTOX® is a nonsurgical cosmetic treatment for moderate to severe frown lines. It has been proven to be a safe and effective treatment for wrinkles.

Medical
BOTOX® is indicated for the treatment of cervical dystonia in adults to decrease the severity of abnormal head position and neck pain associated with spasms of the neck muscles. BOTOX® is indicated for the treatment of abnormal alignment of the eyes and spasm of the eyelids associated with nerve disorders.

"skin-poppers" world wide.) Botulinum toxin type A has other cosmetic and medical uses and is marketed as the well known product – Botox (Box 3.4).

Tetanus toxin acts in a different manner; it is taken up at neuromuscular junctions, transported along axons to synapses; here it acts by inactivating neurons that play a part in inhibiting muscle contraction, resulting in prolonged contraction and a rigid paralysis. Patients typically manifest with a clenched jaw and an arched back due to muscles that are in a sustained state of contraction (Box 3.2).

The **cytotoxins** constitute a larger, more heterogeneous grouping with a wide array of host cell specificities and toxic manifestations. The diphtheria toxin, produced by *Corynebacterium diphtheriae*, is coded for by a gene carried on a lysogenic phage (a virus that infects bacteria, but does not cause cell lysis). The toxin has two functional subunits: the B unit binds to target cells, while the A unit has the toxic activity. It inhibits protein synthesis in many cell types by inhibiting elongation factor 2 (EF 2) in ribosomes, inhibiting peptide chain elongation, and eventually causing cessation of protein synthesis. Inhibition of protein synthesis in a cell eventually leads to cell death (necrosis). In diphtheria damage occurs not only to the cells in the upper airway characterized by a necrotic, adherent membrane seen in the tonsils and pharynx, but it also disseminates in the blood causing cell death in distant tissues, including the heart, muscle, peripheral nerves, adrenals, kidneys, liver, and spleen (see Chapter 25). *Pseudomonas* exotoxin A has a similar mode of action.

The shiga toxin of *Shigella dysenteriae* and the shiga-like toxin of *E. coli* are potent cellular toxins (causing cell death) as well as being enterotoxins (responsible for diarrhea); they inhibit protein biosynthesis at the ribosome leading to cell death. They act specifically on vascular endothelium producing cell necrosis, leading to the bloody stool seen in dysentery. Cell necrosis due to shiga toxin in the gut manifests as an intense inflammatory process of the bowel wall. This is characterized by ulceration of the mucosal surfaces and the characteristic symptoms of bacterial dysentery.

The prototype **enterotoxin** that induces hypersecretion of water and electrolytes from the intestinal epithelium to produce profuse, watery diarrhea is that of *V. cholerae*. It is interesting to note that the labile toxin (LT) of enterotoxigenic *E. coli* is indistinguishable from the cholera toxin in protein structure. They have similar mechanisms of action and produce similar effects on host tissue.

Cholera toxin binds to a specific receptor, monosialosyl ganglioside (GM1 ganglioside) present on the surface of intestinal mucosal cells. It activates adenylate cyclase in cells of the intestinal mucosa; the net effect of the toxin is to cause cAMP to be produced at an abnormally high rate. This stimulates mucosal cells to pump large amounts of chloride (Cl^-) into the intestinal contents. Water, sodium (Na^+), and other electrolytes follow due to the osmotic and electrical gradients caused by the loss of Cl^-. H_2O and electrolytes lost in mucosal cells are replaced from the blood. Thus, the toxin-damaged cells act as pumps for water and electrolytes causing the typical isotonic diarrhea that is characteristic of cholera. The toxic effect is dependent on the organism producing a neuraminidase during the colonization stage which has the interesting property of degrading gangliosides to the monosialosyl form; the specific receptor for the toxin. The exact mechanism of action of the cholera toxin is illustrated in Figure 3.11.

The host relies on locally synthesized IgA that prevents not only bacterial colonization, but also toxin attachment to its receptor. Hence oral cholera vaccines which promote local IgA synthesis are considered far more beneficial than parenteral IgG producing cholera vaccines.

Enzymes

A family of bacterial enzymes that act on tissue matrices and intercellular spaces, promoting spread of the pathogen and often referred to as "**spreading factors**," include hyaluronidase, collagenase, neuraminidase, and kinases.

Hyaluronidase is the prototype spreading factor, produced by the pyogenic streptococci, staphylococci, and clostridia; classically associated with invasive skin and soft tissue infections caused by Group A β–hemolytic streptococci. The enzyme attacks the intercellular cement ("ground substance") of connective tissue by depolymerizing hyaluronic acid.

Collagenase is produced by *Clostridium histolyticum* and *Clostridium perfringens*. It breaks down collagen, the framework of muscles, and is a classic feature of gas gangrene associated with these organisms.

Neuraminidase is produced by intestinal pathogens such as *S. dysenteriae*. It degrades neuraminic acid (also called sialic acid), and intercellular cement of the epithelial cells of the intestinal mucosa.

Streptokinase and **staphylokinase** are produced by streptococci and staphylococci, respectively. Kinase enzymes convert inactive plasminogen to plasmin; this digests fibrin and prevents clotting of blood. The relative absence of fibrin in spreading bacterial lesions allows unchecked spread of the organism through tissue.

Enzymes that cause hemolysis and/or leucolysis usually act on the host cell membrane by insertion of pore-forming proteins that eventually cause cell lysis.

Lecithinases or **phospholipases** act by enzymatic attack on phospholipids destabilizing the cell membrane: **phospholipases**, produced by *C. perfringens* (i.e. alpha toxin), hydrolyze phospholipids in cell membranes. *Candida* species are also able to produce potent phosholipases.

Hemolysins, enzymes that lyse red blood cells, notably produced by staphylococci and streptococci (streptolysin) and various clostridia, may be channel-forming proteins or phospholipases or lecithinases.

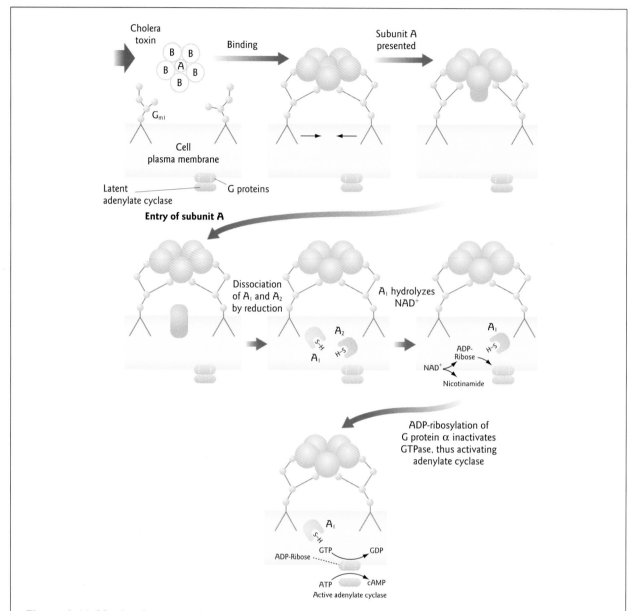

Figure 3.11 Mechanism of action of cholera toxin. Cholera toxin approaches target cell surface. B subunits bind to oligosaccharide of GM1 ganglioside. Conformational alteration of holotoxin occurs, allowing the presentation of the A subunit to cell surface. The A subunit enters the cell. The disulfide bond of the A subunit is reduced by intracellular glutathione, freeing A1 and A2. NAD is hydrolyzed by A1, yielding ADP-ribose and nicotinamide. One of the G proteins of adenylate cyclase is ADP-ribosylated, inhibiting the action of GTPase and locking adenylate cyclase in the "on" mode. Reproduced from Finkelstein R. Cholera, *Vibrio cholerae* O1 and O139, and other pathogenic vibrios. In: *Baron's Medical Microbiology Textbook*, 4th edition, chap 4

Leukocidins, produced by staphylococci, and **streptolysin** produced by **streptococci**, specifically lyse phagocytes and their granules.

Other enzymes such as coagulase, the distinguishing feature of *Staphylococcus aureus*, is a cell-associated and diffusible enzyme that converts fibrinogen to fibrin, promoting clotting. Its virulence potential is controversial: it may be that a walled off staphylococcal lesion encased in fibrin (e.g. a boil or pimple) could make the organism less accessible to phagocytes or antimicrobial agents.

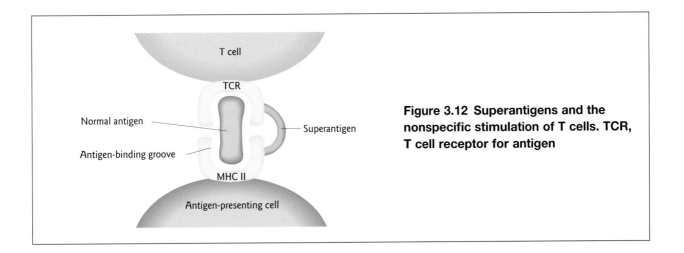

Figure 3.12 Superantigens and the nonspecific stimulation of T cells. TCR, T cell receptor for antigen

Pseudomonas aeruginosa releases **elastases** which inactivate C3a and C4a complement components. Organisms such as gonococci and meningococci produce proteases that split IgA dimers. Many organisms produce drug resistance enzymes which act against antimicrobial agents.

Superantigens

Many bacterial toxins such as the staphylococcal enterotoxins (see Chapter 6) act as superantigens because they stimulate T cells nonspecifically. Superantigens bind directly to class II major histocompatibility complexes (MHC II) of antigen presenting cells outside the conventional antigen binding grove (Figure 3.12). This results in a massive release of cytokines that are responsible for many of the symptoms related to toxin-mediated conditions such as the toxic shock syndrome. Toxic shock syndrome typically begins suddenly with high fever, vomiting, and profuse watery diarrhea, sometimes accompanied by sore throat, headache, and myalgias. The disease progresses to hypotensive shock within 48 hours, and the patient develops a diffuse, macular, erythematous rash with nonpurulent conjunctivitis. Urine output is often decreased, and patients may be disoriented or combative. The adult respiratory distress syndrome or cardiac dysfunction may also be seen. Patients require large volumes of fluid to maintain perfusion and usually require intensive care. In the recovery phase, there is desquamation of at least the palms, soles, or digits, and often of other skin areas as well. Read Box 3.5 for an interesting editorial on toxic shock syndrome in menstruating women.

Endotoxin and the systemic inflammatory response syndrome (SIRS)

In Chapter 1 we discussed the structure of the Gram negative cell wall. The lipopolysaccharide (LPS) component of the outer membrane of Gram negative cell walls is also known as endotoxin. Its structure has been described in detail in Chapter 1. Most of the endotoxin of Gram negative bacteria is released during cell death and degradation, often facilitated by the body's own innate defence mechanism.

When endotoxin enters the bloodstream in significant amounts resulting in endotoxemia or Gram negative septicemia, profound pathophysiological changes are triggered accounting for the classical clinical features of such an infection:

- Fever (the elderly can manifest with hypothermia)
- Tachycardia
- Diminished circulatory volume as evidenced by vasoconstriction, cool extremities, and a narrow pulse pressure
- Increased respiratory rate as the body tries to buffer the metabolic acid load
- Hypotension
- Focal areas of tissue necrosis depending on the site of primary infection

> ## Box 3.5 From an editorial note following reports of toxic-shock syndrome – USA, 1997
>
> A report in 1978, describing seven cases of what was named toxic-shock syndrome (TSS), heralded the apparent emergence of TSS in late 1979 and early 1980. The report about TSS in *MMWR* of May 23, 1980, and the veritable landslide of studies of TSS that followed, demonstrates the speed and effectiveness with which astute clinicians – together with public health officials, epidemiologists, and laboratory scientists – can respond to an "emerging" infectious disease threat.
>
> Cases of TSS in men also occurred during that time but at a low and stable rate. TSS in reproductive-aged women, particularly menstruating women, was reflected in the dramatic data presented in the MMWR report – of the 55 reported cases, 95% occurred among women, and 95% of the cases among women had onset of their illness within the 5-day period following onset of menses. The wave of rapidly completed case-control studies of menstrual TSS that followed clearly demonstrated that use of various brands and styles of tampons was by far the most important risk factor for TSS during menstruation. The most plausible explanation for the "emergence" of menstrual TSS in the late 1970s was the manufacture and widespread use of more absorbent tampons made of a variety of materials not previously used in tampons. There is no evidence to suggest that changes in *Staphylococcus aureus*, the source of the toxin that causes TSS, were responsible for the emergence of menstrual TSS.

- Capillary damage and leakage (leading to bleeding from damaged small vessels in the skin also called a petechial rash; and hypovolemia or low circulatory blood volume and organ perfusion).
- Intravascular coagulation.

Gram negative bacterial infection is an important cause of SIRS. Other infections (Gram positive, fungal, and viral) and noninfectious causes have also been described.

Pathogenesis of SIRS

The term sepsis (in this case Gram negative sepsis) constitutes a spectrum of clinical conditions caused by the immune response of a patient to infection; and is characterized by systemic inflammation and coagulation. Responses can range from SIRS to multiple organ failure and ultimately to death. There are approximately 750 000 cases of septicemia per year in the USA and the mortality rate is between 20% and 50%. Over 210 000 people a year in the USA die from septic shock. Approximately 45% of the cases of septicemia are due to Gram negative bacteria.

We know that the immune response that leads to SIRS is mediated be cytokines. A complex cascade of events, some of which are not fully understood, governs the final outcome in the patient. Patients typically mount a biphasic immunological response in response to sepsis. Initially they manifest an overwhelming inflammatory response to the infection. This is most likely due to pro-inflammatory cytokines: TNF-α, IL-1, IL-12, IFN-γ and IL-6. The body then regulates this response by producing anti-inflammatory cytokines (IL-10), several other soluble inhibitors of TNF, and IL-1. This leads to a relative state of immune depression in the patient, during which time the patient is susceptible to overwhelming intercurrent infections, exacerbating the damage in an already weakened host.

This systemic inflammatory cascade is initiated by various bacterial products, primarily endotoxin (Figure 3.13). LPS molecules released from the outer membrane of the Gram negative cell wall bind to an LPS-binding protein circulating in the blood and this complex, in turn, binds to a receptor molecule, CD14 (CD11/18 may also be involved), found on the surface of macrophages. LPS is a well recognized PAMP (see description of PAMP and phagocytosis earlier); it also binds to specific toll-like receptors

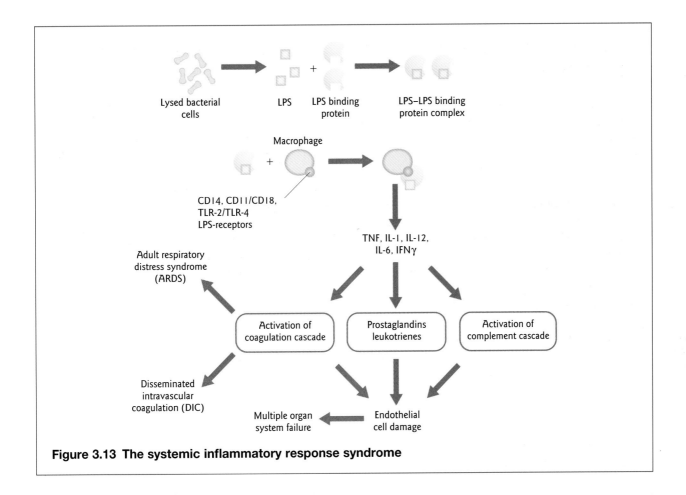

Figure 3.13 The systemic inflammatory response syndrome

(toll-like receptor TLR-2/TLR-4). The relative roles of these receptor molecules in triggering the next stage are not fully understood.

Pro-inflammatory cytokines produced as a result of this trigger (TNF-α, IL-1, -6 and -12, and IFN-γ) act directly to affect organ function or they may act indirectly through secondary mediators. The secondary mediators include nitric oxide (a potent vasodiltaor), thromboxanes, leukotrienes, platelet-activating factor, prostaglandins, and complement. TNF-α and IL-1 (as well as endotoxin) can also cause the release of tissue-factor by endothelial cells leading to fibrin deposition and multiple clot formation. The complex of LPS and LPS binding protein that attaches to CD14 on the surfaces of neutrophils results in release of proteases and toxic oxygen radicals for extracellular killing.

Collectively, cytokines and the secondary mediators cause activation of the coagulation cascade, the complement cascade, and the production of prostaglandins and leukotrienes. Indiscriminate formation of multiple intravascular clots, disseminated intravascular coagulation (DIC), by activation of blood coagulation limits organ perfusion. Concurrent downregulation of anticoagulation mechanisms results in bleeding into tissues leading to hypovolemia. The increased capillary permeability and injury to capillaries in the alveoli of the lungs results in acute inflammation, pulmonary oedema, and loss of gas exchange. This is called acute respiratory distress syndrome (ARDS).

The cumulative effect of this cascade is an unbalanced state, with inflammation dominant over anti-inflammation and coagulation dominant over fibrinolysis. Microvascular thrombosis, hypoperfusion, ischemia, acidosis, and tissue injury result. Collectively, this cascade of events results in irreversible septic shock, multiple system organ failure, and death.

Molecular and genetic basis of virulence

Several well studied bacterial toxin and virulence genes are encoded on chromosomal DNA. Others originate from bacteriophage DNA, plasmid DNA, or transposons located in either the plasmid or the bacterial chromosome. Virulence genes, including those that encode for bacterial drug resistance, are more likely to be transmissible from strain to strain or even between species if they are located on mobile genetic elements (phages, plasmids, and transposons).

The gene for the invasive enterotoxin of *Shigella* species is found in part on a 140-mega-dalton plasmid. Similarly, the gene for the heat-labile enterotoxin (LTI) of *E. coli* is carried on a plasmid; whereas the heat-labile toxin (LTII) gene is found on the chromosome. Other virulence factors are acquired by bacteria following infection by a particular bacteriophage, which integrates its genome into the bacterial chromosome by the process of lysogeny (where infection with a bacteriophage does not cause cell lysis). Examples include diphtheria toxin production by *C. diphtheriae*, erythrogenic toxin formation by *Streptococcus pyogenes*, Shiga-like toxin synthesis by *E. coli*, and production of botulinum toxin (types C and D) by *Clostridium botulinum*. Other virulence factors are encoded on the bacterial chromosome (e.g. cholera toxin, salmonella enterotoxin, and yersinia invasion factors).

Bacterial drug resistance: a major escape mechanism

Bacteria have evolved ingenious ways with which they survive in the presence of antimicrobial agents. Genetic exchange is one mechanism by which bacteria acquire antimicrobial drug resistance (mutation is the other mechanism). Genetic exchange has profound implications for the transmission of drug resistance and the worldwide spread of infections caused by multi-drug resistant organisms.

Bacterial genetic exchange may occur by asexual or sexual processes or by infection with a virus (the bacteriophage). To understand the genetic basis of drug resistance, it is important to describe the methods of genetic exchange that commonly occur in bacteria.

Four important methods are commonly utilized:

- Transformation
- Transduction
- Conjugation
- Transposition.

Transformation

Transformation is a process where bacteria take up naked DNA from the extracellular space. The process of DNA uptake and recombination (integration) into host cell DNA is illustrated in Figure 3.14. Most bacterial cells need to be at a particular stage in their growth cycle or under a particular growth regimen in order to be transformed. Very few species are capable of natural transformation. The pathogenic Gram positive species, namely *S. pneumoniae* and *S. aureus*, are able to take up exogenous DNA. Gram positive strains are capable of taking up both homologous (same species) and heterologous DNA (from other species). Gram negative bacteria that can be transformed by exogenous DNA include *Neisseria meningitis, Neisseria gonorrheae, H. influenzae,* and *E. coli*. Homologous DNA is taken up at a much higher rate than heterologous DNA.

Transduction

Transduction is a process that involves bacteriophages – viruses that specifically infect bacterial cells. When a fragment of donor chromosome is carried to the recipient by a bacteriophage that has been produced in the donor cell, the process of genetic transfer is called transduction. Transduction occurs in Gram positive and Gram negative bacteria and is an important method of transfer of drug resistance genes from cell to cell.

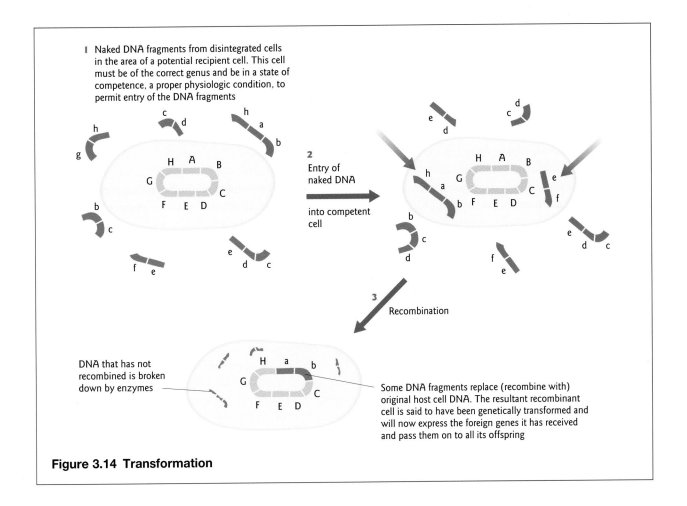

I Naked DNA fragments from disintegrated cells in the area of a potential recipient cell. This cell must be of the correct genus and be in a state of competence, a proper physiologic condition, to permit entry of the DNA fragments

2 Entry of naked DNA into competent cell

3 Recombination

DNA that has not recombined is broken down by enzymes

Some DNA fragments replace (recombine with) original host cell DNA. The resultant recombinant cell is said to have been genetically transformed and will now express the foreign genes it has received and pass them on to all its offspring

Figure 3.14 Transformation

Conjugation

Conjugation is a mating process involving bacteria. It involves transfer of genetic information from one bacterial cell to another, and requires physical contact between the two bacteria involved (Figure 3.15). The contact between the cells is via a protein tube called an F or sex **pilus**. Conjugation begins with the

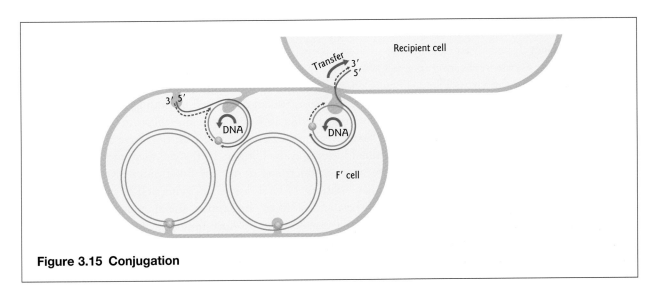

Figure 3.15 Conjugation

extrusion of a sex pilus; the tip of the sex pilus adheres to the recipient bacterial cell surface. Following pilus adherence, the two cells become bound together at a point of direct envelope-to-envelope contact. Transfer of genetic material occurs via plasmids.

Plasmids are small autonomously replicating, extrachromosomal circular pieces of double-stranded DNA. Many of these plasmids also mediate gene transfer; they carry genes for resistance to drugs (called R factors) or virulence factors (genes encoding toxin production) resulting in bacterial strains with unique drug resistance patterns or novel virulence factors. Some conjugative plasmids are able to integrate into the host chromosome. After integration, both chromosome and plasmid can be conjugally transferred to a recipient cell. Plasmids that are able to mobilize chromosomal transfer are called sex factors or F (fertility) factors. Cells that contain the sex factor F are designated F^+ and those that do not contain the factor are F^-.

Transposition

Segments of DNA can move around to different positions in the genome and between chromosomes and plasmids of a single cell. This process is called transposition and the mobile genetic elements are called transposons or "jumping genes." Mobility leads either to mutations or increase (or decrease) in the amount of DNA in the genome.

Many transposons move by a "cut and paste" process: the transposon is cut out of its location and inserted into a new location. This process requires an enzyme – a **transposase** – that is encoded within transposons. Others operate using a "copy and paste" mechanism. This requires an additional enzyme – a **resolvase** – that is also encoded in the transposon. The original transposon remains at the original site while its copy is inserted at a new site. Typically such transposons in bacteria carry genes for one or more proteins that confer resistance to antibiotics. When such a transposon is incorporated in a plasmid, it can leave the host cell and move to another.

Bacteria have thus evolved a highly sophisticated survival mechanism that also has the alarming potential of rapid and unchecked spread within and between communities.

Viruses

Viruses can cause disease either directly by their effects on infected or uninfected cells, or indirectly through the host's immune response to their presence.

Direct viral pathogenesis

Cytopathic effect

By its very nature, a virus replicating in a cell will divert that cell from its normal function into being a production factory for the virus. The cell's cytoskeleton may be disrupted and there may be substantial accumulations of virus particles as inclusion bodies. Many organelles of the cell, including the cell membrane, may become dysfunctional. Cells may fuse together into syncytia. The effects of a particular infection on a particular cell type may have a characteristic appearance in cell culture (where it is referred to as cytopathic effect) or in infected tissues examined histologically. Ultimately, the cell may undergo lysis or apoptosis. As the individual cells of an organ become dysfunctional or die, the function of that organ may be compromised. Many of the organ-specific manifestations of viral disease are generated in this way, e.g. diarrhea associated with norovirus and rotavirus, the skin lesions of chickenpox, the anemia associated with parvovirus B19 (also called B19V). Unlike bacteria, viruses seem to produce toxins having distant, tissue specific effects only very uncommonly: HIV-1 Vpr has been demonstrated to have neurotoxic effects but there are few other examples. Rather, the host damage mediated by the virus itself predominantly occurs at the site of viral replication and the more a virus is able to replicate unchecked by the host's immune responses – which is advantageous for the generation of progeny to infect new cells and even new hosts – the more severe the tissue damage to the host. Mechanisms of viral escape from the host immune response are covered in a later section in this chapter.

Viral transformation

Another way in which viruses can directly mediate disease is by cellular transformation. Transformation is the altered morphology, biochemistry and/or growth of a cell that is transformed by a virus.

The many cellular genes directly involved in cell replication control are often called oncogenes because they were first identified in cancer cells in which their expression was abnormal. The products of some oncogenes drive a cell forward into cell division (the DNA synthesis or S phase of the cell cycle) in response to a set of highly regulated extracellular and intracellular signals. Conversely, the products of other oncogenes function to hold the cell in the growth phase of the cell cycle and prevent its advance into S phase. Viral transformation of cells is mediated *either* by viral interaction with cellular oncogenes *or* by cellular oncogene homologs of viral origin. Accordingly, virus transformed cells usually contain all or part of the viral genome and express at least some viral genes. Most transforming viruses are either DNA viruses or retroviruses.

The oncogenes of adenoviruses, papovaviruses, and herpesviruses each encode proteins that are associated with cell transformation. For example, human papilloma virus (HPV) genotypes are highly associated with carcinoma of the cervix, herpes viruses with certain lymphomas.

Retrovirus transformation can occur in three different ways:

- A cellular oncogene is activated by insertion into the host genome ("cis-activation"), e.g. Murine Leukemia Virus.
- A viral oncogene drives synthesis of cytokines from the infected cell and it is these cytokines, functioning normally but produced to excess, that activate a cellular oncogene ("trans-activation"), e.g. when human T-cell leukemia/lymphoma virus (HTLV-1) integrates into a lymphoid cell, the protein product of the *Tax* gene causes the cell to synthesize an excess of IL-2 and IL-2 receptor α, these are normal drivers for T cell proliferation.
- The viral genome encodes a v-*onc* gene which, originally stolen from infected cells many eons ago, is homologous to a cellular oncogene: the cell's growth regulatory system is short circuited, causing the cell to proliferate uncontrollably. Examples are Kaposi's sarcoma-associated herpes virus or human herpes virus 8 (KSHV/HHV8) which encodes a receptor that drives angiogenesis (profuse growth of small blood vessels) and cell proliferation.

For most transforming viruses, the enhancement of cell division is just one step towards the loss of all cell cycle control that is characteristic of cancer growth – probably multiple mutation events also play a role – and infection by no means inevitably results in tumor formation.

Immune-mediated viral pathogenesis

For many viral infections, it is clear that certain manifestations of those infections are caused by the host's immune response rather than viral replication per se. Examples include, the immune response to primary EBV infection that results in the disease called infectious mononucleosis; HIV seroconversion illness; the rash and arthralgia of parvovirus B19 infection; the rash illness of measles; and postinfectious encephalomyelitis (also known as acute disseminated encephalomyelitis or ADEM). In some instances, the mechanisms of immune-mediated tissue damage have been further elucidated.

Cytokine-mediated disease

Many nonspecific manifestations of viral infection, such as fever, malaise, anorexia, and myalgia, are probably caused by cytokines released in response to viral infection. The influenza-like side-effects commonly seen during therapy with alfa-interferons are evidence of this. In some viral infections, such as Ebola viral hemorrhagic fever and Dengue shock syndrome, cytokine cascades spiralling out of control may account for some of the clinical manifestations.

Bystander damage

This is the term given to the incidental damage to uninfected cells mediated by the host immune response directed at infected cells. The hepatitis associated with hepatitis B virus (HBV) is a classic example of a clinical illness caused by the host's cell-mediated immune response: HBV-specific cytotoxic T lymphocytes (CTLs) induce apoptosis in uninfected as well as infected hepatocytes. Bystander CTL effects are also thought to play a role in the pathogenesis of HTLV1-associated myelopathy/tropical spastic paraparesis. On the other hand, vasculitic phenomena associated with immune-complex deposition are associated with the host's humoral response to certain infections such as hepatitis C virus (HCV), HBV, and parvovirus B19. Doubtless NK cell activity and antibody dependent cellular cytotoxicity, ADCC, also contribute to bystander damage associated with some viral infections.

Viral superantigens

A protein of the retrovirus mouse mammary tumor virus has been clearly shown to function as a superantigen: the protein binds to the MHC class II molecules of a particular subset of T cells, activates the cells and, through apoptosis, causes clonal deletion. However, there is limited evidence of any human viral infections having superantigen effects: the nucleocapsid of rabies virus may have this property.

Autoimmunity

Acute rheumatic fever is thought to result from an immune response directed at certain group A streptococcal epitopes that cross-react with a self-antigen in heart valve tissue. It has been hypothesized that "molecular mimicry" underlies this phenomenon, and the same process, occurring in response to viral infection, has been implicated in a number of autoimmune diseases: multiple sclerosis (MS), systemic lupus erythematosis (SLE), and diabetes mellitus.

Mechanisms of viral immune avoidance and escape

The strategies by which viruses avoid elimination by the host's immune response are of two types. Firstly, viruses may encode specific products which interfere with the surveillance mechanisms of the host's immune response: immune avoidance. Alternatively, viruses may alter their antigenic phenotype so as to escape a specific adaptive immune response.

Immune avoidance
Location, location, location
Virus-specific neutralizing antibodies can prevent cellular infection, usually at the attachment/penetration stage. However, because viruses are obligate intracellular parasites, once intracellular infection has been established, the virus will no longer be vulnerable to elimination by an antibody-mediated response. Some viruses, such as those infecting the upper respiratory tract, are not exposed to the systemic humoral response because they cause infection at or very close to the viruses' portal of entry. Other viruses, including herpesviruses (HSV), HIV-1, HTLV-1 and measles virus, are able to infect new cells while avoiding antibody exposure by spreading cell to cell. Certain viruses are tropic for cells in a "sanctuary site" tissue that is compartmentally separate from the host's systemic immune responses. Examples include varicella zoster virus (VZV) and HSV in neural ganglia and HIV in the brain.

Avoidance of exposure to the host response by virus-infected cells
One of the ways in which a virus can avoid the host immune response is by remaining hidden from immune surveillance. Herpes simplex virus (HSV) blocks presentation of viral peptides to MHC class I-restricted cells and conceals itself from HSV-specific CTLs. Human cytomegalovirus (HCMV) protein US6 seems to have the same action. Adenovirus protein E3 prevents expression of newly synthesized MHC class I molecules.

Immunosuppressive viral proteins

An alternative method for avoiding the host immune response is by interference with immune effector mechanisms. For example, pox viruses encode multiple homologues of human immune regulatory gene products that are presumed to counter the complement and cytokine cascades of the host's defence.

Some viruses express immunosuppressive viral proteins on the surface of infected cells or on the virus particles themselves:

- Although decreased MHC class I surface expression reduces T cell receptor-mediated activation of antiviral CD8$^+$ T cells, it concomitantly diminishes engagement of NK cell inhibitory receptors, rendering infected cells vulnerable to NK cell attack. To foil NK cell activation whilst globally downregulating MHC class I molecules (see above), HCMV encodes an MHC class I homolog, UL18, that may provide a decoy ligand for inhibitory NK cell receptors.
- The E2 protein of HCV viral envelope binds to the inhibitory NK receptor CD81 and suppresses both cell cytotoxic and cytokine NK effector activities.
- Measles virus is able to induce apoptosis of uninfected lymphocytes following contact with infected cells.

There are also many examples of virus-encoded proteins which, released from infected cells, have distant immunosuppressive effects:

- Ebola virus encodes two proteins, VP35 and VP24, which respectively, suppress the secretion and the antiviral action of interferon.
- A highly conserved peptide within the retroviral envelope protein of HIV-1 has been found to suppress numerous immune functions, to the advantage of the virus.
- In HBV-infected pregnant women, maternally derived HBeAg crossing the placenta results in immune tolerance by elimination of T-helper cells that are responsive to HBeAg/HBcAg. The result is persistent perinatal infection.
- Several extracellular HIV-1 products – Tat, gp120, Nef, Vpu – are capable of inducing apoptosis in uninfected lymphocytes and this phenomenon may account for much of the CD4 T-helper cell loss that is characteristic of chronic HIV infection.

It is noteworthy that as the uninfected immune effector cells killed by exposure to HIV and measles virus products are not exclusively HIV or measles virus specific, these phenomena probably make a major contribution to the generalized immunosuppression associated with both of these infections.

Immune escape

There are several ways in which viruses alter the antigenic phenotype that they present to the host's immune system. The same mechanisms, mostly involving genotypic changes, can enable viruses to escape the actions of antiviral drugs.

Point mutation

Transcription of any genome always carries the risk of base substitution errors. For huge, complex, multisystem organisms with very prolonged generation times and extremely few progeny, such point mutations are highly likely to compromise viability and need to be avoided. Human DNA and RNA polymerases therefore are very high fidelity enzymes. Viruses, on the other hand, have the potential for generating vast numbers of progeny from a single virion, they have very short intergeneration times, and their phenotype is subjected to a test for survival as soon as they come into existence. For viruses then, there is less to lose from genome mutation and much to gain.

Predictably, the genomes of viruses that rely on their human hosts' nucleic acid replicative machinery – DNA viruses which replicate in the nucleus – will tend to be highly stable and conserved. Conversely, RNA viruses have to encode their own RNA dependent RNA polymerase, and as these enzymes are invariably considerably more error-prone than human DNA dependent DNA or RNA polymerases, these viruses readily accumulate sequence changes. When, in influenza viruses, mutations in the genes encoding the envelope proteins neuraminidase and hemagglutinin alter the antigenic phenotype, the process of accumulating point mutations is referred to as "**antigenic drift**."

The RNA dependent DNA polymerases of retroviruses, more often known as reverse transcriptases, are particularly error-prone, being without any exonuclease proof-reading ability. The reverse transcriptase of HIV-1 has an estimated mutation rate of 3.4×10^5 per base pair per cycle and, when coupled with massive viral turnover, single point mutations might occur many thousands of times per day in infected individuals. The result is the rapid establishment of extensive genotypic variation within a single infected person. Amongst an HIV-infected individual's swarm of viral variants, or "quasispecies," there will inevitably be some variants with a survival advantage that cause significant antigenic changes no longer recognized by the host's adaptive immune response. This evasion of the host response by continuous genotypic variation of antigenic targets is highly effective. In a similar way, HIV can rapidly evolve variants that are drug resistant: chance mutations in a viral enzyme which is the target of a particular drug confer survival advantage when they prevent binding of the drug without significantly compromising normal enzyme function.

In hepatitis B virus (HBV) infection, the production of anti-HBe (antibody specific for HBeAg) is vital to control the virus and prevent further replication. Certain mutations of the precore and core promoter regions of the HBV genome prevent or reduce eAg expression without unduly compromising viral replication.

Reassortment

As described in Chapter 1, some virus families have segmented genomes. If a single host cell is simultaneously infected with two different strains of the same virus, some of the viable progeny generated may contain complementary genome segments from both parent strains. This phenomenon is known as genetic reassortment.

Orthomyxoviruses carry seven or eight segments. In influenza viruses A and B, the envelope proteins neuraminidase and hemagglutinin are each encoded on a separate genome segment, and there are many different variants of each among the multitude of strains infecting humans and animals. Consequently, in an individual infected with two strains of the same virus, segmental ressortment can result in novel combinations of neuraminidase and hemagglutinin. This phenomenon, which can generate novel viral strains to which a population has little or no herd immunity, is called "**antigenic shift**". It is thought that antigenic shift resulting in reassortants between human and animal/bird strains of influenza A may be the source of human pandemics. This is discussed in more detail in the Chapter 20.

Rotaviruses, members of the Reoviridae, have 10 segments in their genomes and there is certainly evidence that reassortment serves as a crucial evolutionary mechanism. Likewise, reassortment amongst strains of the bunyavirus, Sin Nombre virus, the cause of Hanta Pulmonary Syndrome (HPS) in the Western USA, may contribute to the success of the virus in persisting in the rodent host population.

Recombination

Recombination is in effect a similar phenomenon to reassortment, but involving two strains of an unsegmented virus. It has been shown to occur commonly in many RNA viruses, including HIV, norovirus, HCV, and dengue virus, and seems also to occur, although probably less frequently, in some DNA viruses such as HBV, HSV, and VZV. As with reassortant viruses, recombination may result in viral progeny having a biological advantage of some sort over one or both parents, e.g. an antigenic phenotype that differs significantly from that of the virus most commonly infecting the host population (and to which there is herd immunity).

Protozoa and helminths

Protozoa and helminths are biologically complex entities that are well adapted for survival in human hosts who are immunologically competent. Why are such hosts unable to mount an effective defence strategy

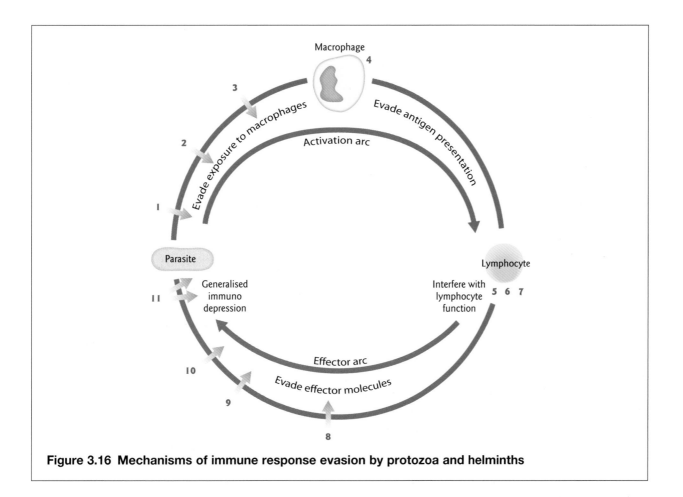

Figure 3.16 Mechanisms of immune response evasion by protozoa and helminths

against even the simplest protozoan parasites? Because there is little evidence of immunologic protection against parasitic infections, adaptive specific immunity has been disputed for a long time. Microorganisms to a certain extent evade immune responses by rapid multiplication. Parasites, because of their complex lifecycles, require time for multiplication and therefore they have evolved various methods of evasion – so successful that parasites can survive in immune hosts for many years.

The many ways in which parasites block normal microbicidal mechanisms is illustrated in Figure 3.16.

1 When parasites such as the *Plasmodium* species (causing malaria) become intracellular and enter the liver, or when metacercariae which do not multiply in the host get embedded in the eye or the brain, they escape the immune mechanism.

2 Similarly when parasites reside and thrive solely in the gut lumen there is little contact with the immune system unless tissue invasion occurs. Helminths within the gut and *Giardia lamblia* are common examples of this phenomenon.

3 Other organisms such as the schistosomes disguise themselves with host antigens. Schistosomes exhibit glycoprotein/glycolipid antigens derived from host red blood cells as the parasites penetrate through the skin. Hence, host responses are not directed to these worms, only to newly entered schistosomulae. This phenomenon has been termed concomitant immunity.

4 *Toxoplasma gondii* and *Trypanosoma cruzi* live within phagocytic cells. *T. gondii* inhibits phagosome-lysosome fusion. *T. cruzi* escapes from the phagosome to lie dormant in the cell cytosol.

5–7 Trypanosomes, leishmania and malaria parasites live within lymphocytes, they inactivate host lymphocytes and cause polyclonal B cell stimulation. This results in an abundance of ineffective and directionless antibodies.

8 Helminths such as *Ascaris lumbricodes* and *Strongyloides stercoralis* migrate around the body stimulating various responses and then move away from an established response, escaping their consequence by entering the gut.

9 The malaria parasite exhibits stage and species specific antigens, shedding antigens at every stage. *Entamoeba histolytica* also regularly sheds its surface antigens confusing the immune system even more.

10 Antigenic variation is the best known example of the evasion tactic. *Trypanosoma brucei* is particularly successful at this gambit. These organisms display several glycoprotein surface coats each with a variable antigen type. When a response is mounted against one type, another one is manifest requiring a whole new set of antibodies.

11 Several parasites inhibit cell or antibody binding, cause depletion of antigen sensitive B cells, and generalized immunodepression. *T. brucei*, *T. gondii*, *Plasmodia* species and *E. histolytica* are a few examples of parasites that cause generalized immunodepression.

The **host's response** to parasitic infections is not totally nonexistent. Innate or natural immunity plays an enormous role as evidenced by the fact that of all the protozoa (animal and human) that man comes into contact with, only a few are pathogenic to humans. **Genetic factors** also play a role in host susceptibility to parasitic disease.

Antibody-mediated immunity is only partially effective and only in some cases. **Premunition** is a term used to describe a controlled level of parasitemia, as in malaria, which results from antibody action. The sporozoite and merozoite stages of plasmodium evoke antibody responses that mediate premunition. The immunoglobulin IgE represents an important line of defence. A series of IgE molecules have been found to coat worms and lead to eosinophil degranulation. The major basic protein (MBP) released produces worm damage and other vasoactive amines enhance a local inflammatory response.

Cellular immunity via T cytotoxic cells does not appear to play a predominant role. However, T cell related lymphokines help activate the formidable macrophage, which is important in the intracellular killing of parasites such as *T. gondii*, *Leishmania* sp., and *T. cruzi*. Parasites have held sway over the human host, in addition, by producing damaging immunopathologic reactions such as liver granulomata and autoimmune cardiac disease. The overall impact of host–parasite interaction seems thus to swing in favor of the parasite. This is evidenced by the finding that all attempts at successful vaccination against parasites have so far failed.

Further reading

Delves PJ, Martin S, Burton D, Roitt I. *Roitt's Essential Immunology*, 11th edition. Oxford: Blackwell Publishing, 2006

Chapter 4
Diagnosis of microbial infection

N. Shetty, M. Wren, E. Aarons, J. Andrews

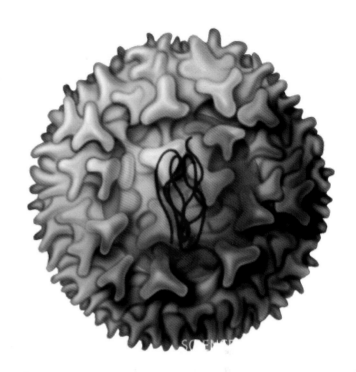

The specimen: collection and transport
Preliminary examination: microscopy
Beyond microscopy
Culture-based diagnostic techniques
  The cultivation of bacteria: growth requirements
    and culture media
  Routine and selective culture
  Cultures of sterile body sites
  The importance of anaerobic culture
  Cultures of sites with a resident normal flora
  Culture of fungi
  Diagnostic identification of bacteria
  Biochemical reactions
  Diagnostic identification of fungi
  Viral culture and diagnostic identification

Non-culture-based diagnostic techniques
  Detection of microbial products
  Detection and application of antigen–antibody
    reactions
  Detection of microbial nucleic acids
Automation in the clinical laboratory
Tests for antimicrobial susceptibility
  Bacterial (and some fungal) susceptibility
    and resistance to antimicrobial agents
  The determination of viral susceptibility
    and resistance to antiviral agents
Diagnosis of protozoal and helminth infections
Other aspects of laboratory diagnosis
  Assessing a new test
  Quality control and quality assurance

Robert Koch laid down the first principles of bacteriology when he formulated the postulates (Box 4.1) that underpin the investigation of an infectious disease. Timely and accurate diagnosis of microbial infection should be the aim of the diagnostic microbiology laboratory. Delay has consequences for both the patient and those in close attendance to him, particularly when such delay results in failure to give appropriate therapy or the patient is infected with an organism with infection control significance.

Results of laboratory investigations not only reflect the accuracy of the investigations performed but also reflect on the standard of specimens taken and their quality. Great care is required when taking specimens for bacterial culture. Avoidance of contamination from the environment, both from the patient's own normal flora whenever possible and from the natural environment surrounding the patient, is paramount. Contamination of a valuable sample may make interpretation difficult and sometimes, at worst, impossible.

Box 4.1 Koch's Postulates

Robert Koch performed some of the most seminal and influential research on anthrax and tuberculosis (TB) in the 19th century. In an attempt to define what an infectious disease actually is, he formulated his eponymous postulates and set out to prove them.

Four criteria are required to establish that an organism causes a disease. The postulates were first set forth by J. Henle in 1840. At that time, however, it was not possible to prove them:

1 The organism must be demonstrated to be present in all animals with the disease, but not in healthy animals.
2 The organism must be isolated from a diseased animal and grown in pure culture.

3 The pure culture must cause the disease in susceptible animals.
4 The organism must be recovered from (3) and re-grown in pure culture.

There are implicit assumptions in steps two and three, (i) the organism is cultivable in the laboratory and (ii) the susceptible animal mentioned in step three, would produce disease similar to the original host (if human).

These steps do not apply to all infectious disease. *Mycobacterium leprae*, the organism that causes leprosy, cannot be cultured in the laboratory. However, **leprosy** is still recognized as an infectious disease.

The laboratory testing of the specimen can only be as good as the sample sent for investigation. For bacteriology, it is important to recognize that, if possible, aspiration of fluid or pus or the deep tissue is the optimum sample. However, this may not always be possible to achieve and, although less desirable, taking a swab sample may be the only option. Swabs, however, are not the optimal sample since they carry only a relatively small amount of material and hence only small numbers of bacteria. Moreover, swabs are more easily prone to contamination. Anaerobiosis is much harder to maintain with swab samples than with a larger volume of fluid or pus (20 ml or more).

The specimen: collection and transport

Proper collection, speed of delivery to the laboratory, and the subsequent handling of the specimen make for a correct and timely microbiological diagnosis. Delay in getting the sample to the laboratory may allow bacteria within the sample to begin to multiply and the sample no longer contains the bacteria in their original state. It is no longer representative of the lesion from which it came and fastidious organisms may be overgrown by more rapidly growing bacteria present in the sample.

Immediate processing is obviously the gold standard but where this is impossible consideration should be given to refrigeration until the sample can be transported. If a cell count is to be useful it should be performed within one to two hours of collection. Swabs must be sent in the appropriate transport medium so as to prevent desiccation of the material and to maintain bacterial/viral viability. Dry swabs do not provide optimal conditions, particularly when there may be a delay in processing. Stuart's or Amie's transport media are the two bacterial transport media most frequently used.

Viral Transport Medium (VTM) is a buffering solution containing antibiotics to prevent the growth of any contaminating bacteria. The tip of the swab bearing the clinical material is broken/cut off into the VTM bottle. Alternatively, the swab is swirled vigorously in the liquid and squeezed against the inside of the bottle before being discarded and the bottle recapped for dispatch to the laboratory. VTM should never be used to moisten swabs **prior** to specimen collection as the medium contains fetal calf serum.

Nasal swabs give the best yield when the anterior nares are swabbed in a circular motion with a swab moistened with saline. Yield is improved when both nares are swabbed.

Throat swabs are taken from the tonsillar fossae with the posterior pharyngeal wall visible by the use of a tongue depressor and in good light.

Sputum is best collected from the first cough in the morning or by the help of a physiotherapist. Clear 60 ml containers are best used as this enables visualization of the sample and provides obvious evidence that the sample is a true sputum sample. Delivery to the laboratory should be prompt so as to avoid overgrowth of the normal salivary flora that is inevitably included in coughed sputum. Refrigeration of sputum samples should be avoided since primary pathogens such as pneumococci and haemophili are sensitive to the cold. In cases of suspected tuberculosis three consecutive early morning samples should be submitted for investigation.

For virological investigation, a **nasopharyngeal aspirate** (NPA) is preferred to sputum. A sample is readily collected from infants and small children by aspiration into a trap. For older children and adults, nasopharyngeal washings (as an alternative to NPA) can be obtained from a seated patient by instilling a few milliliters of saline into the nares using a syringe whilst the head is tilted backwards. The patient then "snorts" the material into a collection pot.

Urine requires immediate delivery to the laboratory, or refrigeration if delay is anticipated; it is a good medium for bacterial growth. General opinion is that a properly collected midstream urine is the best sample. Patients may require instruction on how to provide a good sample and instruction cards should be available in the clinic for them to read.

Feces should be freshly collected in a large clear 60 ml container or in a container devised for the purpose that contains a spoon. **Rectal swabs** are unacceptable for the diagnosis of enteric disease and in patients with diarrhea there should be no difficulty in obtaining a specimen of feces.

Pus and wound exudates are preferred for the diagnosis of infection. Swabs are always second best. When possible 10−20 ml of pus or fluid is preferred since this provides ample material for performing multiple cultures and for direct tests of value such as gas liquid chromatography (GLC) for early detection of anaerobic infection. Moreover, when a large volume of material is present macroscopic examination may reveal characteristics typical of some infections. For example, the "sulfur granules" typical of actinomycosis can be visualized in pus samples. This is impossible on swabs.

For the viral diagnosis of a vesicular rash, vesicular fluid is the ideal specimen. If there are local electron microscopy facilities, then a glass slide can be touched onto a drop of fluid released from a freshly punctured vesicle, the preparation allowed to air-dry and transported to the laboratory for processing. Even better, a scraping of material from the base of a deroofed vesicle is smeared onto a slide.

Samples of other **fluids** (e.g. pleural fluid, joint fluid, ascites, aqueous/vitreous humor from the eye) should generally be obtained by needle aspiration after skin decontamination to avoid contamination which, when it happens, makes interpretation of the cultures erroneous. Fluids taken at operation should be obtained using aseptic technique. Specimens taken from drainage bags that have been standing at room temperature for hours are useless.

Eye swabs are taken from the gently pulled down surface of the lower eyelid using a small swab. If the patient is a neonate and the presence of chlamydia is suspected then a specialized swab used for this purpose should be available. **Corneal scrapings** are performed by the ophthalmic physician. Media should be provided ready at the bedside when these are taken so as to provide immediate culture for these important samples.

Samples of **cerebrospinal fluid** (CSF) are obtained by lumbar puncture. Sufficient volume of sample should be taken to allow for all the likely examinations that are required. At least 2 ml is required for bacterial culture and this should be increased to 10 ml when tuberculosis or fungal infection is suspected. Generally the rule is the more the better. Although not always possible, CSF should be taken before the administration of antibiotics. It is impossible to visualize and grow bacteria from CSF when antibiotic is present in the sample, even after a single dose.

Blood cultures are taken in an endeavor to grow organisms from the blood of patients with septicemia or bacteremia. Skin decontamination is absolutely essential before taking samples since skin contaminants may grow in the very rich media used for these samples and can lead to diagnostic confusion. Ideally 20−30 ml of blood should be drawn for the best yield.

Biopsy samples are generally taken in the operating theatre using full asepsis. For bacteriological investigation, they should be placed in a **dry** sterile container. Even sterile saline is detrimental to most bacteria. If histopathological investigation is also required the sample should be divided into two, the second half being added to formalin. Delivery to the microbiology laboratory should be as rapid as possible to prevent desiccation of the sample. If virological investigation is required, a portion of the biopsy should be sent to the virology laboratory in VTM.

Samples of **clotted and EDTA-anticoagulated blood** are the preferred specimens for the detection of infection-specific antibody responses and for the quantification of blood borne viruses respectively.

The diagnosis of disease caused by **fungi** has become increasingly important in recent years owing to the introduction of aggressive therapies, both antimicrobial and medical/surgical, and to the occurrence of diseases that affect the immune system such as HIV/AIDS. Because of the variety of infections caused by fungi in various sites of the body any of the above sample types may be cultured for fungi when there is a clinical suspicion of their involvement in disease, especially when the treatment of the patient involves the use of immunosuppressive drugs.

Preliminary examination: microscopy

Examination of stained smears of the sample should precede culture. This serves two purposes. Firstly, it will give the examiner an idea of the types and proportions of the microbes present and the presence of inflammation revealed by the presence of white cells (Figures 4.1 and 4.2). Secondly, it may be used as a guide for further procedures. For example, the presence of yeast cells may be an indication to add specific

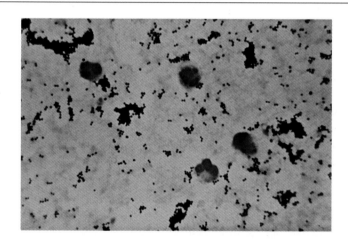

Figure 4.1 Gram stain of a smear (1000×) from pus showing numerous polymorphs and Gram positive cocci in clusters (e.g. *Staphylococcus aureus*)

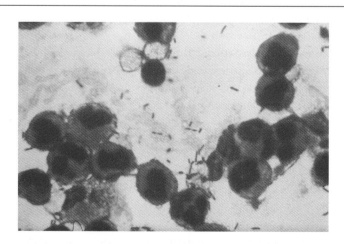

Figure 4.2 Gram stained smear of urine (1000×) showing polymorphs and Gram negative rods (e.g. *Escherichia coli*)

Box 4.2 The Gram stain

The Gram stain procedure was developed by Danish physician Hans Christian Gram in 1884. In brief, the procedure involves the application of crystal violet or gentian violet to a heat fixed smear followed by a solution of iodine (potassium iodide). This procedure stains the cytoplasm of the bacterial cell with a violet–iodine dye complex. The cells are then decolorized with 95% ethanol or a mixture of acetone and alcohol. The difference between Gram positive and Gram negative bacteria lies in the permeability of the cell wall to these violet-iodine dye complexes when treated with the decolorizing solvent. Gram positive bacteria retain violet–iodine dye complexes even after treatment with the decolorizing agent; Gram negative bacteria do not retain the dye complexes when decolorized. Decolorized Gram negative bacteria take up the counter stain, usually a red dye such as safranin or dilute carbol fuchsin, and stain pink in color. The Gram stain provides evidence of the nature of the cell wall of the stained bacterial cell; indirectly it also provides early information on the nature of antimicrobial that may be used in treatment. Commonly used antibiotics such as penicillin act specifically on the Gram positive cell wall.

culture media targeted at these organisms. Moreover, failure to grow organisms seen in the stained smear may indicate a problem with the culture media or the regimen used and this needs further investigation.

Gram stain is the single most useful preliminary diagnostic tool for the assessment of numbers and types of bacteria (Box 4.2).

The initial investigation may be enhanced by the use of specific stains such as acid-fast stains for mycobacteria (Box 4.3) or calcofluor white for fungi (Box 4.4).

Other staining techniques such as capsule and flagella stains add very little additional information at this stage and are difficult to perform. Spore stains may help but only in the identification stages when a pure culture is being investigated.

Direct examination for fungal elements in samples is generally helpful for the detection of the presence of dermatophytes. Dimorphic fungi are more difficult to diagnose by direct examination, but attempts should always be made to do so since early diagnosis of these diseases are important. Unstained wet preparations often yield the causative fungus. The use of such preparations with phase contrast microscopy allows easy visualization of fungal elements.

Immunofluorescence microscopy is very useful for the rapid diagnosis of herpesvirus infection as a cause of a vesicular rash or of respiratory virus infection. Virus specific antibody labeled with a fluorescent dye is applied to a smear of fixed cells on a slide, and the preparation is then examined using a fluorescence microscope. The labeled antibody binds viral antigen in infected cells so that these cells then fluoresce with a pattern that is characteristic of the particular viral antigen targeted (Figure 4.3; also see the section "Immunohistological techniques" below).

If available, electron microscopy (EM) of diarrheal stool or skin vesicle fluid can often enable a specific virological diagnosis to be made rapidly (Figures 4.4 and 4.5). For detection, at least 10^6 particles per ml of sample must be present. However, sensitivity can be enhanced by the pre-treatment of samples with antibody: either a monoclonal directed against a particular viral species or pooled immune serum from recovered patients. This is called immune-EM. Aside from virus-specific immune-EM, the particular value of EM in general is that the technique, unlike culture or antigen/nucleic acid-specific methods, is an entirely nonselective means of detecting *any* virus.

Beyond microscopy

For further bacteriological and fungal investigation, culture remains the basic methodology. However, "first generation" culture-based techniques are progressively being supplemented by "second generation" methods

Box 4.3 Ziehl–Neelsen and auramine stains

The distinctive property of the mycobacterial cell wall is that it is lipid-rich with mycolic acids and relatively impermeable to various basic dyes unless the dyes are combined with phenol. This property is exploited by the Ziehl–Neelsen and auramine staining methods. Once stained the cells resist decolorization with acidified organic solvents and are therefore called **acid fast**. The ability to retain arylmethane dyes such as carbol fuchsin (pink staining in the figure on the right, above) and auramine-rhodamine (orange fluorescence in the figure on the right, below), despite washing with alcohol or weak acids, is a primary feature of this genus. Certain other bacteria which contain mycolic acids, such as *Nocardia*, can also exhibit this feature. The exact method by which the stain is retained is unclear but it is thought that some of the stain becomes trapped within the cell and some forms a complex with the mycolic acids. This is supported by the finding that shorter chain mycolic acids or mycobacterial cells with disrupted cell walls stain weakly acid-fast.

Fluorochrome (auramine rhodamine) staining has advantages and disadvantages over Ziehl–Neelsen staining. One advantage is that the smear is examined under a lower magnification with a dry objective allowing a much larger area of the smear to be examined in a shorter time. One of the disadvantages of auramine staining is that organisms that are dead or rendered noncultivable by chemotherapy may still fluoresce positive. This disadvantage is caused by the superiority of the fluorochrome stain over the carbol fuchsin stain

to bind intensely with the mycolic acids. Many laboratories confirm an auramine positive smear with Ziehl–Neelsen staining.

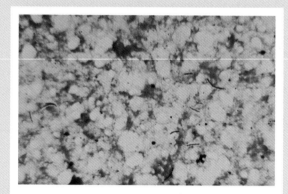

Acid-fast stain of *M. tuberculosis* (1000×)

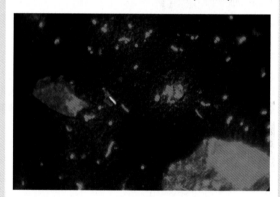

Auramine stain for Mycobacteria (1000×)
Image provided by Ronald W. Smithwick.
Courtesy of the Centers for Disease Control and Prevention; from CDC website:
http://phil.cdc.gov/phil/details.asp

that detect major components of the infective agent or the products of its replication and, more recently, by "third generation" methods which are nucleic acid-based technologies that detect genetic sequences specific to an infectious organism. The latter molecular methods are proving especially valuable where treatment has already begun and culture has subsequently failed to reveal the infecting pathogen, or where the invading organism is difficult to detect by conventional means. Meanwhile, for virological diagnosis, such molecular techniques are increasingly becoming the methodological mainstay alongside "second generation" methods for detection of the virus-specific immune response. Viral culture is in rapid decline. As far as parasitology is concerned, i.e. the diagnosis of protozoan and helminth infections, microscopic examination of appropriate samples is the basic means of investigation: culture is largely irrelevant, and serological and molecular diagnostic techniques are available only in specialist laboratories.

All of these culture and nonculture diagnostic methods will be discussed in detail in the course of this chapter.

Box 4.4 Calcofluor white stain

Calcofluor white stain may be used for direct examination of most specimens using fluorescent microscopy. The cell walls of the fungi bind the stain and fluoresce blue-white or apple-green depending on the filter combination used (see figure right). The use of calcofluor white (CFW), a fluorescent brightener used in the textile industry, with the addition of potassium hydroxide (KOH) will enhance the visualization of fungal elements in specimens for microscopic examination. The CFW nonspecifically binds to the chitin and cellulose in the fungal cell wall and fluoresces a bright green to blue. A substantial amount of nonspecific fluorescence from human cellular materials and natural and synthetic fibres may also occur. The CFW highlights suspicious structures but the interpretation of the structures relies on traditional fungal morphologic features.

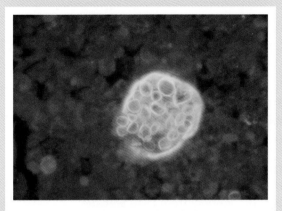

Calcofluor stain. Spherule of *Coccidiodes immitis* with endospores
Provided by Mercy Hospital, Toledo, OH/Brian J. Harrington. Courtesy of the Centers for Disease Control and Prevention; from CDC website: http://phil.cdc.gov/phil/details.asp

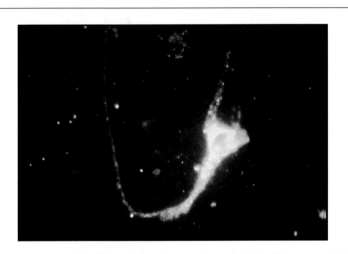

Figure 4.3 Using immunofluorescent stain, it was revealed that this brain tissue sample tested positive for herpes simplex virus (40×). Provided by Dr Craig Lyerla. Courtesy of the Centers for Disease Control and Prevention; from CDC website: http://phil.cdc.gov/phil/details.asp

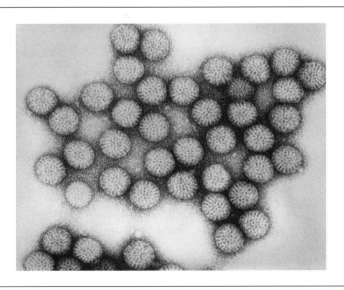

Figure 4.4 Transmission electron micrograph of intact rotavirus particles, double-shelled. Provided by Dr Erskine Palmer. Courtesy of the Centers for Disease Control and Prevention; from CDC website: http://phil.cdc.gov/phil/details.asp

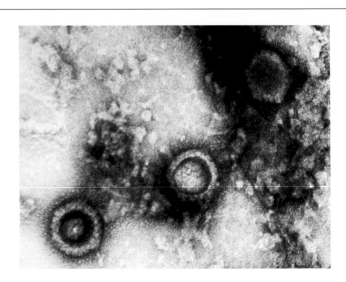

Figure 4.5 Transmission electron micrograph from a pelleted specimen depicting three icosahedral-shaped herpes virus virions. Provided by Dr John Hierholzer. Courtesy of the Centers for Disease Control and Prevention; from CDC website: http://phil.cdc.gov/phil/details.asp

Culture-based diagnostic techniques

The cultivation of bacteria: growth requirements and culture media

Nutrition

The chemicals required to support microbial growth are referred to as nutrients. The requirements for various nutrients may vary with the type of bacterium and, indeed, some nutrient requirements may be specific. Not all nutrients are required in the same amounts, and macronutrients and micronutrients are descriptive terms to illustrate this. The major macronutrients are nitrogen, a source for the building of amino acids and hence proteins, and carbon, the backbone of all biological compounds. Most bacteria obtain their nitrogen from ammonia or nitrate. Carbon is obtained from carbon dioxide and also assimilated from organic carbon sources in culture media such as glucose.

Other macronutrients essential for bacterial growth include phosphorus, sulfur, potassium, magnesium, calcium, and sodium. The construction of the amino acids methionine and cysteine is particularly dependent on a source of sulfur usually in the form of sulfate or sulfide.

Iron plays a major role in respiration and particularly in electron transport mechanisms. Siderophores are enzymes that are used by some bacteria to extract iron from various sources and transport it into the cell. Under conditions of iron limitation a few bacteria will elicit complex siderophores (e.g. enterobactins) without which infection could not occur.

Micronutrients, commonly trace elements, are also important for cell function. Many are metals and pay a role in the functions of enzymes. The requirement for such trace elements is small and hence it is often unnecessary to add them to complex culture media where agar is used as the base and thus already contains these in small concentrations. Such complex media also contain other growth factors that are essential, such as vitamins, amino acids, purines, and pyrimidines. Table 4.1 lists the growth factors required.

Culture media

Culture media are the nutrient solutions or solid forms of nutrient mixtures used to grow bacteria in the laboratory. Most media used in diagnostic microbiology are undefined media (i.e. composition not completely defined) that utilize a complex array of substances tailored to grow medically significant bacteria.

Solid media are constructed using agar as the solidifying agent. Enriched by the use of blood, generally defibrinated horse blood, at a concentration of 7–10%, blood agar will grow medically important bacteria

Table 4.1 Growth factors required by bacteria

Macronutrients	Micronutrients	Growth factors
Carbon	Chromium	p-Aminobenzoic acid
Hydrogen	Cobalt	Biotin
Oxygen	Copper	Cobalamin
Nitrogen	Manganese	Lipoic acid
Phosphorus	Molybdenum	Niacin
Sulfur	Nickel	Pantothenic acid
Potassium	Selenium	Riboflavin
Magnesium	Tungsten	Thiamine
Sodium	Vanadium	Vitamin B_6
Calcium	Zinc	Vitamin K group
Iron		Hydroxamates

with little difficulty. Blood agar is additionally a good media to detect the type of hemolysis a particular organism produces. For example, there are streptococci that produce β hemolysis; this results in complete lysis of red cells in the media, producing a clear zone around the colony. Other streptococci produce α or partial hemolysis resulting in greening around the colony due to residual hemoglobin (Figure 4.6a–c).

Such media can be rendered selective, usually by the addition of chemicals, most often antibiotics, so that the isolation of a particular organism or group of organisms can be recovered from a mixture. Addition of chemicals or carbohydrates and pH indicators to a basic agar medium can be used to differentiate different groups of similar organisms (hence the term differential media).

Indicator media such as MacConkey's agar can also be classified as differential media as they are useful in detecting pH changes due to lactose fermentation by certain organisms (Figures 4.7a–c). They are helpful in the preliminary stages when mixtures of bacteria are being investigated.

Liquid media are often used as enrichment media where they are used to encourage the growth of bacteria from small innocula. However, great care should be taken when using liquid media since one organism accidentally introduced from the environment may contaminate the culture and make diagnosis very difficult.

Other growth requirements include optimum temperature, humidity, pH and aerobic/anaerobic or micro-aerophilic (contains 10% carbon dioxide) atmospheres.

Chromogenic media are agar-based culture media containing various chromogens (substrates that change color on breakdown). Chromogens are incorporated into the medium for the specific detection of certain bacteria, for example *Staphylococcus aureus*, *Candida* species, and certain urinary pathogens. Colonies growing on these media utilize the substrate releasing color. The bacterial species are identified by the color of the colony growing on the agar plate (Figure 4.7d).

Routine and selective culture

The laboratory will have a set protocol for the culture of clinical samples which sets out the minimum standard for each sample type. However, it is impossible to lay down strict routines for all types of specimens because the investigation of a sample may alter or develop as the investigation progresses. The use of a mixture of enriched media and selective media is the usual rule.

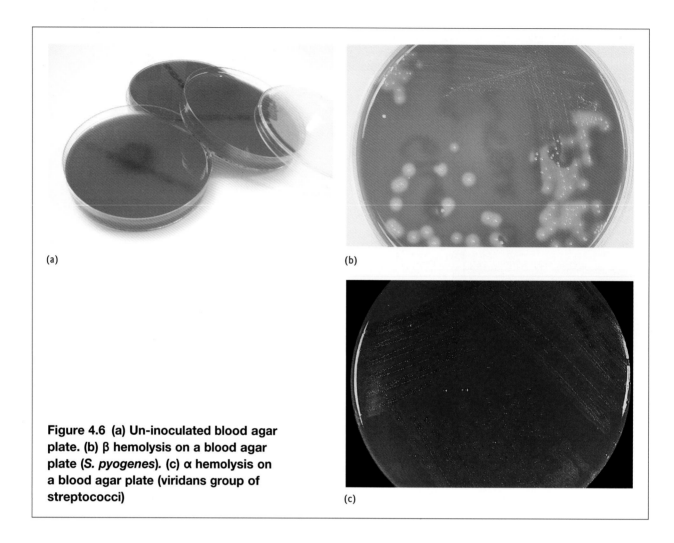

(a)

(b)

Figure 4.6 (a) Un-inoculated blood agar plate. (b) β hemolysis on a blood agar plate (*S. pyogenes*). (c) α hemolysis on a blood agar plate (viridans group of streptococci)

(c)

General rules are easier to apply to specimens taken from body sites that would normally be expected to be sterile. The use of a rich blood agar medium for culture both in air plus 10% carbon dioxide and a parallel plate incubated under anaerobic conditions is the minimum requirement. Incubation times are important, generally the longer the better, but it is important to try to make a diagnosis as rapidly as possible; plates are read at 24 hours and incubated for a further 24 hours. The anaerobic plate is incubated for up to 5 days. It is important that the media used should be able to grow the widest range of pathogens as possible and the range of media may be increased with the used of fluid media to enrich bacteria if they are present in small numbers. The direct Gram stain of the sample may be helpful in making these decisions.

Selective culture media greatly increase the chance of isolation of pathogens from samples taken from body sites that harbor normal flora. The agent used for selectivity may be an antibiotic, a disinfectant, or other chemical compound. Additionally a different incubation temperature may be used to favor the growth of the target organism. Similarly the use of anaerobic conditions may be helpful in selecting bacteria with certain properties such as *Streptococcus pyogenes*, where anaerobiosis favors the production of or enhances the beta-hemolysis (streptolysin O, the major producer of this hemolysis, is oxygen labile).

The use of selective media however is not a complete answer. Some bacteria may be sensitive to the agent used to select them and some agents may often inhibit the target organism when it is present in small numbers. Selective media should never be used on their own as no growth on such media leads to difficulties in interpretation. It cannot be known whether the sample is badly taken or is truly sterile unless a blood agar without any selective agent is also used.

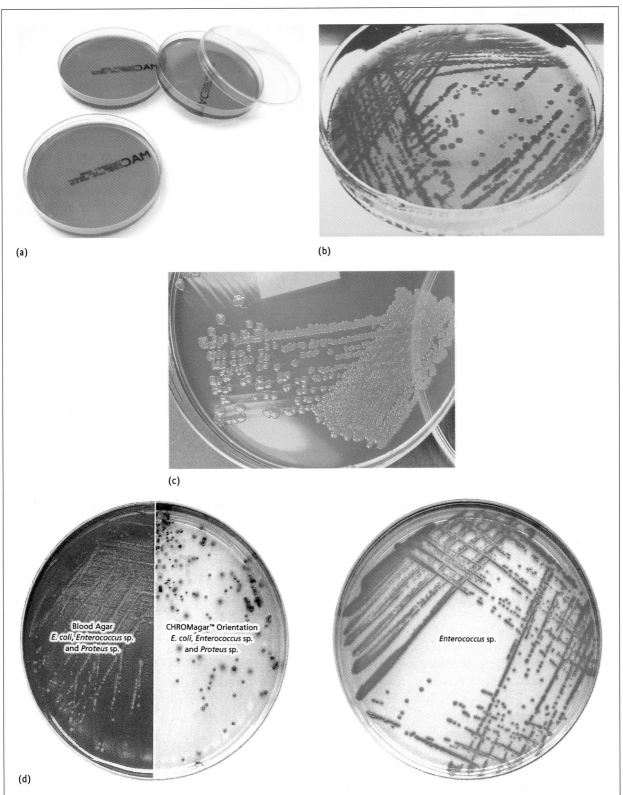

(a)

(b)

(c)

Blood Agar
E. coli, *Enterococcus* sp.
and *Proteus* sp.

CHROMagar™ Orientation
E. coli, *Enterococcus* sp.
and *Proteus* sp.

Enterococcus sp.

(d)

Figure 4.7 (a) Un-inoculated MacConkey agar. **(b)** MacConkey agar showing lactose fermenting colonies of *E. coli* (note pink color due to pH change as a result of lactose fermentation). **(c)** MacConkey agar showing nonlactose fermenting colonies of salmonella (note pale color due to no lactose fermentation, minimal pH change). **(d)** Colored colonies help identify the bacterial species *E. coli* and *Enterococcus* spp. using Chromagar

Cultures of sterile body sites

Any bacterium recovered from a body fluid which is normally sterile should be regarded as a potential pathogen. The aim of the culture is to recover any human pathogen. When a microbe previously considered to be harmless has been recovered from such samples it must not be dismissed lightly as a contaminant. All isolates should be identified to genus level and in most cases to the level of species. This is not unduly difficult as most often the organism will have been recovered in pure culture. Mixed infections, however, do occur, especially in pleural and peritoneal fluid, and care should be taken not to miss slowly growing anaerobic bacteria. Certain groups of patients (i.e. the immunocompromised, cancer or AIDS patient) may also be susceptible to mixed infections at any site.

The submission of frank pus for investigation is evidence in itself of infection or at least an active inflammatory process, and in patients who are not on antibiotic therapy a Gram stain of a thinly made smear will reveal the infecting organisms with ease. The absence of organisms may be an indication to go on to the use of specific stains such as an acid-fast stain for mycobacteria. The failure to detect organisms in such smears may prompt the use of additional culture media such as a broth medium used for the enrichment of bacteria when present in small numbers that may be beyond the detection limits of stained smears.

The importance of anaerobic culture

In the laboratory diagnosis of infection the use of methods to culture anaerobic bacteria is of paramount importance since, depending upon specimen type, anaerobes may account for from about 30% to 80% or so of all bacterial isolates. The provision of an anaerobic atmosphere should be achieved within one hour of the seeding of specimens to agar plates. Anaerobic bacteria are at their most susceptible to the deleterious effects of oxygen at this stage, and the holding of anaerobic cultures until large batches of plates are ready for incubation is anathema. The initial period of incubation should be for 48 hours before examination (unless an anaerobic chamber is in use in which case plates can be examined under continuous anaerobic conditions daily). Further incubation until a total of 5 days (14 days for *Actinomyces* species) has elapsed is recommended before discarding cultures as negative.

Cultures of sites with a resident normal flora

The examination of specimens taken from sites where there is normal flora presents the microbiologist with a dilemma. A detailed list of the entire microbial flora in such a sample cannot be produced without expending considerable time and resources. Such a list may only serve to confuse the attending physician, yet he will need to know whether the sample contains any specific pathogens in quick time.

There are thus two options open to the microbiologist. He can either choose to identify all species present to a superficial level or he may limit the investigation to the examination of known pathogens whilst making no attempt to identify the rest of the flora. It should be borne in mind, when reading such cultures, that a note should be made if the normal flora has changed from the expected pattern. If no primary pathogen is found suspicion may fall on the bacteria that were previously thought harmless especially if the balance of the resident flora has been altered.

Hence investigation may take one of four types: (i) exclusion of known pathogens; (ii) exclusion of known pathogens plus investigation of the normal flora; (iii) full investigation of clinically unusual infections; and (iv) full investigation of all bacteria cultured. Most laboratories will take the first option and perform this investigation as thoroughly as possible, since its reliability influences the well-being of the patient and those exposed to the risk of infection from him. The use of direct stained smears of such specimens serves very little purpose.

Diagnostic identification of bacteria

Detailed identification of species of bacteria is required on many occasions, either for epidemiological purposes or to add weight to the clinical diagnosis (e.g. the identification of *Streptococcus pneumoniae* from a sputum sample of a patient with lobar pneumonia). However, some bacteria take a long time to identify and the diagnostic laboratory is obliged to use methods that are both speedy and accurate. Tests that give accurate identification but take days to reach a result serve little purpose in diagnostic microbiology.

Preliminary information is usefully gained from the Gram stain morphology and colonial morphology. Hemolytic streptococci, staphylococci, and coliform organisms are easily recognized in this way. The consistency of colonial characteristics, effects on the surrounding medium, and the developed color on any indicator media are additional useful pieces of information.

Additional rapid tests further enhance the identity of species. Slide coagulase testing for *S. aureus*, butylase for *Moraxella catarrhalis*, and the spot indole test for *E. coli* are but a few examples. There is a move in the manufacturing of commercial kits towards the development of rapid strip methods that will, where possible, determine bacterial identity within 4–6 hours.

Biochemical reactions

The biochemical activities of bacteria allow different species within a genus or different genera to be delineated. Fermentation or oxidation of carbohydrates or other substrates, or the production of various preformed enzymes, allow this differentiation to be achieved and is made easy by the use of ready-made commercial kits linked with the application of computer generated profiles and databases.

Commercial kits used for identification involve the use of batteries of biochemical tests in a convenient format, the results of which can be translated into a numerical profile which is entered into a computer program containing a database of profiles given by strains of the different bacterial genera and species.

Both colorimetric and fluorimetric reactions may be used depending on the system used. Such systems may make use of carbohydrate fermentation reactions, carbohydrate utilization, or carbon sources utilization. A recent development is the use of preformed enzyme reactions enabling identification to be achieved within 4 hours. However, preformed enzyme profiles may differ according to the growth medium used and, therefore, the manufacturer's recommendations must be followed exactly.

Commercial systems do have certain limitations. Databases should be updated on a regular basis. The accuracy of any system is limited to the manufacturer's claims and the current edition of the database. Furthermore, a strict policy must be agreed on what to do with or how to resolve questionable results or an unexpected result, especially if the identity is paired with a susceptibility result. It is important to have a backup system available to resolve such problems.

Finally profiles of closely related species may make it difficult for the system to separate them. However, this may not affect patient clinical outcome. Clearly an assessment should be made each time this occurs.

The **API rapid identification system (bioMerieux, USA)** is an example of a commercial kit designed to identify microorganisms using a carefully selected set of biochemical tests (Figure 4.8). The wells of this plastic strip have dried ingredients for each test. The wells are inoculated with bacterial suspension and left to incubate overnight, at 37°C. The tests are designed to produce clear results by dramatic color changes (e.g. pH indicators or chromogenic substrates).

Biochemical tests are generally used in various groups to identify bacteria. Hugh and Leifson (Oxidation-Fermentation) medium has traditionally been used to differentiate those organisms which oxidize glucose from those that ferment glucose. This, together with the oxidase reaction and a test for motility, can provide a broad differentiation between the pseudomonads, acinetobacters, alkaligenes, and the Enterobacteriaceae. This is relatively rapid and clinically expedient. Full biochemical identification can then be performed almost always using a commercial kit.

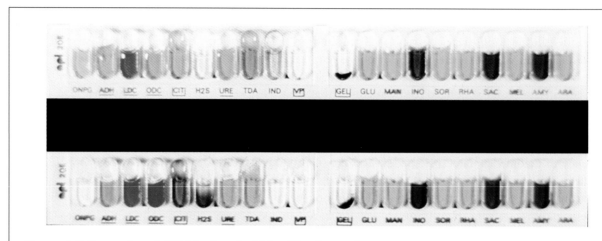

Figure 4.8 Examples of API biochemical identification strips

The use of Lancefield grouping, now performed using latex kits, is still the preferred method for identifying the beta-hemolytic streptococci, although cross-reactions may occur and unusual isolates may give confusing results (e.g. *Streptococcus porcinus*, a rare isolate in humans, will give a positive latex test with Group B streptococcus). It is wise to confirm any unusual grouping result with biochemical tests. Grouping of streptococci is not foolproof and use of grouping only may very occasionally lead to serious errors of identification.

The major problem with alpha-hemolytic streptococci is the differentiation of *Streptococcus pneumoniae* from the rest. Optochin sensitivity has been the traditionally used method, however, optochin resistance in the pneumococcus is known as is sensitivity to this compound among the oral streptococci. Bile solubility should, therefore, be used as a confirmatory test where optochin results are difficult to interpret or are suspiciously abnormal.

Coagulase testing is still the gold standard for identifying *Staphylococcus aureus* but it is not wholly accurate. Meticillin resistant strains of *S. aureus* may give negative results, and false positivity has been noticed with *S. lugdunensis*, *S. intermedius*, and *S. sciuri*. Similar problems occur with the recently developed latex tests. The use of DNAse agar may help to resolve some of these problems but resort to full biochemical identification may be necessary with some aberrant strains.

Diagnostic identification of fungi

The identification of fungi in the diagnostic laboratory involves the use of microscopy to which one must have some experience, coupled with the use of specialized media, carbohydrate utilization tests (especially for yeasts), and other conventional biochemical testing such as urea hydrolysis. Identification of the dermatophytes and some other mold fungi is mainly microscopic and the use of slide culture enhances the ability to recognize specialized structures. For yeasts the tests used may vary from simple tests such as the germ tube test for *Candida albicans* through to assimilation tests which are now much easier to perform owing to the availability of commercial assimilation panels. Corn Meal Agar is also used for identification of the yeasts as typical morphological features, varying with the species, can be seen.

Culture of fungi

Fungal cultures generally require longer incubation than those for bacteria (with a few exceptions). Most dermatophyte fungi will be visible within 10–14 days. The pattern of macroconidia and microconidia (Figures 4.9 and 4.10), together with colonial morphology and color, are the major observations for the recognition of this group. Other fungi and yeasts require specialized methods for their identification.

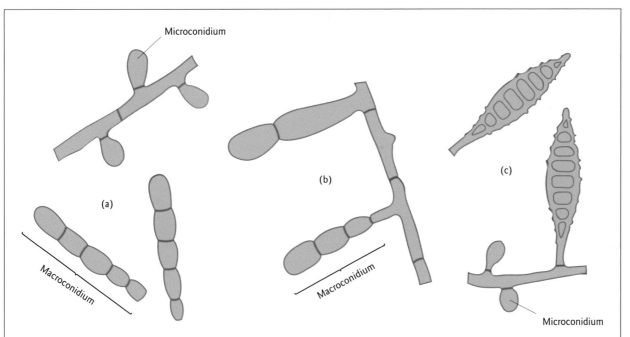

Figure 4.9 Spores of the three common genera of dermatophytic fungi. (a) Macroconidia (about 50 μm long) and microconidia (about 4 μm) of *Trichophyton* spp. (b) Macroconidia of *Epidermophyton* spp., which do not produce microconidia. (c) Spindle-shaped macroconidia and microconidia of *Microsporum* spp. Reproduced from: Deacon J. *Fungal Biology*, 4th edition. Oxford: Blackwell Publishing, 2006. © Jim Deacon

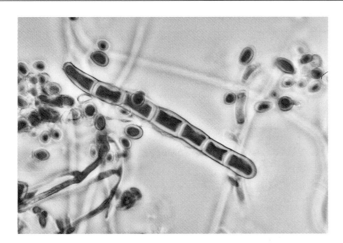

Figure 4.10 Spindle-shaped macroconidia, and microconidia, of *Microsporum* spp. (phase contrast microscopy). Reproduced from: Deacon J. *Fungal Biology*, 4th edition. Oxford: Blackwell Publishing, 2006. Reproduced by courtesy of the Canadian National Centre for Mycology; http://www2.provlab.ab.ca/ bugs/webbug/mycology/dermhome.htm

The identification of the dimorphic fungi relies on the ability to obtain cultures in both yeast and mold phase. The mold phase provides the diagnostic features which will help to make a final identification. Great care must be taken when converting to the mold phase in the laboratory. Many of the dimorphic fungi are Category 3 pathogens and all manipulations should be carried out in a Class I microbiology safety cabinet within a Category 3 laboratory.

The final decision about the identity of a fungus, however, often involves the use of specialized texts or referral to a reference laboratory.

Viral culture and diagnostic identification

The cultivation of viruses requires the use of living cells since viruses cannot grow on inanimate media. Viral culture techniques are increasingly being supplanted by molecular methods. There are three main systems:

1 Tissue culture (*in vitro* cell culture).
2 Chick embryo culture – rarely used.
3 Culture in laboratory animals – rarely used.

Tissue culture is the cultivation of viruses in a single layer (monolayer) of actively metabolizing cells adherent to a glass/plastic surface. The cells are grown in a balanced and buffered nutrient medium with antibiotics to prevent bacterial contamination.

A variety of different cell types can be employed for tissue culture. Primary cells, such as Rhesus monkey kidney cells, are derived directly from mammalian tissues and can be sustained in tissue culture for only a limited number of passages. Semi-continuous cells (e.g. Human Embryonic Lung cells) are capable of 30–50 passages following their isolation from embryonic tissues. Continuous cells are immortalized cell lines which can be grown *in vitro* almost indefinitely. Examples include Vero cells, originally obtained from African green monkey kidney, and HeLa cells derived from cancerous human cervix.

Following inoculation of a tissue culture with an infected sample, viral replication causes the development of morphological changes in the cell monolayer: cytopathic effect (CPE). The appearance of this CPE in a particular type of cell culture together with its timecourse of development may be more or less characteristic of a particular virus (Figure 4.11a and b). The particular diagnosis can then be confirmed by hemadsorption (adherence of erythrocytes to the infected cells is typical of certain viral infections, as with influenza and measles viruses, because the viral antigens expressed include a hemagglutinin) or by immunofluorescence using virus specific antibody labeled with a fluorescent dye.

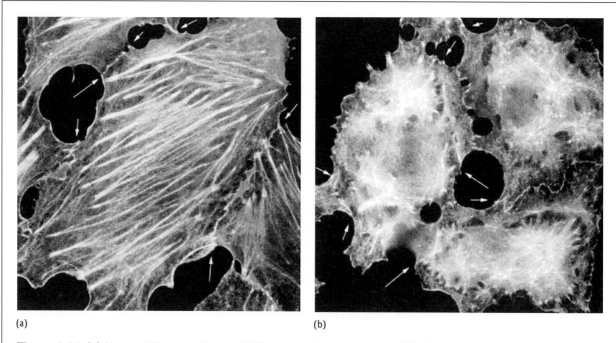

(a)   (b)

Figure 4.11 (a) Normal tissue culture. (b) Tissue culture showing CPE. Reproduced from Wagner et al. (2008), with permission from Blackwell Publishing

Non-culture-based diagnostic techniques

Detection of microbial products

Bacterial growth results in the production of excess materials such as metabolites, lipopolysaccharide, and capsular material during the logarithmic growth phase and these may be detected in the specimen using various methods.

The detection of metabolic short chain fatty acids in body fluids for the rapid detection of anaerobic infection has been used successfully for many years. Moreover, as the acids remain within the fluid for up to 5 days when refrigerated, the technique can be used retrospectively and can be useful when anaerobes have failed to grow. A simple procedure of acidification and extraction using sulfuric acid followed by ether will provide the material for injection into a gas–liquid chromatograph (GLC). The detection of short chain fatty acids in the sample is a sensitive method for the indication of the presence of anaerobic infection.

In some circumstances it is more rapid and specific to detect the presence of bacterial toxin than to go through the lengthy process involved in isolation and identification, and may be the preferred option for infection control purposes. Using a rapid test to detect the presence of vero toxin in feces rather than the lengthy culture regimen for the various serotypes of *Escherichia coli* is an example. Similarly, toxin detection is the preferred method for the detection of *Clostridium difficile* diarrhea, with culture being reserved for suspected outbreaks where isolates are required for typing (see section on "Detection and application of antigen–antibody reactions" below).

As viruses do not metabolize independently of their host cell, diagnosis can never be based on detection of viral metabolites. However, viral infections invariably result in the synthesis of virus-specific proteins, some of which have enzymic functions not seen in normally functioning human cells. The detection of such enzymes has occasionally been exploited for diagnostic purposes, as is the case for reverse transcriptase assays in the diagnosis of retroviral infection.

The use of direct tests for fungal specific metabolites and structural components has been reported with varying sensitivities and specificities.

For bacteria that are difficult to culture such as mycoplasmas and rickettsiae, diagnosis is dependent on detection of specific antigen/nucleic acid or of the host's specific immune response. Similarly, where culture is especially slow, as with TB, nucleic acid detection may be very useful. These same general diagnostic methods are fundamental to clinical virology and there has been an exponential growth in the use of nucleic acid tests for diagnosis and monitoring in recent years.

Detection and application of antigen–antibody reactions

Much of this section will be devoted to the clinical laboratory applications of antigen–antibody interactions. These interactions form the basis of many important diagnostic tests in clinical infectious diseases.

The application of antigen–antibody reactions in the diagnosis of infectious diseases is based on a simple concept: antigen–antibody reactions are specific. Antibodies usually react only with the antigen that stimulated their production in the first place. As a result it is possible to detect either unknown microbial antigen or the antibody elicited in response to it in clinical specimens such as serum or CSF. We can use known antiserum, i.e. antibody (prepared by animal inoculation or monoclonal antibody technology), to identify the presence of antigens of suspected microorganisms; alternatively we can use known antigen to detect antibody in clinical specimens.

Classically antigen–antibody reactions have been broadly classified into:

- Precipitation
- Agglutination
- Complement fixation

- Immunoassay using labeled reagents
- Cytokine immunoassays (e.g. ELISPOT).

Modern diagnostic laboratories rarely use precipitation, tube agglutination or complement fixation tests. This section will focus on those tests most commonly used for laboratory diagnosis of infection.

(i) Direct agglutination

In this simple direct technique, a cell or insoluble particle is agglutinated directly by antibody. An example is the agglutination of group A red cells by anti-A sera in a simple slide agglutination test. In this way several species of bacteria (grown on culture) can be directly agglutinated and thus definitively diagnosed by specific antibody using a slide agglutination reaction. Slide agglutination reagents are available to group pathogenic streptococci and to detect somatic (O) and flagellar (H) antigens of enteric pathogens.

(ii) Indirect or passive agglutination

Soluble antigens can be adsorbed to a variety of carrier particles; animal red cells, latex and gel particles are commonly used in the diagnostic laboratory. As with tube agglutination, the addition of a standardized quantity of antigen-bearing carrier particles to serial dilutions of serum permits quantification of the titer of specific antibody. *Treponema pallidum* particle agglutination assay is an example of a commercial passive agglutination assay. Tests for HIV antibody and for heterophile antibodies in acute EBV infection are also available in this format.

Commercial latex particle agglutination tests for the identification of cultured bacterial colonies have been available for many years. Some of these reagents can be used on primary patient samples such as blood, urine, or CSF. The titer of a specific antigen, such as cryptococcal antigen, present in a patient's serum or CSF can be determined by serial dilution of the sample.

Immunoassay using labeled reagents

The enzyme-linked immunosorbent assay (ELISA or EIA) is based on the simple principle that enzyme-labeled antibodies can convert a colorless substrate into a colored product. Furthermore, the reaction can be quantified by measuring the density of color using a colorimeter. Commonly used enzyme labeled antibodies and their respective color substrate complexes are given in Table 4.2.

Figure 4.12a illustrates a generic ELISA system. Variants on the format can be used to detect class specific antibodies (IgG, IgM, IgA, or IgE) by using the appropriate second antibody (Figure 4.12b) or to detect specific antigen by using the appropriate antibody to "capture" the target antigen (Figure 4.12c). In the latter case, because the target antigen is "sandwiched" between capture and conjugate antibodies, these assays are sometimes called "sandwich" immunoassays.

The ELISA/EIA and its many variations are widely used in diagnostic microbiology, especially in clinical virology (Table 4.3).

When immunoassays were first developed in the 1960s for the detection and quantification of small amounts of antigen present in biological samples, the detector antibodies were labeled by means of conjugation to the radioactive isotope I^{131}. Later, relatively safer isotopes such as I^{125} and P^{32} became

Table 4.2 Enzyme labeled antibodies with respective substrate complexes

Antibodies conjugated to	Substrates
Horseradish peroxidase	Hydrogen peroxide + ortho phenylene diamine
Alkaline phophatase	*p*-Nitrophenyl phosphate
β-Galactosidase	*o*-Nitrophenyl-β-D-galactopyranoside

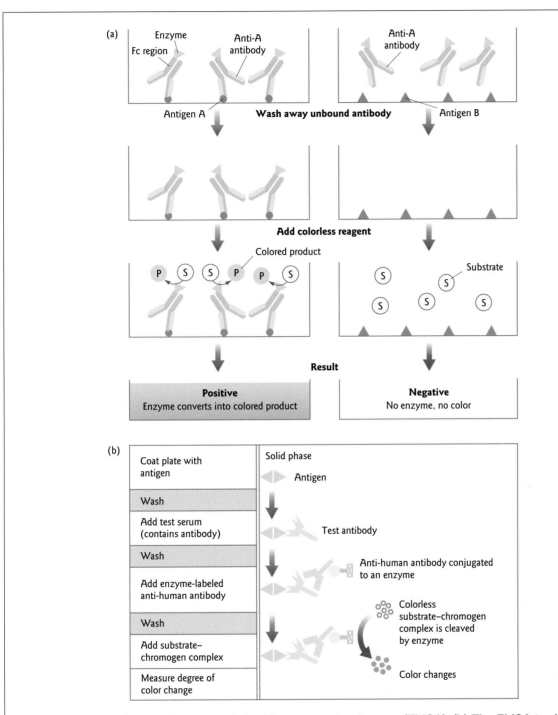

Figure 4.12 (a) The generic enzyme linked immunosorbent assay (ELISA). (b) The ELISA to detect antibody. (c) The ELISA to detect antigen. (a) Reproduced from Wagner EK, Hewlett MJ, *Basic Virology*, 2nd edition. Oxford: Blackwell Science Ltd, 2004, figure 7.9, with permission from Blackwell Publishing Ltd

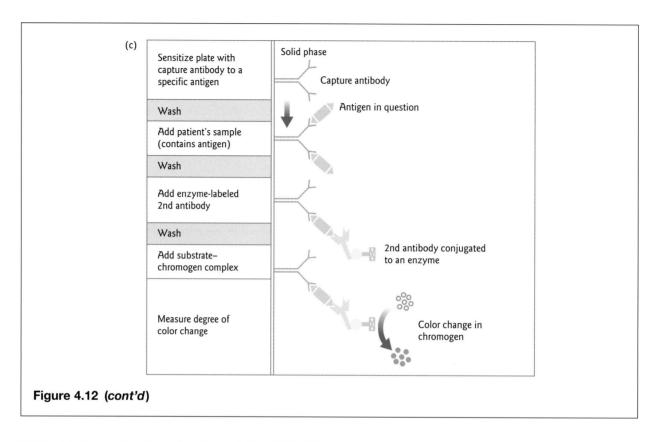

(c)

| Sensitize plate with capture antibody to a specific antigen |
| Wash |
| Add patient's sample (contains antigen) |
| Wash |
| Add enzyme-labeled 2nd antibody |
| Wash |
| Add substrate–chromogen complex |
| Measure degree of color change |

Solid phase
Capture antibody
Antigen in question
2nd antibody conjugated to an enzyme
Color change in chromogen

Figure 4.12 (*cont'd*)

Table 4.3 Examples of applications of the ELISA/EIA

For antigen detection:
Hepatitis B surface and e (a part of the viral core antigen) antigens: HBsAg and HBeAg
HIV-1 p24 antigen
For antibody detection:
Antibodies to hepatitis B core and surface antigens: anti HBc and anti-HBs
Antibodies to *Treponema pallidum*
Antibodies to toxoplasma
Antibodies to HIV 1 and HIV 2
Antibodies to rubella

available. However, these radio-immunoassays (RIA) required the procurement of expensive emissions counters and carried the risk of exposing their users and the environment to unnecessary radiation, whilst the labeled reagents had a limited shelf life due to radioactive decay. Consequently, when the safer more flexible enzyme immunoassay technique came into use in the late 1970s RIA was gradually supplanted. EIAs of various formats continue to be important for rapid diagnosis and have considerable commercial significance. However, since the 1980s, several nonisotopic, nonenzymic reagent labeling and detection methods have been developed. Examples include fluorescence polarization and time resolved fluorescence assays (Box 4.5). Such fluorescence-based methods are very sensitive, very rapid, and highly amenable to incorporation into automated systems. Thus, these may in turn supplant EIAs at least for certain diagnostic applications.

Box 4.5 Fluorescence-based immunoassay techniques

Fluorescence is the production of light that occurs when absorption of radiation at one wavelength (excitation) is followed by nearly immediate re-radiation (emission), usually at a different wavelength.

The fluorescence polarization assay (FPA) is based on the rotational differences between a small soluble antigen molecule in solution (labeled with a fluorochrome) and the same labeled antigen molecule when complexed with its antibody. A small molecule rotates randomly at a rapid rate, resulting in rapid depolarization of light, while a larger complex molecule rotates more slowly and depolarizes light at a reduced rate. The change in rate of depolarization can be measured.

Time resolved fluorescence assays (TRFA) rely on the principle that the fluorescence emissions of chelates of certain rare earth metals, lanthanides (e.g. Europium), are relatively long-lived. Consequently, when fluorescence intensity is measured at a delayed time after excitation, background fluorescence, which has a fast decay time, is almost completely eliminated. Lanthanide chelates can be conjugated to antibody or antigen molecules so as to create labeled reagents.

Immunochromatography (Immunocard tests)

Immunoassays have been used in a variety of commercially available immunocard tests. These tests use the principle of immunochromatography (Box 4.6 and Figure 4.13). Such tests are simple and quick to perform. Several have been developed as point of care tests (POCT) that can be performed at the patient's bedside. Examples include tests for malarial antigens, *Clostridium difficile* toxins A and B, *Helicobacter pylori* fecal antigens, and for HIV antibodies.

Immunoblotting (Western blots)

Western blots are used to detect antibody targeted to individual antigenic determinants in a crude whole cell antigen mixture or viral culture supernatant. Initially, the antigen mixture is subjected to electrophoretic separation in a gel using, for example, sodium dodecyl sulfate polyacrylamide gel electrophoresis (SDS–PAGE). The separated protein bands are then transferred by transverse electrophoresis ("electro-blotting") onto nitrocellulose or nylon membranes, where they bind nonspecifically. These membranes are

Box 4.6 Immunochromatography

The disposable device is composed of a base membrane such as nitrocellulose. A detector reagent (an antigen or antibody conjugated to a colored indicator) specific to the target analyte is impregnated at one end of the membrane. A capture reagent is coated on the membrane at the test region. When the specimen is added to the sample pad, any target analyte present in the specimen binds to the detector reagent and is carried along the membrane by capillary action. As the specimen passes over the test region coated with capture reagent, the analyte-detector reagent complex is immobilized. A colored band proportional to the amount of analyte present in the sample develops. The excess unbound detector reagent moves further up the membrane and is immobilized at the control band by an anti-detector antibody and a second colored line appears. Thus, two colored lines on the test stick indicate the presence of analyte. In the absence of analyte in the patient's sample, only the control band appears. Color must always be seen at the control line. If no color is seen, the test has failed and must be repeated.

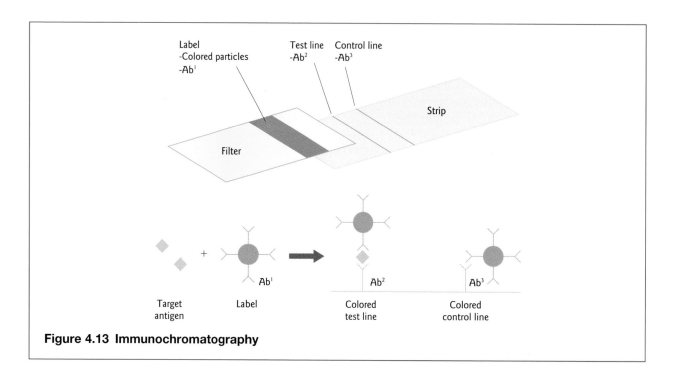

Figure 4.13 Immunochromatography

then incubated with the patient's serum, whereupon any antibodies present will bind to their individual protein antigens. Bound human antibody is then detected using radioisotope- or enzyme-labeled antihuman immunoglobulin, much like the system used in an EIA (Figure 4.14).

The recombinant immunoblot assay (RIBA) used for the diagnosis of hepatitis C uses the Western blot principle: serum is incubated on nitrocellulose strips onto which four recombinant viral proteins are blotted. Control proteins are also included on each strip. Color changes indicate that antibodies have adhered to the proteins and the immunoblot is considered positive if two or more viral proteins show reactivity.

Immunohistological techniques

Immunofluorescence is essentially a technique for detection and localization of antigens in histology or cytology specimens. Fluorescent dyes such as fluorescein and rhodamine can be coupled to antibodies without destroying their specificity. Such conjugates can combine with antigen present in a tissue section and the bound antibody can be visualized by means of a fluorescence microscope. In this way the distribution of antigen throughout a tissue and within cells can be demonstrated.

Immunofluorescence tests can be either direct or indirect (Figure 4.15a and b). In a **direct immunofluorescence** test, the antibody to the target antigen is itself conjugated with the fluorescent dye and applied to tissues or cells fixed on a slide (Figure 4.15a).

The **indirect immunofluorescence** test is a double layered technique (Figure 4.15b). The unlabeled target-specific antibody is applied to the cell or tissue preparation. The preparation is then treated with an anti–human immunoglobulin labeled with a fluorescent dye. After washing away unbound label, the preparation is inspected under a fluorescence microscope. The bound, labeled anti-globulin fluoresces, emitting light of a characteristic color. Immunofluorescence techniques can be used to detect both antigen and antibody in clinical material. Examples of clinical applications of immunofluorescence are given in Table 4.4.

Cytokine immunoassays

Detecting an immune response to the pathogen has been a successful method of diagnosis of infection for many years. However, there are a number of limitations to using antibody detection for the diagnosis of

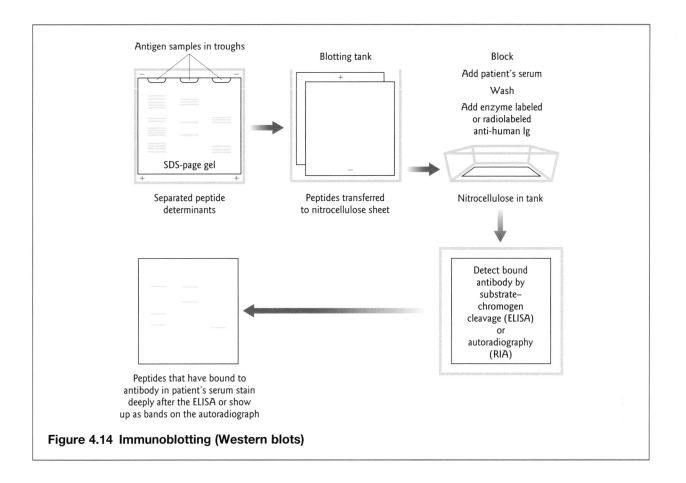

Figure 4.14 Immunoblotting (Western blots)

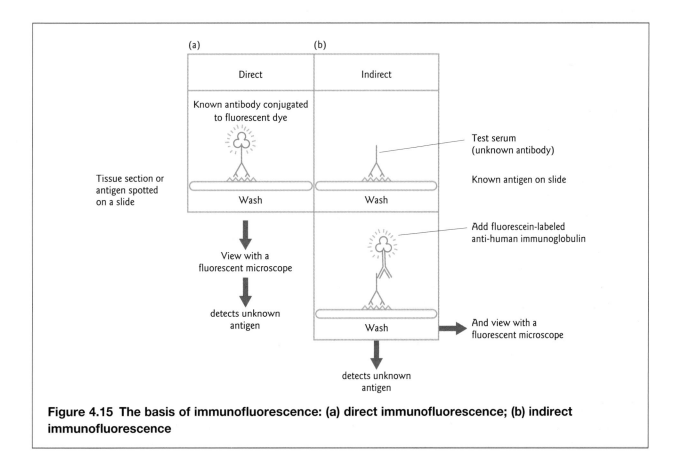

Figure 4.15 The basis of immunofluorescence: (a) direct immunofluorescence; (b) indirect immunofluorescence

Table 4.4 Clinical applications of immunofluorescence

Identification of T and B cells in blood
Detection of immunoglobulins in tissues
Detection of complement components in tissues
Rapid identification of microorganisms in tissue or culture, e.g. *Chlamydia trachomatis*
Detection of specific viral antigens in infected cells (see section "Immunohistological techniques" on p. 106)
Identification of transplantation antigens

acute infection: even using IgM serology it may be difficult to differentiate past infection from acute current infection, and sometimes the antibody response is insufficient and cannot be used as a diagnostic method. A classical example is tuberculosis (TB) where antibody detection has not played a role in diagnosis.

Our understanding of the immune response mechanisms tells us that antibodies are invariably formed with T cell help. So where there are antibodies there must also be activated T cells. T cells, in particular, control the fight against intracellular pathogens such as *M. tuberculosis*, viruses, and tumour antigens. Until recently, specific T cells have been difficult to detect other than with sophisticated flow cytometric equipment.

When white cells from the patients' blood are exposed to a specific antigen (e.g. *M. tuberculosis* antigen), the T lymphocytes produce γ interferon as a result of activation by antigen. This γ interferon is captured by antibody to γ interferon which is pre-coated in wells of a micro-titer plate. By a modification of the ELISA method the captured γ interferon is detected by a second anti-γ interferon antibody conjugated to a suitable substrate–indicator complex. Cytokine immunoassays are being developed for a number of other viral and tumour antigens. The γ interferon assays for tuberculosis are sensitive and specific, are able to detect active and latent TB in immunocompetent as well as immunosuppressed individuals, and do not cross-react with BCG.

Detection of microbial nucleic acids

Nucleic acid-based technologies that detect genetic sequences specific to an infectious agent are revolutionizing clinical laboratory practices. These techniques rely on hybridization: the process of complementary base-pairing between two single-stranded molecules of DNA or of DNA and RNA. All involve specific oligonucleotide probes or primers which bind to target genetic sequences that can be DNA or RNA depending on the particular methodology. They can be divided into two categories: (i) target amplification methods, in which the target sequence is amplified by means of a nucleic acid-processing enzyme such as a polymerase or ligase, and (ii) signal amplification methods in which there is no amplification of the target sequence but the signal generated by the presence of the target is amplified.

Nucleic acid-based tests are inherently highly sensitive and their lower limits of detection range from approximately 10 to 10 000 target molecules in biological samples. Precisely because of this sensitivity, these assays are vulnerable to false positivity arising from sample contamination. Conversely, the hybridization and amplification processes can be inhibited by substances present in biological samples, resulting in false negatives. Thus any laboratory undertaking molecular methods must employ the most rigorous controls in order to establish consistent sensitivity and specificity. Nucleic acid-based tests are also relatively quick to perform, particularly in comparison to conventional culture. With some techniques, such as real-time PCR, it is possible to generate results within a few hours of sample receipt.

Nucleic acid-based methods have been used to detect numerous bacteria, fungi, parasites, and viruses. New infectious agents are being identified at regular intervals using these techniques (e.g. SARS, coronavirus, and human metapneumovirus) and the nonculturable organisms are particularly appropriately detected using nucleic acid-based tests.

Target amplification methods

Polymerase chain reaction (PCR)

This technique is based on a three step, temperature dependent process involving the denaturing of double-stranded DNA into single strands, annealing oligonucleotide primers to the single strands, and finally extending the primers that are complimentary to the single-stranded templates (Figure 4.16). After the primers are annealed to the denatured DNA the single strand becomes the template for the extension reaction. Excess nucleotides are present in the reaction mixture and are enzymatically polymerized by thermostable *Taq* polymerase to form the copy DNA sequences.

During the second and subsequent cycles (up to about 40 cycles) the original DNA strand and the newly generated complementary DNA strand both become templates. Hence the number of DNA strands is doubled after each cycle. In the reaction tube a million copies or more of the original target DNA are present at the end of the PCR reaction.

Other PCR-based methods of target amplification

Modification of the basic PCR method has led to the development of assays with differing properties, and some of these assays can be used in conjunction with one another. Reverse transcriptase (RT)-PCR enables the detection of an RNA rather than DNA target: prior to conventional PCR amplification, a

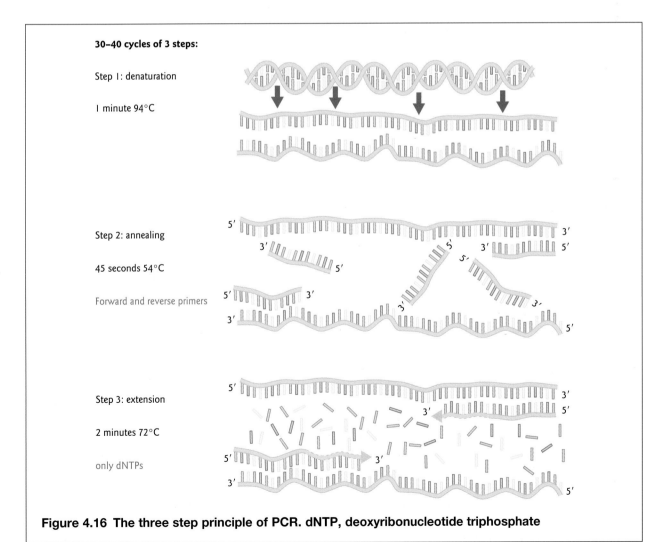

30–40 cycles of 3 steps:

Step 1: denaturation

1 minute 94°C

Step 2: annealing

45 seconds 54°C

Forward and reverse primers

Step 3: extension

2 minutes 72°C

only dNTPs

Figure 4.16 The three step principle of PCR. dNTP, deoxyribonucleotide triphosphate

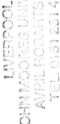

reverse transcriptase-mediated step is used to transcribe the RNA target into copy DNA. In nested PCR, the sensitivity and specificity for the target DNA sequence is enhanced by performing a second round of PCR on the product of the first round. The primer pair used for the second round is targeted to the sequence of the first round product, i.e. nested within it. Multiplex PCR involves the simultaneous use of multiple primer pairs so as to amplify more than one target in the same reaction mix. In degenerate PCR, each of the two primers is a mixture of related oligonucleotides, their variation determined according to the anticipated variability of the target sequence. This strategy makes it possible to identify novel species/strains by targeting conserved sequence motifs and then sequencing the amplified product.

Real time PCR

Conventionally, detection of an amplified PCR product (amplicon) is achieved by agarose or polyacrylamide gel electrophoresis. Ethidium bromide incorporated into the gel binds to the amplified DNA product which then can be visualized using UV light. The appearance of a DNA band of the expected molecular size indicates that the target genetic sequence must have been present in the original sample. However, this gel-based detection is very cumbersome, besides which, ethidium is highly mutagenic. In "real time PCR," the amplification of product generates a fluorescent signal which is monitored in the closed reaction tube as the PCR proceeds. The lack of post-PCR manipulation means that real time PCR assays require less hands-on time, and are therefore simpler and quicker to perform. Moreover, the risk of contamination of samples or sample extracts with PCR amplification products is virtually eliminated.

There are a number of alternative technologies for generating the fluorescent signal. One of the simplest is the use of SYBR Green, the fluorescence of which increases greatly on incorporation into double-stranded (ds) DNA: the amount of fluorescence is directly proportional to the amount of ds DNA present in the reaction tube. However, although this method is sensitive and inexpensive, it is not specific as the presence of any dsDNA (including primer dimers) will cause increased fluorescence. This problem can be partially overcome with the use of post PCR melting curve analysis, thereby confirming that the amplicon has a melting point consistent with the length and base composition of the intended PCR product.

More specific real time PCR assays can be designed through the use of fluorescence-labeled oligonucleotide "probes." A dual-labeled (or Taqman™) probe is an oligonucleotide selected as being complimentary to a short stretch of amplicon sequence, the 5′ end of which is bound to a "reporter" fluorophore molecule whilst the 3′ end is bound to a molecule of "quencher" fluorophore. The fluorescence of the reporter moiety is quenched by the proximity of the quencher moiety by means of Fluorescence (or Förster) Resonance Energy Transfer (FRET): a process whereby energy is passed between molecules separated by 10–100 Å (1–10 nm) that have overlapping emission and absorption spectra. However, following hybridization of the probe to target DNA during PCR, the 5′ → 3′ exonuclease activity of *Taq* DNA polymerase sequentially cleaves the 5′ nucleotides from the probe, so releasing free reporter molecules. FRET no longer occurs so the signal from unquenched reporter molecules accumulates and is detected by continuous monitoring.

Molecular Beacons are similar to dual-labeled probes but their ends are designed to be complimentary. Therefore, at low temperatures the ends of the probe anneal to each other creating a stem–loop structure that causes FRET quenching. When the target specific area of the probe (i.e. the loop) hybridizes to its complimentary DNA target sequence in the amplicon, the reporter and quencher are forced apart, resulting in fluorescence.

"Kissing" (or Lightcycler™) probes are pairs of oligonucleotide probes which hybridize adjacently. The upstream oligonucleotide is labeled with a 3′ donor fluorophore and the downstream oligonucleotide is labeled with a 5′ acceptor fluorophore. When both probes hybridize adjacent to one another on the target amplicon, the two fluorophores are brought together resulting in FRET and, in turn, the generation of a fluorescent signal from the acceptor fluorophore.

Relative quantification is inherent in the real time PCR process: the earlier the PCR cycle at which fluorescent signal (corresponding to amplicon production) appears in the reaction mix, the more template

DNA must have been present in the first place. Thus, with the use of standards containing known copy numbers of target DNA, absolute quantification is readily achieved.

Alternative methods for detection of PCR products

Gel electrophoresis and real time PCR methods are not the only ways of detecting PCR products. In an enzyme-linked oligonucleotide assay (ELONA), the first step is the immobilization of the double-stranded DNA amplicon in the microplate well. This is typically achieved by utilizing the extremely high binding affinity of streptavidin (a naturally occurring protein) for biotin, an essential co-enzyme in many biological systems. The microplate well is coated with streptavidin and therefore "captures" any amplicon that has been labeled with biotin via the incorporation of a biotinylated primer in the preceding PCR. After denaturation of the amplicon into single-stranded DNA, an enzyme-conjugated oligonucleotide probe that hybridizes to a specific DNA sequence is then used to determine whether or not the expected PCR product is present, by means of a color change in a suitable enzyme substrate. Variants on this method involve the use of anti-double-stranded DNA antibody for either capture or detection of the amplicon.

Non-PCR methods of target amplification

Non-PCR-based target amplification methods that have been used successfully in a variety of commercial kit forms for detecting infectious agents include nucleic acid sequence-based amplification (NASBA) and its variant, transcription mediated amplification (TMA) (Figure 4.17). Sensitivity and specificity of these methods are similar to PCR and, in some cases, have advantages for certain applications. Furthermore, these techniques are adaptable to all nucleic acid targets, have multiplex capabilities, and can be both qualitative and quantitative. The products of these amplification methods are single-stranded nucleic acids and hence do not require denaturation before hybridization. These amplification methods are therefore isothermal.

NASBA

NASBA involves the use of three enzymes (avian myeloblastosis virus reverse transcriptase, RNAse H, and T7 RNA polymerase) together with two DNA oligonucleotide primers specific for the target of interest, producing a tenfold amplification product based on primer extension and RNA transcription in an isothermal reaction that can be instrument free. Continuous cycles of reverse transcription and RNA transcription to replicate an RNA target using a double-stranded DNA template intermediate are achieved.

Signal amplification methods
Branched DNA hybridization assay (bDNA)

This assay relies on signal amplification rather than target amplification for its sensitivity. Target nucleic acid is captured onto a microwell by a set of specific oligonucleotide capture probes. A set of target probes hybridize to the captured target. The target probes are designed to have a free end that is complementary to amplifier probes consisting of multiply enzyme-labeled branched DNA molecules. The signal amplification is linear. The technology is both sensitive and quantitative, and has been successfully applied to quantification of HIV and hepatitis B and C viruses.

Capture of RNA:DNA hybrids

This is another signal amplification method that has been employed commercially for diagnostic tests in clinical virology. Specimens containing the target DNA hybridize with an RNA probe mix specific to the target (HBV or HPV for example). The resultant RNA:DNA hybrids are captured onto the surface of microplate wells coated with antibodies specific for RNA:DNA hybrids. Immobilized hybrids are then detected by enzyme-labeled anti-hybrid antibody EIA. Because multiple enzyme molecules are conjugated to each antibody and because multiple conjugated antibody molecules bind to each hybrid, substantial signal amplification occurs.

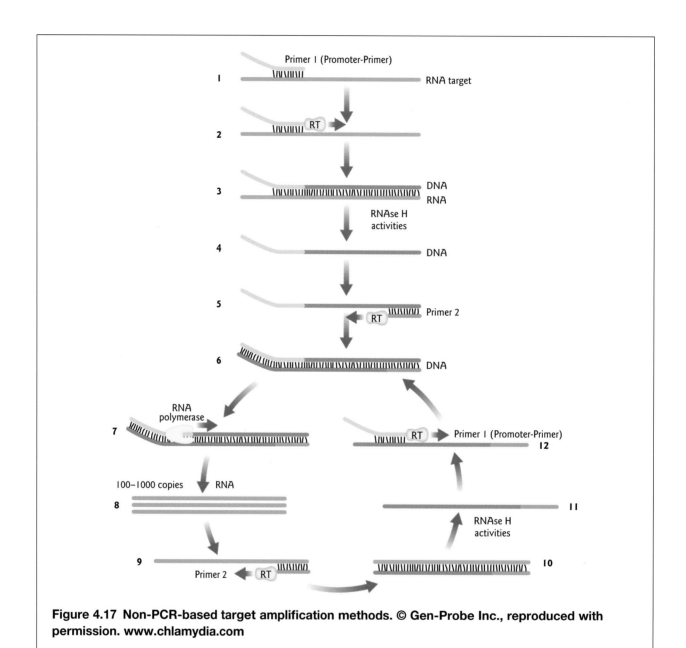

Figure 4.17 Non-PCR-based target amplification methods. © Gen-Probe Inc., reproduced with permission. www.chlamydia.com

Future developments in nucleic acid testing
Microarrays

Microarrays consist of arrays of single-stranded DNA oligonucleotide probes spotted onto specific locations on a small glass slide, membrane or coated quartz microchip surface. Tens of thousands of spots can be contained on one microarray. By extracting, amplifying and labeling nucleic acids from experimental samples, and then hybridizing those labeled nucleic acids to the array, the amount of label can be monitored at each spot, thereby indicating whether or not the complementary nucleic acid sequence was present in the original sample. At present, microarrays are a research tool rather than in routine laboratory usage, but in future it is likely that they will be developed for the simultaneous detection of multiples of infectious agents in individual patient samples. By detecting specific target sequences, not only should they be able to detect the presence of a specific pathogen but also to determine whether that pathogen demonstrates genotypic drug resistance (see below).

Automation in the clinical laboratory

Automated methods in the bacteriology laboratory will ultimately succeed if they are proficient at screening out the negative specimens and leaving the positive samples for further investigation by cultural methods. Blood cultures and urines submitted for culture are examples of large numbers of specific types of specimen that would benefit from such automated methods.

Automated, continuous monitoring blood culture systems involve the incubation of vials containing the patient's blood in a highly enriched nutrient medium, each bottle being monitored every 10–15 minutes depending upon the system used. The signal from each bottle (measured using either colorimetric or fluorimetric methods) is transmitted to the system's computer which analyzes and files positive readings. The system can be interrogated and growth curves can be examined and stored for future reference. Positives may be flagged as early as 2–4 hours after the initiation of incubation.

Urine analyzers also vary in type but the major consideration with these machines is the capability of handling large numbers of samples with a fast turn around time. The aim is to rapidly identify those samples that are negative for white cells and bacteria, leaving the scientist to investigate the likely positive samples more thoroughly. This same day reporting of negative urines has real advantages for the busy laboratory.

The different machines available use either particle counting, automated microscopy, adaptation of flow cytometry, or stained sediment analysis, and may express the result numerically or visually. Decisions as to which application to use are local and made on space and financial considerations.

Serological assays are highly amenable to automation. Several different biotechnology companies have developed random-access immunoassay autoanalysers that, preloaded with all the required reagents and controls, will perform a wide variety of different serological tests. The patient blood samples, barcoded for specific identification, are fed into the analyzer on a conveyer belt and the test(s) required for each sample are individually programd in. The test results data can be electronically downloaded into the Laboratory Information System so the opportunity for human error is truly minimized. These autoanalysers offer the possibility of very high throughput, rapid turnaround time, and processing that requires minimal technician time and almost no expertise.

With the use of highly sophisticated robotics, the component processes of molecular assays – extraction of nucleic acid, real time PCR reaction set-up, amplification, and detection – can also be automated. Thus, it is possible for a single machine to perform a specific diagnostic nucleic acid test on a patient sample and deliver the result without any technical expertise being required at all. Such "black boxes" may come into common use in the future, perhaps not only in diagnostic laboratories but also in physicians' offices to enable immediate "Point of Care" testing for common infections.

Tests for antimicrobial susceptibility

Bacterial (and some fungal) susceptibility and resistance to antimicrobial agents

There are few diseases where there is a single bacterial cause of the infection and it is always susceptible to a given antibiotic. The one exception to this is the susceptibility of *Streptococcus pyogenes* to penicillin.

The need for the laboratory control of antimicrobial therapy is a widely desirable target but unfortunately the practice falls short of the theory. The laboratory would normally aim to issue a susceptibility report within 24 hours of obtaining a pure culture of the organism under test. For those patients already on therapy the result will confirm the usefulness of the treatment or, if not, will suggest alternative agents for those patients where the therapy will be of no use due to resistance of the infecting organism.

Susceptibility testing of antibiotics in the laboratory is fraught with difficulty since many factors influence the result. These limiting factors include inoculum size of the test organism, the nature of the test medium, the pH of the medium, and the incubation time.

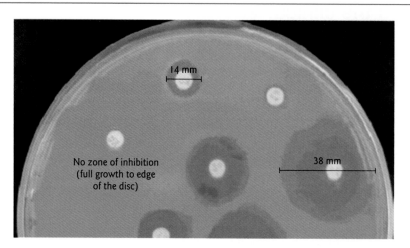

Figure 4.18 The Kirby-Bauer disc diffusion method of antibiotic susceptibility testing

Standardized disc diffusion methods are the goal aimed at by many laboratories and institutions and some are now in use in many laboratories but they vary from country to country and from method to method (e.g. CLSI, BSAC, or DIN methods see below). All manual methods are labor intensive. Commercially produced automated methods have been developed over the years to eliminate the labor element involved. Generally they work very well on fully susceptible organisms, but there are still some difficulties of interpretation when organisms with unusual sensitivity patterns occur. Vancomycin resistant enterococci (VRE) present particular difficulties with automated methods.

Manual disc methods

The most commonly utilized method of antibiotic susceptibility testing is the Kirby-Bauer Method using Mueller-Hinton agar (Figure 4.18). An inoculum giving semi-confluent growth of colonies after overnight incubation is used. An inoculum too dense will result in reduced zone diameters and one too light will have the reverse effect. The correct inoculum is generally achieved by comparison to a standard (called the McFarland standard) followed by an appropriate dilution. Discs impregnated with a standardized concentration of antibiotics are placed onto the lawn. Discs may be placed on the plate by hand or using a distribution device. Several antibiotics may be tested at once (one per disc). The antibiotic will diffuse into the agar of the plate where it interacts with the bacteria. After incubation, antibiotics that are effective will have areas around the disc where the lawn no longer grows. These areas are called "zones of inhibition." Measuring the diameter of the zone (in mm) in relation to the disc helps determine the amount of effectiveness that the antibiotic may provide. Appropriate control strains are set up each day to validate the test method. A standard table of antibiotics and measurements is used. There are three results: **susceptible (S), intermediate (I)**, or **resistant (R)**. Each tested organism is rated using these criteria. The Clinical and Laboratory Standards Institute (CLSI) for susceptibility testing has set up a list of guidelines that if followed should produce an accurate susceptibility response.

Manual minimum inhibitory concentrations (MIC) of antibiotic agents for a particular organism may be determined by using a commercial E-test (Figure 4.19). These consist of a plastic strip to which has been added an antibiotic in such a way as to provide a concentration gradient along the strip. The elliptical zone of growth that is obtained intersects the strip. The point of contact between the zone edge and the strip is read off as the MIC. E-tests may be used for both antibacterial and antifungal agents. They are a convenient method of obtaining an MIC very quickly but they are expensive. E-tests are available for a wide range of antibacterial agents and some antifungal agents.

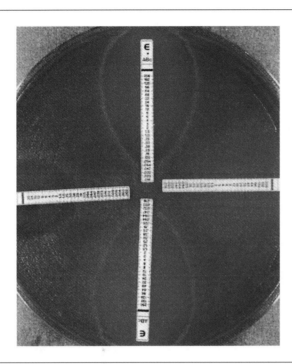

Figure 4.19 The E-test

Automated sensitivity methods

There are a number of automated sensitivity methods available for use. All work on a similar application whereby a standardized suspension is placed into a card pre-charged with set concentrations of antimicrobial agents. Incubation occurs after loading onto the machine and the growth rate measured in the control well by laser or light scatter. When sufficient growth has occurred in the control wells the other wells are scanned for growth. Reports are generated giving sensitive, resistant or intermediate results together with a predicted MIC based on a breakpoint calculation. Final results are generated by expert software.

Such methods have the advantage of speed (results can be available within 6 hours) and high throughput (up to 120 investigations in each run), but this has to be tempered by their expense and the fact that problems still exist with certain organism–antibiotic combinations such as enterococci and glycopeptides. Some of these methods will also provide identification cards but these will obviously double the expense.

The determination of viral susceptibility and resistance to antiviral agents

Many antiviral drugs are "designer drugs" targeted specifically to interfere with essential viral functions that differ significantly from or are not found within the host. Where antivirals have been developed and are extensively used – for HIV, hepatitis B, and influenza – there is always the potential that resistant mutants may arise, leading to limitation of the drug's usefulness. Determination of phenotypic resistance, by culturing virus in the presence of the drug, would be extremely labor intensive and slow. However, sequencing of the viral gene encoding the target of the drug is fairly readily undertaken with modern molecular technology and will demonstrate where the gene differs from the wild-type drug-sensitive sequence. Database information on the association of the particular mutations observed with phenotypic resistance *in vitro* and/or with treatment failure in patients can be used to infer the genotypic sensitivity or resistance of a particular patient's virus: particular mutations are consistently associated with resistance to specific drugs. For example, a mutation that results in a switch from methionine (ATG) to valine (GTG) at codon 184 in the HIV reverse transcriptase gene invariably causes high level resistance to lamivudine and a number of other nucleoside reverse transcriptase inhibitors. Genotypic resistance testing has become a vital component in the management of HIV infection.

Diagnosis of protozoal and helminth infections

The diagnosis of protozoal and helminthic infections will be considered separately to highlight important differences when compared to bacterial, fungal and virological diagnostic methods.

When considering a possible parasitic infection in a patient it is important that the clinician shares information such as the patient's symptoms and travel history with the diagnostic laboratory. This is to ensure that appropriate specimens are taken, handled correctly and pathogens present in that geographical region are looked for. In general protozoal and helminthic infections may be diagnosed by examining intestinal, blood or tissue specimens. Sputum, urine and vaginal specimens may also be important in specific situations. Culture is less important in diagnosis of protozoal and helminth infections; due to their complex lifecycles most are unable to grow in simple media. Specialist laboratories may provide limited culture for infections with organisms such as *Strongyloides stercoralis* and *Leishmania* spp. Serological and molecular diagnostic techniques are available in specialist laboratories. Antimicrobial testing is rarely available again because of culturing difficulties, however reference-based laboratories may provide services for organisms with important resistance patterns such as *Plasmodium falciparum*.

Intestinal specimens

Intestinal specimens include fecal, duodenal and sigmoidoscopy samples. Multiple fecal samples may be required as a single sample may not contain parasitic material due to irregular shedding of cysts or eggs by organisms. Fecal specimens should be examined macroscopically to reveal consistency, color and presence of visible components such as proglottids. Several procedures are used for the microscopic examination of stools, including direct wet mounts, concentration methods, and preparation of permanently stained smears. Direct wet saline mounts are particularly useful to detect the presence of motile protozoan trophozoites, protozoal cysts, and helminth eggs. Iodine may be added to saline to emphasize glycogen masses and nuclear material (Figure 4.20). Concentration techniques are designed to remove as much background debris as possible. Protozoal trophozoites cannot survive this process, although cysts, larvae and eggs do. Formalin-ether acetate-based kits are generally used by most laboratories for concentration purposes. Stained smears, such as the trichrome or iron-hematoxylin, are used to detect protozoan trophozoites and cysts. In a properly stained slide structures such as nuclear detail and internal organelles can be seen and used for identification purposes (Figure 4.21). Use of a modified acid-fast or fluorescent stain will enable detection of cysts of *Cryptosporidium parvum* and *Isospora belli* in particular.

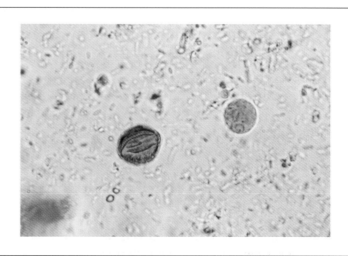

Figure 4.20 Direct wet saline mount showing *Entamoeba histolytica* cysts with addition iodine staining. From CDC website: http://www.dpd.cdc.gov/dpdx/HTML/

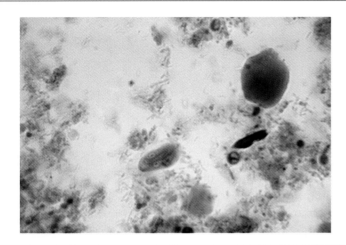

Figure 4.21 Trichrome stain of *Giardia lamblia* cyst. From CDC website: http://www.dpd.cdc.gov/dpdx/HTML/

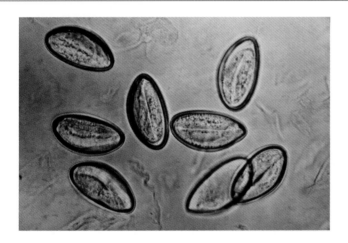

Figure 4.22 Eggs of the human parasite *Enterobius vermicularis*, or "human pinworm," captured on cellophane tape taken from the perianal region. From CDC website: http://www.dpd.cdc.gov/dpdx/HTML/

Duodenal aspirates specimens are especially useful in cases of suspected strongyloidiasis or giardiasis when stool examination has been negative. Specimens obtained by sigmoidoscopy may be used to diagnose amebiasis or cryptosporidiosis. Cellophane tape preparation is used for the diagnosis of *Enterobius vermicularis* infection as the lifecycle of the pinworm includes the female laying eggs in the perianal region. Cellophane tape is placed on the perianal region and then on a microscope slide and scanned at low power for the classical shaped eggs (Figure 4.22).

Blood specimens
Examination of blood smears that have been stained with a Giemsa- or Wright-based stain is the most common method of diagnosing *Plasmodium* sp., *Trypanosoma* sp., and many infections associated with microfilaria (Figure 4.23). Further information on taking, preparation and interpretation of thick and thin blood smears for malaria diagnosis are discussed in Chapter 17.

Biopsy specimens
Tissue specimens are usually required to diagnose *Leishmania* spp. infections as the organisms are intracellular. The tissue samples can be obtained from samples such as skin, liver, spleen, and bone marrow (Figure 4.24). Appropriate staining of biopsy samples can also be useful to diagnose other parasitic infections including schistosomiasis, strongyloidiasis, and toxoplasmosis.

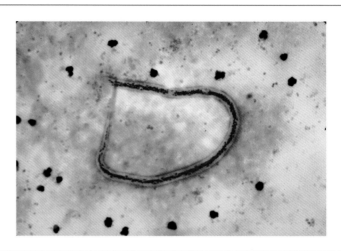

Figure 4.23 *Wuchereria bancrofti* microfilaria blood smear stained using Giemsa. From CDC website: http://www.dpd.cdc.gov/dpdx/HTML/

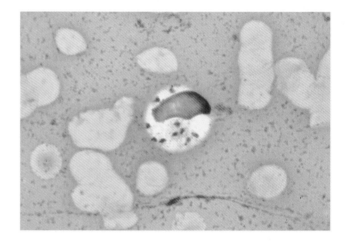

Figure 4.24 *Leishmaina donovani* in a bone marrow smear. From CDC website: http://www.dpd.cdc.gov/dpdx/HTML/

Other specimens

Sputum wet mounts can be examined for the presence of eggs from infections such as *Paragonimus westermani* and larvae from infections such as *Strongyloides stercoralis*. Urine investigation is the specimen of choice for diagnosing *Schistosoma haematobium* infection as characteristic eggs can be seen after filtering urine (Figure 4.25). Trophozoites of *Trichomonas vaginalis* and eggs of pinworm can also be visualized by examining urine, and *T. vaginalis* can be seen in vaginal or urethral discharge. Liver and other cyst aspiration and examination of contents is useful for the diagnosis of infections such as *Echinococcus granulosus* and *Entamoeba histolytica*. (See CDC website: http://www.dpd.cdc.gov/dpdx/HTML/.)

Immunological diagnosis

Serological methods are used far less commonly in the diagnosis of protozoal and helminth infections because of difficulties in obtaining antigen for assays and cross-reactivity between organisms. Routine commercial tests are available using ELISA- or FTA-based technology for the diagnosis of infections with organisms such as *Toxoplasma gondii* and extra-intestinal *E. histolytica*. Fluorescent antibody techniques using monoclonal antibodies are commonly used to detect *Cryptosporidium parvum* oocysts in feces and a commercial ELISA is available for the detection of *E. histolytica*. Specialized laboratories may also have in house assays for diagnosis of other infections including schistosomiasis, hydatid disease and strongyloidiasis.

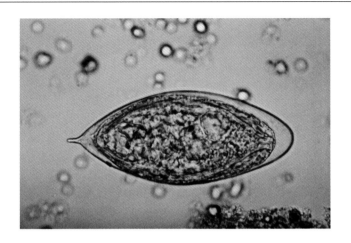

Figure 4.25 *Schistosoma haematobium* egg from filtered urine sample. From CDC website: http://www.dpd.cdc.gov/dpdx/HTML/

Molecular techniques

PCR has been introduced into most laboratories for the rapid diagnosis of malaria in patients. It is highly sensitive and can detect down to five parasites per microliter of blood; it has the advantage of being able to speciate easily as well. The disadvantage of using PCR for routine diagnosis of plasmodium infection is the expense of this technique. Other molecular methods have been introduced to reference laboratories according to local specialized expertise.

Other aspects of laboratory diagnosis

Assessing a new test

When any test is used to make a decision there is some probability of drawing an erroneous conclusion. This divides results into four categories:

- True positives (a + c)
- True negatives (b + d)
- False positives (b)
- False negatives (c).

		Gold Standard test	
		Positive	Negative
New test	Positive	a	b
	Negative	c	d

The **diagnostic sensitivity** of a new test is the proportion of true positives (as defined by a gold standard test) correctly identified by the new test. Sensitivity = a/a + c

The **diagnostic specificity** is the proportion of true negatives (as defined by a gold standard test) correctly identified by the new test. Specificity = d/b + d

The **positive predictive value (PPV)** of the new test is the proportion of individuals showing a positive result with the new test who actually have the disease. PPV = a/a + b

The **negative predictive value (NPV)** of the new test is the proportion of individuals showing a negative result with the new test who do not actually have the disease. NPV = d/c + d

Quality control and quality assurance

Quality control (QC) and quality assurance (QA) practices are now an essential part of the modern laboratory. QC involves the control of every step of the analysis of a patient's sample. This will include checks at all stages of the laboratory procedure from receipt of the sample to issue of the final laboratory report. The performance of culture media, stains, identification tests, and the performance of antibiotic sensitivity testing are controlled and monitored by the use of known positive and negative control materials. These materials may be known control organisms or clinical material, the results of which are already established.

Laboratories generally have an internal QC program which covers all aspects of an analysis and are also expected to take part in an external QA program run by an independent organization from the laboratory (e.g. the AAB system in the USA or the UKNEQAS system in the UK). Material of unknown content is sent to the laboratory every month to be analyzed and a full report issued within a certain time frame.

All of these stages make up the QA program which essentially ensures that every stage of the analytical process is controlled and that the analysis can be completed to an acceptable standard. QA programs will also include staff training programs, regular audits of performance, and an annual assessment of the laboratory's overall performance.

Test yourself

Case study 4.1
A surgical wound is infected, the wound is swabbed and sent to the laboratory.

? 1. Report on the Gram stain.

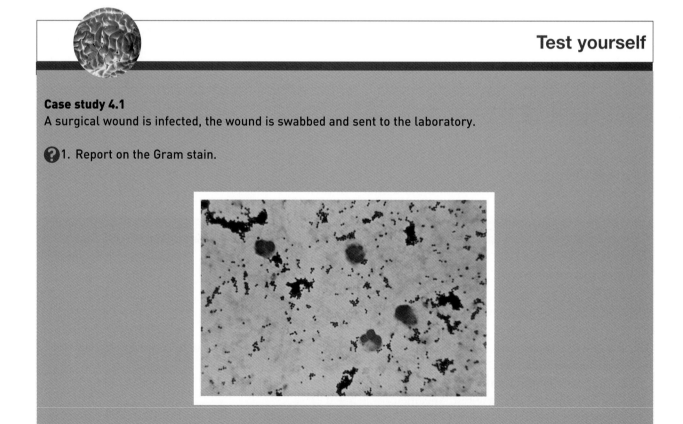

? 2. Culture on blood agar. Report your culture findings.

Test yourself

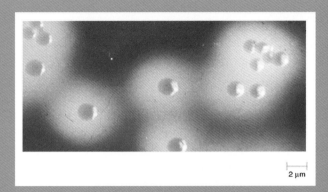

2 µm

Biochemical reactions: coagulase positive; DNAse positive.
Antibiotic susceptibility results: resistant to penicillin, erythromycin, oxacillin.

?3. Identify to genus and species level.

Case study 4.2
An 80-year-old man with cough, chest pain, and fever. Sputum is coughed into a sterile container and sent to the laboratory.

?1. Report on the Gram stain.

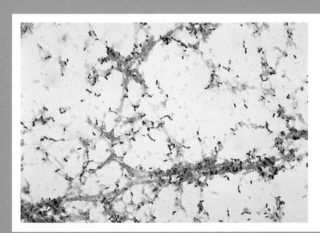

Courtesy: CDC/Dr. Mike Miller

?2. Blood agar. Report your culture findings.

Biochemical reactions: optochin sensitive; bile soluble.
Antibiotic susceptibility results: susceptible to penicillin.

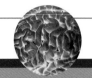

Test yourself

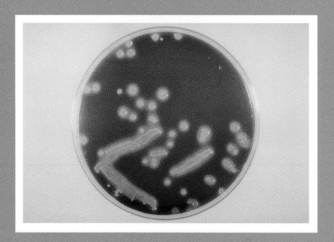

?3. Identify to genus and species level.

Case study 4.3
A 30-year-old woman complains of frequency and pain when passing urine. A midstream sample of urine is sent to the laboratory

?1. Report on the Gram stain.

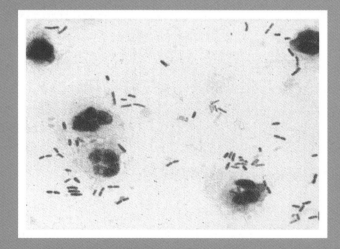

?2. Culture on MacConkey agar. Report your culture findings.

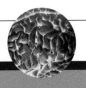

Test yourself

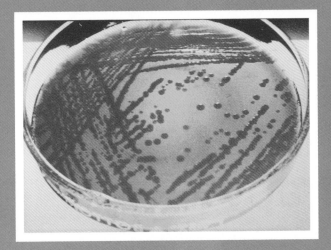

Biochemical reactions: spot indole positive; oxidase negative.
Antibiotic susceptibility: susceptible to cotrimoxazole, ciprofloxacin, resistant to amoxicillin.

3. Identify to genus and species level.

Further reading

de la Maza LM, Pezzlo MT, Shigei JT, Peterson EM. *Color Atlas of Medical Bacteriology*. New York: ASM Press, 2004

Dismukes WE, Pappas PG, Sobel JD (eds). *Clinical Mycology*. Oxford: Oxford University Press, 2003

Forbes BA, Sahm DF, Weissfeld AS. *Bailey and Scott's Diagnostic Microbiology*, 11th edition. St Louis, MO: Mosby, 2002

Mandell GL, Bennett JE, Dolin R. *Principles and Practice of Infectious Diseases*, 6th edition. Edinburgh: Elsevier/Churchill Livingstone, 2005

Murray PR, Baron EJ, Jorgenson EH, Faller MA, Yolken RH (eds). *Manual of Clinical Microbiology*, 8th edition. New York: ASM Press, 2003

O'Grady F, Lambert HP, Finch RG (eds). *Antibiotic and Chemotherapy*, 7th edition. New York: Churchill Livingstone, 1997

Ryan KJ, Ray CG. *Sherris Medical Microbiology, An Introduction to Infectious Disease*. New York: McGraw Hill, 2004

Stokes EJ, Ridgway GL, Wren MWD (eds). *Clinical Microbiology*, 7th edition. London: Edward Arnold, 1993

Chapter 5

General principles of antimicrobial chemotherapy

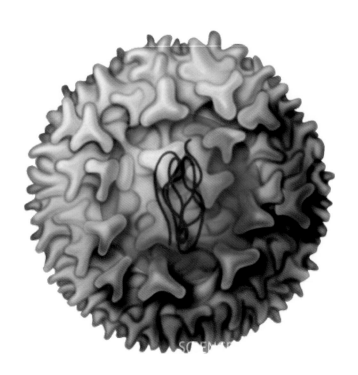

N. Shetty, E. Aarons, J. Andrews

What are antibiotics?
Mechanisms of antimicrobial resistance
The major classes of antibiotics
  β-lactams
  Glycopeptides
  Macrolides, lincosamides, and streptogramins
    (the MLS group)
  Other agents with narrow spectrum Gram
    positive activity
  Fluoroquinolones
  Aminoglycosides
  Miscellaneous antibiotics

Antifungal agents
Drugs for the treatment of protozoal and
helminth infections
  Antiprotozoal drugs
  Antihelminth medications
Antiviral drugs
  Drugs active against herpesviruses
  Anti-retroviral compounds (active against HIV
    and/or HBV)
  Anti-influenza virus compounds
  Drugs active against other viruses

The discovery of antibiotics has been hailed as one of the wonders of modern medicine; its use has had dramatic effects on the wider practise of all branches of medicine. From poultice administration and chicken soup the management of infection has advanced to a highly evolved and scientific "evidence-based" subject; forging an alliance between healthcare workers and industry in the pursuit of the randomized double blind controlled trial as the true gold standard. However, the subject has been fraught with media hype, myth, and frustration as the spectre of the untreatable organism looms as the harbinger of a latter day Armageddon (Figure 5.1).

As research and development into antibiotics has made unprecedented advances, so has the volume of information students are expected to assimilate before making rational decisions on antibiotic use. It is physically (and intellectually) impossible to grasp everything there is to know about antimicrobial agents, which is why a simple checklist of questions often helps to distil the essential features of a particular agent. These are listed in Box 5.1.

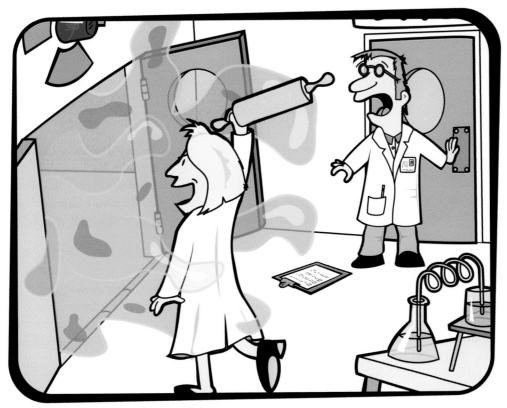

'What a breakthrough – we've bred the first germ we can attack with everyday household objects!'

Figure 5.1 The untreatable organism

Box 5.1 The checklist

✓ Mechanism of action
✓ Spectrum: is it active against Gram positive/Gram negative and/or anaerobic organisms?
✓ Route of administration: can it be administered oral/intravenous/other
✓ Dosing regimen: once, twice or three times a day; compliance becomes a serious issue when it is four times a day!
✓ Penetration: across the blood–brain barrier into the cerebrospinal fluid; bone and joint; intracellular

✓ Side-effects: allergic reactions; toxicity to the liver, kidney, bone marrow; can it be used in pregnancy, for children?
✓ Resistance: innate or acquired, how widespread geographically?
✓ Clinical uses: is it the drug of choice (alone or in combination) as recommended by American or other guidelines for the management of specific infectious diseases such as meningitis or community acquired pneumonia?
✓ Cost
✓ Mechanism of microbial resistance

Before a decision on antimicrobial choice is made, look at:

- Gram reaction of pathogens causing common community acquired infections ie are some infections caused largely by Gram positive /negative organisms; are others polymicrobial in origin (i.e. Gram positive + Gram negative+anaerobes)?
- Gram reaction of constituents of normal flora at various sites in the body; constituents of normal flora translocated to sterile sites can cause infection. For example, the mouth streptococci (Gram positive cocci) can be the cause of infective endocarditis when they flood the bloodstream.

Box 5.1 outlines the questions you demand answers to before you make any decisions. Conversely, if you know the answers to these questions then you know the essential features of the antibiotic! This checklist can be used for antiviral and antiparasitic agents as well. If you have a clinical situation you can use as a peg to hang your antibiotic on, you are more likely to remember its functions. Infectious disease case scenarios in the chapters that follow will deal with the broad clinical indications of antibiotics for specific infections.

What are antibiotics?

The first antibiotics were compounds, extracted from other microorganisms, that demonstrated anti-infective potential; they are therefore distinguished, by definition, from the synthetic anti-infective agents such as the sulphonamides. The classical example of an antibiotic is penicillin, which was originally extracted from the mold penicillium. Often the term antibiotic or antimicrobial is used loosely to include microbial and synthetic antimicrobial agents.

As antibiotic therapy evolved it became quite clear that an antibiotic was a true "magic bullet" if it could target microbial cellular constituents leaving the host cell unharmed – the very desirable quality of selective toxicity. It was therefore necessary to understand the mechanisms of action of antibiotics. This understanding, underpins many of the answers to the questions in Box 5.1, so here is where we start our discussion on antibiotics. Figure 5.2 illustrates the mechanisms of action of common antibacterial agents.

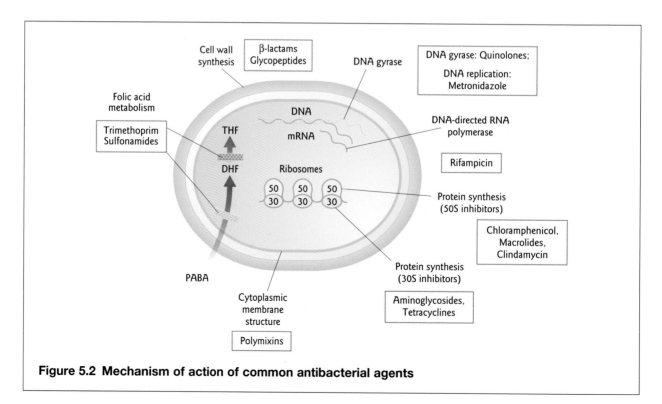

Figure 5.2 Mechanism of action of common antibacterial agents

When an agent achieves bacterial kill it is termed a **bactericidal agent**, if it merely stops multiplication allowing the organisms to be alive but dormant it is said to be a **bacteriostatic agent**. The "cidal" or "static" action of an agent is dependent on many factors other than the organism alone: it depends on dose, site of infection, and underlying disease to name just a few.

Mechanisms of antimicrobial resistance

How do microbes escape the action of antimicrobial agents and become resistant?

Most **Gram positive** organisms escape antibiotic action by utilizing one or both of the underlying mechanisms:

1 Enzymatic inactivation. Gram positive organisms such as the staphylococci produce **β-lactamase** which inactivates the β-lactam family of drugs (e.g. penicillin) by cleaving the β-lactam ring (Figure 5.3).

2 Altered target site. β-lactamase stable antibiotics are designed to block enzymatic access to the β-lactam ring. Some Gram positive organisms, notably staphylococci, have evolved secondary mechanisms to mediate resistance.

Resistance to semisynthetic penicillins (methicillin and other β-lactamase stable antibiotics) is mediated by the synthesis of novel penicillin binding protein (PBP 2a) by bacteria, these have reduced affinity for methicillin. Since methicillin cannot bind, it is unable to act on the cell wall.

Gram positive organisms have a peptide chain attached to the *N*-acetyl muramic acid of peptidoglycan; it consists of the amino acids L-alanine, D-glutamine, L-lysine, and one or two D-alanines (see Figure 2.2a). Vancomycin has high affinity to D-Ala-D-Ala pentapeptide side chain leading to inhibition of cell wall synthesis. Vancomycin-resistant bacteria, due to a mutation, express an altered target, i.e. D-Ala-D-lactate, so that there is low affinity binding to vancomycin, allowing cell-wall synthesis to proceed. Genes for vancomycin resistance are coded on a plasmid and are liable to spread by conjugation and transposition (see Chapter 3).

Gram negative organisms have evolved three important mechanisms that mediate antimicrobial resistance.

1 Permeability barriers. Penicillin is not effective against Gram negative bacteria because it cannot penetrate its outer membrane to reach its target site on the peptidoglycan. Gram negative bacteria have outer membrane pore proteins called porins which allow passage of nutrients and other molecules into the cytosol of the cell. Porin mutations may confer resistance against the extended spectrum penicillins and carbapenems because they use specific porins in the membrane to gain entrance into the cell. This type of "impermeability" may act alone or in combination with other resistance mechanisms.

2 Efflux pumps. Antibiotic efflux pumps that pump out antibiotic as quickly as it comes in have been seen in many Gram negative (and some Gram positive) bacteria. The bacterium produces transporter molecules in the cytoplasmic membrane capable of an energy-driven efflux that pumps the antibiotic back out of the bacterium.

Table 5.1 Gram positive and Gram negative β-lactamases

Gram positive β-lactamase	Gram negative β-lactamase
Primarily found in staphylococci	Found in many Gram negative species with large spectrum of activity
Secreted into the extracellular space	Secreted into the periplasmic space
Plasmid-mediated	Chromosomal or plasmid mediated; extended spectrum β-lactamases (ESBLs); are also cephalosporinases – point mutation extends spectrum dramatically. When transferred by conjugative plasmids, large outbreaks have occurred

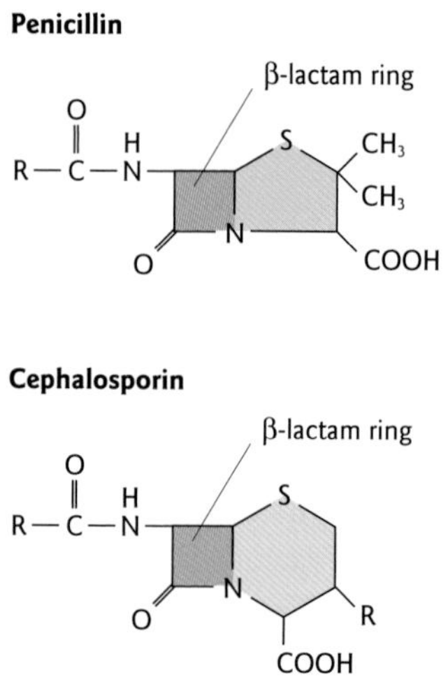

Figure 5.3 Basic structure of the β-lactam antibiotic

3 Enzymatic degradation. A huge complement of plasmid and chromosomally encoded conventional and extended spectrum β-lactamases (ESBLs) play an important part in mediating Gram negative resistance to β-lactam drugs. Table 5.1 describes the main differences between Gram positive and Gram negative β-lactamases. The extended spectrum β-lactamases described in Table 5.1 also inactivate the cephalosporins and are sometimes called cephalosporinases.

The major classes of antibiotics

β-lactams

The β-lactams are so called because of their common β-lactam ring structure (Figure 5.3). These include penicillins and β-lactamase inhibitor combinations, carbapenems, cephalosporins, and monobactams.

(a) Penicillins

Penicillins are classified according to their spectrum of activity (Table 5.2). Progression towards the carbapenems is characterized by increasing Gram negative (including antipseudomonal) activity.

Mechanism of action; mechanism of resistance

The penicillins are prototype β-lactam antibiotics that act by inhibiting bacterial cell wall synthesis. Peptidoglycan is a major component of the bacterial cell wall: layers of peptide chains comprising alternating molecules of N-acetylglucosamine and N-acetylmuramic acid are cross-linked by smaller peptides to form a rigid meshwork. Cross-linking is catalyzed by enzymes (trans-, carboxy- and endopeptidases) which are collectively named the penicillin binding proteins (PBPs) because these proteins are also binding sites for the penicillins. Penicillins act by interrupting cross-linkages (transpeptidation) that stabilize the peptidoglycan matrix within the cell wall of the bacterium (see Figure 2.3). There are at least seven penicillin binding proteins, and the various penicillins have different affinities for each of the PBPs. Because penicillins inhibit cell wall synthesis they are most effective on rapidly multiplying cells, a phase during which most of the cell wall proteins are synthesized.

Mere inhibition of cell wall synthesis does not account for the rapid lethality of penicillins on bacterial cells. Important mediators of cell death after exposure to a β-lactam are the endogenous autolysins. Bacterial

Table 5.2 Classification of penicillins

β-lactamase susceptible narrow spectrum penicillins	β-lactamase resistant penicillins	β-lactamase susceptible broad spectrum penicillins	Penicillins with β-lactamase inhibitors	β-lactamase susceptible extended spectrum penicillins (anti-pseudomonal activity)	Carbapenems
Penicillin V Penicillin G	Flucloxacillin Oxacillin★ Methicillin★ Nafcillin	Ampicillin Amoxicillin	Amoxicillin + clavulanic acid Ampicillin + sulbactam Piperacillin + tazobactam (anti-pseudomonal)	Carbenicillin Ticarcillin Azlocillin Piperacillin	Imipenem Meropenem Ertapenem (not an anti-pseudomonal)

As the generations escalate there is increasing activity against various Gram negative bacteria, including the pseudomonads; Gram positive activity remains static

★ Not used clinically

cells contain enzymes that synthesize peptidoglycan and autolysins that help break it down. Penicillins appear to upset this delicate control of cell wall synthesis by autolysins, leading to excessive autolysis and cell death. Organisms that lack endogenous autolysins are inhibited by penicillin but not killed by it – a phenomenon called tolerance. Penicillin tolerance has been described in many bacterial species, including *Streptococcus pneumoniae* and *Staphylococcus aureus*.

Resistance is mediated by enzymatic inactivation (coded for by genes carried on transposons or plasmids) and by altered PBPs (both chromosomal and plasmid mediated).

Oral penicillin V (phenoxymethyl penicillin)

Penicillin V is a narrow spectrum Gram positive agent that is stable in the acid pH of the stomach and is readily absorbed from the gastrointestinal tract. After oral administration peak serum levels are obtained within half and hour to one hour. There is considerable variation in the oral absorption of penicillin from patient to patient, for reasons unexplained. Patients with malabsorbtion syndromes do not absorb the drug very well. Peak serum levels are three times higher if the dose is taken an hour before food rather than after. Interstitial tissue distribution of the drug is poor because it is extensively protein bound, however it readily diffuses into pleural, pericardial and ascitic fluid and passes into fetal circulation. There is very little penetration into the CSF if the meninges are uninflammed and poor penetration into maxillary sinus secretions.

Penicillin G

Penicillin G is available as an injectable drug either as highly soluble sodium or potassium salts (benzyl or crystalline penicillin), or the less soluble procaine and benzathine penicillins, the latter two are long acting or depot preparations. Penicillin G is destroyed by acid in the stomach and is therefore given parenterally, the soluble salts can be given intravenously. High serum levels are achieved soon after parenteral administration, and the drug diffuses readily into body fluids and inflamed tissues. The drug readily penetrates the inflamed meninges; however penetration into uninflammed tissues and human polymorphonuclear leukocytes is poor. The drug crosses the placenta and produces adequate concentrations in the fetus and the amniotic fluid.

About 20–40% of the dose (penicillin V and G) is excreted unchanged in the urine during the first 6 hours. This urinary excretion of most penicillins can be partially blocked by probenecid. Very small amounts of these agents are excreted in the bile.

β-lactamase resistant penicillins

Methicillin, oxacillin, nafcillin, and flucloxacillin are some examples of β-lactamase resistant penicillins. Methicillin and oxacillin have been replaced by the latter two for clinical use because of issues of tolerability. Nafcillin is the preferred drug in the USA and has become the drug of choice for a variety of soft tissue infections. Nafcillin can be administered both orally and parenterally. It penetrates well in pus and bone in patients with soft tissue, bone and joint infections. It crosses the placenta and is excreted in breast milk. Its penetration into normal CSF, vitreous humor and polymorphonuclear leukocytes is poor, though penetration across the inflamed meninges is thought to be adequate.

These penicillins are mainly excreted in the urine and to a lesser extent by the biliary tract.

β-lactamase susceptible broad spectrum penicillins

The earliest drugs in this group to become therapeutically useful were ampicillin followed by amoxicillin. Both agents have a broader range of activity compared to the earlier penicillins, being active against Gram positive and negative organisms. They can be administered orally and parenterally. Absorption of amoxicillin by the oral route is considerably more efficient as compared to ampicillin. Both drugs can also be administered parenterally and adequate tissue levels are attained throughout the body. Like the other penicillins penetration into CSF is adequate only if the meninges are inflamed. Both agents cross the placenta and reach therapeutic concentrations in the amniotic fluid and fetal tissues.

Amoxicillin and ampicillin are excreted by the kidney and additionally they can be detected unchanged in the bile at concentrations that are therapeutic for many susceptible organisms.

Extended spectrum penicillins

Earlier agents such as carbenicillin and ticarcillin have now been replaced by broad spectrum acylaminopenicillins such as azlocillin and piperacillin. These agents have added antipseudomomal activity; they can only be administered parenterally. Tissue distribution and excretion of these drugs is similar to ampicillin and amoxicillin.

Penicillin β-lactamase inhibitor combinations

Clavulanic acid, sulbactam, and tazobactam are β-lactam compounds that have little intrinsic antibacterial activity. They function by binding irreversibly to and inactivating β-lactamases produced by a variety of bacteria. They are sometimes called "suicide" β-lactams. Clavulanic acid with amoxicillin is available as an oral and parenteral agent, ampicillin-sulbactam and piperacillin-tazobactam are available in parenteral formulations only. In addition they have considerable anti-anaerobic activity and piperacillin-tazobactam, because of piperacillin action, is also a potent antipseudomonal drug.

Tissue distribution and excretion of these compounds are similar to those described for the extended spectrum penicillins, penetration into CSF is poor.

Carbapenems

Like other β-lactam antibiotics, carbapenems are bactericidal and act by inhibiting cell wall synthesis. Imipenem and meropenem possess extensive Gram negative (including *Pseudomonas* spp.) and Gram positive (except MRSA) activity and potent anti-anaerobic effects. Three properties account for the extraordinarily broad antibacterial properties of the carbapenems: ease with which they penetrate bacterial cell walls, a high affinity for PBP 2, a protein essential for cell wall stability, and resistance to hydrolysis by most β-lactamases. Two compounds currently available for use are characterized by their antipseudomonal activity: imipenem co-administered with cilastatin which inhibits renal degradation of the drug and the preferred single agent, meropenem, which does not suffer this disadvantage. Both drugs are given parenterally and are widely distributed in body fluids, meropenem has better penetration into the CSF.

The third and more recent carbapenem, ertapenem, is distinguished by the complete absence of activity against pseudomonads and *Acinetobacter* spp. Its main role in therapy is for the treatment of infections caused by ESBL producing Enterobacteriaceae. Recently newer carbapenems such as doripenem are available for use. Minor differences exist when compared with entapenem.

Excretion is primarily through the kidneys and they penetrate readily into amniotic fluid and fetal tissues.

Side-effects and tolerability

The most important side-effects, common to all the penicillins, relate to hypersensitivity and rarely anaphylaxis. Most often it is a delayed reaction characterized by maculopapular eruptions, fever, or both; eosinophilia may also be present. Immune complexes can produce serum sickness and antibodies to β-lactam antibiotics can cause hemolytic anemia. Many patients with vague histories of penicillin allergies are not truly hypersensitive. A careful history is the best way to establish true drug allergy. A recollection of rash, urticaria, arthralgias, wheezing, or anaphylaxis confirms the diagnosis of hypersensitivity, whereas treatment failure, diarrhea, vaginitis, other superinfections, and other vague symptoms do not. Skin tests have a limited role in predicting true penicillin allergy and may even be dangerous. Patients who are allergic to one penicillin should be considered allergic to all penicillins including carbapenems. This generalization may not be true for some children who contract infectious mononucleosis and develop a rash after taking ampicillin or amoxicillin. Why this happens is not clear, the rash does not indicate allergy to penicillin, if unrecognized the patient is greatly disadvantaged by an incorrect "allergic to penicillin" label. Empiric treatment in cases of doubt should therefore involve prescription of an alternative oral penicillin such as penicillin V. Patients who are allergic to penicillin have a 10–12% likelihood of having an allergic reaction to a cephalosporin antibiotic. All cephalosporins are best avoided in patients who give a history of severe hypersensitivity to penicillin. Apart from the risk of hypersensitivity reactions, penicillins have a wide safety margin and can be prescribed in pregnancy.

Penicillin G is conjugated with sodium or potassium salts to form a soluble substance and cation intoxication is a rare possibility with massive doses of these salts. Very high levels of penicillin G in the CSF could cause convulsions. Imipenem but not meropenem is also known to be associated with epileptiform convulsions.

The orally administered penicillins are associated with transient bouts of nausea and diarrhea and all penicillins carry the risk of causing antibiotic associated colitis.

If the number and range of penicillins completely confound you, construct your own profiles for the penicillins you encounter most often. Box 5.2 is a profile constructed for amoxicillin.

Box 5.2 Profile a penicillin

Using the checklist in Box 5.1 construct a profile for amoxicillin:

✓ Mechanism of action: *inhibit peptidoglycan or cell wall synthesis; enhance autolysins*
✓ Spectrum: *Gram positive and Gram negative; no anti-anaerobic action*
✓ Route of administration: *oral and IV*
✓ Dosing regimen: *three times a day*
✓ Penetration: *penetrates most tissues including into the CSF in meningitis*
✓ Side-effects: *rule out penicillin allergy; safe in pregnancy and in children*

✓ Resistance: *over 80% of staphylococci are resistant; S. pneumoniae resistance in the USA, Spain; gonococcal resistance worldwide*
✓ Clinical uses: *drug of choice for listeria, streptococcal disease except when used empirically for a sore throat (see interaction between amoxicillin and infectious mononucleosis in text)*
✓ Cost: *inexpensive*
✓ Mechanism of microbial resistance: *production of β-lactamase and alteration of penicillin binding proteins*

Table 5.3 Classification of cephalosporins

First generation	Second generation	Third generation	Fourth generation
Cephalexin (prototype of this generation) Cephalothin Cefazolin Cefadroxil	Cefuroxime (prototype of this generation) Cefotetan Cefomandole	Cefotaxime Ceftriaxone Ceftazidime – anti *Pseudomonas aeruginosa*	Cefipime

As the generations escalate there is increasing activity against various Gram negative bacteria, Gram positive activity remains static

→

(b) Cephalosporins

The first member of this the second series of β-lactams was isolated in 1956 from extracts of *Cephalosporium acremonium*, a sewer fungus. Like the penicillins, cephalosporins are classified, according to increasing spectrum of activity, into generations (Table 5.3). A few important examples in each of the cephalosporin classes are listed in Table 5.3. Too many cephalosporins exist all beginning with "ceph/cef. . .". It becomes humanly impossible to remember and recall the finer differences between this bewildering group of antibiotics. We advise students to choose the ones they use in their practice and study them using the checklist in Box 5.1. See Box 5.3 for an example of the clinical use of a cephalosporin.

Cephalosporins being β-lactam drugs have a similar mode of action to penicillins.

In general many gut-associated anaerobes are not susceptible to cephalosporins. They have no activity against methicillin resistant *S. aureus*. High concentrations can be recovered from the urine within a few hours after the first dose. Cephalosporins, like penicillins, have been used in pregnancy without any apparent evidence of fetal damage. All cephalosporins have been implicated in *Clostridium difficile* colitis and in the emergence of serious infections with enterococci.

Box 5.3 Which cephalosporin do I use?

A young woman comes into the emergency department and is diagnosed clinically with possible acute meningitis. As pharmacologist you are asked to advise on the suitability of ceftriaxone.

Using the checklist in Box 5.1 let us construct a profile for ceftriaxone:

✓ Mechanism of action: *inhibit peptidoglycan or cell wall synthesis; enhance autolysins*
✓ Spectrum: *Gram positive and Gram negative; no anti-anaerobic action; will cover meningococcus, pneumococcus, and Haemophilus influenzae – the commonest causes of acute bacterial meningitis*
✓ Route of administration: *available IV*
✓ Dosing regimen: *once a day*

✓ Penetration: *excellent penetration into the CSF in meningitis*
✓ Side-effects: *rule out penicillin allergy, safe in pregnancy*
✓ Resistance: *not a particular issue for the meningococcus or H. influenzae, concerns about resistance in the pneumococcus*
✓ Clinical uses: *drug of choice for empiric management of meningitis (may be combined with other agents to counter pneumococcal resistance)*
✓ Cost: *expensive*
✓ Mechanism of microbial resistance: *alteration of penicillin binding proteins*

Ceftriaxone is the most suitable cephalosporin

First generation cephalosporins

Agents belonging to this generation have a spectrum similar to that of amoxicillin with some resistance to the Gram positive β-lactamases. However, their activity against staphylococci is unpredictable and none of the cephalosporins are active against methicillin resistant strains. They are active against susceptible streptococci causing upper respiratory tract infections but have no useful activity against the *Neisseria*, *Haemophilus*, or *Corynebacterium* species. Most are only available orally, some agents, such as cefazolin, can be administered parenterally.

They are active against a range of enterobacteria causing urinary tract infections, including some amoxicillin resistant *Escherichia coli*, though they are degraded by many enterobacterial β-lactamases. They have been used successfully to treat urinary tract infections in pregnancy. Gram negative organisms commonly encountered in the hospital environment such as *Citrobacter*, *Enterobacter*, indole-positive *Proteus*, and *Serratia* species are all resistant to first generation cephalosporins.

Second generation cephalosporins

Cefuroxime is the prototype second generation cephalosporin. Although available in oral formulation, it has much better tissue penetration when given parenterally. Much of the description of first generation cephalosporins is applicable to cefuroxime, however being up a generation it has *in vitro* activity against a wider range of Gram positive bacteria (including *S. pneumoniae*, *S. pyogenes*, and *S. aureus*); and many of the enteric Gram negative organisms responsible for upper and lower urinary tract infections; it is stable in the presence of β-lactamases of Gram positive and certain Gram negative bacteria. Activity against *Haemophilus influenzae* (including amoxicillin resistant strains) and *Neisseria gonorrhoeae* (including penicillinase producing strains) have made it a contender for the treatment of these infections.

Cefuroxime is excreted by the kidneys over an 8 hour period, resulting in high urinary concentrations. Tissue penetration into sputum, pleural fluid, bone, joint fluid, and bile is adequate; however other cephalosporins have replaced cefuroxime for the management of meningitis. Cefoxitin (classed as a cephamycin, because it was originally extracted from a *Streptomyces* spp.) is the only one that has anaerobic activity.

Many hospital acquired Gram negative infections with *Morganella morganii*, *Enterobacter cloacae*, *Citrobacter* spp., *Pseudomonas*, *Acinetobacter* spp., most strains of *Serratia* spp., and *Proteus vulgaris* are resistant to most first and second generation cephalosporins.

Third generation cephalosporins

The third generation cephalosporins are characterized by three clinically important features:

* Increased activity against *E. coli*, *Klebsiella* spp., indole-positive *Proteus*, and *Enterobacter* spp.
* Activity against *P. aeruginosa*
* High concentrations in the CSF.

Ceftazidime is the only antipseudomonal cephalosporin and is resistant to a wide variety of entero β-lactamases. However, it is degraded by the extended spectrum β-lactamases. Cefotaxime and ceftriaxone, though not antipseudomonal, are valuable as first line agents for the empiric management of meningitis as they are found in high concentrations in the CSF. Ceftriaxone has a long half life and is amenable to once a day dosing. It is also used widely for multiply resistant *N. gonorrhoeae* infections.

Fourth generation cephalosporins

Cefepime is an injectable fourth generation cephalosporin that has a broader spectrum of antibacterial activity than the third generation cephalosporins and is more active *in vitro* against Gram positive aerobic bacteria (except MRSA). The fact that cefepime is stable to hydrolysis by many of the common plasmid and chromosomally mediated β-lactamases, and that it is a poor inducer of chromosomally mediated β-lactamases, indicates that cefepime may be useful for treatment of Gram negative infections resistant to earlier cephalosporins. Cefepime also has activity against *Pseudomonas* spp.

Monobactams

Aztreonam, the first marketed monobactam, has activity against most aerobic Gram negative bacilli including *P. aeruginosa*. It is not active against Gram positive or anaerobic organisms. The drug is not nephrotoxic, is weakly immunogenic, and has not been associated with disorders of coagulation. Its major advantage is that it is structurally different from older β-lactams and possesses different adverse drug reaction profiles. Cross-hypersensitivity between aztreonam and other β-lactams is rare, which makes the drug a useful therapeutic alternative in those allergic to penicillin. However, hypersensitivity to aztreonam does occur.

Aztreonam may be administered intramuscularly or intravenously; the primary route of elimination is urinary excretion. Patients with renal impairment require dosage adjustment. Aztreonam is used primarily as an alternative to aminoglycosides and for the treatment of aerobic Gram negative infections. It is often used in combination therapy for mixed aerobic and anaerobic infections. Approved indications for its use include infections of the urinary tract or lower respiratory tract, intra-abdominal and gynecologic infections, septicemia, and cutaneous infections caused by susceptible organisms. Concurrent initial therapy with other antimicrobial agents is recommended in patients who are seriously ill or at risk for Gram positive or anaerobic infection.

Glycopeptides

Glycopeptides are a class of narrow spectrum (act against Gram positive organisms only) antibacterial agents derived from the organism *Streptomyces* spp. Two glycopeptides are used in the treatment of infections: vancomycin and teicoplanin.

Older preparations of vancomycin were referred to as "Mississippi Mud," alluding to their origins from soil microorganisms. These preparations were more toxic because of the various impurities; newer agents are less impure and consequently less toxic.

Mechanism of action; mechanism of resistance

These agents act by inhibiting cell wall synthesis, at a different site to that of β-lactams. Gram positive organisms have a peptide chain attached to the *N*-acetyl muramic acid of peptidoglycan; it consists of the amino acids L-alanine, D-glutamine, L-lysine, and one or two D-alanines (see Figure 2.2a). Glycopeptides have high affinity for the D-Ala-D-Ala pentapeptide side chain. Binding at this site, they inhibit the action of transglycosidase and transpeptidases, the enzymes that cross-link chains of peptidoglycan building blocks into the rigid mesh that forms the cell wall.

Vancomycin-resistant bacteria contain mutations that have resulted in the altered D-Ala-D-lactate target site, so that there is low affinity binding to vancomycin thereby allowing for cell wall synthesis. Genes for vancomycin resistance are coded on a plasmid and are liable to spread by conjugation and transposition (see Chapter 2).

Route of administration

Vancomycin can only be given intravenously. If given orally, it is not absorbed systemically and so has been used to treat some infections that are limited to the gastrointestinal tract, i.e. *C. difficile* causing antibiotic associated colitis. Teicoplanin can be given intravenously or intramuscularly.

Side-effects and tolerability

Glycopeptides are potentially toxic to the kidneys (similar to the aminoglycosides). If the drug is infused too rapidly, a reaction known as "red man syndrome" may occur; this manifests with severe flushing of the face and neck, and possibly itching and a drop in blood pressure, and occurs because of increased histamine release. Glycopeptide allergy has also been documented. Teicoplanin is not nephrotoxic.

Clinical uses

Glycopeptides are expensive and potentially toxic; they are really only used for severe infections, or for infections with organisms that are resistant to other antibiotics. They are also sometimes used if a patient is allergic to penicillin. Infections with methicillin resistant *S. aureus* (MRSA), some enterococcal species, and prosthetic and intravascular catheter infections caused by coagulase negative staphylococci are some examples where glycopeptide usage is justified. Penetration into the CSF is poor. However, given in high doses, vancomycin is used for the treatment of bacterial meningitis due to penicillin and cephalosporin resistant *S. pneumoniae*.

Macrolides, lincosamides, and streptogramins (the MLS group)

Macrolides, lincosamides, and streptogramins belong to the MLS group of antibiotics (Table 5.4) because they share similar binding sites on the bacterial cell and hence similar modes of action.

Mechanism of action; mechanism of resistance
The MLS group of antibiotics act by inhibiting protein synthesis (Figure 5.4). They bind to the 50S subunit of the ribosome and prevent its movement along m-RNA. Resistant organisms have a modified target binding site, as a result the drug fails to bind. This is common to all macrolides, lincosmides, and streptogramins (MLS group), organisms thus resistant to one drug in the group display cross-resistance to others. In addition, macrolides, streptogramins, lincosamides, and chloramphenicol have antagonistic pharmacological action as their mode of action is similar.

Macrolides are products of actinomycetes (soil bacteria) or semi-synthetic derivatives of them. Erythromycin, the first orally effective macrolide, was discovered in 1952 in the metabolic products of a strain of *Streptomyces erythreus*, originally obtained from a soil sample. They are bacteriostatic except at high concentrations. Quinupristin-dalfopristin is a synergistic bactericidal combination of two streptogramins. Both are water-soluble derivatives of streptogramins produced by *Streptomyces pistinaespiralis*.

Route of administration
Erythromycin is available in oral and intravenous formulations; the oral is preferred as intravenous preparations cause severe thrombophlebitis. Clarithromycin and azithromycin are tolerated orally and parenterally as is the lincosamide, clindamycin. Clarithromycin has a half-life in serum of 4.7 hours (three times that of erythromycin), and azithromycin has a much longer half-life (several days).

Quinupristin-dalfopristin is an intravenous drug only.

Side-effects and tolerability
Erythromycin commonly causes dose-related gastrointestinal (GI) tract disturbances, including nausea, vomiting, and diarrhea. These adverse effects are less common with clarithromycin and azithromycin. Clindamycin can cause antibiotic associated colitis (caused by *C. difficile*), which can be severe.

Clinical uses
After oral or parenteral administration, these drugs diffuse well into body fluids, except CSF. Excretion is mainly in the bile, and dose adjustments are not required when renal failure is present.

A macrolide is the drug of choice in *Mycoplasma pneumoniae* and *Legionella* infection, in *Corynebaterium diphtheriae* carriers, and in *Bordetella pertussis*. Severe *Campylobacter* enteritis is also treated with erythromycin.

Erythromycin is active against Gram positive cocci (including anaerobes), with the exception of enterococci; but many *S. aureus* strains are now resistant and it should not be used in serious

Table 5.4 Drugs in the MLS group of antibiotics

Macrolides	Lincosamides	Streptogrammins
Erythromycin Clarithromycin Azithromycin	Clindamycin	Quinupristin-dalfopristin

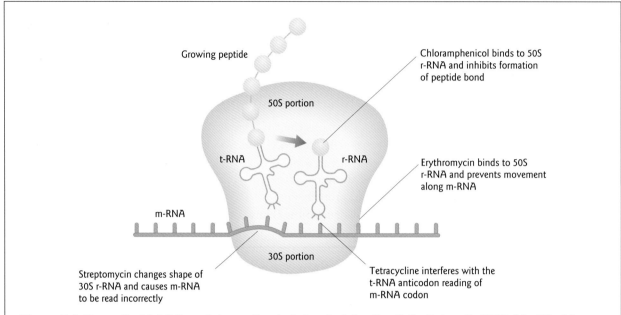

Growing peptide

Chloramphenicol binds to 50S
r-RNA and inhibits formation
of peptide bond

50S portion

t-RNA

r-RNA

Erythromycin binds to 50S
r-RNA and prevents movement
along m-RNA

m-RNA

30S portion

Streptomycin changes shape of
30S r-RNA and causes m-RNA
to be read incorrectly

Tetracycline interferes with the
t-RNA anticodon reading of
m-RNA codon

Figure 5.4 Drugs that inhibit protein synthesis in bacterial cells. © C. Ophardt, 2003. Modified from http://elmhurst.edu/%7Echm/vchembooks/654antibiotic.html

S. aureus infection. It is, however, commonly used as an alternative in penicillin allergic individuals for the treatment of staphylococcal and streptococcal infections in general practice. It is also used as an alternative to the tetracyclines for the treatment of chlamydial infections in pregnancy and in children. Because of GI intolerance to erythromycin, clarithromycin and azithromycin are often used as substitutes, although they are much more expensive. Clarithromycin and azithromycin have an antibacterial spectrum similar to that of erythromycin. In addition, they have enhanced activity against *H. influenzae* and activity against *Mycobacterium avium-intracellulare*. Clarithromycin is used in combination with other drugs for the treatment of *H. pylori* infections. Azithromycin is used in a single dose for *Chlamydia trachomatis* urethritis and cervicitis.

Clindamycin has a spectrum similar to that of erythromycin, except that it has poor activity against some *Mycoplasma* spp. The major advantage of clindamycin over erythromycin is the much greater activity against anaerobic bacteria, especially *Bacteroides* spp. (including *B. fragilis*). It is useful for serious respiratory tract infections such as empyema, aspiration pneumonitis, and lung abscess; serious skin and soft tissue infections; intra-abdominal abscess (typically resulting from anaerobic organisms resident in the normal GI tract); infections of the female pelvis and genital tract such as endometritis, nongonococcal tubo-ovarian abscess, pelvic cellulitis, and postsurgical vaginal cuff infection. It also has activity against toxoplasma and pneumocystis when used in combination with other drugs. Clindamycin penetrates well into bone and joint cavities and also into large abscesses. Clindamycin cannot be used in central nervous system infections because penetration into the brain and CSF is poor.

Quinupristin-dalfopristin is active against most Gram positive bacteria. Its clinical usefulness relates to the treatment of MRSA, penicillin resistant pneumococci, *Enterococcus faecium* infections including strains which are resistant to ampicillin and vancomycin. However, it is not active against *Enterococcus faecalis*.

Other agents with narrow spectrum Gram positive activity

Linezolid

Mechanism of action; mechanism of resistance
Linezolid is a synthetic antibiotic belonging to a new class of antimicrobials called the oxazolidinones. Linezolid disrupts bacterial growth by inhibiting the initiation process in protein synthesis. This site of inhibition

occurs earlier in the initiation process than in other protein synthesis inhibitors (e.g. chloramphenicol, clindamycin, aminoglycosides, and macrolides) that interfere with the elongation process. Because the site of inhibition is unique to linezolid, cross-resistance to other protein synthesis inhibitors has not yet been reported. It has been demonstrated that linezolid is bacteriostatic against enterococci and staphylococci, and bactericidal for the majority of streptococci. Resistance to linezolid has been reported; specific mutations have been sequenced in resistant organisms that are thought to be responsible for conferring resistance.

Route of administration
Linezolid is highly absorbed when administered orally, with a bioavailability of approximately 100%. This allows conversion from intravenous to oral therapy as soon as the patient is clinically stable.

Side-effects and tolerability
Thrombocytopenia, defined as a decrease in platelet count below 75% of normal, may be associated with the higher dose or treatment duration exceeding 2 weeks. In addition, cases of myelosuppression (anemia, leukopenia, and pancytopenia) and peripheral neuropathy have been reported. It is recommended that the patient's complete blood count is monitored weekly, especially in those receiving therapy longer than 2 weeks' duration. Clinical data in other special patient populations (i.e. children, pregnant women, or breastfeeding mothers) are limited. The safety and efficacy, and an appropriate dosage, have not been established.

Clinical uses
Linezolid is indicated for infections with vancomycin-resistant *Enterococci* (VRE) and invasive MRSA infections that have not responded to or cannot be treated with conventional therapy using glycopeptides. Linezolid has good tissue penetration, particularly to the skin and soft tissues and the CSF.

Daptomycin
Daptomycin, a fermentation product of *Streptomyces roseosporus*, is a cyclic lipopeptide antibiotic with potent bactericidal activity against most Gram positive organisms including multiple antibiotic resistant and susceptible strains. Its mechanism of action is unclear, it is thought to act by insertion of the lipophilic daptomycin tail into the bacterial cell membrane, causing rapid membrane depolarization and a potassium ion efflux. This is followed by arrest of DNA, RNA, and protein synthesis, resulting in bacterial cell death. It is available only as an intravenous drug. Daptomycin does not cross the blood–brain barrier and does not penetrate the cerebrospinal fluid of normal individuals. It has poor penetration into alveolar lining fluid and should not be used to treat pneumonias. Experience with daptomycin is limited to skin and soft tissue infections caused by staphylococci (including MRSA), streptococci, and enterococci (including VRE). Recently it has been approved for use in right sided *S. aureus* endocarditis. The risk of myopathy is the only documented serious adverse effect; monitoring of creatine kinase is recommended.

Fluoroquinolones

The fluoroquinolones are synthetic antimicrobial agents effective in the treatment of selected community acquired and nosocomial infections. Earlier agents (ciprofloxacin, norfloxacin, ofloxacin) had predominantly Gram negative activity, the newer quinolones (i.e. levofloxacin and moxifloxacin) are broad spectrum agents with enhanced activity against many Gram positive organisms.

Mechanism of action; mechanism of resistance
Quinolones are bactericidal agents that target bacterial DNA gyrase (main target in Gram negative bacteria) and topoisomerase IV (main target in Gram positive bacteria), enzymes essential for DNA replication and transcription. Although this major mechanism of action requires cell division, quinolones have other mechanisms of action which they use to act against bacteria that are not actively replicating. They cross the outer membrane of Gram negative bacteria via porins. Resistance is mediated by mutation of target

enzymes, porin impermeability, and efflux of drug. Resistance to one fluoroquinolone generally means resistance to all.

Route of administration

Most quinolones are available for oral and intravenous usage and are widely distributed in most body tissues and fluids; and penetrate intracellularly.

Side-effects and tolerability

Serious adverse reactions are uncommon. There is some concern that tendinitis, including rupture of Achilles tendon, is associated with fluoroquinolone use. Seizures are rare, but these drugs should be avoided in patients with convulsive or other CNS disorders. The fluoroquinolones are currently not licensed for use in children and pregnant women, but further research is ongoing.

Clinical uses

Quinolones are widely distributed throughout the body. Tissue penetration is higher than the concentration achieved in plasma, stool, bile, prostatic tissue, and lung tissue. Intracellular concentration is exceptional in neutrophils and macrophages. Quinolones also penetrate well in urine and kidneys when renal clearance is the route of drug elimination. Penetration into prostatic fluid, saliva, bone, and cerebrospinal fluid does not exceed serum drug levels. Because cerebrospinal fluid levels of quinolones are predictably poor, these agents are inadequate for first-line treatment of meningitis.

Ciprofloxacin is widely used to treat genitourinary infections, sexually transmitted infections, and enteric fever when susceptible organisms are implicated. When indicated they are also empiric first choice drugs for the treatment of bacterial diarrhea (especially traveler's diarrhea) except when *C. difficile* is suspected. However, there is widespread resistance among campylobacters, a common cause of bacterial diarrhea. Ciprofloxacin is widely used as a prophylactic agent for adult contacts of patients with *Neisseria meningitidis* infection.

Because ciprofloxacin is active against a wide range of enteric Gram negative bacteria including *P. aeruginosa*, it is a common choice for serious Gram negative sepsis in patients who cannot tolerate the β-lactam drugs. Ciprofloxacin has no anti-anaerobic activity.

Fluoroquinolones have excellent bactericidal activity against many mycobacteria and achieve effective serum, tissue, and intracellular levels following oral administration and have relatively few adverse effects. Ofloxacin and ciprofloxacin have shown good clinical efficacy against several mycobacterial diseases, especially tuberculosis and leprosy. The fluoroquinolones are also being effectively used in combination regimens for the treatment of multiple drug resistant tuberculosis. Disseminated infections caused by *Mycobacterium avium* complex (MAC) are often seen in patients with advanced AIDS. Although they have demonstrated only modest *in vitro* activity against MAC, the fluoroquinolones have been used in regimens to treat infections due to this organism usually in combination with macrolides, ethambutol, rifampin, or amikacin.

Ciprofloxacin should not be used to treat community acquired pneumonia because of its poor activity against *S. pneumoniae*.

As mentioned the major limitation for the use of the fluoroquinolones in respiratory infections has been their poor activity against *S. pneumoniae* and anaerobic bacteria. The newer quinolones like levofloxacin and moxifloxacin are active against *S. pneumoniae* and appear to be effective for the treatment of community acquired pneumonia including that caused by multidrug resistant *S. pneumoniae*. Major advantages of these newer quinolones are their oral availability, their effectiveness against the "atypical" agents such as *Mycoplasma pneumoniae* and their good *in vitro* activity against the penicillin resistant pneumococci.

Ciprofloxacin, ofloxacin, and the newer fluoroquinolones achieve exceptional intracellular concentrations. Moxifloxacin and levofloxacin, have excellent activity against *Legionella*, *Chlamydia*, *Mycoplasma*, and *Ureaplasma* species. Intracellular respiratory pathogens such as *Chlamydia pneumoniae*, *Mycoplasma pneumoniae*, and *Legionella pneumophila* are predictably susceptible to the newer fluoroquinolones, making these drugs attractive as single agents for the treatment of community acquired pneumonia, particularly in areas where penicillin resistance in *S. pneumoniae* is a problem. The newer quinolones have no activity against *Pseudomonas* spp.

Box 5.4 Can I recommend using ciprofloxacin?

The nurse at a family practice calls you to say she is advising a family of four, two adults and two children, who are travelling to Southeast Asia. They would like to take a supply of antibiotics to treat traveler's diarrhea and have read that ciprofloxacin is widely used. They would like you to comment on its suitability for this purpose.

Using the checklist in Box 5.1 construct a profile for ciprofloxacin:

✓ Mechanism of action: *inhibits DNA gyrase*
✓ Spectrum: *Gram positive and Gram negative organisms including pathogens that cause traveler's diarrhea*
✓ Route of administration: *available oral (also IV, though not applicable here)*
✓ Dosing regimen: *twice a day*
✓ Penetration: *excellent penetration into bowel lumen and for intracellular pathogens (salmonellae)*

✓ Side-effects: *rare, reports of tendonitis. Not recommended in children and in pregnant women*
✓ Resistance: *campylobacter resistance to ciprofloxacin is widespread*
✓ Clinical uses: *drug of choice for empiric management of moderate to severe traveler's diarrhea in adults provided resistance is not an issue*
✓ Cost: *inexpensive*
✓ Mechanism of microbial resistance: *altered target enzymes, porin impermeability, and efflux of drug*

Though ciprofloxacin is the drug of choice in adults, it is not licensed for use in children. Azithromycin, a macrolide, is recommended for children. Go ahead and profile it. See Chapter 21 for more information on traveler's diarrhea.

One disadvantage of the new quinolones is that they have a broad spectrum of activity including activity against Gram negative organisms and some anaerobes; their widespread use can result in increasing incidence of antibiotic associated colitis due to *C. difficile*. Test yourself regarding the appropriate use of ciprofloxacin by attempting the exercise in Box 5.4.

Aminoglycosides

The aminoglycosides used for systemic infections include gentamicin, amikacin, netilmicin, tobramycin, and streptomycin. Neomycin and kanamycin have a limited antibacterial spectrum and are more toxic than the other aminoglycosides. The latter two drugs are only used topically or orally.

Mechanism of action; mechanism of resistance

The aminoglycosides are bactericidal antibiotics that bind to the 30S ribosomal unit and inhibit bacterial protein synthesis (Figure 5.4). They are active only against aerobic Gram negative bacilli and staphylococci. Activity against streptococci and anaerobes is poor. Aminoglycosides may be used in combination with a penicillin in staphylococcal, streptococcal and especially enterococcal endocarditis, as in combination they display significant antimicrobial synergy.

Enzymatic modification is the most common type of aminoglycoside resistance (Box 5.5). Over 50 different enzymes have been identified. Enzymatic modification results in high level resistance. The genes encoding for aminoglycoside-modifying enzymes are usually found on plasmids and transposons. Most enzyme-mediated resistance in Gram negative bacilli is due to multiple genes.

A large and diverse population of aminoglycoside-modifying enzymes exist and act at virtually every susceptible position on aminoglycoside structures. By testing the susceptibility of isolates against a range of clinically available and experimental aminoglycosides, a pattern of resistance emerges that is unique to a specific enzyme. This method has been referred to as interpretative reading (Table 5.5).

Box 5.5 The three types of aminoglycoside modifying enzymes

- *N*-Acetyltransferases (AAC) – catalyzes acetyl CoA-dependent acetylation of an amino group. Several subtypes of AAC exist (Table 5.5)

- *O*-Adenyltransferases (ANT) – catalyzes ATP-dependent adenylation of hydroxyl group
- *O*-Phosphotransferases (APH) – catalyzes ATP-dependent phosphorylation of a hydroxyl group

Table 5.5 Aminoglycoside resistance phenotypes of *Enterobacteriaceae* spp., including *E. coli* (excluding *Serratia* spp. and *Klebsiella* spp.)

	Phenotype						
	Classical	**AAC(3)I**	**AAC(3)II**	**AAC(3)IV**	**AAC(6′)**	**ANT(2′)**	**APH(3′)**
Gentamicin	S	R	R	R	S/r	R	S
Netilmicin	S	S	R	R	R	S	S
Tobramycin	S	S	R	R	R	R	S
Amikacin	S	S	S	S	R	S	S
Kanamycin	S	S	R	r	R	R	R
Neomycin	S	S	S	R	R	S	R

Classical, no aquired resistance; S, Susceptible; R, resistant; r, reduced zones but likely to remain susceptible at standard breakpoints.

Route of administration

All of the aminoglycosides are poorly absorbed orally and are only available as injectable drugs for systemic infection. They are well absorbed from the peritoneum, pleural cavity, joints, and from denuded skin as in burns. When instilled into these areas, therapeutic levels need to be monitored for toxicity.

After injection, the aminoglycosides are distributed mainly in the extracellular fluid and blood. They are water soluble drugs; they do not penetrate lipids and lipid cell membranes and consequently will not penetrate fatty tissue, cross the blood–brain barrier, or penetrate intracellularly. The major exceptions are urine, middle ear fluid, and renal cortical tissue, which selectively bind aminoglycosides. Therefore aminoglycosides must not be relied upon to treat meningitis, intracellular infections such as typhoid fever, and infections in the eye or the respiratory tract.

Side-effects and tolerability

All aminoglycosides have similar toxicity profiles: they are nephrotoxic and ototoxic.

Aminoglycosides are excreted unchanged into the urine by glomerular filtration. To avoid toxicity, the maintenance dosages of aminoglycosides in patients with renal insufficiency must be modified by either decreasing the dose or increasing the interval between doses or both.

Clinical uses

With the exception of streptomycin, which has a more limited antibiotic spectrum, all aminoglycosides have good activity against Gram negative aerobic bacilli but lack activity against anaerobes. Gentamicin, tobramycin, amikacin, and netilmicin have excellent activity against *P. aeruginosa*. The aminoglycosides are active against staphylococci but not against streptococci including *S. pneumoniae*.

Streptomycin has limited uses because of resistance. It is used for brucellosis, tularemia, and plague. It is used in combination with isoniazid and rifampin in the treatment of tuberculosis.

Neomycin and kanamycin are limited to oral or topical (eye, ear) use because of toxicity. They are used orally for bowel preparation before surgery or in the treatment of hepatic coma to reduce GI bacterial populations and thus ammonia production.

Gentamicin, tobramycin, amikacin, and netilmicin are used in the treatment of serious Gram negative bacterial sepsis, usually as adjuvant to other antibiotics such as β-lactams or quinolones. Gentamicin is also used as an adjuvant to a penicillin or vancomycin in the treatment of streptococcal, enterococcal, or *S. aureus* endocarditis or in prophylaxis of endocarditis.

Resistance of Gram negative bacilli to aminoglycosides has occurred in some hospitals. The resistance is most commonly due to a plasmid-mediated enzymatic alteration of the aminoglycoside.

Amikacin has the same spectrum of activity as gentamicin and tobramycin but is less susceptible to enzymatic inactivation. Therefore, amikacin is valuable in managing infections caused by Gram negative bacilli resistant to gentamicin, netilmicin, and tobramycin, and should probably be reserved for use in these cases.

Miscellaneous antibiotics

Tetracyclines

Tetracyclines are closely related bacteriostatic antibiotics and have similar antibacterial spectrum and toxicity. They bind to the 30S subunit of the ribosome and thus inhibit bacterial protein synthesis (Figure 5.4). Bacterial resistance to one tetracycline indicates likely resistance to the others.

Of all the tetracyclines, doxycycline is the most well absorbed orally and the most widely used. Tetracyclines penetrate into most tissues and body fluids. However, CSF levels are not reliably therapeutic. Doxycycline is excreted mainly in the feces.

Doxycycline is used primarily for treating sexually transmitted infections due to *C. trachomatis* (penicillinase-producing gonococci are relatively resistant to tetracyclines), rickettsiae, *Vibrio* species, Lyme disease, brucellosis, and granuloma inguinale, and as alternative therapy to penicillin in syphilis. Doxycycline is used for chemoprophylaxis of malaria caused by chloroquine resistant *Plasmodium falciparum*.

All tetracyclines can cause staining of teeth, hypoplasia of dental enamel, and abnormal bone growth in children younger than 8 years and in the fetuses of pregnant women. Therefore, tetracyclines should be avoided after the first trimester of pregnancy and in children less than 8 years old.

Sulfonamides

The sulfonamides are synthetic bacteriostatic antibiotics with a wide spectrum against most Gram positive and many Gram negative organisms (except pseudomonas). Sulfonamides inhibit multiplication of bacteria by acting as competitive inhibitors of p-aminobenzoic acid in the folic acid metabolism cycle. Bacterial susceptibility is the same for the various sulfonamides; and resistance to one sulfonamide indicates resistance to all.

Most sulfonamides are readily absorbed orally; injectable formulations cause inflammation of local tissues. The sulfonamides are widely distributed throughout all tissues. High levels are achieved in pleural, peritoneal, synovial, and ocular fluids. Although these drugs are no longer used to treat meningitis, CSF levels are high in meningeal infections. Their antibacterial action is inhibited by pus.

Sulfonamides are currently used in combination with pyrimethamine in the treatment of toxoplasmosis, in ulcerative colitis (as sulfasalazine), and in combination with trimethoprim (see below).

Adverse reactions include hypersensitivity reactions and Stevens–Johnson syndrome; crystalluria, oliguria, and anuria; kernicterus (jaundice in the newborn) can result from administration of sulfonamides to the mother at term or to the newborn. Sulfonamides displace bilirubin from albumin in the newborn; therefore pregnant women near term and newborns should not be given sulfonamides.

Broad spectrum (enhanced Gram negative activity) tetracyclines such as tigecycline have recently been introduced.

Co-trimoxazole; trimethoprim

Co-trimoxazole is the combination of trimethoprim-sulfamethoxazole (TMP-SMX) in a 1 : 5 fixed ratio respectively and is usually bacteriostatic. Both drugs block folic acid metabolism in bacterial cells and display *in vitro* synergistic bacterial activity in combination when compared to either agent alone. Sulfonamides act on incorporation of *p*-aminobenzoic acid into the metabolic pathway; trimethoprim prevents reduction of dihydrofolate to tetrahydrofolate. TMP-SMX is active against most Gram positive and Gram negative organisms but is inactive against anaerobes and the *Pseudomonas* spp.

Co-trimoxazole is well absorbed orally and is excreted into the urine. It penetrates well into tissues and body fluids, including the CSF.

Co-trimoxazole is the first line drug for treatment of urinary tract infections in women. It is the drug of choice for *Pneumocystis jirovecii* pneumonia and in prophylaxis of this infection in AIDS patients, and in children and adults with malignancies. It has been used worldwide for the treatment of typhoid fever, especially when ampicillin and chloramphenicol cannot be used and when other agents are not available or too expensive. It is also the drug of choice against *Nocardia*.

Trimethoprim alone is commonly used for prophylaxis and treatment of urinary tract infections in women and children in many parts of the world.

The adverse reactions for co-trimoxazole are the same as those listed above for sulfonamides. Trimethoprim causes identical adverse reactions to SMX but less commonly. When it does, nausea, vomiting, rash, and folate deficiency (resulting in macrocytic anemia) most likely occur. For this reason trimethoprim is not used for the treatment of urinary tract infections in the first trimester of pregnancy.

Chloramphenicol

Chloramphenicol is primarily a bacteriostatic drug. It binds to the 50S subunit of the ribosome and inhibits bacterial protein synthesis (Figure 5.4). It has a wide spectrum of activity against Gram positive and Gram negative organisms including anaerobes and rickettsiae. Chloramphenicol is well absorbed orally and is available as an intravenous formulation to treat serious infections. The drug is distributed widely in body fluids and therapeutic concentrations are achieved in CSF. Chloramphenicol is metabolized in the liver to the inactive glucuronide. Both chloramphenicol and the glucuronide metabolite are excreted in the urine.

Chloramphenicol, once the drug of choice for typhoid fever, has now been replaced by other agents due to emerging resistance. It is still the alternative for meningitis caused by susceptible *H. influenzae*, meningococci, or pneumococci when a β-lactam antibiotic cannot be used (as in cases of severe allergy); for brain abscess where streptococcal and anaerobic cover is required; and for rickettsial infections not responding to tetracycline or in which tetracycline cannot be used.

Two types of bone marrow depression may be caused by chloramphenicol: a reversible dose-related interference with iron metabolism and an irreversible idiosyncratic form of aplastic anemia. The reversible form is likely to occur with high doses, a prolonged course of treatment, and in patients with liver disease. Irreversible idiosyncratic aplastic anemia occurs in < 1 : 25 000 patients given chloramphenicol.

The gray baby syndrome, which is often fatal, occurs in newborns. It is related to high blood levels resulting from an inability of the immature liver to metabolize chloramphenicol and occurs with standard doses.

Metronidazole

Metronidazole is active only against strictly anaerobic bacteria and protozoa, such as *Giardia lamblia*, *Entamoeba histolytica* and *Trichomonas vaginalis*. It is not active against aerobic or microaerophilic bacteria. Its selectivity for anaerobic bacteria is a result of the ability of these organisms to reduce metronidazole to its active form intracellularly. The electron transport proteins necessary for this reaction are found only in anaerobic bacteria. Reduced metronidazole then disrupts DNA's helical structure, thereby inhibiting bacterial nucleic acid synthesis. This eventually results in bacterial cell death. Metronidazole is equally effective against dividing and nondividing cells.

Metronidazole is absorbed well when given orally; intravenous formulations are also available. It is distributed widely in body fluids and penetrates into the CSF in high concentrations. Metronidazole and its metabolites are excreted mainly in urine.

Metronidazole is used primarily for the treatment of intra-abdominal and pelvic infections caused by anaerobes, particularly *Bacteroides fragilis*, and protozoal infections. It is effective in treating meningitis and brain abscess when caused by susceptible anaerobes. It is the drug of choice in *Clostridium difficile* colitis. Metronidazole is also the drug of choice for bacterial vaginosis.

It can cause a metallic taste and dark urine and has caused cancer in mice and rats, but the risk to humans is unknown. It is not recommended for use in pregnancy. A disulfiram-like adverse reaction may occur if alcohol is ingested.

Rifampicin

Rifampicin is an antibiotic that inhibits DNA-dependent RNA polymerase, leading to suppression of RNA synthesis. It is bactericidal and has activity against most Gram positive bacteria and *Mycobacterium* sp. Because of rapid emergence of resistant bacteria, use is restricted to treatment of mycobacterial infections and a few other indications. Resistance occurs due to modification of RNA polymerase and is not inhibited by the drug.

Rifampicin is well absorbed when taken orally and is distributed widely in body tissues and fluids, including the CSF. It is metabolized in the liver and eliminated in bile and, to a much lesser extent, in urine.

Rifampicin, isoniazid, ethambutol, and pyrazinamide are used in combination for the treatment of TB. Rifampicin is also used to treat atypical mycobacterial infection and leprosy. Rifampicin is one of the drugs of choice for eradication of the meningococcal and *H. influenzae* type b carrier state in prevention of meningitis caused by these organisms. It may also be useful in combination with a penicillin, cephalosporin, or vancomycin in treatment of staphylococcal endocarditis and staphylococcal osteomyelitis. Addition of rifampicin to erythromycin may be helpful in treating *Legionella* infections. It is also used with vancomycin in treatment of pneumococcal meningitis.

The most serious side-effect is hepatitis, which occurs much more often when isoniazid and rifampin are used together than when either is used alone. The urine, saliva, sweat, sputum, and tears are stained red-orange by rifampicin.

Nitrofurantoin

Nitrofurantoin is used orally for the treatment or prophylaxis of lower UTI. It is active against *Escherichia coli*, *Klebsiella/Enterobacter* spp., staphylococci, and enterococci, but *Pseudomonas* and most strains of *Proteus* are resistant. It is absorbed well when given orally but does not produce antibacterial blood levels. However, urinary levels are high. It is not recommended for use in the last trimester of pregnancy as it may cause neonatal hemolysis. Nitrofurantoin is *contraindicated* in patients with renal insufficiency, because serious toxicity is possible and adequate urinary concentrations may not be attained.

Fusidic acid

Fusidic acid inhibits bacterial protein synthesis by interfering with amino acid transfer from aminoacyl-tRNA to protein on the ribosomes. It is effective against pathogenic staphylococci, including β-lactamase producing and methicillin resistant strains. It is much less active against streptococci and has no activity against Gram negative organisms. It is used largely in the oral form or topical form as parenteral formulations cause tissue irritation.

Concentrations adequate for bactericidal activity against staphylococci have been demonstrated in pus, exudate, soft tissue, bone tissue, synovial fluid, aqueous humour, vitreous body, burn crusts, intracranial abscess, and sputum.

It is therefore used in the treatment of localized as well as generalized staphylococcal infections (e.g. abscesses, furunculosis, wound infections, pneumonia, peritonitis, osteomyelitis, and septic arthritis). When administered systemically, fusidic acid is always used in combination with other anti-staphylococcal agents such as flucloxacillin, rifampicin, and the glycopeptides. Monotherapy results in rapid development of resistance.

Drugs for the treatment of **tuberculosis** will be described in Chapter 16.

The common antimicrobial agents used in clinical practice and their activity is summarized in Table 5.6.

Table 5.6 A summary of the common anti-microbial agents and their activity

Anti-microbial	Major class	Spectrum	Mechanism of action
Penicillin V and G	β-lactam-penicillin	Gram positive bacteria	Inhibits cell wall synthesis; is **not** β-lactamase stable
Cloxacillin/nafcillin	β-lactam-penicillin	Gram positive bacteria	Inhibits cell wall synthesis; is β-lactamase stable
Amoxicillin/ampicillin	β-lactam-penicillin	Gram positive and Gram negative bacteria	Inhibits cell wall synthesis; is **not** β-lactamase stable
Co-amoxiclav	β-lactam-penicillin + inhibitor combination	Gram positive and Gram negative bacteria + anaerobes	Inhibits cell wall synthesis; is β-lactamase stable
Piptazobactam	β-lactam-penicillin + with inhibitor combination	Basic Gram positive action and extended Gram negative action (including pseudomonas) + anaerobes	Inhibits cell wall synthesis; is β-lactamase stable
Carbapenems	β-lactam-penicillin	Basic Gram positive and extended Gram negative action (including pseudomonas) + anaerobes	Inhibits cell wall synthesis; is β-lactamase stable
I generation cephalosporin, e.g. cephalothin	β-lactam-cephalosporin	Gram positive and Gram negative bacteria	Inhibits cell wall synthesis; is stable to Gram positive β-lactamase only
II generation cephalosporin, e.g. cefuroxime	β-lactam-cepahlosporin	Gram positive and Gram negative bacteria	Inhibits cell wall synthesis; is stable to Gram positive β-lactamase only
III generation cephalosporin, e.g. ceftriaxone	β-lactam-cephalosporin	Gram positive and Gram negative bacteria	Inhibits cell wall synthesis; is stable to Gram positive β-lactamase only
III generation cephalosporin, e.g. ceftazidime	β-lactam-cephalosporin	Gram positive and broader Gram negative action (including pseudomonas)	Inhibits cell wall synthesis; is stable to Gram positive β-lactamase only
IV generation cephalosporin, e.g. cefipime	β-lactam-cephalosporin	Gram positive and broader Gram negative action (including pseudomonas)	Inhibits cell wall synthesis; is stable to Gram positive β-lactamase only
Aztreonam	Monobactam	Gram negative bacteria including pseudomonas	Inhibits cell wall synthesis
Vancomycin/teicoplanin	Glycopeptide	Gram positive bacteria; especially MRSA	Inhibits cell wall synthesis at a site different from the β lactams
Erythromycin/clarithromycin	Macrolide	Gram positive bacteria and agents of "atypical" pneumonia: mycoplasma/legionalla	Inhibits protein synthesis (acts of 50S subunit of ribososme)
Clindamycin	Lincosamide	Gram positive bacteria + anaerobes	Inhibits protein synthesis (acts of 50S subunit of ribososme)

Table 5.6 (*cont'd*)

Anti-microbial	Major class	Spectrum	Mechanism of action
Linezolid	Oxazolidinone	Gram positive bacteria; especially MRSA and GRE	Inhibits initiation of protein synthesis
Daptomycin	Lipopeptide	Gram positive bacteria; especially MRSA and GRE	Unclear; multiple sites of action – cell membrane and protein synthesis
Ciprofloxacin	Fluoroquinolone	Gram positive (less) and broader Gram negative action (including pseudomonas)	DNA gyrase
Levofloxacin/moxifloxacin	Fluoroquinolone	Gram positive (more) and less Gram negative action (not anti-pseudomonal)	DNA gyrase and topoisomerase
Gentamicin/amikacin and others	Aminoglycoside	Gram positive and Gram negative action (including pseudomonas)	Inhibits protein synthesis (acts of 30S subunit of ribososme)
Doxycycline	Tetracycline	Gram positive and Gram negative action (not antipseudomonal); intracellular pathogens: *Rickettsia. Ehrlichia. Borellia*	Inhibits protein synthesis (acts of 30S subunit of ribososme)
Trimethoprim	Diaminopyrimidines	Gram positive and Gram negative bacteria (not antipseudomonal)	Folate metabolism
Co-trimoxazole	Anti-folate	Gram positive and Gram negative bacteria (not antipseudomonal)	Folate metabolism
Chloramphenicol		Gram positive bacteria (not anti-pseudomonal) + anaerobes	Inhibits protein synthesis (acts of 50S subunit of ribososme)
Metronidazole	Nitroimidazole	Anaerobes/protozoa	DNA helix
Rifampicin	Rifamycins	Gram positive bacteria + mycobacteria	RNA polymerase
Nitrofurantoin	Nitrofurans	Gram positive and Gram negative bacteria (not anti-pseudomonal)	Unclear
Fusidic acid	–	Gram positive bacteria	Protein synthesis, acts on t-RNA

MRSA, methicillin resistant *S.aureus*; GRE, Glycopeptide resistant enterococci.

Antifungal agents

As fungi are eukaryotic organisms, antibacterial agents have no action against them. Specialized antifungal drugs have been developed for use. Knowledge of the structure of fungal cells and of fungal biosynthetic pathways are essential for understanding how antifungal agents work. The homology of mammalian and fungal cells creates problems for designing drugs that act selectively on fungal cells alone without causing significant toxicity to host human cells. To minimize toxicity issues superficial lesions are often *treated* with topical agents but deeper mycoses may need prolonged treatment with intravenous agents. The spectrum of activity of the main classes of antifungal agents in common use is briefly covered in Table 5.7.

Antifungal agents currently available for the treatment of fungal infection may have actions on four target sites in fungi.

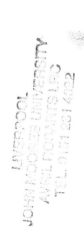

Table 5.7 Spectrum of activity of antifungal agents against some common pathogenic fungi

Fungi	Polyenes	Azoles	Flucytosine	Allyamines	Echinocardins
Candida albicans	+	+	+	−	+
Cryptococcus neoformans	+	+	+	+/−	−
Dermatophytes	−	+	−	+	−
Aspergillus species	+	+*	−	+	+
Dimorphic fungi (e.g. *Blastomyces/Histoplasma*)	+	+	−	+	−

+, good activity; −, no activity.
* Itraconazole and voriconazole only.

Fungal cell membrane

Ergosterol is the main sterol component in fungal cells rather than cholesterol, which is the predominant sterol found in human host cells. This difference in sterol composition has been exploited in the design of several classes of commercially available antifungal therapies used to treat mycoses, including the **azoles, polyenes**, and **allyamines**.

Polyene antifungals such as **amphotericin B** and **nystatin** act by binding to ergosterol, resulting in depolarization of the cell membrane, pore formation, leakage of essential metabolites, and ultimately cell death. They are broad spectrum antifungal agents. Nystatin is often prescribed orally for treating mucous membrane candida infections. Systemic amphotericin B is used for the empiric treatment of deeper mycoses, including disseminated aspergillosis, candidiasis, and infections caused by dimorphic fungi.

Toxicity is a significant problem with systemic polyenes, for example, stimulation of host cells can cause release of inflammatory cytokines resulting in rigors, nausea, myalgia, and headache during intravenous infusions. Amphotericin B, especially at higher concentrations, may bind to cholesterol in mammalian cell membranes leading to variety of toxicity problems, the most clinically relevant being nephrotoxicity. Various pharmaceutical methods have been employed with the aim of reducing toxicity of amphotericin B. Lipid-complexed colloidal formulations or phospholipid vesicles (liposomes) have allowed higher doses of the drug to be delivered to the site of infection without causing increased toxicity.

Azole antifungals such as clotrimazole (an imidazole) and **fluconazole, itraconazole** and **voriconazole** (triazoles), inhibit the fungal enzyme 14-α demethylase, inhibiting the synthesis of ergosterol (see Figure 2.13). With reduced ergosterol synthesis there is accumulation of toxic precursor sterols, increased membrane permeability, leading eventually to cell death. 14-α demethylase is a cytochrome P450 dependent enzyme and azole agents are capable of inhibiting several similar mammalian P450 dependent enzymes. Although in general less toxic than polyene agents, azole drugs are thus susceptible to many drug interactions with other medications (such as rifampicin) metabolized through the P450 pathway. New azoles such as posaconazole have similar activity.

Imidazoles such as clotrimazole are most commonly used for topical application in superficial fungal infections. Triazole agents have a broader spectrum of activity and are used for the oral treatment of superficial infections and for many forms of systemic mycoses. Itraconazole and voriconazole exhibit better activity than fluconazole against *Aspergillus* species and *Candida krusei* and *C. glabrata* infections.

Allyamines such as **terbinafine** act at an earlier point in the ergosterol pathway inhibiting another P450 dependent enzyme squalene expoxidase. Therefore the allyamines also have the potential for clinically significant interactions with other medications that are metabolized by the P450 pathway. It is nearly completely absorbed when given orally and accumulates in keratin, where it persists even after treatment has stopped. Terbinafine is the drug of choice for dermatophyte toenail infections and other refractory dermatophyte infections where systemic treatment is required.

Fungal cell wall

Mammalian cells lack a cell wall and thus the fungal cell wall provides a highly selective target for antifungal agents. Disruption in the synthesis and construction of fungal cell walls leads to cell death via osmotic lysis due to structurally defective walls.

Echinocandin agents such as caspofungin, anidulafungin, and micafungin are glucan synthesis inhibitors, which prevent cell wall synthesis by inhibiting the enzyme 1,3-β-glucan synthase (see Figure 2.13). As these agents are specific they have limited toxicity issues and are well tolerated. Echinocandins have no action against the yeast *Cryptococcus neoformans*.

DNA and protein synthesis

DNA and protein synthesis have been difficult targets for the development of selectively toxic antifungal therapy as both fungal and mammalian cells share similar biosynthetic pathways. Only one agent, **flucytosine** (or 5-flurocytosine), a pyrimidine analog, is currently available but in the future advances in molecular science may highlight differences between fungal and host cells that could be exploited for the development of new agents.

Flucytosine is transported into fungal cells by a specific enzyme cytosine permease and converted in the cytoplasm to 5-fluorouracil and then phosphorylated. Phosphorylated 5-fluorouracil is incorporated into RNA where it causes miscoding and prevents protein synthesis. Also phosphorylated 5-fluorouracil can be converted into its deoxynucleoside which inhibits DNA synthesis. The most common toxicities of flucytosine are dose related nausea, diarrhea, and bone marrow suppression and thus drug assays are sent when patients are on treatment. Flucytosine has considerable activity against yeasts but no useful activity against molds. The drug can be given orally and systemically but resistance develops rapidly, for this reason it is usually co-administered with amphotericin B.

Fungal cell mitosis

Griseofulvin is believed to inhibit fungal cell mitosis by disrupting mitotic spindle cell formation. Use of this agent is limited to the treatment of dermatophyte infections of the skin, nail, or hair. Griseofulvin is well absorbed when given orally and serious side-effects are uncommon.

Drugs for the treatment of protozoal and helminth infections

The pharmacological treatment of infections caused by protozoa or helminths is complex and reference from specialist centers should be sought when dealing with most patients. There are some general principles when prescribing for these parasitic infections. Firstly, some of the drugs currently available have unreliable efficacy or safety profiles and thus the decision to initiate treatment should not be taken lightly. Secondly, many people, predominately in the developing world, are infected with one or more species asymptomatically. Most do not require treatment and indeed it would not be cost effective to recommend mass treatment. When re-infection from the environment or other community members is highly likely it may also prove a waste of valuable resources to treat infection. With their complex lifecycles, at some stages the protozoal or helminthic organism may not be susceptible to a particular agent because it is in a nonaccessible site or in a resting state. For several protozoal infections such as *Cryptosporidium parvum* and *Microspora* species, reliable chemotherapy regimens have not yet been elucidated.

Antiprotozoal drugs

Antiprotozoal drugs are most often classified according to the organisms being treated rather than the drug group they belong to. The categories covered in this chapter include:

- Antimalarials (covered in Chapter 17)
- Amebicides
- Trichomonicides
- Antigiardial drugs
- Drugs for toxoplasmosis
- Leishmanicides.

This is not an exhaustive list and treatment for infections not discussed here can be sought by reference to specialist textbooks.

Amebicides

Drugs commonly used: metronidazole, tinidazole, diloxanide furoate.

The anti-anaerobic medication metronidazole discussed under miscellaneous antibiotics is the drug of choice for acute invasive amebic dysentery and liver abscesses caused by *Entamoeba histolytica*, it is given usually for 5–10 days. The exact mechanism of action of metronidazole is not completely understood, it is reduced to an unidentified polar compound in the cell and this compound acts by disrupting DNA and nucleic acid synthesis. Aspiration of liver and other abscess collections may be indicated if the collection is large or if no clinical improvement has been made after 72 hours of treatment. Metronidazole and tinidazole (a related nitroimidazole) have only limited activity against the cyst form of *E. histolytica*, and thus a drug called diloxanide furoate is given for 10 days following initial treatment with metronidazole. As this drug is relatively free from toxic effects is it also prescribed to asymptomatic cyst carriers.

Trichomonicides

Drugs commonly used: metronidazole, tinidazole.

Metronidazole for 5–7 days is the treatment of choice for urogenital trichomonas infection. Sexual contacts should be screened and treated simultaneously. If metronidazole is ineffective, tinidazole may be used as an alternative.

Anti-giardia drugs

Drugs commonly used: metronidazole, tinidazole.

Metronidazole is the treatment of choice for *G. lamblia* infections, given for 3–5 days, alternative treatment is with tinidazole given as a single dose. Resistance to these two agents is extremely uncommon

Drugs for toxoplasmosis

Drugs commonly used: pyrimethamine and sulfadiazine; pyrimethamine and clindamycin; spiramycin.

The majority of infections associated with *T. gondii* are self-limiting and do not require treatment. Situations that may warrant treatment include infections in patients who are immunocompromised, those with eye involvement, and infections in pregnant women or neonates. First line treatment is a combination of pyrimethamine and sulfadiazine given for several weeks. Pyrimethamine is a potent folate antagonist and thus folinic acid supplements are always co-prescribed and weekly blood counts should be performed. Pyrimethamine and clindamycin combinations have also been used successfully. Spiramycin, a macrolide agent, is given to women who acquire toxoplasmosis in pregnancy as it has been shown to reduce the risk of transmission of maternal infection to the fetus.

Leishmanicides

Drugs commonly used: sodium stibogluconate, amphotericin, pentamidine isethionate.

Most cutaneous leishmaniasis lesions resolve spontaneously and treatment is not indicated. Treatment for extensive lesions is the same as for visceral leishmaniasis (VL). Sodium stibogluconate, an organic antimony compound, is the first line treatment of VL and it is administered by intramuscular or intravenous injection. The dosage and treatment length varies with different geographical regions and local expert advice should be sought.

Amphotericin can be used alone, in combination with or after an antimony compound for VL, the liposomal preparation (which carries the drug into macrophages) has been shown to be as effective with fewer side-effects.

Pentamidine isethionate, an agent which works by inhibiting polyamine metabolism, is used in patients with VL resistant to antimony-based medications.

Antihelminth medications

Enterobius vermicularis is the only common helminth infection seen in the USA, other helminthic infections should be treated with reference to expert advice. Some of the drugs used to treat important helminth infections are described in Table 5.8.

Table 5.8 Drugs for other helminth infections

Helminth	Drugs	Comments
Trichuris trichiura	Mebendazole Albendazole	Mebendazole works by inhibiting β-tubulin in worms
Ascaris lumbricoides	Levamisole Piperazine Mebendazole Albendazole	Levamisole is considered the drug of choice although it may be difficult to obtain
Ankylostoma duodenale/Necator americanus	Mebendazole Albendazole	
Strongyloides stercoralis	Thiabendazole Mebendazole Albendazole Ivermectin	Thiabendazole is the drug of choice
Wuchereria bancrofti	Diethylcarbamazine (DEC)	
Loa loa	DEC	
Onchocerca volvulus	Ivermectin	This agent works as a GABA antagonist (β-aminobutyric acid). Repeated treatments at 3- to 6-monthly intervals may be required
Schistosoma species	Praziquantel	This medication interferes with calcium homeostasis
Paragonimus westermani	Praziquantel	
Echinococcus granulosus	Albendazole Praziquantel	Drugs are used in conjunction with surgery to remove cysts
Taenia solium/saginatum	Niclosamide Praziquantel	Niclosamide is the most commonly used agent

Drugs for *Enterobius vermicularis*

Drugs commonly used: mebendazole, piperazine

Mebendazole is the drug of choice for treating threadworm infection in all patients over the age of 2 years of age. Its mechanism of action is inhibition of β-tubulin and it works against most of the intestinal nematodes. It is given as a single dose but often a second dose is given after 2 weeks. All family members should be treated and strict hygienic measures (handwashing, scrubbing nails) should be adhered to so as to break the cycle of auto-infection. Piperazine is an alternative treatment and can be given to children less than 2 years of age. It works by causing worm paralysis and its spectrum of activity covers other intestinal roundworms.

Treatment for other helminth infections is tabulated in Table 5.8.

Antiviral drugs

Because viruses are obligate intracellular parasites, any putative chemotherapeutic agent must first enter the host cells, and therefore carries the inherent potential for cellular toxicity. The strategy for development of antiviral drugs has therefore been to target viral proteins and processes that are not found within the host. Table 5.9 illustrates the diversity of virus-specific functions targeted. Most of the 40 or so compounds that have been officially approved for clinical use have been licensed only within the last 5 years. At least half of

Table 5.9 Mechanisms of action of antiviral drugs

Process inhibited	Viral component targeted	Agent(s)*
Attachment	HIV co-receptor on host cell	CCR5 and CXCR4 antagonists
	HIV envelope protein, gp120	HIV attachment inhibitors
Penetration	HIV fusion protein, gp41	Enfuvirtide
Disassembly	M2 protein of influenza A	Amantadine, rimantadine
	Enteroviral capsid protein	Pleconaril
Transcription	Reverse transcriptase of HIV	NRTIs and NNRTIs (see below)
	Regulatory proteins or their binding sites	HIV *tat* inhibitors
	Mediators of RNA transcript processing	Ribavirin
Translation	mRNA	Interferons Fomivirsen and other antisense oligonucleotides
Replication	HIV integrase	Integrase inhibitors
	Herpesvirus DNA polymerases	Nucleoside analogs, e.g. aciclovir
	Reverse transcriptase of HBV	NRTIs
	Viral RNA replicases	Replicase inhibitors
Assembly	Viral proteases mediating post translational cleavage	HIV protease inhibitors, HCV protease inhibitors
Release	Influenza virus neuraminidase	Neuraminidase inhibitors

★ Those drugs which are in clinical or preclinical development are shown in purple rather than black.

them are used for the treatment of HIV infections. Many more agents, some with novel mechanisms of action, are in development.

Drugs active against herpesviruses

Aciclovir

Mechanism of action
Aciclovir is a nucleoside analog that is not active until it has been triply phosphorylated. The first phosphorylation step requires the action of herpesvirus encoded **thymidine kinase** (TK) such that the drug is only activated in virus-infected cells and remains inactive in uninfected cells. Following two further phosphorylations by host cell enzymes, the active nucleotide triphosphate form of the drug selectively inhibits viral DNA polymerase. Moreover, once incorporated into the nascent DNA chain, because the acyclic sugar moiety lacks a 3′ −OH group for linkage to the next sugar, the molecule acts as a **chain terminator**.

Mechanism of resistance
Viral resistance can arise from mutation of either the TK gene or the DNA polymerase gene.

Activity range
Viral thymidine kinase is required to initiate drug activation. As this enzyme is specific to HSV-1, HSV-2, and VZV, aciclovir is active only against these three viruses. The DNA polymerase of VZV is significantly less sensitive to inhibition by aciclovir triphosphate than the DNA polymerases of HSV-1 and 2. Therefore higher drug doses are required for treatment of VZV. The enzyme in cytomegalovirus (CMV) that is analogous to TK in function, CMV-encoded protein kinase (PK), does not monophosphorylate aciclovir effectively and hence the drug has little activity against this virus.

Indications
HSV-1 and 2 infections including herpes labialis ("cold sores"), genital herpes, herpetic keratitis (i.e. infection of the cornea), neonatal herpes, and herpetic encephalitis. VZV infections including varicella ("chickenpox") and zoster ("shingles").

Major side-effects
Because it is only activated inside herpesvirus-infected cells and because human DNA polymerase is resistant to the inhibition, aciclovir is remarkably nontoxic.

Drugs related to aciclovir
Valaciclovir is the valine ester of aciclovir and serves as the oral prodrug. **Penciclovir** has an almost identical mechanism of action to aciclovir and **famciclovir** is its oral prodrug. The mechanism of action of **ganciclovir** is essentially the same as for aciclovir but it is much more readily monophosphorylated by CMV PK than is aciclovir, hence its far greater activity against CMV than aciclovir. Unfortunately, it is quite toxic to the bone marrow and commonly causes neutropenia. **Valganciclovir** is its oral prodrug. **Cidofovir** is a cytosine analog that acts as a chain terminator but targets the viral DNA polymerase of many more different viruses: papilloma-, polyoma-, adeno- and poxviruses, as well as herpesviruses. Unfortunately, it is also highly nephrotoxic, which limits its clinical use.

Foscarnet

Mechanism of action
This pyrophosphate analog interferes with the binding of pyrophosphate to its binding site of the viral DNA polymerase during the DNA replication process.

Activity range
The drug is active against all the herpesviruses and also against HIV.

Indications and major side-effects
The drug is notably toxic, commonly causing gastrointestinal disturbance and renal impairment. Consequently, its indications are limited to severe CMV disease and severe infections with aciclovir-resistant HSV or VZV.

Fomivirsen

Mechanism of action
This antisense oligonucleotide is complementary in base sequence to the CMV immediate early 2 (IE2) mRNA. It therefore hybridizes specifically with this mRNA, preventing its translation.

Activity range and indications
The drug is active only against CMV and is licensed only for intraocular administration in the management of CMV retinitis (in AIDS patients).

Anti-retroviral compounds (active against HIV and/or HBV)

There are four classes of drugs in current usage: nucleoside reverse transcriptase inhibitors (NRTIs), non-nucleoside reverse transcriptase inhibitors (NNRTIs), protease inhibitors, and viral entry inhibitors. For treatment of HIV infection, these drugs are usually used in combinations of three or more agents in order to avoid the development of drug resistance. This combination treatment is referred to as Highly Active Antiretroviral Therapy: HAART (see also Chapter 18).

Nucleoside reverse transcriptase inhibitors: NRTIs

Mechanism of action
Zidovudine (azidothymidine: AZT) was the first of these to be licensed for the treatment of HIV infection. These drugs are nucleoside analogs that target the reverse transcriptase (RT) of HIV and act as chain terminators. **Didanosine** (DDI), **zalcitabine** (DDC), **stavudine** (D4T), **lamivudine** (3TC), **abacavir**, and **emtricitabine** are also NRTIs.

Mechanism of resistance
Characteristic mutations in the RT gene arise readily when zidovudine is used alone or if drug levels fall to a subtherapeutic level. These mutations reduce the affinity of the enzyme for the drug such that the altered enzyme is able to function normally even in the presence of the drug. To a variable extent the mutations that confer resistance to zidovudine also confer resistance to other NRTIs.

Activity range and indications
These drugs are active against HIV-1 and -2, and are usually used in combination with other anti-HIV agents in the treatment of HIV infection. **Lamivudine** and **emtricitabine**, being active against the RT of HBV, are also used in the treatment of chronic HBV infection.

Major side-effects

NRTIs are quite diverse in their side-effects, which however often include gastrointestinal disturbance. Hematological toxicity is notable for zidovudine and peripheral neuropathy for stavudine, zalcitabine, and didanosine.

NRTI-related drugs: nucleotide reverse transcriptase inhibitors

These drugs are phosphorylated nucleosides that function in exactly the same way as NRTIs. For oral administration they have to be given as the esterified prodrug. **Tenofovir** is used to treat HIV-1 and -2, and **adefovir** is used for HBV.

Non-nucleoside reverse transcriptase inhibitors (NNRTIs)

Mechanism of action

These drugs – **efavirenz**, **nevirapine** and **delavirdine** – inhibit HIV reverse transcriptase by targeting an allosteric "pocket" in the nonsubstrate binding site of the enzyme.

Mechanism of resistance

Characteristic mutations in the RT gene arise readily when NNRTIs are used singly or if drug levels fall to subtherapeutic levels. These mutations tend to confer cross-resistance with other NNRTIs. There is no cross-resistance between NRTIs and NNRTIs.

Activity range and indications

This class of drugs is not active against the RT of HIV-2 and therefore is indicated only in the management of HIV-1 infection, where these drugs are used in combination with other anti-retroviral agents.

Major side-effects

Rashes, which can be severe and even life-threatening (Stevens–Johnson syndrome), are the most notable major side-effect of the drugs in this class. Efavirenz quite commonly causes CNS disturbances such as sleeplessness, intense dreams, altered mood, and anxiety.

Protease inhibitors (PIs)

Mechanism of action

These complex drug compounds act as peptidomimetic inhibitors of HIV protease and so block post-translational processing of viral products and hence viral assembly. **Saquinavir, ritonavir, indinavir, nelfinavir, amprenavir, lopinavir,** and **atazanavir** are all PIs.

Mechanism of resistance

Characteristic mutations in the protease gene arise readily when any PI is used alone or if drug levels fall to a subtherapeutic level. These mutations reduce the affinity of the protease enzyme for the drug such that the altered enzyme is able to function normally even in the presence of the drug. Some of these mutations confer cross-resistance to other PIs.

Activity range and indications

These drugs are active against HIV-1 and -2, and are used in combination with other anti-HIV agents in the treatment of HIV infection.

Major side-effects

These drugs commonly cause gastrointestinal symptoms such as diarrhea, nausea, vomiting, abdominal pain, and flatulence.

Viral entry inhibitors

Mechanism of action
Enfuvirtide (T-20) is a 36-aminoacid peptide, corresponding to residues 127–162 of the HIV-1 envelope glycoprotein gp41. It binds to its homologous gp41 region in a coil–coil interaction and prevents it from undergoing the conformational change that mediates fusion between the viral envelope and cell membrane. Other related drugs are in development (for a summary and a link to a helpful video showing the mechanism of action of T-20, see: http://www.hiv.ch/rubiken/news/roche280503.htm).

Mechanism of resistance
Mutations in the *env* gene alter the sequence of amino acid residues in the gp41 glycoprotein such that enfuvirtide no longer binds.

Activity range and indications
Enfuvirtide has reduced activity against HIV-2. Because it has to be given by subcutaneous injection – the polypeptide is broken down by digestive enzymes if administered orally – this drug tends to be used only in salvage HIV-1 therapy where there is extensive resistance to other classes of drugs.

Major side-effects
Reactions at the injection site almost always occur but are usually not serious.

Anti-influenza virus compounds

Synthetic primary amines

Mechanism of action
These drugs, **amantadine** and **rimantadine**, block the M2 ion channel in the capsid of the influenza A virus preventing the influx of H^+ ions necessary for viral uncoating.

Mechanism of resistance
Mutations that stop these drugs from binding to the M2 protein arise readily and are now widespread, worldwide amongst human influenza A viruses.

Activity range and indications
These drugs are active only against influenza A but, although they can be used for prophylaxis and treatment of infection with this virus, they are rarely used now because of their side-effects and easily generated resistance.

Major side-effects
Both drugs, but amantadine especially, can cause nausea and anxiety.

Neuraminidase inhibitors

Mechanism of action
Viral neuraminidase is responsible for the cleavage of *N*-acetylneuraminic acid (also called sialic acid) from the influenza virus receptor so that progeny virions can be released from infected cells. The neuraminidase inhibitors **zanamivir** and **oseltamivir** are sialic acid analogs that inhibit the viral enzyme and keep the virus trapped on the infected cells.

Mechanism of resistance
Mutations of the viral neuraminidase gene that confer drug resistance arise only rarely, and are usually associated with reduced viral infectivity. However, recently, during 2007–08, human seasonal influenza

(H1N1) viruses have arisen that are naturally resistant to oseltamivir. Research is currently ongoing as to the possible origins of these oseltamivir-resistant viruses.

Activity range and indications
These drugs are used for prophylaxis and treatment of influenza A and B virus infections.

Major side-effects
Significant side-effects are uncommon. There is a small risk of bronchospasm with zanamivir as this drug has to be administered by inhalation.

Drugs active against other viruses

Ribavirin

Mechanism of action
The drug is a nucleoside analog, structurally related to guanosine, which requires phosphorylation for activity. Its principal target is IMP dehydrogenase, an enzyme that converts IMP (inosine monophosphate) to XMP (xanthosine 5′-monophosphate) which is a key step in the *de novo* biosynthesis of guanosine triphosphate (GTP). Further mechanisms of action are not entirely understood. It appears to interfere with viral mRNA synthesis both by inhibiting some viral RNA polymerases and by reducing RNA capping efficiency.

Mechanism of resistance
This is not well understood.

Activity range and indications
The drug is active against a wide range of viruses including arena-, flavi-, orthomyxo-, paramyxo-, picorna-, and poxviruses. It is given as inhaled treatment for severe respiratory syncytial virus (RSV) bronchiolitis in infants and children, and as an oral therapy (alongside injected interferon – see below) for chronic hepatitis C infection. It is also effective in Lassa fever if given early enough.

Major side-effects
Ribavirin can cause severe anemia. It is teratogenic and must be avoided in pregnancy.

Interferons (see Chapter 3)

Mechanism of action
Interferons induce an antiviral state by prompting the synthesis of multiple other proteins that inhibit viral replication. The induced enzymes include:

- A dsRNA-dependent protein kinase (PKR) that phosphorylates and inactivates a cellular initiation factor eIF-2α, thus preventing formation of the initiation complex required for viral protein synthesis
- An oligonucleotide synthetase (OAS) that catalyzes the synthesis of a family of oligoadenylates, the binding of which to a latent endonuclease, RNAseL, activates this enzyme to degrade mRNA
- Mx protein guanosine triphosphatases (GTPases) that bind to viral nucleoproteins and prevent their transport to the usual intracellular site at which viral transcription takes place. Mx proteins are induced by α/β interferons but not by γ interferon.

Interferons also mediate indirect antiviral effects through upregulation of MHC antigen expression that enhances the cellular immune response.

Mechanism of resistance

As the mechanisms of antiviral action of interferons are diverse, the mechanisms of resistance must be correspondingly diverse. There is some evidence that certain HCV proteins interact with and inhibit various interferon-induced enzymes.

Activity range and indications

Interferons inhibit the replication of a wide variety of viruses *in vitro* but their clinical utility is relatively limited, not least by the need to give these agents by injection and by their side-effects. α Interferon preparations are used in the treatment of chronic hepatitis B and hepatitis C infections.

Major side-effects

They almost invariably cause influenza-like symptoms. Depression is not uncommon.

Further reading

Brooks GF, Butel JS, Morse SA. *Jawetz, Melnick, & Adelberg's Medical Microbiology*, 23rd edition. New York: McGraw-Hill Medical, 2004

Koonin EV. Virology: Gulliver among the Lilliputians. *Curr Biol* 2005;15(5):R167–R169

The Sanford Guide to Antimicrobial Therapy, 35th edition. Florida: US Biomedical Information Systems, 2005

Timbury MC, McCartney AC, Thakker B, Ward K. *Notes on Medical Microbiology*. London: Churchill Livingstone, 2004

Chapter 6

Basic concepts of the epidemiology of infectious diseases

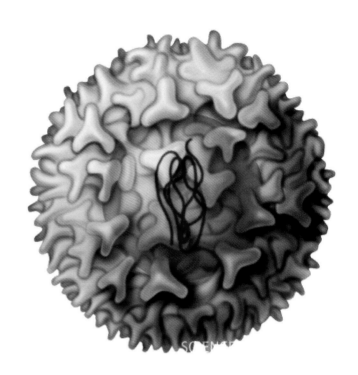

N. Shetty

Definition of an infectious disease
Global burden of infectious disease: six deadly killers
Emerging and resurgent infectious diseases
Why study epidemiology?
Terms used in epidemiology

Natural history of disease
Transmission
Vaccination programs and herd immunity
Investigation of an outbreak
How to investigate an outbreak

The study of epidemiology of infection has undergone major changes since its infancy when it was largely a documentation of epidemics. It has now evolved into a dynamic phenomenon involving the ecology of the infectious agent, the host, reservoirs and vectors, as well as the complex mechanisms concerned in the spread of infection and the extent to which this spread occurs. The understanding of epidemiologic principles has its origins in the study of the great epidemics. Arguably the most powerful example of this is the study of that ancient scourge of mankind, the so-called Black Death or Plague. A study of any of the plague epidemics throughout history has all the factors that govern current epidemiologic analysis: infectious agent, host, vector, reservoir, complex population dynamics including migration, famine, fire and war; resulting in spread followed by quarantine and control.

Definition of an infectious disease

The following definition, though wordy, describes the classic triad of agent (and its reservoir), host, and environment that comprise the complex dynamics of infectious disease:

An infectious disease is defined as an illness due to a specific infectious agent or its toxic product/s that arises through transmission of that agent or its products from an infected person, animal, or reservoir to a susceptible host. It may be transmitted directly or indirectly through an intermediate plant or animal host, vector, or the inanimate environment.

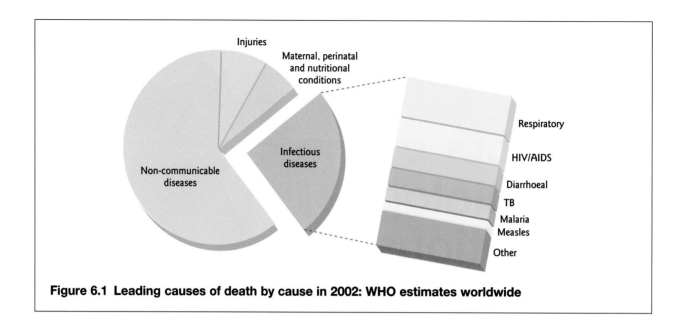

Figure 6.1 Leading causes of death by cause in 2002: WHO estimates worldwide

Global burden of infectious disease: six deadly killers

The World Health Report 1996 – "Fighting disease, fostering development," stated that infectious diseases were the world's leading cause of premature death. Into the millennium infectious diseases still account for more than 25% of deaths (Figure 6.1) and up to 63% of deaths in children under 4 years of age worldwide. In addition new and emerging infections pose a rising global threat.

No more than six deadly infectious diseases – pneumonia, tuberculosis, diarrheal diseases, malaria, measles, and more recently HIV/AIDS – account for half of all premature deaths, killing mostly children and young adults (Figure 6.2).

Emerging and resurgent infectious diseases

Since 1991 resurgent and emerging infectious disease outbreaks have occurred worldwide. In addition many diseases widely believed to be under control, such as cholera, dengue, and diphtheria, have re-emerged in many areas or spread to new regions or populations throughout the world. A growing population and increasing urbanization contribute to emerging infectious disease problems. In many parts of the world, urban population growth has been accompanied by overcrowding, poor hygiene, inadequate sanitation, and unclean drinking water. Urban development has also caused ecologic damage. In these circumstances, certain disease-causing organisms and some of the vectors that transmit them have thrived, making it more likely that people will be infected with new or re-emerging pathogens. The existing public health infrastructure is already overtaxed and ill-prepared to deal with new health threats. Breakdown of public health measures due to civil unrest, war, and the movement of refugees have also contributed to the re-emergence of infectious diseases (Table 6.1). Examples of new and resurgent infections include: Ebola, dengue fever, rift valley fever, diphtheria, cholera, Nipah virus infection, severe acute respiratory syndrome (SARS), and avian influenza.

International travel and commerce have made it possible for pathogens to be quickly transported from one side of the globe to the other (Figure 6.3). The SARS outbreak of 2003 is a typical example. SARS, a viral respiratory illness caused by a coronavirus, called SARS-associated coronavirus (SARS-CoV) was first reported in Asia in February 2003. Over the next few months, the illness spread to more than two dozen countries in North America, South America, Europe, and Asia before the SARS global outbreak of 2003 was contained.

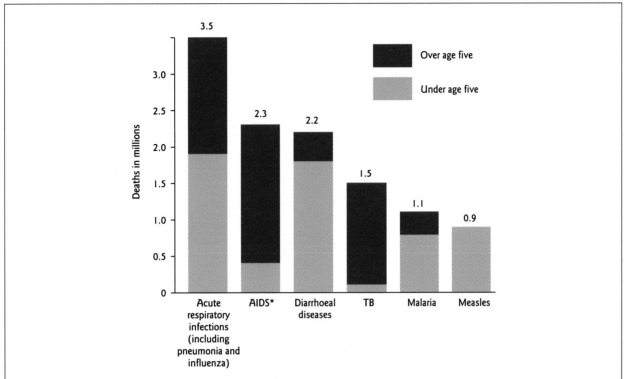

Figure 6.2 Leading infectious killers (millions of deaths, worldwide, all ages, 1998). * HIV-positive people with TB have been included among AIDS deaths. Source: WHO 1998

Table 6.1 Factors in emergence and re-emergence of infectious diseases

Categories	Specific examples
Societal events	Economic impoverishment; war or civil conflict; population growth and migration; urban decay
Healthcare	New medical devices; organ or tissue transplantation; drugs causing immunosuppression; widespread use of antibiotics
Food production	Globalization of food supplies; changes in food processing and packaging
Human behavior	Sexual behavior; drug use; travel; diet; outdoor recreation; use of child care facilities
Environmental changes	Deforestation/reforestation; changes in water ecosystems; flood/drought; famine; global warming
Public health	Curtailment or reduction in prevention programs, infrastructure; inadequate communicable disease surveillance; lack of trained personnel (epidemiologists, laboratory scientists, vector and rodent control specialists)
Microbial adaptation	Changes in virulence and toxin production; development and change of drug resistance; microbes as cofactors in chronic diseases

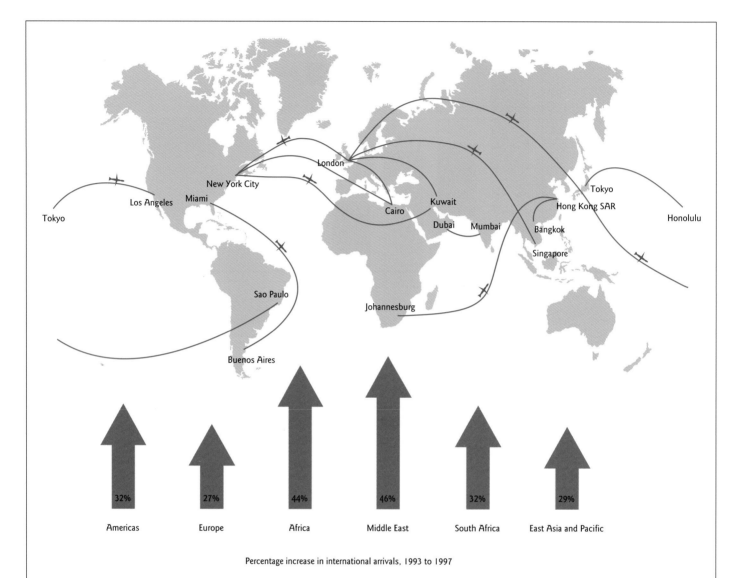

Figure 6.3 is annotated with the following map labels: Tokyo, Los Angeles, Miami, New York City, London, Cairo, Kuwait, Dubai, Mumbai, Hong Kong SAR, Bangkok, Singapore, Tokyo, Honolulu, Sao Paulo, Johannesburg, Buenos Aires.

| Americas | Europe | Africa | Middle East | South Africa | East Asia and Pacific |
| 32% | 27% | 44% | 46% | 32% | 29% |

Percentage increase in international arrivals, 1993 to 1997

Figure 6.3 Most popular air routes between continents, 1997. Sources: World Tourism Organizations and Civil Aviation Organization

Why study epidemiology?

The standard textbook definition of epidemiology is: "The study of the distribution and determinants of disease." Epidemiology is both a field of knowledge and a study of the dynamics of investigating and determining the health status of communities. Therefore epidemiology is both descriptive and analytical as a scientific method.

Major concepts in the epidemiology of infectious diseases are:

- The Epidemiology Triangle or Triad (agent–host–environment)
- Natural History of Disease
- Person–Place–Time approach to investigating outbreaks.

The epidemiology triad will be described along with each of the infectious diseases in detail. This chapter aims to provide the student with a basic understanding of the general concepts of epidemiology as related to infectious diseases.

Terms used in epidemiology

Prevalence is a measure of a disease state in a given population at a particular point in time. It is a measure of *existing cases*. Prevalence data are usually collected initially in order to plan health interventions.

Incidence is a measure of the number of new cases of a particular disease state in a given population at risk during a specified period of time. Incidence data are useful in determining the etiology of disease states.

Mortality and morbidity rates:

    Mortality rate is the annual number of deaths (from a disease or from all causes) per 1000 people.

    Morbidity rate accounts for the number of people who have a disease compared to the total number of people in a population.

    The **infant mortality rate** is a common index that is used to compare the health status of different countries. It is the annual number of deaths of children less than 1 year old per thousand live births.

    Pandemic refers to the worldwide spread and occurrence of a disease.

    Epidemic refers to the presence of disease states at a higher level than normal for the area being described.

    Endemic refers to the constant occurrence of a disease state within a population.

Natural history of disease

Patterns of infection and disease

The progression of an individual from infection to disease and beyond is illustrated in Figure 6.4.

Following entry of an infectious agent into a susceptible host, a period of latency occurs during which there is a rise in the abundance of the infectious agent in the host. The latent period can vary from a few days to many years depending on the infectious agent. In the infectious period there is rapid multiplication of the infectious agent and therefore the greatest risk of transmission. If recovery has followed the host may either have short or long-term immunity, again depending on the nature of the infectious agent.

The host manifests with symptoms during the period of illness (green bar in Figure 6.4). It is important to note that the host can be infectious before he manifests with an illness, i.e. during the incubation period, during the period of illness (symptomatic period), and after symptoms have subsided depending on the infectious agent. There are therefore two factors to consider when addressing the risk of transmission from a potentially infected individual. For the specific infection that you suspect the host to have:

- What is the incubation period?
- What is the period of communicability?

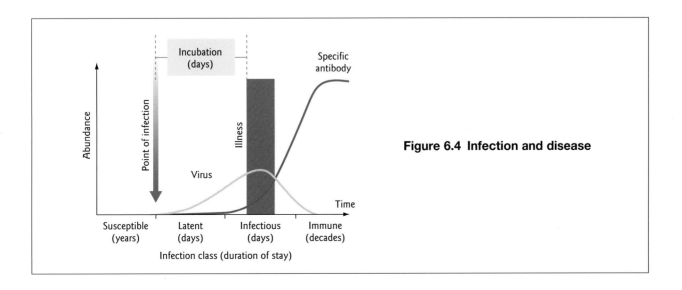

Figure 6.4 Infection and disease

For example, the host infected with HIV is infectious right through the latent and symptomatic periods. In chicken pox the host is infectious only 2–3 days before the period of illness (at the end of the incubation period) and during the illness. An individual remains infectious (to the mosquito – see Chapter 17) after symptoms have subsided when the sexual stages of the organism are present in the peripheral blood, as in malaria. These time periods are critical when advising patients and their contacts about periods of quarantine.

Transmission

The infectiousness of an infective agent is the ease with which it is transmitted to another host and this is closely associated with mode of transmission. As illustrated above, the duration of infectiousness is an important determinant of transmissibility. Virulence is the measure of severity of disease that may result from an infection. Virulence is modulated by the infectious agent to achieve the requisite level of transmissibility. It is not in the interest of the organism to kill off every host it infects, the chain of transmission would be interrupted and the disease would die out.

Transmission of infection can be direct or indirect

Direct – examples are fecal–oral (enteric pathogens and hepatitis A), kissing and droplet spread (Epstein–Barr virus and other upper respiratory tract infections, including diphtheria), sexual (gonorrhoea, chlamydial and trichomonas infections)

Indirect – occurs in a variety of ways:

- Vehicle – food, water (most enteric pathogens are transmitted in this way), needles (spread of HIV, hepatitis B).
- Vector – mechanical (the housefly carries fecally excreted pathogens such as salmonella and shigella and can contaminate food); biological (the mosquito is an essential part of the lifecycle of the malarial parasite).
- Airborne – suspended in the air (varicella zoster virus).

Transmission in infectious diseases is a dynamic process. Therefore infectiousness of a disease in a population depends on:

- Factors unique to the organism:
  - When a case becomes infectious and for how long
  - Probability of transmission given contact between infectious and susceptible person (infectiousness of organism).
- Characteristics of the environment:
  - Type and number of contacts between infectious and susceptible individuals in a population. For an infection that is directly transmitted, there will be many opportunities for effective contact, while for a sexually transmitted infection opportunities are fewer.
- Characteristics of the individuals in the population:
  - Variations in individual behavior, social and cultural factors.

Transmission probability

The continued transmission of an infectious agent in a population is dependent on the number of infective and susceptible individuals present and on the effective contact between these individuals. A critical number of susceptible individuals are required for the continuous transmission of an infectious agent in a population.

If sufficient individuals are immune to a particular infectious agent, the remaining susceptible individuals may be protected by this population characteristic, known as herd immunity.

The rates at which infective contacts occur depend on population size and behavior. Populations do not mix randomly hence complex contact patterns exist. Persistent infections circulate better in small

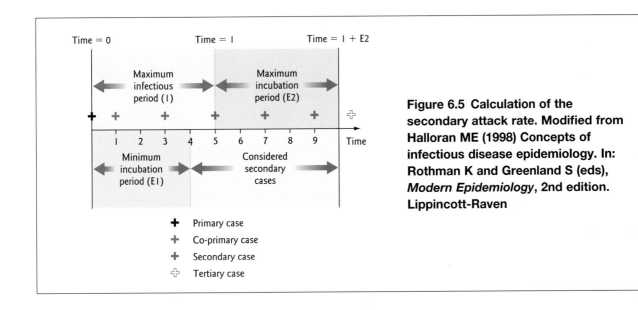

Figure 6.5 Calculation of the secondary attack rate. Modified from Halloran ME (1998) Concepts of infectious disease epidemiology. In: Rothman K and Greenland S (eds), *Modern Epidemiology,* **2nd edition. Lippincott-Raven**

communities as the infection will remain long enough to infect subsequent generations of susceptible individuals.

What type of contact the host makes and with whom has an influence on the transmission of an infectious agent in a population. There is increased transmission of sexually transmitted infections in sex workers; much less than in the general population.

The spread of an infectious disease in a population is therefore dependent on the duration of infectiousness of each case and the transmission probability.

Transmission probability – the probability that a susceptible individual will become infected given contact with an infective source – depends on factors relating to:

- Infective source (case, vector, vehicle)
- Infectious agent
- Susceptible host.

Estimation of transmission probability (Figure 6.5) is achieved by **calculating the secondary attack rate (SAR)** (Box 6.1).

If it is not possible to get accurate numbers of exposed susceptible individuals, all exposed individuals are taken. Since contact increases with overcrowding, SAR is not an absolute measure; it is relative to the conditions in which it was calculated.

If time = 0 (Figure 6.5) is the beginning of the period of infectiousness of the primary case, we plot the minimum incubation period of the disease (E1). Secondary cases as a result of contact with the primary case **(the black +)**, can only occur after E1. If we add the maximum infectious period of the primary case to the maximum incubation period of the secondary case (I + E2), we know that any secondary case (the blue +) should have occurred before this period (between E1 and I + E2). Any cases occurring before this time are called co-primary cases (the red +) and are not included in the numerator or denominator for the calculation

Box 6.1 SAR = number of exposed susceptible individuals who develop disease ÷ total number of exposed susceptible individuals

---

Box 6.2 Assumptions underlying SAR calculations

- That each secondary case is derived from a single primary case
- All cases of successful transmission are symptomatic

- All individuals in the denominator are equally susceptible.

---

of SAR as they are not susceptible to getting infection from the primary case. Cases occurring outside I + E2 are called tertiary cases as they are not as a result of contact with the primary case; they are not included in the numerator of the equation, but they should be included in the denominator as they belong to the susceptible pool of individuals who could have been infected by the primary case. It is important to understand that there are certain basic assumptions that underscore SAR (Box 6.2) calculations, if these assumptions are not met, the calculations may be erroneous.

Another way to measure the spread of infectious disease is to estimate the **basic reproductive rate**, i.e. to calculate the average number of secondary cases produced by each primary case (Box 6.3).

The basic reproduction rate (R_o) is the average number of infective secondary cases produced by each infective case in a totally susceptible population. This can be represented by the number of successful transmissions per case (assuming the entire population is susceptible). R_o is not a constant for a specific agent, rather it reflects the transmission potential of a specific agent within a specific host population and at a specific point in time.

R_o assumes that all contacts are with susceptible persons. Where the population is not totally susceptible, for example some are immune having already contracted and recovered from the infection, transmission will not occur and the average number of secondary cases will be lower. We then calculate the **net reproductive rate (R)** (Box 6.4). R is the average number of secondary infective cases produced by each primary case in a population where some of the individuals are not susceptible. If all individuals mix together at random, so that infectious cases are likely to make contact with susceptible as well as immune individuals, then R is the product of R_o times the proportion of the population that are susceptible (x).

Box 6.3 Basic reproductive rate (R_o)

R_o = average number of new infective cases produced by each infective case in a totally susceptible population

$R_o = c \times p \times d$

Where:

c = number of contacts per unit time
d = duration of infectiousness of the case
p = transmission probability

Box 6.4 Net reproductive rate (R)

Where not all the individuals are susceptible:

$R = R_o \times$ the proportion that are susceptible (x)
$R = R_o x$
$R_o = R/x$

Seroprevalence (prevalence of specific antibody in population studies) is one way of establishing susceptibility

If $R_o = 10$ and the proportion of susceptible persons in a population is 80%, then $R = 10 \times 0.8 = 8$. So every infectious case will produce 8 new cases in such a population. If the disease is endemic, where the average incidence and prevalence of the infection is stable, $R = 1$; i.e. each primary case leads to one new case:

As $R = R_o x$
$1 = R_o x$
or $R_o = 1/x$

In these circumstances, R_o is equal to the reciprocal of the population susceptible to the disease.
Where seroprevalence surveys are not possible:

- If disease is endemic ($R = 1$) that so each case leads to one new case, and
- If the population is stable; births balancing deaths, and
- If the disease results in life long immunity, and
- If no one in the population is vaccinated.

In these circumstances, one can calculate

$x = a/L$ or $R_o = L/a$

where: x = proportion of susceptible individuals in the population; L = average life expectancy; a = average age of infection (e.g. measles on average occurs at 5 years of age).

Uses of reproduction rates

The reproduction rate is a central concept in infectious disease epidemiology. It provides a measure of the way an infectious agent may spread within a population. It can be used to predict the success of public health interventions on the transmission of an infectious agent in a population.

It is important to understand that these calculations assume that transmissibility is constant (that there are no super spreaders within the community) and that there is random and homogeneous mixing within the population. It is worth noting that in reality communities seldom mix homogeneously, people tend to cluster within their own groups and this can have a significant impact on transmission within a community.

Vaccination programs and herd immunity

Mass vaccination programs can reduce transmission of infection by reducing the proportion of susceptible individuals within a population (x) and increasing the proportion of the immune ($1 - x$).

The term **herd immunity (HI)** is used when an individual, though not vaccinated, is protected because everyone around him/her is immune. Vaccination reduces the proportion of susceptible individuals who may acquire infection and pose as a transmission risk to other susceptible hosts. The higher the herd immunity the less likely an infected case is to make contact with another susceptible host and transmit infection. At a certain threshold called the **herd immunity threshold (HIT)** each case will only be able to transmit the infection to one other case.

Herd immunity threshold (Box 6.5) is thus the proportion of the population that needs to be immune ($1 - x$) for the disease to become stable, or for R to equal 1.

We can therefore use the information on R_o to estimate the proportion of the population that will have to be immune to ensure that the disease becomes stable.

This calculation is useful for disease control or eradication programs.

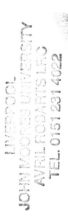

Box 6.5 Herd immunity threshold (HIT)

We can calculate HIT if we know the R_0 for the disease in that population:

Given that $R = R_0 x$ and $HI = (1 - x)$

$x = R/R_0$

Where $R = 1$ at threshold: $HIT = 1 - (1/R_0)$

$HIT = R_0 - 1/R_0$

Investigation of an outbreak

Concept of risk refers to the probability an event will occur within a specified time period.

Person, **place**, and **time** are three factors central to analyzing epidemiologic data.

The **person** refers to the characteristics of the people affected by illness. Commonly used characteristics are gender, age, occupation, and other socioeconomic factors such as income and education levels.

Place refers to the geographical distribution of disease states.

Time refers to the changes over time (temporal clustering) in disease states and includes such factors as clustering of cases within a definite time span.

Besides the well defined outbreak that occurs in a definite time period, temporal clustering can be seasonal or cyclical. Seasonality implies that disease occurrence is related to changes in climate. Reasons for seasonal variation of infections could be related to temperature, humidity, vector density, migration, or population behavioral patterns. For example, meningitis is common in the winter in temperate regions, and during the dry season in the tropics. In the tropics malaria increases sharply during the wet season; stagnant water is the breeding ground for the anopheles mosquito. Outbreaks of shigella dysentery occur during the wet season, and are related to an increasing fly population.

Cyclic changes in disease occurrence may be related to a number of events that are related to periodicity: market visits, seasonal migration patterns for labor, and school terms. An increase in measles is seen every 2 years and is related to an increase in the pool of susceptible newborn babies who lack immunity.

How to investigate an outbreak

In investigating an outbreak, speed is essential, however valuable information may be lost if the investigation is not methodical. Health professionals have devised a systematic approach using 10 important steps. (Box 6.6).

These steps are not necessarily in order, several steps may overlap. For example, control measures that intervene to curb spread should be implemented as soon as possible and may be the first task to be performed.

Box 6.6 Outbreak investigation in 10 easy (!) steps

1. Background information
2. Establish the existence of an outbreak
3. Define and identify cases
4. Collect preliminary data
5. Describe and orient the data in terms of time, place, and person
6. Formulate a provisional hypothesis
7. Evaluate hypothesis
8. Refine hypothesis and carry out additional studies
9. Recommend and/or implement interventions and control measures
10. Communicate findings

Step 1: Background information

This includes gathering information on clinical presentation of the disease, diagnostic tests; ascertaining incubation period, and period of communicability. It also involves preliminary study into the main transmission routes, the most vulnerable in the population, and the occurrence of previous outbreaks of the same nature in the area.

Step 2: Establish the existence of an outbreak

One of the first tasks as a field investigator is to verify that a suspected outbreak is indeed a real outbreak. We do this by determining whether the observed number of cases exceeds the expected number for the area in the given time frame.

Depending on the sources of data this is done by comparing the current number of cases with the number from the previous few weeks or months, or from a comparable period during the previous few years. If this is not available, we can use estimates using data from neighboring states or national data.

Step 3: Define and identify cases

To do this we need to develop a case definition and verify the diagnosis. An ideal case definition should be sensitive enough to identify most of the actual cases and specific enough to avoid too many false positives.

This is achieved by reviewing the clinical findings within the time period and within the geographic area. A confirmatory laboratory result will sharpen the case definition. To this we may be able to add an epidemiologic focus such as a particular food or water source. Remember case definitions may evolve and become more focused as the investigation progresses. If there are discrepancies between clinical features and laboratory results these need to be checked again.

Keep it objective and simple: for example you could define a case as three or more loose bowel movements per day, among those who went to a restaurant, over the weekend. This definition uses a clinical feature set to a particular geographic venue within a specific time period. And most importantly use it consistently.

Step 4: Collect preliminary data

Cast the net wide to determine the true size and geographic limits of the outbreak. Use appropriate data gathering instruments: telephone interviews, letters, health records, the media, and house to house field workers. Develop a suitable questionnaire that can be used easily and is unambiguous.

Regardless of the particular disease you are investigating, you should collect the following types of information about every person affected:

- **Identifying information:** This may include name, address, and telephone number. Addresses and post codes allow you to map the geographic extent of the problem.
- **Demographic information:** This may include age, sex, race, and occupation and provides the details that you need to characterize the population at risk.
- **Clinical information:** This information allows you to verify that the case definition has been met. Date of onset allows you to create a graph of the outbreak. Laboratory findings, immunization status, and outcome may supplement this section.
- **Risk factor information:** Information about risk factors will help focus the investigation to the probable cause of the outbreak. For example, in an investigation of gastroenteritis, you would look at exposure to food and eating places.

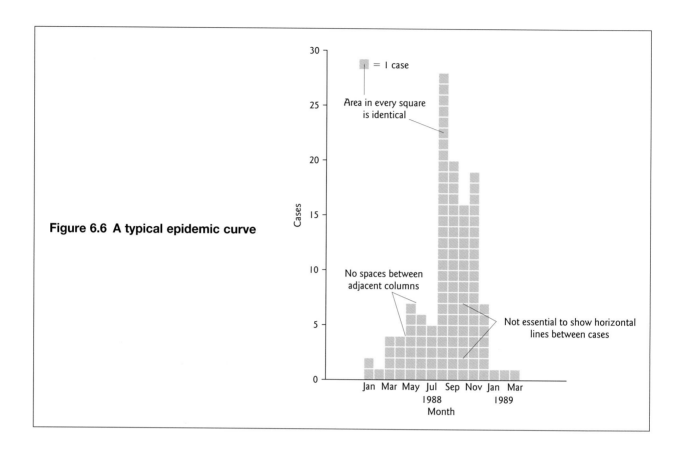

Figure 6.6 A typical epidemic curve

Step 5: Describe and orient the data in terms of time, place, and person

This is the most exciting part of the investigation, as the mystery begins to unravel. It is also the most critical. This process is often referred to as **Descriptive Epidemiology**.

Characterize in terms of time

To visualize the magnitude and time course of an epidemic we draw a histogram (Figure 6.6) of the number of cases (on the *y* axis) by their date/hour of onset (on the *x* axis).

This graph, called an **epidemic curve**, can help establish:

• The type of outbreak
• The time of exposure when the incubation period is known
• The incubation period when the time of exposure is known.

Using an epidemic curve to establish type of outbreak

Look at its overall shape. Figure 6.7 describes a **point source outbreak**. Here the cases are clustered tightly around a single peak. There is a sharp up slope and a trailing down slope. This indicates that they were probably infected from the same source at the same time. The spread of cases around the peak reflects the variation in incubation periods between cases.

Sometimes a point **source outbreak** produces a number of infected individuals who may serve as sources of infection to others. **Secondary cases therefore occur as person–person transmissions** and may appear as an individual wave following a point source by one incubation period (Figure 6.8).

Continuing or extended common source outbreaks may arise from common sources and continue over time (Figure 6.9). The epidemic curve will rise sharply as with a point source. Because of continuing

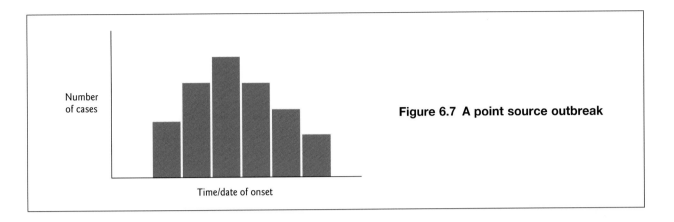

Figure 6.7 A point source outbreak

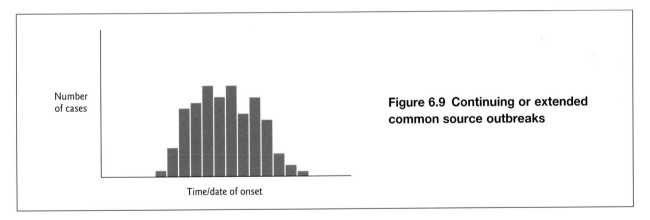

Figure 6.8 A point source outbreak with secondary cases

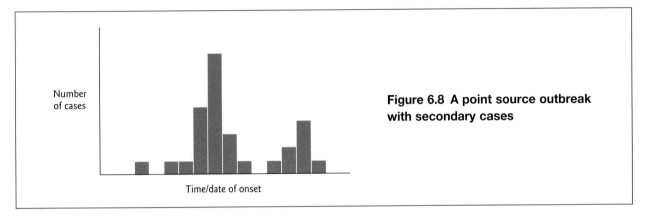

Figure 6.9 Continuing or extended common source outbreaks

exposure to the common source, rather than rise to a peak, this type of epidemic curve will plateau. The down slope may be precipitous if the common source is removed or gradual if it exhausts itself. A good example is when a contaminated public water supply becomes a source of infection and stays a source until it is discovered and shut off.

The **propagated** pattern arises with agents that are communicable between persons either directly or through an intermediate vehicle (Figure 6.10). This pattern has four principal characteristics: (i) it encompasses several clusters of cases occurring in distinct generations; (ii) it often begins with a small number of cases and rises with a gradually increasing upslope; (iii) with time distinct peaks of clusters disappear because generations of cases overlap, the last few cases of one generation overlap with the first few of the next generation; and (iv) after the outbreak peaks, the exhaustion of susceptible hosts usually results in a rapid down slope.

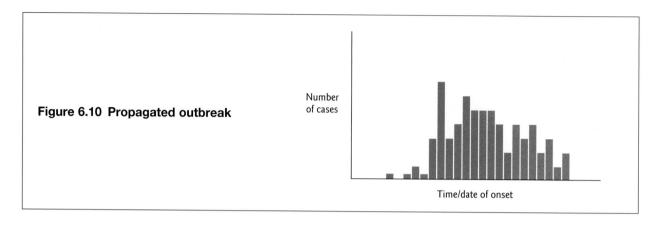

Figure 6.10 Propagated outbreak

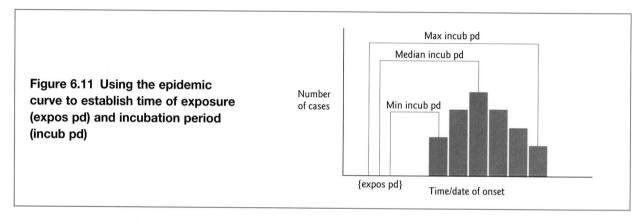

Figure 6.11 Using the epidemic curve to establish time of exposure (expos pd) and incubation period (incub pd)

Using the epidemic curve to establish time of exposure and incubation period

In a point source outbreak of a known disease with a known incubation period, the epidemic curve can be used to identify the most likely time period of exposures to the agent (Figure 6.11). This is critical to asking the right questions to identify the source of the epidemic.

To do this:

- Identify the peak of the outbreak (or the median case) and count back on the *x* axis the number of days constituting the median or average incubation period of the infectious agent.
- Start at the last case and count backwards the number of days constituting the maximum incubation period.
- From the earliest case count backwards the number of days that constitute the minimum incubation period.

Conversely, if you knew the time of exposure you could calculate incubation period ranges for the putative agent and that would help in understanding the pattern of spread of an unidentified agent in an outbreak.

Characterize in terms of place

Assessment of an outbreak by place provides information on the geographic extent of an outbreak and may also show clusters or patterns that provide clues as to the source of the problem. A simple and useful technique for looking at geographic patterns is to plot the location of each case, on a "spot map" of the area.

A spot map of cases in a community may show clusters or patterns that reflect water supplies, wind currents, or proximity to a food outlet.

Characterize in terms of person

This exercise helps describe the populations that are at risk for the disease. We usually define such populations by personal characteristics (e.g. age, ethnic origin, and sex) or by exposures (e.g. occupation, leisure activities, use of medications, tobacco, drugs). These factors are important because they may be related to susceptibility to the disease and to opportunities for exposure. Other characteristics will be more specific to the disease under investigation and the setting of the outbreak.

Step 6: Formulate a provisional hypothesis

At this point in an investigation, we have interviewed affected people, spoken with other health officials in the community, and characterized the outbreak by time, place, and person. It is time to formulate a hypothesis. The hypotheses should address the source of the agent, the mode (vehicle or vector) of transmission, and the exposures that caused the disease. Also, the hypotheses should be proposed in a way that can be tested. Descriptive epidemiology often provides the first clues to developing a hypothesis.

Step 7: Evaluate the hypothesis

The next step is to formally test the credibility of our hypothesis. This is usually done by conducting an **analytical epidemiologic** study using the data collected.

There are two approaches to analytical studies; both use comparison groups to compare exposures and disease outcomes. They are **cohort studies** and **case control studies**. Cohort studies compare groups of people who have been exposed to suspected risk factors with groups who have not been exposed. Case control studies compare people with a disease (cases/patients with an outcome) with a group of people without the disease (controls). The nature of the outbreak determines which of these studies you will use.

Cohort studies

A cohort study is the study design of choice for investigating an outbreak in a small, localized community where it is feasible to collect information on the entire population. For example, we would use a cohort study if an outbreak of gastroenteritis (GE) occurred among people at a conference, or among those attending a social function such as a wedding. In this situation, we would be able to ask every member of the party, the same set of questions about potential exposures (e.g. what foods and beverages they had consumed during the event) and whether they had become ill with gastroenteritis.

With this information we would be able to calculate an attack rate for people who ate or were exposed to a particular item (say shrimp cocktail) and an attack rate for those who did not eat that item (were not exposed). This is done for all possible items on the menu:

$$\text{Attack rate for those who ate the shrimp cocktail} = \frac{\text{No. of GE cases who ate the shrimp cocktail}}{\text{Total no. of persons who ate the same item}}$$

$$\text{Attack rate for those who } \textbf{did not eat} \text{ the shrimp cocktail} = \frac{\text{No. of GE cases who } \textbf{did not eat} \text{ shrimp cocktail}}{\text{Total no. of persons who } \textbf{did not eat} \text{ the same item}}$$

$$\text{Then calculate the relative risk} = \frac{\text{Attack rate in those who ate the shrimp cocktail}}{\text{Attack rate in those who did } \textbf{not eat} \text{ the shrimp cocktail}}$$

Case control studies

In most outbreaks the population at risk is not well defined or too large and cohort studies are not feasible. In these instances, we would conduct a case control study. As with all case control studies the most important decision is whom do we select as the control group. Controls should not obviously suffer the disease or else they would be cases, however they should have come from the same population that produced the cases. Depending on the number of cases we may need to interview one or more controls per case.

To find an association between exposure and outcome in a case control study, we cannot calculate attack rates because we do not know the total number of people in the community who were or were not exposed to the exposure in question.

Instead the measure we use is called the odds ratio. The easiest way to do this is to tabulate the data using a 2 × 2 table (see table immediately below). For example, if we were investigating an outbreak of typhoid in a small town, and we suspected that the source was a local delicatessen, we would question the cases brought to our notice and controls from the same neighborhood about whether they had shopped at the delicatessen. The 2 × 2 table should have the following information:

		Cases	Controls	Total
Shopped at delicatessen?	Yes	a = 26	b = 48	74
	No	c = 12	d = 76	88
Total:		38	124	162

The odds ratio is calculated as:

odds of disease in the "yes" group (a/b) ÷ odds of disease in the "no" group (c/d)

The odds ratio for the delicatessen is (a/b) ÷ (c/d)

In this case the odds ratio for developing infection after shopping at the "deli" is:

(26/48) ÷ (12/76) = 3.43

This means that people who shopped at the "deli" were three times more likely to get typhoid than were people who did not shop there. Even so, we could not conclude that the "deli" was the source without comparing its odds ratio with the odds ratios for other possible sources. It could be that the source is elsewhere and that it just so happens that many of the people who were exposed also shopped at the deli.

This method therefore does not prove that a particular exposure caused the disease; however, it is a very useful method for evaluating possible sources of disease. Odds ratios are usually expressed together with 95% confidence intervals and probability (P) values; indicating whether they are significantly different from an odds ratio of 1.

Step 8: Refine hypothesis and carry out additional studies

When analytical epidemiologic studies do not confirm the hypothesis, we need to reconsider our hypothesis and look for new vehicles or modes of transmission. Laboratory and environmental studies provide evidence for a source of an outbreak. They may also be able to tell us how the contamination occurred.

Step 9: Recommend and/or implement interventions and control measures

Control measures and interventions should be implemented as early as possible in the investigation to protect susceptible members of the population. This may involve withdrawing a food article from the shops, disconnecting a water source, or closing a food outlet if suspicions are high. If the source of an outbreak has been identified, interventions are aimed at specific links in the chain of infection, the agent, the source, or the reservoir. Patient management and containment is important to prevent secondary transmissions. Contact tracing and administration of prophylaxis, whether by medications or vaccinations, are vital components of any control strategy. An outbreak investigation usually prompts ongoing surveillance.

Step 10: Communicate findings

The final task in an outbreak investigation is to communicate findings to all those who may need to know. This may take the form of oral presentations and updates at regular incident control meetings and to health authorities; a written report or a publication in a scientific journal.

A written report or publication serves as a document for potential legal issues, and is a reference facility if other workers encounter a similar situation in the future. A scientific publication also serves the broader purpose of contributing to the knowledge base of epidemiology and public health.

Test yourself

Use what you have learnt to solve these epidemiology problems.

Case study 6.1
A case of chickenpox occurred among children in a nursery school. A total of 20 children attended the school and they were all aged 3–5 years. Two weeks later there were two more cases among the children. Before the outbreak none of the children had any previous exposure to chickenpox and childhood vaccination was not offered in this region. The illness proved difficult to control because the children mixed freely so that all children had contact with the cases in the days before they became ill.

The incubation period for chickenpox is estimated to be 15 days (range 8–21 days), and the infectious period is estimated to be from 2 days before onset of symptoms until ~5 days after onset (7 days in total). Once symptomatic no child attended the nursery.

1. From the list below identify which pieces of information you would need to use in order to directly calculate the secondary attack rate (SAR). Mark all that apply:
   A Exact time of onset of each case
   B Exact time of resolution of each case
   C Number of susceptible people exposed to infection
   D Minimum incubation period
   E Maximum incubation period
   F Minimum infectious period
   G Maximum infectious period
   H Probability of transmission of infection.
2. Calculate the secondary attack rate and list three assumptions for its calculation here.
3. For the following statement state True or False and justify your answer: In the calculation of the secondary attack rate in general, both the co-primary and tertiary cases are excluded from the denominator of the equation.
4. Give a definition of the basic reproduction and net reproduction rates. How do they relate to each other at the start of the epidemic in this nursery?
5. If some of the children in the nursery had been vaccinated previously for chickenpox, how would this affect the SAR and the reproduction rate?

Staff at the nursery are worried and would like to know if there will be any more cases after the most recent case. A child became ill with chickenpox on the May 25th, and was sent home, but was at the nursery on the May 23rd and 24th. There were 17 other children who also attended the nursery on those days, including one who had already had chickenpox and 16 who had never had it. The probability of transmission of infection is 0.7 for someone in contact with a case during the whole of their period of infectivity.

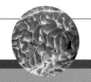

6. Do you think there will be any other cases of chickenpox among these children within the following 2 weeks? If so, how many would you expect?

Case study 6.2
A large gastroenteritis outbreak occurred in staff and children of several nurseries in July 2003 following a party which they all attended. The food was prepared by external caterers and also by staff and parents. The outbreak was notable for the rapid onset of a severe but brief illness, characterized by vomiting in over 70% of cases and diarrhea in over 60%. The primary attack rate was 68%.

1. Use the following data to plot the epidemic curve. What type of outbreak was this? Justify your answer.

	Time since party (12 hour intervals)						
	12–18 hours	18–24 hours	24–30 hours	30–36 hours	36–42 hours	42–48 hours	48–54 hours
New cases reported	2	10	19	22	8	2	0

2. What are the minimum, maximum, and median incubation periods?

Case study 6.3
In a recent outbreak, 80 cases of Chagas disease (South American trypanosomiasis) were detected in a population of 800 people. The following data were collected by questionnaire of the whole population to test whether a range of activities were risk factors for Chagas disease.

Activity	Number with disease	Number without disease	Total undertaking activity in last 6 months
Working in fields	68	590	658
Owning pigs	10	137	147
Washing clothes in the river	15	95	110
Collecting firewood	41	179	220
Owning cattle	24	183	207
Living in a mud hut	27	51	78
All	80	720	800

1. Calculate BOTH the risk and relative risk associated with each activity. On the basis of these results, which activities do you consider to be the most likely risk factors for Chagas disease?

Test yourself

2. All 80 cases were detected using microscopy. During the outbreak a cheaper and quicker novel diagnostic test was used on the 800 population. This novel test had a sensitivity and specificity of 75% and 95% respectively. Use this information to complete a standard 2 × 2 table and then calculate the positive predictive value and negative predictive value.

3. Given that Chagas disease can lead to serious complications if not treated, do you recommend replacing microscopy with the new diagnostic test for determining whether to treat?

Case study 6.4

Following a wedding lunch at a local restaurant, over a third of the guests suffered with diarrhea. A questionnaire survey of all guests showed the following relationships between choice of food eaten at the party and whether or not a guest got diarrhea.

Food eaten	Guests with diarrhea (total = 111)	Guests without diarrhea (total = 188)
Prawns	65	72
Liver pâté	37	44
Pasta and cheese salad	51	79
Chicken and rice	93	162
Green salad	95	37
Chocolate cake	37	82
Mango mousse	8	5

1. Calculate BOTH the risk and relative risk associated with each food type eaten. On the basis of these results, which food do you consider to be the most likely cause of this outbreak?

Further reading

Armstrong BK, White E, Saracci R. *Principles of Exposure Measurement in Epidemiology*. New York: Oxford University Press, 1992

Webber R. *Communicable Disease Epidemiology and Control: A Global Perspective*, 2nd edition. MA: CABI Publishing, 2005

Useful websites

Centers for Disease Control and Prevention. Epidemiologic Case Studies. http://www2a.cdc.gov/epicasestudies/dwnload_case.htm

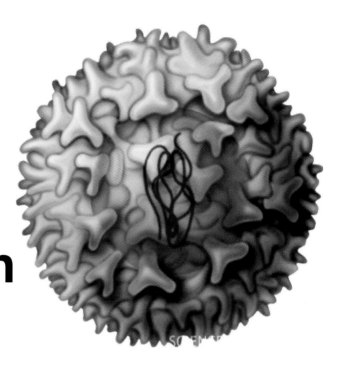

Part 2

A systems based approach to infectious diseases

Chapter 7
Infections of the skin, soft tissue, bone, and joint

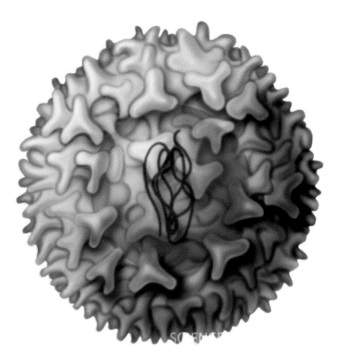

N. Shetty, J.W. Tang

Bacterial infections
  Impetigo, cellulitis, and necrotizing fasciitis
  Folliculitis/abscesses/furuncle/carbuncle
  Toxin associated conditions
  Osteomyelitis
  Septic arthritis
  Hospital acquired infections of skin, soft tissue, bone, and joint
Pathogenesis and virulence of bacterial infections
  Streptococcus pyogenes
  Staphylococcus aureus and coagulase negative staphylococci
  Clostridium species
  Corynebacterium diphtheriae

Viral infections
  Macular and maculopapular rash
  Vesicular lesions
  Hyperplastic lesions
Fungal infections
  The dermatophytes
  Fungal infections involving cutaneous and deeper tissues
  Cutaneous manifestations of systemic fungal disease
Parasitic infections
  Cutaneous leishmaniasis
  Larva migrans and larva currens
  Myiasis
  Scabies

The intact skin is our primary barrier against potential pathogens and most organisms are unable to cross it. The innate defense mechanism of the skin is alluded to in Chapter 3. Many infectious agents require some breach in the skin such as an abrasion or an insect bite before infection can be established. Breaches of the skin by intravascular catheters are an important source of healthcare associated skin infections. Dermatophytic fungi cause a variety of skin infections without a breach in the skin but do not cause more invasive disease because they prefer temperatures below body temperature of 37°C. Sweat glands and sebaceous glands are potential points of entry for *Staphylococcus aureus* which commonly infects the hair follicle and survives despite the protective secretions of sweat and sebum.

Box 7.1 Skin infection at the site of an insect bite

A 5-year-old child returned from holiday and presented to the doctor with red crusted lesions on her arms. Her mother said the child was bitten by mosquitoes while on holiday, leading to severe itching at the bite sites. On examination the lesions were yellow and crusted in the center with surrounding redness. There was no fever and the child was otherwise well. A Gram stain of a swab taken from the lesion showed numerous neutrophils and Gram positive cocci in chains and clusters. Read on and discover how the major causes of skin infection inflict damage, then try and answer these questions:

❓What is the most likely diagnosis?
❓What are the most likely organisms implicated?
❓What is the pathophysiology?

Bacterial infections

The major bacterial etiologic agents for infections of the skin, soft tissue, bone and joint are the Gram positive cocci. Deep infections are often preceded by superficial skin infections (bacterial and fungal) and strategies for diagnosis and management have several common threads (Box 7.1).

Impetigo, cellulitis, and necrotizing fasciitis

Impetigo is a common infection of the superficial layers of the skin and occurs frequently in children. Impetigo often manifests as a dual infection caused by the S. aureus and group A beta-hemolytic streptococci (GABHS, also known as *Streptococcus pyogenes*); even though either organism can cause impetigo on its own. Methicillin-resistant S. aureus (MRSA) acquired either in hospital or in the community is also associated with impetigo. If the patient is infected with community acquired MRSA, it like other methicillin sensitive strains of S. aureus may have the virulence factor Panton-Valentine leukocidin (PVC), which is associated with more purulent and necrotizing skin lesions.

Approximately 30% of the population is colonized in the anterior nares with S. aureus. Colonization of the axillae, groin, and hairline also occurs. Some individuals colonized by S. aureus experience recurrent episodes of impetigo on the nose and lip. Individuals who are permanent carriers serve as reservoirs of the infection for other people. Patients with atopic dermatitis or other inflammatory skin conditions are also likely to be colonized with S. aureus.

While impetigo can manifest as a primary infection of unbroken skin, the patient often gives a history of minor trauma such as cuts and abrasions or insect bites associated with itching. A more serious and generalized form of impetigo is associated with pre-existing skin disease such as eczema or superinfection of chickenpox lesions.

There are two clinical presentations of impetigo: the bullous and nonbullous forms. Bullous impetigo is less common than the nonbullous form and presents as superficial, fragile bullae on the trunk and the extremities (Figure 7.1). Often, only the remnants of ruptured bullae are seen at the time of presentation. The separation of the epidermis is due to an exfoliative exotoxin produced by staphylococci.

Nonbullous forms are more often associated with dual infections caused by S. pyogenes and S. aureus. The lesions initially appear as a single 2–4 mm erythematous macule that rapidly evolves into a vesicle or a pustule. The typical lesions of impetigo are crusted and vesicular (Figure 7.2). The vesicle is fragile and ruptures early, leaving a crusted yellow colored exudate of pus over the superficial erosion. Itching is frequent. Satellite impetigo lesions may develop along scratch lines spreading to contiguous and distal areas through direct inoculation. Transient lymphadenitis occurs, and significant regional lymphadenopathy is characteristic of streptococcal impetigo. Secondary infection of skin conditions, such as eczema and seborrheic dermatitis, results in the development of confluent, purulent, crusted lesions with concomitant lymphatic

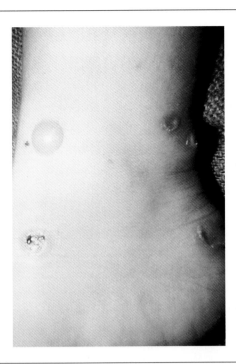

Figure 7.1 Bullous impetigo of the lower limb

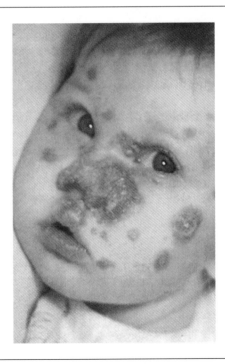

Figure 7.2 Nonbullous impetigo of the face

involvement. Impetigo rarely progresses to systemic infection and the patient may remain systemically well, although poststreptococcal glomerulonephritis is a rare complication of skin infections with *S. pyogenes*.

Ecthyma and hydradenitis is a deeper, ulcerated impetigo infection associated with lymphadenitis.

Cellulitis manifests as a spreading inflammation of the skin and subcutaneous tissues and is associated with local pain, tenderness, swelling, and erythema (Figure 7.3). Patients are often systemically unwell and present with fever, chills, and malaise. Streptococcal bacteremia is not uncommon. People who use intravenous drugs are particularly at risk of developing severe streptococcal cellulitis.

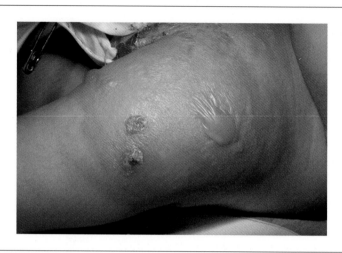

Figure 7.3 Severe spreading cellulitis. Note fluid-filled blebs

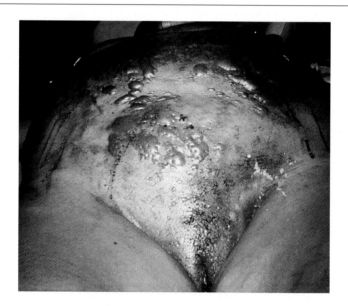

Figure 7.4 Necrotizing fasciitis. Note dusky purple changes on the skin indicating deep necrosis. Reprinted from H.P. Lambert and W.E. Farrar (1982) *Slide Atlas of Infectious Diseases*, **Gower Medical Publishing Ltd. Reproduced with permission of Elsevier.**

Meleney first described streptococcal gangrene in 1924. Now known as necrotizing fasciitis, it is the most rapidly invasive and serious form of infection with *S. pyogenes*. It may arise following minor trauma or from hematogenous spread of the organism from the throat to the site of a wound. Initially, the lesion appears as mild cellulitis, and progresses rapidly to become dusky purple with bullae containing hemorrhagic fluid (Figure 7.4). Rapid necrosis and gangrene of subcutaneous tissue, fat, fascia, and muscle results in a life-threatening systemic illness requiring immediate surgical debridement of all necrotic tissue, intensive care, and high doses of appropriate antibiotics (Box 7.2).

Folliculitis/abscesses/furuncle/carbuncle

Most skin and subcutaneous infections that present as abscesses or well delineated collections of pus are caused by *S. aureus*. The commonest and mildest form is often referred to as a folliculitis, an infection of a hair root (follicle) that produces a slightly painful, tiny white pimple at the base of a hair. Larger staphylococcal skin abscesses (boils, furuncles) are painful collections of pus in the skin or subcutaneous

Box 7.2 Flesh-eating bacteria ate my leg – rare infection apparently spread through a minor cut (Andover, Massachusetts, March 24, 2006)

Public health officials from CDC are investigating the case of a 38-year-old Andover school teacher who is critically ill after a school trip to the local museum.

Barbara Stone, a certified special needs teacher, works at Andover High in Massachusetts. According to investigators, she jammed her toe in the door of the school bus. By the next day, her entire leg was red, hot, swollen, and exquisitely painful.

Stone went to St Joseph's Hospital in Lowell, where doctors gave her local ointments and dressings and sent her home and advised her to take tylenol if the pain became worse. She spent a restless and feverish night. Her husband, Chuck, called the ambulance when she became drowsy and disorientated. At the hospital doctors found that the redness and swelling had spread up to mid-calf. When the dressings were removed Chuck saw the entire foot had gone a dusky purple with blebs of fluid around her toes and ankle.

At St Josephs the surgeons were called in to review and they knew exactly what they were looking at.

"The entire leg, below the knee looks bad," they said to Chuck. "She needs immediate surgery, we may have to amputate her leg. If we don't act soon she may die. Barbara is in shock. All the toxins that the bacterium secretes have entered and poisoned her blood."

Barbara is now in critical care after an amputation that has removed the leg below the knee.

Editorial note: Flesh-eating disease . . . it sounds like a science fiction horror story. *Streptococcus pyogenes* can spread through human tissue at a rate of 3 centimeters per hour. Twenty-five percent of its victims die, and in severe cases the patient is dead within 18 hours. In 1990 it caused the death of Jim Henson, the creator of the Muppets.

The scientific name for this disease is necrotizing fasciitis and it is caused by a bacterium called *S. pyogenes*, or Group A streptococcus (GAS). It is the same bug that causes strep. throat but is much more aggressive.

Each year in the United States, there are 10 million strep. infections. Only about 1000 develop into the flesh-eating condition. According to Centers for Disease Control, it is fatal in about 20% of cases.

tissue. When small furuncles coalesce they form a larger lesion called a carbuncle (Figure 7.5). Multiple points of exit may form and drain pus spontaneously. The lesion is often accompanied by generalized systemic illness including fever, malaise, or rigors. Carbuncles are more common in men and usually occur on the back of the neck. Recurrent folliculitis, furuncles, and carbuncles are associated with diabetes. Those

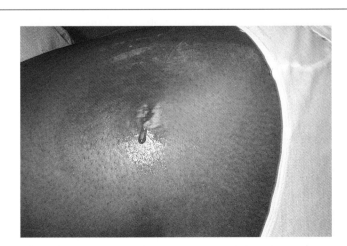

Figure 7.5 Carbuncle

individuals who use intravenous recreational drugs are also prone to recurrent staphylococcal infections, mainly due to poor injection technique.

Staphylococcal breast infections (mastitis) and abscesses typically develop 1–4 weeks after delivery in a lactating mother. The infection is transmitted from the colonized baby (who might also have a staphylococcal umbilical infection) to the mammary glands via cracked nipples (see Chapter 12).

Toxin associated conditions

Erysipelas is an acute, toxin associated condition caused by *S. pyogenes*. The condition usually occurs in children and the elderly. The portal of entry is the skin or outer mucous membrane. Erysipelas is characterized by a typical lesion: a raised, demarcated, bright red area of dermal and subcutaneous inflammation which advances as the disease progresses (Figure 7.6). There may be fluid-filled bullae at the site of the lesion. It is often found affecting the face and orbit; the lesion can be found on the extremities as well. Lymphatic involvement is common.

Scarlet fever occurs because of pyrogenic exotoxin (erythrogenic toxin) released by *S. pyogenes*. The disease is associated with a characteristic fine reticular rash that is diffuse and blanches on pressure. Though diffuse the rash does not involve the palms, soles, and face. Typically the face appears flushed with circumoral pallor. The tongue may be covered with a whitish coating initially; it later develops a florid red color often described as "strawberry tongue" (Figure 7.7). The skin rash fades in a week and is followed by extensive desquamation that lasts for several weeks.

Streptococcal toxic shock is a complication of invasive streptococcal disease. *S. pyogenes* bacteremia, associated with a widespread erythematous rash, early onset of shock, and organ failure, is the classic presentation of streptococcal toxic shock syndrome. These patients usually develop renal failure, acute respiratory distress syndrome, hepatic dysfunction, and a diffuse capillary leak syndrome.

Staphylococcal toxic shock syndrome (TSS) is a toxin mediated syndrome characterized by fever, rash, hypotension, constitutional symptoms, and multi-organ involvement. Almost every organ system can be involved, including the cardiovascular, renal, skin, mucosa, gastrointestinal, musculoskeletal, hepatic, hematologic, and central nervous systems. Todd first described it in 1978 in children, aged 8–17 years, with *S. aureus* infection. In 1981 an epidemic of TSS was associated with tampon use in healthy menstruating

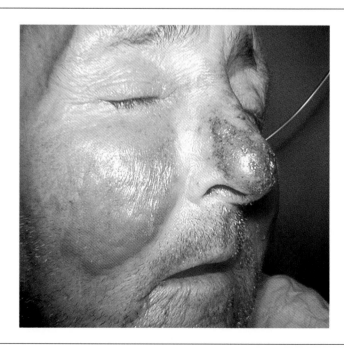

Figure 7.6 Erysipelas. Provided by Dr Thomas F. Sellers. Courtesy of the Centers for Disease Control and Prevention; from CDC website: http://phil.cdc.gov/phil/details.asp

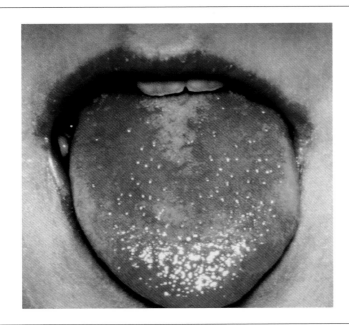

Figure 7.7 Strawberry tongue in scarlet fever

women. The disease is now known to occur in men, neonates, and nonmenstruating women who have a focus of infection with a toxin producing strain of *S. aureus*.

Toxic shock syndrome toxin-1 (TSST-1) is the major toxin implicated in TSS caused by *S. aureus*. The toxin, like the toxins of streptococcal toxic shock, act as potent superantigens and induce the activation of cytokines such as tumor necrosis factor,

Staphylococcal scalded skin syndrome (SSSS) is a syndrome characterized by acute exfoliation of the skin following an erythematous cellulitis (Figure 7.8). SSSS is caused by an exotoxin released by *S. aureus*.

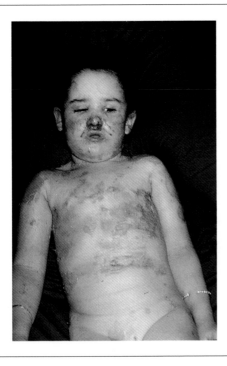

Figure 7.8 Scalded skin syndrome. Reprinted from H.P. Lambert and W.E. Farrar (1982) *Slide Atlas of Infectious Diseases*, Gower Medical Publishing Ltd. Reproduced with permission of Elsevier.

SSSS is also known as Ritter disease. SSSS almost always occurs in infants and in young children; outbreaks in neonatal nurseries or in day care centres have been known. Older children and adults may also develop the disease, particularly if there is a background of renal insufficiency or immunodeficiency (e.g. HIV infection). This is because such patients are unable to excrete the massive toxin load that is associated with SSSS.

The course of infection usually involves colonization of the oral or nasal cavities, throat, or umbilicus. Two epidermolytic toxins (A and B) are implicated in the generalized systemic manifestation of the syndrome. These toxins enter the bloodstream and act at a site remote from the site of colonization. They are responsible for the florid red rash and separation of the epidermis beneath the granular cell layer. Bullae formation leads to diffuse or patchy desquamation of the superficial layers of the skin. Healing typically occurs within 1–2 weeks. Cultures from fluid aspirated from the bullae are usually sterile, and is consistent with hematogenous dissemination of a toxin produced from a remote source, i.e. nose or umbilicus.

Treatment of staphylococcal infections necessitates the use of β-lactam antibiotics that are stable to staphylococcal β-lactamases.

Osteomyelitis

Osteomyelitis is a purulent infection of bone, caused most often by *S. aureus* and sometimes by *Streptococcus* species. In some forms of chronic osteomyelitis, such as those associated with chronic diabetic ulcers, Gram negative organisms belonging to the Enterobacteriaceae may be implicated. When the presence of a prosthetic orthopedic device is a predisposing factor for the development of osteomyelitis, organisms that form part of patient's normal skin flora (the coagulase negative staphylococci, e.g. *S. epidermidis*) are the most commonly implicated causative organisms. Spread of organisms from a distant focus into the bone occurs via two main routes:

1 Via the bloodstream, the hematogenous route where infection is caused by bacterial seeding into bone from the blood. The clinical picture varies with age. In children through the age of puberty the long bones of the extremities are most often involved with the metaphysis as the initial infected site (Figure 7.9). The apparent slowing and turbulence of blood flow as the vessels make sharp angles at the distal metaphyseal end of bone are increased risks for the formation of clots and the subsequent seeding of bacteria. This results in inflammation and necrosis of bone.

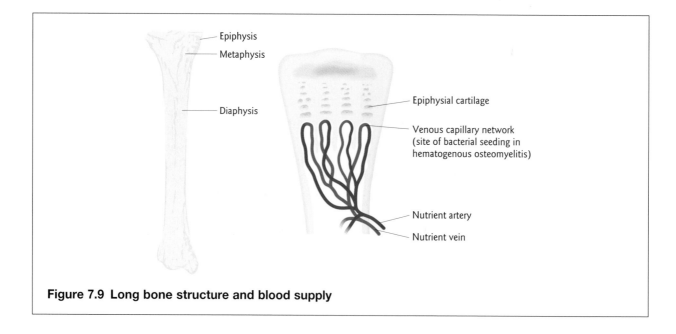

Figure 7.9 Long bone structure and blood supply

In adults, hematogenous osteomyelitis most often affects the spine. The vertebral bodies become more vascular with age and bacteremia may result in bacterial seeding of vertebral bodies preferentially at the more vascular anterior vertebral end plates. In addition, many large lumbar veins communicate freely with pelvic veins; retrograde flow from pelvic tissues (urethra, prostate, bladder) to lumbar vertebrae is a possible route for the spread of pelvic infections to the lumbar vertebrae.

2 In about 25% of patients with osteomyelitis, the predisposing factor is trauma to the bone at or near the site of infection (direct or contiguous osteomyelitis). Bacteria seed directly into bony tissues from a contiguous site of infection or as a result of sepsis after surgery. Infections of the mandible are often due to traumatic dental procedures while the installation of prosthetic devices, such as artificial joints, predisposes to long bone infection. Clinical manifestations of direct inoculation osteomyelitis are more localized than those of hematogenous osteomyelitis and may involve multiple organisms.

Other types of osteomyelitis include chronic osteomyelitis and osteomyelitis secondary to peripheral vascular disease or diabetic ulcers, particularly of the lower extremities. Chronic osteomyelitis persists or recurs, in spite of aggressive intervention, because of a chronic source of soft tissue infection typical of nonhealing ulcers. Many different species of Gram positive, Gram negative and anaerobic organisms may be involved in chronic osteomyelitis. Other predisposing factors for osteomyelitis include sickle-cell disease, acquired immune deficiency syndrome (AIDS), intravenous drug use, alcoholism, chronic steroid use, and chronic joint disease. Here a number of different organisms may be involved besides staphylococci and streptococci, and every attempt must be made to send relevant materials for culture to the microbiology laboratory. In addition, the presence of a prosthetic orthopedic device is an independent risk factor for the development of osteomyelitis; usually caused by coagulase negative staphylococci that form part of the normal flora of the skin.

Septic arthritis

Septic arthritis occurs when there is invasion of the synovial membrane enveloping the joint space by microorganisms. This is accompanied by extension of infection into the joint space. Infection is usually spread hematogenously from a focus elsewhere in the body. In all age groups the most common agent is *S. aureus*, which seeds into the bloodstream from a cutaneous lesion. Several other agents are reported to cause septic arthritis but their incidence is low and will not be discussed here (examples are *Haemophilus influenzae*, particularly in unvaccinated children, mycobacteria, and *Pasteurella* species).

In young adults, the primary infection may be a genital lesion caused by *Neisseria gonorrhoeae* (see Chapter 11).

Infection of prosthetic joint implants

Infection of prosthetic joint implants (artificial hip, knee, or other joints) is complicated by the fact that the patient is likely to have one or more underlying disease conditions that lead to the joint needing to be replaced. These predisposing factors also raise the risk of infection in artificial joints (Table 7.1).

Organisms may lodge in the prostheses either because they were locally introduced or because they gained access via the bloodstream (hematogenous spread). Local contamination of a prosthetic joint could be due to poor surgical technique, wound infection tracking deep into the joint, or via an infected blood clot (hematoma) at the site of the prosthesis. Hemotogenous spread could occur due to any infection at a distant site; for example a diabetic foot ulcer could become infected, the organisms could then gain access into the

Table 7.1 Predisposing factors that increase the risk of infection in prosthetic joint implants

• Prior surgery	• Nutritional status
• Rheumatoid arthritis	• Obesity
• Steroid therapy	• Advanced age
• Diabetes	• Prior infection

bloodstream and seed in the prostheses. Prosthetic infections are prevented by meticulous attention to asepsis during surgery and by the administration of prophylactic antibiotics during surgery. The commonest organisms implicated in prosthetic infections are the coagulase negative staphylococci such as *Staphylococcus epidermidis* and other organisms colonizing the skin, *S. aureus*, various streptococci, and rarely Gram negative aerobic bacilli.

The definitive diagnosis of bone and joint infection involves the direct examination and culture of synovial fluid specimens accompanied by blood cultures.

Treatment of osteomyelitis and septic arthritis consists of initial intravenous administration of appropriate antibiotics followed by a prolonged course of oral antimicrobial agents. Drainage and washout of affected joints is also indicated. Prosthetic joints may need to be removed and replaced after a prolonged course of antibiotics.

Gas gangrene/anaerobic cellulitis

Gas gangrene occurs as a result of infection by bacteria belonging to the genus *Clostridium*. The condition is associated with massive tissue destruction as in war wounds or road traffic accidents. Rarely surgical wounds, diabetic ulcers, and other surface wounds may also be at risk of contamination with clostridia. About a third of cases occur spontaneously. Patients who develop this disease spontaneously often have underlying vascular disease, diabetes, or colon cancer. Under such conditons, spores of clostridia that are ubiquitous in dust, dirt, human and animal waste, can contaminate dead or dying tissue. The spores germinate under the anaerobic conditions of tissue necrosis, produce potent exotoxins, and cause tissue death and associated symptoms typical of gas gangrene. The onset of gas gangrene is sudden and dramatic. Inflammation begins at the site of infection as a red to brown and extremely painful swelling (Figure 7.10). Gas may be felt in the tissue as a crepitant sensation when the swollen area is palpated. The margins of the infected area expand rapidly and the underlying tissue is completely necrosed, often with the marked absence of pus. Progressive and rapid myonecrois (necrosis of underlying muscle) is a characteristic feature. Systemic symptoms develop early in the infection. These consist of sweating, fever, rigors, and tachycardia. If untreated, the individual develops a shock-like syndrome with hypotension, renal failure, and death.

Treatment consists of extensive surgical debridement of the affected area until all the necrotic tissue has been excised. Appropriate anti-anaerobic antibiotics need to be administered without delay. Most clostridia are susceptible to penicillin and metronidazole.

Cutaneous diphtheria

Classic cutaneous diphtheria is an indolent nonprogressive infection characterized by a superficial, necrotic, nonhealing ulcer with a characteristic gray-brown membrane. Patients typically give a history of travel to

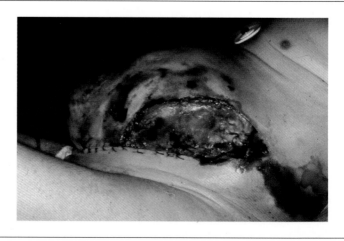

Figure 7.10 Gas gangrene after abdominal surgery

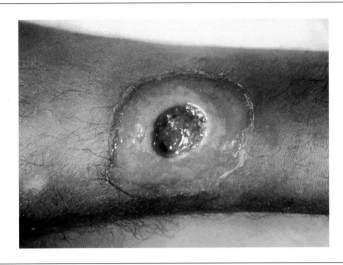

Figure 7.11 Cutaneous diphtheria. Courtesy of the Centers for Disease Control and Prevention; from CDC website: http://phil.cdc.gov/phil/details.asp

tropical/endemic countries; hence the term "tropical" ulcer is often used to differentiate these ulcers from those unrelated to travel. Patients may also present with underlying dermatoses, lacerations, burns, insect bites, or impetigo that have become secondarily infected. Diphtheritic skin infections cannot always be differentiated from streptococcal or staphylococcal impetigo clinically, and they frequently coexist. Cutaneous diphtheria is most often found on the extremities and is associated with pain, tenderness, erythema, and superficial necrosis or slough (Figure 7.11). Cutaneous diphtheria is most often associated with nontoxigenic strains of the organism; however toxigenic strains have also been implicated in a minority of cases.

Cutaneous anthrax (see Chapter 26)

All of the above conditions can be diagnosed in the laboratory; organisms are recovered from tissue samples, wound swabs, blood and fluid cultures using appropriate microscopy and culture methods.

Hospital acquired infections of skin, soft tissue, bone, and joint

See Chapter 14 for discussion on MRSA/GISA/VRSA/VRE.

Pathogenesis and virulence of bacterial infections

Streptococcus pyogenes

Microbiology

S. pyogenes or Group A beta hemolytic streptococcus (GABHS) belongs to a large and diverse group of Gram positive, nonmotile, nonsporing cocci that display a characteristic chain-like arrangement (see Figure 1.3). They grow best on agar medium containing either sheep or horse blood, at 37°C in the presence of 5% carbon dioxide. On blood agar plates they appear as white or grey colonies 1–2 mm in diameter surrounded by zones of complete hemolysis (see Figure 4.6b). Some colonies produce large amounts of hyaluronic acid, giving them a characteristic mucoid appearance on the culture plate.

The cell surface of *S. pyogenes* has been studied exhaustively (Figure 7.12). Historically, the classification of beta hemolytic streptococci has rested on the basis of serologic reactivity of "cell wall" polysaccharide antigens (also known as C substance or group carbohydrate antigen) as originally described by Rebecca Lancefield. Alphabetically named (A through U), 18 group-specific antigens (Lancefield groups) were established. Only Group A beta hemolytic streptococcus (GABHS) or *S. pyogenes* will be discussed in detail.

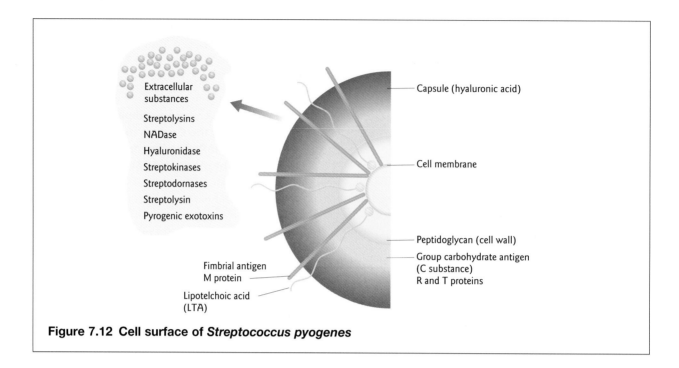

Extracellular
substances

Streptolysins
NADase
Hyaluronidase
Streptokinases
Streptodornases
Streptolysin
Pyrogenic exotoxins

Capsule (hyaluronic acid)

Cell membrane

Peptidoglycan (cell wall)

Group carbohydrate antigen
(C substance)
R and T proteins

Fimbrial antigen
M protein

Lipotelchoic acid
(LTA)

Figure 7.12 Cell surface of *Streptococcus pyogenes*

Groups C and G cause similar infections; they are less frequent and less severe. The cell surface of *S. pyogenes* contains two major classes of proteins called the M and T antigens. Typing of M and T antigens is a useful epidemiologic surveillance tool. Some M and T antigens are implicated in severe disease and others are associated with complications of streptococcal disease.

Virulence mechanisms

The major virulence factor of *S. pyogenes* is the M protein. M protein is a macromolecule present on the cell membrane; it traverses and penetrates the bacterial cell wall (Figure 7.10). M protein is an alpha helically coiled dimer and appears as hair-like projections on the cell wall. M protein helps the organism adhere to human epithelial cells and resist phagocytosis; the latter is achieved by inhibiting activation of alternate complement pathways. After infection, type-specific antibodies develop, M protein activity is neutralized and the immunity is only type-specific but long-lasting. The M proteins of certain M-types are considered **rheumatogenic** as they contain antigenic epitopes that cross-react with mammalian heart muscle; this may lead to the development of an autoimmune rheumatic carditis (rheumatic fever) following an acute infection.

 S. pyogenes produces a number of adhesins that mediate adhesion to various human and animal cell types. These include lipoteichoic **acids (LTA)**, **M protein**, and **fibronectin-binding proteins**. Like the M protein, LTA is anchored to proteins on the bacterial surface. Once adherence has occurred, streptococci resist phagocytosis, proliferate, and begin to invade the local tissues.

Extracellular enzymes and toxins

In addition to virulence factors *S. pyogenes* produces an impressive array of toxins and enzymes. Most strains produce **streptolysin S**, an oxygen-stable enzyme that is toxic to polymorphonuclear leukocytes (a leukocidin) and **streptolysin O**, an oxygen-labile leukocidin. Streptolysin S is a polypeptide protein molecule that causes lysis of a variety of human and animal red and white blood cells and is responsible for the hemolysis observed on blood agar plates used to culture the organism. Streptolysin O is an immunogenic single-chain protein that induces a brisk antibody response. Measurement of antistreptolysin O antibodies is an important clinical test and is used as an indicator of recent streptococcal infection. Other enzymes include streptokinases that cause lysis of fibrin clots; deoxyribonucleases (A–D); and hyaluronidase which digests the hyaluronic acid of connective tissue resulting in the rapid spreading cellulitis characteristic of *S. pyogenes* infection.

Additionally, streptococci produce proteinase, nicotinamide adenine dinucleotidase, adenosine triphosphatase, neuraminidase, lipoproteinase, and cardiohepatic toxin.

Pyrogenic exotoxins

S. pyogenes is capable of producing three **streptococcal pyrogenic exotoxins (SPE)**, i.e. types A, B, and C. Formerly known as **erythrogenic toxin**, these toxins act as **superantigens**; they do not require processing by antigen presenting cells. Rather, they stimulate T cells by binding class II MHC molecules directly and nonspecifically resulting in overwhelming cytokine release which is detrimental to the host (see staphylococcal enterotoxins below). The erythrogenic toxin got its name because of its role in the pathogenesis of scarlet fever which occurs when the toxin is disseminated in the blood. Re-emergence in the late 1980s of exotoxin-producing strains of *S. pyogenes* was associated with a **toxic shock-like syndrome** similar in pathogenesis and manifestation to staphylococcal toxic shock syndrome and to a destructive skin and soft tissue condition called **necrotizing fasciitis**. The rapidly destructive nature of wound infections has led to media interest in the organism which has often been referred to as the "flesh-eating bacteria."

Staphylococcus aureus and coagulase negative staphylococci

Microbiology

S. aureus is a Gram positive coccus, arranged in characteristic grape-like clusters (see Figure 1.4). Staphylococci are differentiated in the laboratory from streptococci by positive catalase and coagulase tests. Colonies are golden yellow and beta hemolytic on blood agar.

Virulence mechanisms

S. aureus is armed with a variety of **virulence determinants** (Figure 7.13):

1 **Surface proteins** such as fibronectin and finbrinogen binding proteins that promote colonization of traumatized host tissues and blood clots.

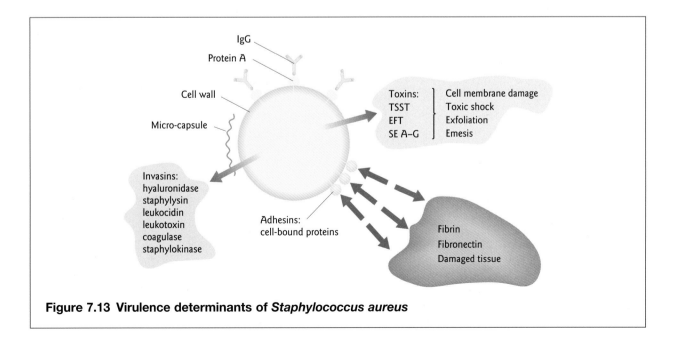

Figure 7.13 Virulence determinants of *Staphylococcus aureus*

2 Toxins (α, β, γ, and δ) that induce bacterial spread and damage a variety of human and animal cell membranes including erythrocytes, platelets, and leukocytes. The classical Panton and Valentine (PV) leukocidin has potent leukotoxicity. The PV leukocidin is associated with severe dermonecrotic lesions and necrotizing abscess formation.

3 Cell surface molecules (**capsule**, **protein A**) bind to the Fc portion of IgG, this is thought to prevent opsonization and inhibit phagocytosis.

4 *S. aureus* expresses several different types of protein **toxins** which are responsible for a number of toxin related symptoms of staphylococcal infection. Some of the toxins of *S. aureus* are also referred to as superantigens. These are the staphylococcal **enterotoxins (SE)**, of which there are six antigenic types (SE-A, B, C, D, E, and G), and the **toxic shock syndrome toxin (TSST-1)**. Staphylococcal enterotoxins are responsible for the symptoms of food poisoning (see Chapter 8). A focus of staphylococcal infection in any part of the body, expressing the TSST-1 gene, results in the systemic manifestation of toxic shock syndrome (TSS). Some enterotoxins can also cause TSS. For example, enterotoxins B and C cause 50% of nonmenstrual cases of TSS.

Staphylococcal enterotoxins and TSST-1 act as superantigens because they stimulate T cells nonspecifically. Superantigens bind directly to class II MHCs of antigen-presenting cells outside the conventional antigen-binding grove (Figure 7.14, also read the section "Superantigens" in Chapter 3). This results in a massive release of cytokines and is directly responsible for the symptoms of TSS.

Exfoliatin toxin (ET) is responsible for the scalded skin syndrome in neonates, which results in widespread blistering and separation of the epidermis. Healing occurs with little scarring though fluid loss and secondary infections are possible complications. There are two antigenically distinct forms of the toxin, ETA and ETB. The toxins have esterase and protease activity and target a protein, desmoglein 1, which is involved in maintaining the integrity of the epidermis.

In contrast to *S. aureus*, little is known about mechanisms of pathogenesis of infections caused by the coagulase negative staphylococci like *S. epidermidis*. Adherence is a crucial step in the initiation of prosthetic infections. Interaction between prosthesis and bacteria is facilitated by the deposition of host proteins on the implanted device – all staphylococci bind to fibronectin.

A characteristic of many pathogenic strains of coagulase negative staphylococci is the production of a slime layer, resulting in "biofilm" formation. The slime is predominantly a secreted teichoic acid, normally found in the cell wall of the staphylococci. This ability to form a biofilm on the surface of a prosthetic device is a significant virulence determinant. The bacteria can be found trapped in slime; furthermore many antibiotics used to treat these infections are unable to penetrate the biofilm.

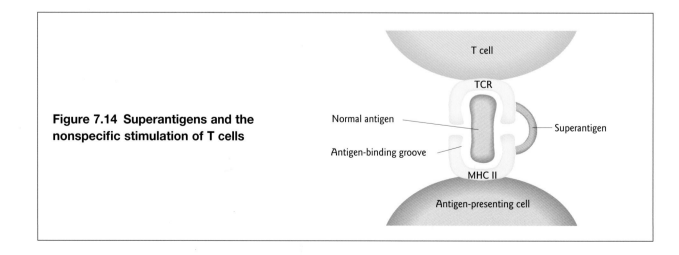

Figure 7.14 Superantigens and the nonspecific stimulation of T cells

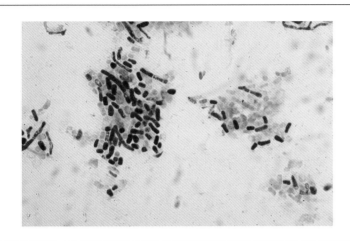

Figure 7.15 Gram stain of *Clostridium* species, note the appearance of nonstaining spores (1000×)

Clostridium species

Microbiology

Clostridia are Gram positive, anaerobic, spore-forming bacilli that are ubiquitous in nature (Figure 7.15). Clostridia are normally found in manure enriched soil as they are normal flora of animal dung. In the human body clostridia can be isolated from normal human colonic flora, skin, and the vagina. Of the 150 *Clostridium* species that have been identified, six have been incriminated in fulminant clostridial gas gangrene. Usually, more than one *Clostridium* species is isolated from clinical tissue specimens of patients presenting with gas gangrene.

Clostridium perfringens, is the most common cause of clostridial gas gangrene and is present in 80–90% of cases. Other clostridial species include *Clostridium novyi* (40%), *C. septicum* (20%), *C. histolyticum* (10%), *C. bifermentans* (10%), and *C. fallax* (5%).

Virulence mechanisms

Although many wounds may be contaminated with clostridia of human or animal origin, invasion and infection requires two conditions to coexist. Organisms must be inoculated deep into the tissues and the oxygen tension must be low enough for the organisms to multiply. These organisms are not strict anaerobes. They are tolerant to about 30% oxygen tension (however at 70% oxygen tension organisms fail to grow) – hence their predilection for deep wounds and massive blast injuries where there is blood loss and tissue damage. Inoculation of organisms into damaged tissues is followed by an incubation period that usually ranges from 12 to 24 hours. As the spores germinate and the organisms multiply, they release exotoxins that result in extensive tissue necrosis.

An impressive array of protein exotoxins and enzymes produced by the clostridia have been studied and characterized. Of the many exotoxins that clostridia produce, four (alpha, beta, epsilon, iota) cause potentially fatal syndromes. The exotoxins of *C. perfringens* are used for species typing (e.g. type A, type B, type C). Clostridia additionally produce many tissue-destroying enzymes, besides which the toxins also display enzymatic activity.

Alpha toxin is a lecithinase and is produced by most clostridia; it also has phospholipase C activity. Lecithinase is a potent toxin and causes lysis of red blood cells, myocytes, fibroblasts, platelets, and leukocytes.

Theta toxin causes direct vascular injury, cytolysis, hemolysis, leukocyte degeneration, and polymorphonuclear cell destruction. The degradation of leukocytes may explain the relatively minor neutrophil reaction that is observed in the tissues of patients with clostridial myonecrosis.

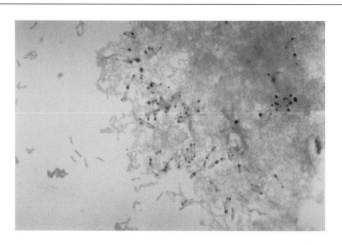

Figure 7.16 *Corynebacterium diphtheriae* **in Chinese letter arrangement. Albert's stain (1000×) Reprinted from H.P. Lambert and W.E. Farrar (1982)** *Slide Atlas of Infectious Diseases***, Gower Medical Publishing Ltd. Reproduced with permission of Elsevier**

Kappa toxin, also produced by *C. perfringens*, is a collagenase that facilitates the rapid spread of necrosis through tissue planes by destroying connective tissue.

Together these toxins are responsible for both the local tissue destruction and the systemic symptoms associated with gas gangrene.

Corynebacterium diphtheriae

Microbiology

Corynebacterium diphtheriae is a Gram positive, aerobic, nonmotile, rod shaped bacterium. The bacilli appear in X and V shaped forms when grown in culture, resembling the characteristic "Chinese letter" arrangement of these organisms. On special stains dark staining granules known as metachromatic granules are visible in the bacilli (Figure 7.16). The granules consist of polymetaphosphate and are a necessary energy source for the toxin activity that is responsible for the pathogenesis of the organism.

Virulence mechanisms

Strains of *C. diphtheriae* that cause cutaneous diphtheria can be either nontoxigenic or toxigenic. Lesions infected with nontoxigenic strains show a local inflammatory response that can be chronic. Systemic toxic manifestation is absent. If the infecting strain is capable of toxin production, the skin lesions absorb toxin slowly and can induce high levels of antibodies that produce natural immunization. These lesions are an important reservoir of infection and can cause respiratory and cutaneous infections in contacts. The toxin is a potent exotoxin and acts by ADP-ribosylation of elongation factor 2, which results in the irreversible inhibition of protein synthesis and cell death. (Also see Chapter 25.)

Viral infections

Viral infections can lead to skin manifestations by a variety of mechanisms, but generally a particular virus will cause a characteristic skin appearance. Some of these viral rash illnesses will be covered in Chapter 15. The viral rashes of childhood (rubella, parvovirus B19, measles, and chickenpox) are generally very infectious, being transmitted between children by infectious aerosols that are inhaled. The transmissibility of these viral infections can be stratified approximately as: measles (rubeola) > chickenpox (varicella zoster virus – VZV) > rubella (German measles) and parvovirus B19 ("fifth" or "slapped cheek" disease) > herpes simplex 1 (HSV-1 causing "cold sores") and herpes simplex 2 (HSV-2 causing genital herpes) – both HSV-1 and HSV-2 are only transmitted by direct contact and not by aerosol transmission. Other nonchildhood viral infections with characteristic skin manifestations are covered in other chapters, such as the viral hemorrhagic fevers (VHFs) and dengue hemorrhagic fever (DHF), as well as West Nile fever, HIV seroconversion illness, and smallpox and monkey pox (see Chapters 22–24).

Diagnosing viral rashes correctly is important both for specific treatment and infection control purposes. The latter is of particular importance when dealing with pregnant women (due to possible viral damage to the fetus) and immunocompromised patients (who may develop life-threatening viral disease) – see Chapters 12 and 13 respectively.

Viral rash illnesses are usually macular, petechial/hemorrhagic, maculopapular, vesicular, or hyperplastic. The most common physical skin appearances of viral rash illnesses are described below.

Macular and maculopapular rash

This type of skin rash is flat ("macules" – not raised above the skin; papules are raised above the skin), and consists of small red ("erythematous") spots. Examples of viruses causing these sorts of skin appearance (Figure 7.17) are rubella (German measles) and parvovirus B19 (also known as "fifth" or "slapped cheek" disease). These rashes may be "blanchable", i.e. they will disappear when they are pressed gently with your finger. These are due to dilated capillaries lying just under the skin, which empty under the finger pressure. Not all of these spots may completely disappear with finger pressure. Sometimes the spots may be larger and different shades of red and purple. These rashes are caused by bleeding or "hemorrhaging" under the skin, known as petechiae (for small patches), or ecchymoses (for larger patches, also the same appearance and

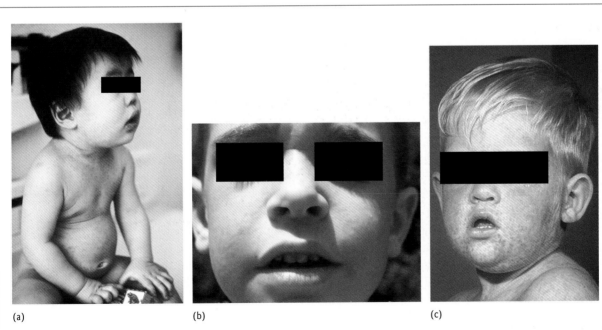

(a)   (b)   (c)

Figure 7.17 (a) An 11-month-old infant with a mild rubella (German measles) rash. Generally rubella rashes are macular, not maculopapular. (b) The face of a boy showing symptoms of parvovirus B19 infection ("fifth" or "slapped cheek" disease). This is a relatively common viral infection that is usually acquired in childhood. (c) This child with measles ("rubeola") is displaying the characteristic red, blotchy pattern on the fourth day of the rash. A red blotchy rash appears around day 3 of the illness, first on the face and then becoming generalized. Courtesy of the Centers for Disease Control and Prevention; from CDC website: http://phil.cdc.gov/phil/details.asp

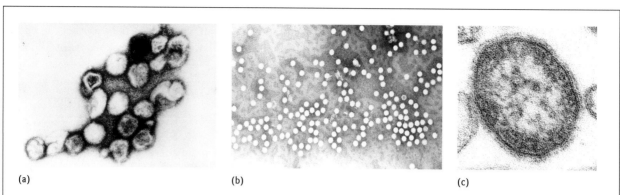

Figure 7.18 Electron micrographs of (a) rubella (a single-stranded RNA virus), (b) parvovirus B19 (a single-stranded DNA virus), and (c) measles (single-stranded RNA virus). Rubella and measles are enveloped viruses, whereas parvovirus is nonenveloped. Courtesy of the Centers for Disease Control and Prevention; from CDC website: http://phil.cdc.gov/phil/details.asp

mechanism as bruises). Viruses that cause this appearance are those that can cause bleeding under the skin, such as the viral hemorrhagic fevers (VHFs), including dengue and dengue hemorrhagic fever (DHF) (see Chapters 22 and 24). This type of rash can also be seen with meningococcal meningitis.

A "maculopapular" rash means a red rash that is raised above the surrounding surface of the skin. This sort of rash is commonly seen in measles. The rash of measles (also known as "rubeola") differs from that of rubella, in that it is more patchy, more red, blotchy and "angry"-looking, and the rash can be felt to be raised above the level of the surrounding skin (Figure 7.17). Such viral rash illnesses are systemic and the patient (most often children) will have fever, general malaise, and feel miserable – this is particularly true of measles. Rubella and parvovirus B19 usually cause milder systemic illness in children. Electron photomicrographs of rubella virus, parvovirus, and measles virus are shown in Figure 7.18.

The diagnosis of these childhood viral rash infections is usually by serology (IgG and IgM antibody detection), with culture and molecular testing (for the virus nucleic acid) being performed in reference laboratories for further characterization of these viruses, particularly in outbreak situations. Treatment is usually supportive and in most cases takes place at home, rather than in hospitals, unless there are complications. There is no specific antiviral treatment for these three common rashes of childhood, but there is a very effective vaccine for measles and rubella (the MMR vaccine – see Chapter 15).

Vesicular lesions

These lesions are raised, fluid-filled blisters (the fluid and surrounding skin contain the virus), which can be epidermal (superficial skin layer) or dermal (deeper skin layer). Epidermal vesicles are relatively delicate and easy to burst, and are typical of varicella zoster (VZV causing chickenpox and shingles) and herpes simplex virus (HSV-1 causing cold sores, HSV-2 causing genital herpes) infections (Figure 7.19). The blisters are generally preceded by an itchy or painful maculopapular rash before becoming vesicular. The characteristic rash of chickenpox has different spots becoming vesicular at different times, so a mixture of spots at different stages of blister development can be seen at any one time in an infected individual. Occasionally, serious cases of hemorrhagic chickenpox show a typical chickenpox skin rash at first, which then becomes more confluent and starts to bleed. Such cases can become rapidly fatal without appropriate antiviral treatment. Chickenpox can be distinguished from smallpox by three characteristics. Firstly, the chickenpox rash tends to affect the trunk more than the face and limbs (a "centripetal" distribution), whereas smallpox lesions tend to be found in greater numbers on the face, arms, and legs. Secondly, the rash of chickenpox shows lesions in various forms of development at the same time (macular, maculopapular, vesicular, and scabbing over), whereas smallpox lesions are all at the same stage. Thirdly, the vesicles of chickenpox are epidermal and

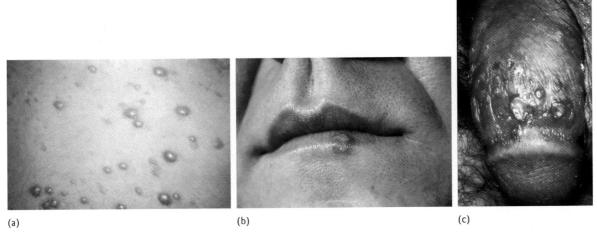

(a)   (b)   (c)

Figure 7.19 (a) This vesicular rash is typical of chickenpox (varicella zoster virus – VZV). The fluid-filled blisters are preceded by an itchy, erythematous (red), maculopapular rash. The VZV remains in the body after chickenpox and can reactivate to re-emerge as painful "shingles" in a particular patch of skin, during times of physical or emotional stress, or immunocompromise. (b) A "cold sore" caused by herpes simplex 1 (HSV-1) on the lower lip. (c) Herpes simplex 2 blisters on the penis. Occasionally, HSV-1 can cause genital herpes and HSV-2 can cause cold sores. When the blisters burst, the resulting ulcer can be very painful to touch and may get infected secondarily with bacteria. Left alone, these epidermal blisters will dry up and heal with relatively little or no scarring. Courtesy of the Centers for Disease Control and Prevention; from CDC website: http://phil.cdc.gov/phil/details.asp

relatively fragile and easily burst, whereas those of smallpox are in the deeper dermis and are tougher and less easily broken.

Shingles is a problem normally seen in older patients who have previously had chickenpox. After chickenpox, the VZV stays latent or dormant in nerve cells in the spinal cord, then during times of stress and reduced immunity (e.g. during physical or emotional stress, in the elderly, or during immune suppressive conditions), the same VZV that caused chickenpox in that individual reactivates and reappears on the skin as blisters, called "shingles." Shingles can be very painful, even after the skin rash heals, as the VZV damages the nerves and this pain is called "post-herpetic neuralgia," which can be very difficult to treat.

The skin appearances of herpes simplex virus infections (HSV-1 and HSV-2) have the same appearance, and are similar to those of chickenpox, being vesicular – fluid-filled blisters. With both chickenpox and herpes, the skin rash appearances can change in immunocompromised patients (e.g. congenital immunodeficiency, those with cancer on chemotherapy or in transplantation or HIV/AIDS patients, and those on steroid therapy).

Diagnosis of VZV and HSV infections are often from fluid and skin samples from the lesions themselves, using viral culture, immunofluorescence viral antigen staining, and sometimes molecular tests for the viral DNA. Microscopic characteristics of these viruses are shown in Figure 7.20. For VZV, an IgM and IgG antibody test can give an indication of an acute infection, i.e. chickenpox (if IgM is positive and the IgG is positive or negative), or previous infection with current immunity (if IgM is negative and IgG is positive). For HSV, serology is not usually used in standard diagnostic laboratories because seroconversion after primary HSV infection can be very slow (as long as 6–8 weeks). Investigating the HSV serological status can be misleading in some situations (Boxes 7.3 and 7.4). Most primary HSV-1 and HSV-2 infections are asymptomatic, and it may be a reactivation of the virus that causes the first lesions noticed by the individual. Both VZV and HSV can cause more serious infections and damage to the central nervous system (brain and spinal cord) that may result in paralysis and even death from encephalitis if not recognized and treated early

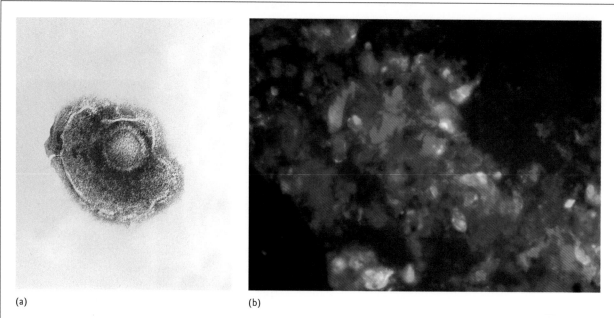

(a)   (b)

Figure 7.20 (a) An electron micrograph (EM) of varicella zoster virus (VZV) that causes chickenpox and shingles. The herpes simplex viruses (HSV-1, HSV-2) look virtually identical to VZV under EM. Courtesy of the Centers for Disease Control and Prevention; from CDC website: http://phil.cdc.gov/phil/details.asp. (b) Specific immunofluorescence staining can be used to identify VZV, HSV-1 and (in this image) HSV-2. Cells with the green fluorescence are those infected with HSV-2. Courtesy of the Department of Microbiology, The Chinese University of Hong Kong, Prince of Wales Hospital

Box 7.3 Herpes simplex 2 infections: viral latency or partner infidelity?

A common scenario facing a couple in a sexually transmitted disease (STD) clinic is the diagnosis of one member of the couple with HSV-2 – genital herpes. This may be due to HSV-2 vesicular lesions being found on the vulva or penis. If the other partner is tested, using HSV-2 serology, and found to be negative, it may be asked from where the HSV-2 infection was acquired – have they been unfaithful?

Of course this may be true in some cases, but another explanation may be that that partner acquired the HSV-2 infection with a previous partner, before meeting his/her current one. Many people do not realize that after primary (first-time) infection, the herpes viruses remain in the body for life, and the primary infection may have occurred many years previously. The virus can then reactivate during times of illness or stress, when the lesions may be seen for the first time. Many primary HSV-2 infections are asymptomatic, with no lesions seen at the time of infection. Without knowing this, it is natural for the HSV-2 negative

partner to assume that if there are visible lesions (especially on the genitals, though HSV-2 can also cause cold sores around the mouth), then the infection must have been acquired recently, suggesting infidelity.

This scenario is important for another reason. If the male partner is found to be HSV-2 positive, and the female partner is not, but they are trying to have a baby, or if she is already pregnant, then there may be a risk to the baby if the man infects her with HSV-2. Primary HSV-2 infection during pregnancy, particularly in the last trimester (last 13 weeks), can be transmitted to the baby during delivery and cause serious infection, as the mother may have no maternal antibody against HSV-2 to pass onto the baby for protection. So, the moral here is new genital lesions do not necessarily mean infidelity, but of course this cannot be excluded. Secondly, if there is a discordant HSV-2 status between the partners and they are considering pregnancy, then obtain expert advice about how to manage this.

Box 7.4 Herpes simplex 2 infections in children: sexual abuse or innocent transmission?

A 9-year-old girl is seen in the emergency room with her mother, with a 1-week history of painful vesicular and ulcer lesions on her vulva. On questioning the mother, she says that she is now divorced with no current boyfriend and she just lives with her two daughters (there is another daughter of 5 years old with her at the time). She, herself, has never had genital herpes as far as she can remember and also that none of her previous male partners have had any noticeable genital lesions or any previous diagnosis of "genital herpes" infections as far as she was aware. She also said that she occasionally gets cold sores, particularly when she gets "the flu" in the winter months, but these lesions have never been tested in a laboratory. The 9 year old goes to primary school and the 5 year old goes to kindergarten all day. She drops them off at around 8 am each morning and collects them at around 5 pm each afternoon. She works as a librarian at the local public library and her employer has given her some flexibility for her childcare. As far as she knows, the children seem happy and have no problems at school with the other children or teachers. She does everything for her children, including cooking, cleaning, bathing, etc., as she cannot afford any other domestic help on her relatively low income. Upon questioning the two children, separately, they seem to support their mother's account, appearing to be happy contented girls. Neither of them report any events suggestive of sexual abuse by anyone, and also neither of them have complained of any previous similar lesions around the mouth or "down below."

Laboratory testing of swabs from the lesions confirms that HSV-2 is present by both culture and molecular testing for viral DNA from the 9-year-old girl's swabs. Serum samples are taken for HSV serology and both the mother's and the 9-year-old daughter's results come back as both HSV-1 and HSV-2 IgG positive. Upon receiving this result, the mother consents to have her other 5-year-old daughter tested who has not had any genital or other lesions previously. She turns out to be HSV-1 IgG positive, but HSV-2 IgG negative. The clinical virologist suggests that, given this history and laboratory test results, it is possible that the mother's cold sores may be caused by HSV-2 reactivation, and that kissing contact with her 9-year-old daughter has inadvertently transmitted

HSV-2 to her, sometime ago. It is difficult to ascertain the time-frame of such a transmission event as both the mother and child are HSV-2 IgG positive now; however, it is possible that the younger 5-year-old daughter may still be seroconverting to HSV-2 IgG positivity (it may take 6–8 weeks for the HSV-2 IgG to become positive after infection).

The mother agrees to further followup testing, a month later. However, perhaps due to the stress of this situation, she calls the clinical virologist a week later, saying that she has one of her typical cold sores on her lower lip, and would they like to test her now? She is seen again in the emergency room when a swab is taken from the cold sore. This indeed tests positive for HSV-2 by both culture and DNA detection methods, which is a great relief to the mother, not because she is HSV-2 infected, but because it offers an innocent explanation for this situation. It seems that the clinical virologist's hypothesis is correct. Although it is still impossible to absolutely exclude any possibility of child sexual abuse, it seems much less likely now. The appointment for 1 month later is still kept and the 5-year-old daughter's serum is taken to check for HSV-2 IgG seroconversion then. The test result comes back as HSV-2 IgG positive (low but definitely more positive than the previous test result). A further followup test, another month later, confirms that the younger daughter is definitely HSV-2 IgG positive, although there have been no clinical symptoms (e.g. no genital lesions) in her yet.

Thus, HSV infections may be asymptomatic in both adults and children, even during reactivation, when the virus is present in the saliva or genital secretions. In this way, HSV infections can be innocently transmitted by kissing, sexual intercourse, and also during the delivery of a baby, without the infected person being aware that he/she is infected or that there is any risk that he/she may transmit this infection to others. This characteristic, of viral latency and asymptomatic primary infection with HSV, therefore makes it difficult to ascertain the nature of transmission events, in some situations. Both clinical and laboratory evidence has to be weighed, but in the end, the final sequence of transmission events may only be the most likely rather than the true scenario.

enough. Hence, where treatment is necessary, VZV and HSV viral infections can be treated with specific antiviral drugs, including aciclovir and its related drug formulations.

Examples of dermal vesicular-like skin lesions are also caused by the orthopoxviruses, such as smallpox and monkeypox, both of which are described in chapters elsewhere in this book. Another poxvirus infection causes molluscum contagiosum, producing skin lesions that are similar to those caused by orthopoxviruses, though they are far fewer in number and more localized to one area of the body. In immunocompromised patients, particularly those with HIV/AIDS, molluscum contagiosum can become more widespread and quite disfiguring, particularly if they appear on the face. Diagnosis of poxvirus infections is most rapidly made using electron microscopy (EM), as the appearance is distinctive and specialists can even distinguish between the different types of poxvirus using EM. Poxviruses can also be cultured, but for smallpox, Biosafety Level 4 (BSL-4) facilities are required, which are not available to many healthcare institutions. Suspected cases of smallpox need to be referred urgently to the CDC in Atlanta for expert advice and diagnostic testing (see Chapter 28). Other tests include molecular detection of the viral DNA and possibly antigen and serological testing. The poxviruses are DNA viruses and it has been shown *in vitro* that an antiviral drug, cidofovir, may be effective against them. This has been investigated, particularly for smallpox. For monkeypox and molluscum contagiosum, these are usually self-limiting infections in immunocompetent individuals and rarely need specific antiviral treatment (though there is limited data on the effectiveness of antiviral therapy for these particular poxviruses).

Enteroviruses may also cause a variety of skin lesions, including maculopapular and vesicular with a surrounding erythematous (red) base (Figure 7.21). In hand-foot-and-mouth disease (HFMD), a relatively

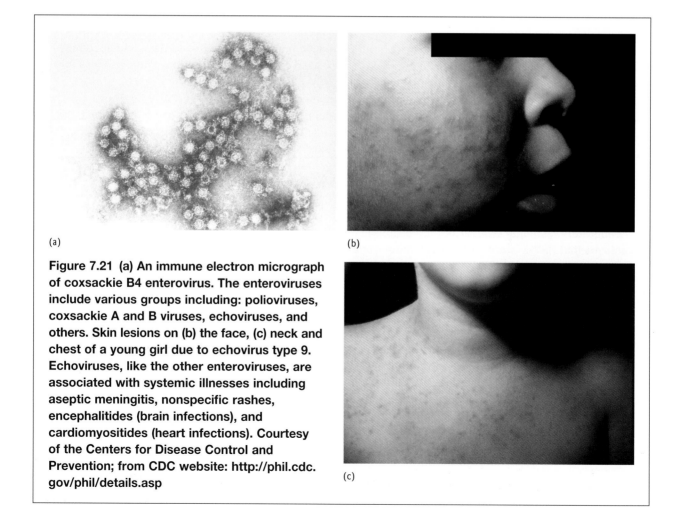

(a)

(b)

Figure 7.21 (a) An immune electron micrograph of coxsackie B4 enterovirus. The enteroviruses include various groups including: polioviruses, coxsackie A and B viruses, echoviruses, and others. Skin lesions on (b) the face, (c) neck and chest of a young girl due to echovirus type 9. Echoviruses, like the other enteroviruses, are associated with systemic illnesses including aseptic meningitis, nonspecific rashes, encephalitides (brain infections), and cardiomyositides (heart infections). Courtesy of the Centers for Disease Control and Prevention; from CDC website: http://phil.cdc.gov/phil/details.asp

(c)

common childhood enterovirus infection, the lesions can appear anywhere on the child's skin, but distinctively they can appear on the palms of the hands and soles of the feet, where other viral rash lesions are few or unusual. The lesions for HFMD are also painful to touch and pressure. The diagnosis is usually made by culture of the virus from swabs or skin scrapings from the lesion, or from other systemic sites (as enterovirus is a systemic infection), such as throat swabs and stool samples where the virus is also shed. Nowadays, molecular tests for the enteroviral RNA can also be performed on these samples, and serological testing can be used to diagnose recent or previous infections, as well as for typing the specific enterovirus species involved by "neutralization" assays. This assay uses the patient's convalescent serum antibodies to prevent the growth of that particular enterovirus type in *in vitro* cell culture, thereby providing its specific identity. Enterovirus infections are also one of the commonest causes of aseptic or lymphocytic meningitis, but usually these are self-limiting, with perhaps just a few days of headache and fever. Generally, most enterovirus infections are self-limiting and do not require treatment, but they can cause epidemics amongst children (especially HFMD), as they have little previous exposure and immunity to these viruses. Currently, there is no licensed specific anti-enterovirus drug, though there is one drug (called pleconaril), which is available for the rare life-threatening enterovirus infections (such as enterovirus myocarditis and meningoencephalitis, especially in children) on a special request basis. There is no vaccine licensed for enteroviruses, at present.

Hyperplastic lesions

This describes warty skin lesions often found on the hands and genital areas (Figure 7.22) caused by the human papilloma viruses (HPVs; see Chapter 11). There are many different types of this virus, some are more often associated with warts on the hand or genital areas, and some are now known to be causal for cervical cancer in women, particularly types HPV 16 and 18. These lesions are produced by overactive replication of the skin epidermis induced by HPV. Diagnosis is usually clinical, but can be confirmed by biopsy and molecular detection and typing. For HPV, culture is difficult and serological tests are either

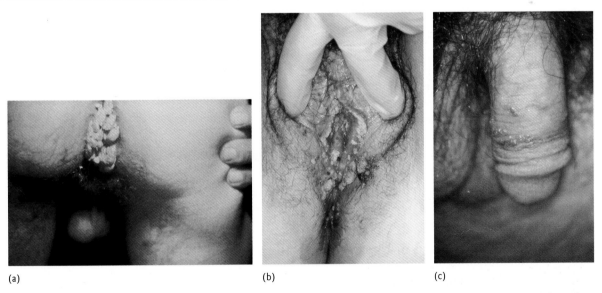

(a) (b) (c)

Figure 7.22 (a) Anal (b) vulval and (c) penile genital warts (also known as condylomata acuminata) is a sexually transmitted disease caused by human papilloma virus. The virus causes excessive growth of the epidermal skin cells resulting in these hyperplastic lesions. They can be removed by a variety of means, and can occasionally transform into cancerous growths. Courtesy of the Centers for Disease Control and Prevention; from CDC website: http://phil.cdc.gov/phil/details.asp

unreliable and/or difficult to interpret. In some cases, specific HPV typing is required, particularly in the case of suspicious cervical lesions where some high-risk HPV types (e.g. 16, 18, 52, 58) have been strongly associated with cervical carcinoma. Most HPV infections are normally confined to the skin and are more disfiguring and inconvenient than life-threatening. These can often be removed by cryotherapy (freezing the lesions with liquid nitrogen), surgery or chemotherapy. However, the few HPV types that are associated with human cancers, such as HPV types 16, 18, 52, and 58 for cervical cancer and HPVs 6 and 11 for laryngeal papillomatosis, a warty tumour of the larynx, may require more urgent intervention with surgery and/or chemotherapy.

Apart from the physical removal of HPV lesions, there is no specific antiviral drug for treating HPV at present. However, recent advances in HPV research have lead to the development of a vaccine against the high-risk HPV types (HPV 16 and 18) for preventing cervical carcinoma. Other vaccines to protect against other HPV-induced diseases are currently under investigation.

So it can be seen that most viral infections that result in skin rashes produce a characteristic appearance that can give a good clinical indication of the causative virus. Further discussion of viral infections, their skin rashes, and the consequences of infection are given in the chapter on rashes of childhood (see Chapter 15) and other chapters in this book.

Fungal infections

Fungal infections of the skin can be divided into three major groups, described under the headings below:

The dermatophytes

The **dermatophytes** exclusively infect superficial layers of the skin, hair, and nails; areas rich in keratin. They do not invade deeper tissues and the diseases they produce are known as "tineas" or ringworm. Ringworm is transmitted from person to person by close contact, either by direct contact with infected hosts (human or animal) or contact with infected exfoliated skin or hair in combs, hair brushes, clothing, furniture, bed linen, towels, and carpets to name just a few. Some species of dermatophytes are viable in the environment for up to 15 months. Susceptibility to infection increases with pre-existing injury to the skin in the presence of excessive humidity.

Clinically, the dermatophytes are divided into three important genera:

1 *Microsporum* species infect hair and skin
2 *Epidermophyton* species infect skin and nails
3 *Trichophyton* species infect skin, hair, and nails.

In the laboratory they are diagnosed by the pattern of macro- and microconidia on stained slides and by culture and biochemical characteristics (see Further reading).

Figure 7.23 shows some examples of some macro- and microconidia of the three important genera above.

Important characteristics of the more common dermatophyte infections are described in Table 7.2.

Fungal infections involving cutaneous and deeper tissues

An important group of fungal infections in this category is called **Mycetoma**. This is a clinical syndrome consisting of localized deforming, swollen lesions, and sinuses involving skin, subcutaneous tissue, fascia, and bony tissues. It occurs usually on the hands and feet and results from the traumatic implantation of organisms from the soil and vegetation into tissues. The classic triad of swelling, draining sinuses, and characteristic fungal granules are diagnostic. The infectious agents causing mycetoma can be fungal or bacterial. Fungal agents associated with mycetoma (sometimes known as Madura foot) are many and include the *Madurella* spp.

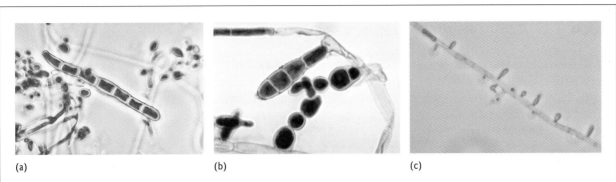

Figure 7.23 Microscopic characteristics of some of the common dermatophyte species in the three genera (phase contrast microscopy). (a) *Microsporum canis*: **long, rough, thick walled macroconidia, few pyriform microconidia. (b)** *Epidermophyton floccosum*: **blunt, smooth, thin walled, club-shaped macroconidia in clusters, no microconidia. (c)** *Trichophyton rubrum*: **few pyriform, lateral microconidia, macroconidia uncommon. Reproduced from National Centre for Mycology, Microbiology & Public Health, University of Alberta Hospitals, Edmonton, Alberta, Canada; http://www2.provlab.ab.ca/bugs/ webbug/mycology/dermhome.htm#Introduction and CDC website: http://phil.cdc.gov/phil/details.asp**

Table 7.2 Common dermatophyte infections

Clinical disease (Figure 7.24)	Affected area	Manifestation	Fungal species
Tinea pedis (athlete's foot)	Feet Webs of toes Soles	Mild to chronic scaling with inflammation	*Trichophyton* spp. *Epidermophyton* sp. *Candida* spp.★
Tinea unguium (onychomycosis)	Fingernails Toenails	Discoloration and pitting of the nail surface with lifting of the nail bed	*Trichophyton* spp. *Candida* spp.★
Tinea corporis	Superficial; most layers of the skin	Characteristic ringworm lesions with some scaling and erythema (redness and inflammation)	Most dermatophytes (commonly *Trichophyton* and *Microsporum* spp.)
Tinea cruris (jock-itch)	Groin Perineum Perianum	Raised erythemetous spreading scaly lesions with itching if the lesions are wet and weeping	*Epidermophyton* sp. *Trichophyton* spp. *Candida* spp.★
Tinea capitis	Scalp Eyebrows Eyelashes	Scaly erythematous lesions, hair loss, may be ulcerated	*Microsporum* sp. *Trichophyton* spp.

★ *Candida* spp. are not one of the dermatophyte agents, however they are included here because they cause similar lesions.

Infections caused by the **bacterial** actinomycetes are clinically similar to the fungal mycetomas (Box 7.5). Diagnosis is established by histology and culture. For further information on the mycetomas and for their management see Further reading.

Sporotrichosis is another subcutaneous fungal infection that is characterized by the development of nodular lesions in skin, subcutaneous tissue, and lymph nodes. These lesions are hard and freely movable and may ulcerate and discharge pus. Often the initial lesion develops on the fingertip or wrist and progresses up

Box 7.5 Actinomycetomas and actinomycosis

A 41-year-old male laborer presented complaining of a diffuse swelling with multiple discharging nodules on the thenar eminence (next to the thumb) of the right palm involving the first web space and back of the right hand for 6 years (see photograph right). The patient could not recollect any history of trauma. Bacterial culture grew *Streptomyces* spp.

Actinomycetomas are caused by **aerobic**, Gram positive partially acid-fast actinomycetes belonging to the genera *Nocardia*, *Streptomyces*, and *Actinomadura*.

By contrast, actinomycosis is a subacute-to-chronic bacterial infection caused by filamentous, Gram positive, **anaerobic/microaerophilic** bacteria, the *Actinomyces* spp., which are not acid fast. Actinomycosis is characterized by spreading lesions that discharge pus; multiple abscesses and sinus tracts may discharge yellow "sulfur" granules. The most common clinical forms of actinomycosis are of the face and jaw (i.e. lumpy jaw), the thorax, and the abdomen. In women, pelvic actinomycosis is possible.

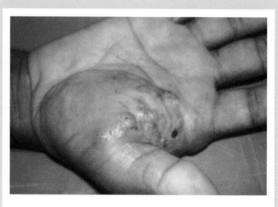

From Rai VM, Balachandran C. *Indian J Dermatol Venereol Leprol* 2006; 72: 178

the arm over a period of weeks to produce a chain of interconnected swollen lymph nodes. The agent responsible for this condition is *Sporothrix schenckii*, a common fungus of soil, wood, and plants. Infection occurs by trauma to the skin. Because it has been so commonly associated with gardening, and trauma related to rose thorns, it has been known as the rose gardener's disease. Diagnosis is established by histology and culture. For further information on management see Further reading.

Cutaneous manifestations of systemic fungal disease

Many systemic fungal infections also manifest with skin and subcutaneous lesions. Among those that are common in the Americas are:

Blastomycosis: a chronic granulomatous and pus forming disease that begins primarily as a lung infection, and may spread to skin, bone, and other body sites. Skin lesions are crusty granulomas that can ulcerate. It is caused by *Blastomyces dermatidis*, a soil fungus endemic along the Mississippi and Ohio rivers.

Coccidioidomycosis, caused by *Coccidioides immitis*, is endemic in some areas of the South-Western United States and Mexico and manifests as a chronic pulmonary infection with granulomas and abscesses in the skin and other organs.

Paracoccidioidomycosis is caused by *Paracoccidioides brasiliensis*, a systemic lung infection with disseminated skin lesions, and is endemic in South and Central America.

Almost any fungus can cause skin lesions in the **immunocompromised host**; patients with diabetes, burns and trauma victims, neutropenic hosts (those that have no or reduced numbers of circulating white blood cells), and AIDS patients are particularly vulnerable. Among those reported are *Cryptococcus neoformans*, *Aspergillus* spp., *Trichosporon beigelii*, and *Fusarium* spp.

For further information on all of the above conditions see Further reading.

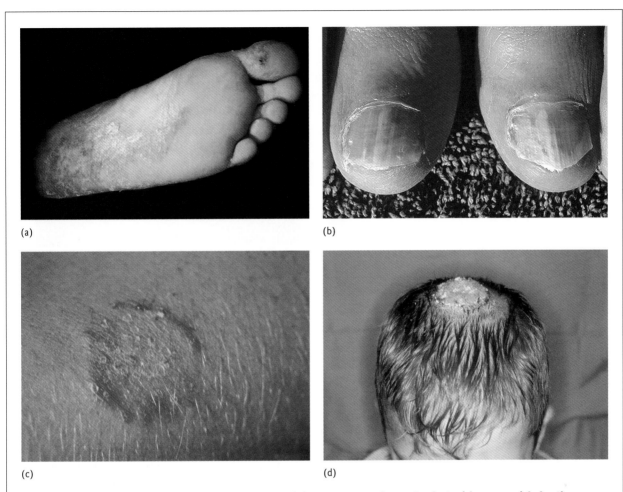

Figure 7.24 Clinical characteristics of some of the common dermatophyte (ringworm) infections. (a) Tinea pedis (athlete's foot) caused by *T. rubrum*. (b) Tinea unguium (onychomycosis) caused by *T. rubrum*. (c) Tinea corporis caused by *Trichophyton* sp. (d) Tinea capitis caused by *Microsporum* sp. Reproduced from National Centre for Mycology, Microbiology & Public Health, University of Alberta Hospitals, Edmonton, Alberta, Canada; http://www2.provlab.ab.ca/bugs/webbug/mycology/ dermhome.htm#Introduction

Parasitic infections

A wide range of parasitic infections can involve the skin and subcutaneous tissues.

Depending on the species of parasite, this involvement may be transient, the parasite merely passes through the skin on its migration to the bloodstream and so to a specific target organ, or the infection may be localized to the skin. This section will discuss the most common parasitic infections of the skin and refer you to other more specialized texts for more detail (see Further reading). See also Chapter 21 for an overview of travel related infections worldwide.

Cutaneous leishmaniasis

Commonly recognized species include *Leishmania tropica* (Oriental sore), *L. braziliensis* (Espundia), and *L. mexicana* (Chiclero ulcer). The geographical distribution of cutaneous leishmaniasis is worldwide: Africa, the Middle East, the Mediterranean, Southeast Asia, Asia, and Latin America. The lesions are typically single or few in number, while in some forms of the disease lesions tend to be diffuse. In cutaneous leishmaniasis,

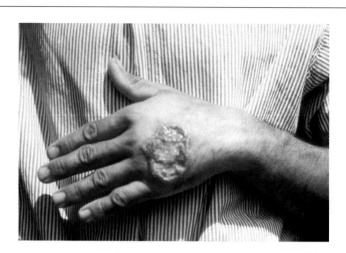

Figure 7.25 Cutaneous leishmaniasis. Provided by Dr. D.S. Martin Courtesy of the Centers for Disease Control and Prevention; from CDC website: http://phil.cdc.gov/phil/details.asp

the lesions tend to eventually heal but leave extensive and disfiguring scarring (Figure 7.25). See Chapter 2 for a description of the lifecycle and transmission of *Leishmania* spp.

Larva migrans and larva currens

The dog and cat hookworms (*Ancylostoma braziliense, A. caninum*, etc.), accidentally infect the human host; they almost never mature into the adult form. The larval form enters through the skin and wanders aimlessly in an alien host. This causes serpiginous itchy tunnel-like lesions in the skin and is also called cutaneous larva migrans or creeping eruption and can last for weeks or months.

Larval forms of *Strongyloides stercoralis* (a type of round worm) can cause similar lesions (**larva currens** rash) while penetrating the skin. The rash lasts a few days before disappearing as the infective larvae of the *Strongyloides* enter the circulation to perpetuate the infection. Such larva currens rashes may occur at irregular intervals for months or years after the patient leaves the endemic region. See Further reading for the lifecycle and transmission of *Strongyloides* spp.

Adult worms of *Onchocerca volvulus* and *Loa loa* produce an intense granulomatous tissue reaction as they migrate through the skin and subcutaneous tissue. In onchocerciasis nodular skin swellings tend to be commoner on the head in Latin America and around the groin ("hanging groin") in Africa. In loaiasis a range of allergic symptoms are seen including nodules in the skin called "Calabar swellings". Calabar swellings can occur anywhere on the body but are most common on the face, arms, and hands. For more information on these parasitic infections see Further reading.

Myiasis

The putsi (or tumbu) fly of tropical Africa and the human botfly (*Dermatobia hominis*) of central and tropical South America are interesting because they can invade normal human skin. The putsi fly lays its eggs on clothing laid out to dry on the ground while *D. hominis* lays its eggs on female mosquitoes or ticks. The eggs hatch as a result of the warmth from the human body when the clothes are worn or when the tick or mosquito feeds. The maggots develop in pustular, boil-like skin lesions for about 7–10 days, after which the fully developed larva emerges, drops to the ground and pupates, eventually emerging as the adult fly. Mostly these skin lesions are benign, although scarring can result when the maggot drops out. Sometimes, however, serious complications or even death may result when a maggot on the head penetrates the skull and invades the brain. Maggots can also be good for you – see Box 7.6.

Box 7.6 Creepy crawlies make wonderful medicine

Imagine going to a doctor for a leg wound that just won't heal. Instead of prescribing antibiotics, the doctor suggests a treatment of maggots! Maggot therapy is now standard practice in many hospitals worldwide.

The year 1995 remains a landmark in the history of maggot therapy when the first controlled prospective trial showed a significant improvement in the rate of healing associated with maggot therapy for treating pressure ulcers in patients with injuries to their spinal cord. Results demonstrated that maggot therapy was more effective and efficient at debriding (cleaning) many types of infected and gangrenous wounds than the commonly prescribed treatments in the control groups. Maggots act in several ways. Moving over the surface of wounds, maggots secrete a rich mixture of proteolytic enzymes, which liquidizes dead tissue. Maggots then ingest

this and, by raising the pH of wounds and secreting chemicals, can prevent the growth of some bacteria.

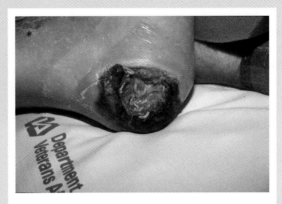

Heel pressure ulcer, undergoing maggot debridement, c. 1992 at VA Medical Center in Long Beach, CA. Photo by R.A. Sherman. © BTER Foundation

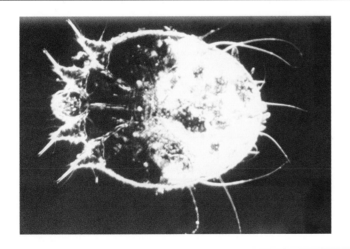

Figure 7.26 *Sarcoptes scabiei* var. *hominis* or "itch mite," associated with the transmission of human scabies. Provided by Joe Miller/Reed and Carnrick Pharmaceuticals, Courtesy of the Centers for Disease Control and Prevention; from CDC website: http://phil.cdc.gov/phil/details.asp

Scabies

Scabies is the most important ecto-parasitic (parasites that infect external surfaces) infection of humans. It is caused by the human scabies mite, *Sarcoptes scabiei* (Figure 7.26). Clinical features of scabies involve two components – tunnels in which the mites live (these occur predominantly in the web spaces of the fingers, wrists, elbows, ankles, and the inner aspect of the thighs) and an allergic rash (Figure 7.27). The mite lesions itch unbearably and the rash tends to cover the body, but spare the face. Thus as a diagnostic rule of thumb, any person presenting with an itchy rash which covers the body but spares the face can be considered to have scabies until proven otherwise. Scabies is transmissible from person to person by skin to skin contact. Box 7.7 describes a rare form of scabies in the immuno-compromised.

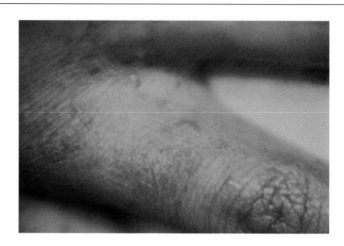

Figure 7.27 The pimple-like rash in the webbing between the fingers of this adult's hand due to *Sarcoptes scabiei* var. *hominis*. Courtesy of the Centers for Disease Control and Prevention; from CDC website: http://phil.cdc.gov/phil/details.asp

Box 7.7 Norwegian or crusted scabies

Norwegian scabies differs from regular scabies in the number of mites present. In regular scabies patients are infested, on average, with 10–15 mites at any one time. Persons with Norwegian scabies harbor thousands to millions of mites. Consequently, their skin manifestations are much more severe with thick, hyperkeratotic (thickened superficial skin) crusts that can occur on almost any area of the body including the head and face. The type of mite is exactly the same in both presentations. The difference lies with the host; patients with Norwegian scabies have severely compromised immune systems; before the advent of antiretroviral therapy Norwegian scabies was a common opportunistic infection of AIDS patients.

Test yourself

Case study 7.1

This lady came to casualty with a painful, red lesion on her face, as shown in the photograph. She gave a history of sustaining an insect bite during a recent holiday. The bite became red and inflamed, but subsided over time. She was febrile with pain and swelling over the left eye. The rash had begun to blister with clear fluid. There was no abscess formation and she was otherwise well. She also complained of aches and pains in her joints, and pain in her throat. In casualty, blood and throat cultures were taken (see Gram stain and culture on agar to the right of the photograph), and she was admitted for observation.

1. What is your diagnosis?
2. What is the causative organism (give genus and species)?
3. Name one other toxin associated condition as a result of infection with this organism.
4. Name one potentially life-threatening infection with this organism.

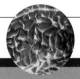

Test yourself

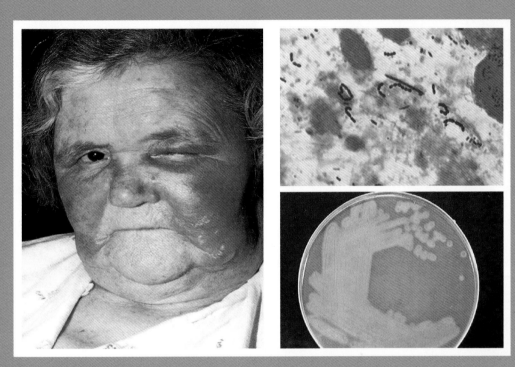

Case study 7.2

A 50-year-old man with a longstanding history of insulin dependent diabetes mellitus developed a boil on his left shoulder. His diabetes was increasingly difficult to control and he developed a spreading lesion at the site of the original boil, shown in the photograph below. On examination he had a fever, the lesion was tender and inflamed with pus formation. See Gram stain from the pus (image below at 1000× magnification).

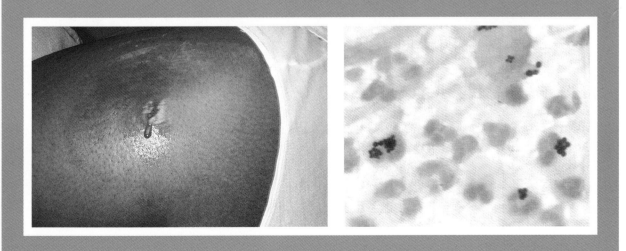

Test yourself

1. What is the lesion called?
2. Based on the Gram smear, what is the most likely causative organism (give genus and species)?
3. Name two toxin mediated conditions caused by this organism.
4. Why would it not be appropriate to treat this organism with amoxicillin?

Case study 7.3

A young boy sustained an injury to his shin during a hockey match. The surface wound became infected, but healed eventually. Several weeks after the initial infection he still complained of pain while playing hockey. He presented to the clinic with low grade temperature, occasional loss of energy, and pain over his lower leg (especially on exercise). He was unable to sustain regular hockey training, and needed pain killers. He was admitted when he became increasingly febrile and the pain became considerably worse. An X-ray of his lower leg was taken and the surface wound examined (Gram stain at 1000× magnification).

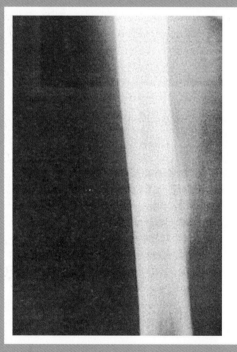 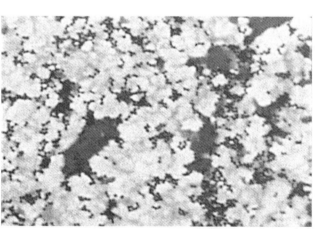

1. What is the most likely clinical diagnosis?
2. What is the most important organism implicated in this condition (give genus and species)?
3. Name one microbiological investigation you would send before commencing empirical treatment.
4. Describe the pathophysiology of this condition.

Further reading

Carneiro SC, Cestari T, Allen SH, Ramos e-Silva M. Viral exanthems in the tropics. *Clin Dermatol* 2007;25(2):212–220

Chiodini PL, Moody A, Manser DW. *Atlas of Medical Helminthology and Protozoology*, 4th edition. London: Churchill Livingstone, 2001

Dyer JA. Childhood viral exanthems. *Pediatr Ann* 2007;36(1):21–29

Guidelines from the Infectious Diseases Society of America. Practice Guidelines for the Diagnosis and Management of Skin and Soft-Tissue Infections. *Clin Infect Dis* 2005;41:1373–1406. http://www.journals.uchicago.edu/CID/journal/issues/v41n10/37519/37519.html

Pickering LK, Baker CJ, McMillan J, Long S (eds). *Red Book*, 27th edition. Bk Grove Villlage, IL: American Academy of Pediatrics, 2006, 992pp

Useful websites

CDC website on infectious disease. http://www.cdc.gov/ncidod/diseases/

Dermatology Information Service. http://dermis.multimedica.de/dermisroot/en/list/all/search.htm

An online dermatology atlas with photographs of most rash appearances, though you need to know the name of the rash illness you are looking for (or suspecting)

Hardin MD. Childhood Skin Rashes. http://www.lib.uiowa.edu/hardin/md/skinrashes.html

Another useful site combining text and images with multiple links to other relevant websites, but you still have to know the name of the rash you are looking for (or suspecting)

The Mycoses. http://www.doctorfungus.org/mycoses/human/other/mycetoma.htm

Patient UK. Common Childhood Rashes. http://www.patient.co.uk/showdoc/40000396/

A useful website for both patients and doctors to differentiate and recognize different childhood rashes (but no photographs)

World of Dermatophytes: A Pictorial. http://www2.provlab.ab.ca/bugs/webbug/mycology/dermhome.htm#Introduction

Chapter 8
Gastroenteritis

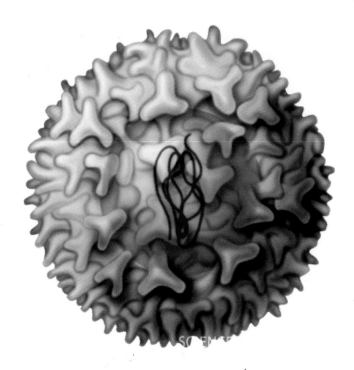

N. Shetty, J.W. Tang

Food and waterborne diarrhea
  Salmonellae
  Campylobacter jejuni
  Bacillus cereus
  Staphylococcus aureus
  Clostridium perfringens
  Escherichia coli O157
  Shigella spp.
Viral diarrheas

Pathophysiology of diarrheas
  Bacterial diarrheas
  Viral diarrheas
Parasitic diarrheas
  Giardiasis
  Cryptosporidiosis
  Amebiasis
Principles of management of diarrheal disease

The pathophysiology of infections of the gastrointestinal tract is a complex mechanism involving interaction between food, humans, animals, and microbes. To clarify the multifactorial issues that underpin the disease syndrome that is broadly and loosely termed "infectious diarrhea," we begin our discussions with a simple classification. Table 8.1 illustrates the threads that comprise the various clinical and epidemiologic scenarios that relate to the discussion on gastroenteritis. These categories do not constitute water tight compartments as some organisms may be in more than one clinico-epidemiologic scenario. For example *Salmonella* spp. is an important foodborne pathogen; it is also transmitted from person to person via fecal–oral contamination. As with all enteric pathogens the attack rate and severity of symptoms depends on the dose ingested. Read the rest of the chapter and try and answer the questions in Box 8.1.

For traveler's diarrhea including cholera, see Chapter 21.

Food and waterborne diarrhea

According to the WHO, 1.8 million people (mostly children) die every year from diarrheal diseases (including cholera). Globally infectious diarrhea remains one of the most common diseases afflicting children under five years of age and accounts for 15–30% of deaths in children under five years of age. The number

Table 8.1 An overview of agents implicated in gastroenteritis

Food borne diarrhea	Viral diarrheas	Parasitic diarrheas	Traveler's diarrhea (see Chapter 21)	Antibiotic associated colitis
Salmonellae *Campylobacter* spp. *Bacillus cereus* *Staphylococcus aureus* *Clostridium perfringens* *Escherichia coli* O157 *Shigella* spp. Noroviruses	Rotavirus Human caliciviruses (e.g. norovirus "winter-vomiting disease" Enteric adenoviruses (serotypes 40 and 41) Astroviruses	*Giardia lamblia* *Cryptosporidium* spp. *Cyclospora* *Isospora belli* *Balantidium coli* *Entamoeba histolytica*	**Invasive:** *Shigella* spp. Enteroinvasive *E. coli* *E. coli* O157 Enteropathogenic *E. coli* Salmonellae *Campylobacter* spp. **Secretory** *Vibrio cholerae* and other species Enterotoxigenic *E. coli*	See Chapter 14

Box 8.1 Food-borne infections

A 2-year-old boy is referred to the pediatricians with a 24-hour history of vomiting and diarrhea. He is floppy and listless. He is normally a happy and playful child and is up to date with immunizations. No one else in the family is unwell. His mother has recently introduced soft-boiled eggs into his diet.

On examination he is mildly dehydrated and his temperature is 37.5°C. Ear, nose, and throat examination is normal, and his chest is clear. His abdomen is soft, and he complains of a mild tenderness in the lower quadrants. A fecal sample has been sent to the laboratory. Read on to answer these questions.

- What is the most likely organism (to genus level) that may have caused these symptoms?
- Describe the pathophysiology of disease by this group of organisms?
- What control of infection measures are necessary?

of episodes per year among these children varies according to the area and country, and is reported to be between two and four. The lowest reports come from East Asia and the highest from South Asia (Bangladesh). Diarrhea remains a disease of poverty afflicting malnourished children in crowded and contaminated environments. Efforts to provide safe water and adequate sanitation facilities, and to encourage mothers to exclusively breastfeed infants through 6 months of age, can blunt an increase in diarrhea morbidity and mortality. Unsafe water supply, inadequate sanitation, and hygiene contribute to 88% of diarrheal disease.

Preventive strategies to limit the transmission of diarrheal disease need to go hand in hand with national diarrhea disease control programs that concentrate on effective diarrhea case management and the prevention of dehydration (Box 8.2). The WHO has shown that improved sanitation can reduce diarrhea morbidity by 32%; hygiene interventions including hygiene education and promotion of hand washing can lead to a reduction of diarrheal cases by up to 45% and improvements in drinking-water quality through household water treatment, such as chlorination at point of use, can lead to a reduction of diarrhea episodes by between 35% and 39%.

In the USA, current Public Health Service records estimate that there are approximately 76 million people who suffer foodborne diarrheal disease annually, with 300 000 hospitalizations and 5000 deaths. Special risks of death exist in the elderly, the immunocompromised, or pregnant. Notification of foodborne diarrheal disease cases to a Central Public Health Authority such as the Centers for Disease Control (CDC) is

Box 8.2 What would you vote for as the top medical advance since 1840?

Think about the interventions that have had the greatest impact on human health. Here are the results, ranked in order of importance, of a global vote conducted by the *British Medical Journal* (BMJ) in 2007.

1. Sanitation	6. Germ theory
2. Antibiotics	7. Oral contraceptive pill
3. Anesthesia	8. Evidence based medicine
4. Vaccines	9. Medical imaging
5. Discovery of DNA structure	10. Computers

The competition was tough as is evident from the list above. Clean water and sewage disposal gathered the most votes in an online poll that asked voters to rank the top 15 milestones, as selected by a panel of the BMJ's editors and advisers.

The editorial comments that followed state:

Believing that diseases were caused by air contaminated by poor urban drainage, governments built new sewage disposal and water supply systems. This revolutionized public health in Europe, and mortality from infectious diseases fell dramatically. Nowadays we know that better water supply and sanitation can cut diarrhea among children in developing countries by about a fifth. The 19th century "sanitary revolution" shows that effective intervention does not always need accurate knowledge, that environmental measures may be more effective than changing individual behavior, and that universal measures may be better than targeted measures in reducing health inequalities.

mandatory in most countries where facilities exist. Table 8.2 provides an overview of the more common causes of foodborne diarrhea in the developed world. Study the chapter and fill in the last column with the most common incriminating foodstuff.

Salmonellae

Salmonellosis is an important cause of foodborne diarrhea worldwide, including the USA. According to the FDA and CDC there are an estimated 2–4 million cases of salmonella diarrhea annually, with more than 500 deaths per year. Salmonella gastroenteritis has classically been associated with eating raw eggs or foods prepared with salmonella infected raw eggs such as mayonnaise and mousse. The CDC estimates that 75% of *Salmonella* outbreaks are linked to raw or inadequately cooked Grade A whole shell eggs. Infected hens deposit the organism in the yolk prior to shell deposition.

Raw eggs like any other raw food of animal origin should be stored and handled properly. According to the CDC eggs should be refrigerated until they are needed because refrigeration prevents any *Salmonella* present in the egg from multiplying. Other guidelines from the CDC to reduce infection include:

- Cook eggs thoroughly until the yolk and white are firm.
- Discard cracked or dirty eggs.
- Wash hands and cooking utensils with soap and water after contact with raw eggs.
- Eat eggs promptly after cooking. Do not keep eggs warm for more than 2 hours.
- Refrigerate unused or leftover egg-containing foods.

Outbreaks of salmonella food poisoning have also been linked with a variety of foods such as raw meats, poultry, milk and dairy products, fish, frog legs, yeast, coconut, peanut butter, chocolate, and environmental sources such as water, insects, pets, and kitchen surfaces. The typical route of infection for humans is by ingesting *Salmonella* from an animal source, i.e. eggs and poultry (zoonoses). However, *Salmonella* can also

Table 8.2 The foodborne diarrhea ready reckoner (read on and list the foodstuffs most commonly implicated with each organism)

Organism	Pathogenesis	Incubation period (h)	Vomiting	Diarrhea	Abdominal pain	Fever	Foods?
Salmonellae	Multiplication of organisms in small and large intestines causing epithelial cell damage	16–48	Slight	Moderate, may be bloody	Frequently present	Often present	
Campylobacter spp.	Multiplication of organisms (?) release of enterotoxin in gut	16–48	Nausea rarely vomiting	Profuse and often bloody	Often severe	Often present	
Bacillus cereus	Emetic enterotoxin in food or diarrheogenic enterotoxin	0.5–6	Profuse	If toxin present	Absent	Absent	
Staphylococcus aureus	Heat stable enterotoxin in food	1–6	Profuse	Slight	Absent	Absent	
Clostridium perfringens	Multiplication of organisms and release of enterotoxin in gut during sporulation	12–24	Absent	Moderate	Colicky pain	Absent	
Escherichia coli O157	Multiplication of organisms, and release of cyto entero-toxins	16–48	Absent	Bloody	Cramps	Often present	
Human calicivurses (e.g. Norovirus "winter-vomiting disease")	Precise mechanisms of diarrhea and vomiting unknown, but may involve transient malabsorption of fat due to decreased activity of enzymes in intestinal mucosa	12–24	Frequent, can be projectile	Moderate, nonbloody	Cramps	Often present, low grade	

Note: Pure toxins such as botulism, scrombotoxin, and shellfish poisoning may also be considered as agents of food poisoning.

Box 8.3 Pet turtles and salmonellosis (report from *MMWR* July 6, 2007/56(26);649–652)

On February 20, 2007, a female infant aged 3 weeks with a 1-day history of poor feeding and lethargy was evaluated in an emergency department at a Florida hospital. The patient was transferred immediately to a tertiary-care pediatric hospital; on arrival, she was febrile and in septic shock. Antibiotics were administered. She died on March 1. Cultures of cerebrospinal fluid and blood samples yielded *Salmonella* serotype Pomona.

The parents of the patient were interviewed by the Florida Department of Health. A family friend had purchased a small turtle with a carapace of 1.25 inches and gifted it as a pet to the patient's family in late January 2007. After the death of the infant, laboratory testing of the turtle and its environment was performed by the Florida Bureau of Laboratories. A fecal sample from the turtle yielded *S.* Pomona. The *S.* Pomona isolates from the patient and the turtle were indistinguishable by a molecular typing method.

Editorial: Despite a federal law prohibiting the sale or distribution of small turtles as pets, such sales still occur. *Salmonella* can be transmitted to humans by direct or indirect contact with a turtle or its feces. No reliable methods are available to guarantee that a turtle is free of *Salmonella*. Most turtles are colonized with *Salmonella* and shed the bacteria intermittently in their feces. In addition, water in turtle bowls or aquariums can amplify any *Salmonella* shed by turtles. For these reasons, all turtles, regardless of carapace size, should be handled as though they are infected with *Salmonella*.

---

be transmitted by food handlers who are chronic carriers of the infection, by using contaminated water for cleaning utensils, by houseflies who flit from excrement to foodstuffs, or by eating shellfish or vegetables grown in contaminated water or soil. This latter mode is commonly seen in travelers who return from endemic areas where there is poor water and sanitation. A recent multi-state outbreak of the serotype *Salmonella* Agona caused much concern because it was the first outbreak of *Salmonella* spp. in a commercial cereal product. Between April and May 1998, a total of 11 states in the USA reported an increase in cases of *S.* Agona infections. Over 200 cases were reported and nearly 50 people were hospitalized.

Salmonella infections can also be acquired from nonfood sources such as close contact with animals and pets. Reptiles (lizards, snakes, and turtles), baby chicks and ducklings, dogs, cats, birds (including pet birds), horses, and farm animals can pass *Salmonella* in their feces (Box 8.3).

Campylobacter jejuni

Campylobacter jejuni is a leading cause of bacterial foodborne illness in the USA as in most of the western world. In the USA, more than 2 million cases occur annually, with an estimated death toll of 200–500 per year. Peak incidence occurs in children below 1 year of age and in young adults (15–24 years old). Campylobacteriosis is a zoonotic infection, the animal reservoir and foodstuff most commonly implicated is chicken. In many countries *Campylobacter* diarrhea is a seasonal illness associated with summer barbecues, where the risk of ingesting inadequately cooked barbecued chicken is high. In the USA a secondary peak is seen in the late fall. Humans also acquire the infection via unpasteurized milk or improperly treated water.

In resource poor countries where campylobacter infections are hyperendemic, fecal–oral and person to person transmission is more common. Symptomatic disease occurs in young children and persistent, asymptomatic carriage in adults.

Bacillus cereus

Bacillus cereus is described as a true poisoning as the illness is associated with ingesting a pre-formed toxin or toxins (Box 8.4). Between 1972 and 1986, 52 outbreaks of foodborne disease associated with *B. cereus* were

Box 8.4 Gastrointestinal illness in diners at a restaurant – a report from CDC

Reported by J Vandeloski, Portland City Health Department; KF Gensheimer, MD, State Epidemiologist, Maine Department of Human Services; Enteric Diseases Br., Division of Bacterial Diseases, Center for Infectious Diseases, CDC
On September 22, 1985, the Maine Bureau of Health was notified of a gastrointestinal illness among patrons of a Japanese restaurant. The customers exhibited symptoms of illness while still on the restaurant premises.

A case was defined as anyone who had vomiting or diarrhea within 6 hours of dining at the restaurant. All 11 patrons affected reported nausea and vomiting; nine reported diarrhea; one reported headache; and one reported abdominal cramps. Onset of illness ranged from 30 minutes to 5 hours (mean 1 hour, 23 minutes) after eating at the restaurant.

Analysis of the association of food consumption with illness was not instructive, since all persons consumed the same food items: chicken soup; fried shrimp; stir-fried rice; fried zucchini, onions and bean sprouts; cucumber, cabbage, and lettuce salad; ginger salad dressing; hibachi chicken and steak; and tea.

According to the owner, all meat was delivered two or three times a week from a local meat supplier and refrigerated until ordered by restaurant patrons. Appropriate sized portions for a dining group were taken from the kitchen to the dining area and diced or sliced, then sautéed at the table directly in front of restaurant patrons. The fried rice served with the meal was reportedly customarily made from leftover boiled rice. It could not be established whether the boiled rice had been stored refrigerated or at room temperature. Read the rest of the chapter to answer these questions:

❓What is the most probable bacterial cause of this incident? State your reasons.
❓Elaborate on the toxin mechanisms responsible?
❓What food/s due you think is/are most likely to be the culprit?
❓How could the restaurateur have prevented this from happening?

reported to the CDC. *B. cereus* infection is characterized by two clinical syndromes: an emetic syndrome with profuse vomiting and abdominal cramps has an incubation period of 0.5–6 hours; and a diarrheic form presenting with abdominal cramps and diarrhea with an incubation period of 8–16 hours. Diarrhea may be a small volume or profuse and watery.

B. cereus food poisoning occurs year-round and has a worldwide distribution. The emetic syndrome is most often associated with fried rice that has been cooked and then held at warm temperatures for several hours; and is almost always linked with fried rice served in Oriental restaurants. Interestingly, a recent, well documented outbreak of the emetic syndrome of *B. cereus* in a British prison implicated beef stew. This was thought to be caused by adding vegetables that were cooked a day earlier to freshly cooked meat.

The diarrhoeic *B. cereus* food poisoning is frequently associated with stored cooked meat or vegetable-containing foods. The bacterium has been isolated from 50% of dried beans and cereals and from 25% of dried foods such as spices, seasoning mixes, and potatoes. One outbreak of the long-incubation form was traced to a "meals-on-wheels" program in which food was held above room temperature for a prolonged period.

The short-incubation or emetic form of the disease is diagnosed by the isolation of *B. cereus* from the incriminated food. The long-incubation or diarrheal form is diagnosed by isolation of the organism from stool and food. In both cases quantitative cultures are needed to demonstrate gross contamination. This is because *B. cereus* is a ubiquitous organism found in cereals, spices, and dried foods; in addition, 14% of healthy adults have been reported to have transient gastrointestinal colonization with *B. cereus*. Infection can be prevented by keeping cold food cold and hot food hot (bacteria grow best at temperatures ranging from 40 to 140°F).

Staphylococcus aureus

Staphylococcal food poisoning is a major concern worldwide since staphylococcal contamination of foods and staphylococcal carriage in food handlers is widespread. The true incidence of staphylococcal food poisoning is unknown as the condition is often misdiagnosed. In the USA 7–10 outbreaks are reported annually involving hundreds of cases. Staphylococcal food poisoning can be severe and distressing if the foods or the food handler harbors a strain that carries the gene for the enterotoxin. The onset of symptoms in staphylococcal food poisoning is usually rapid, within 0.5–6 hours. Like *B. cereus* emetic food poisoning, it is a true intoxication, the individual having consumed foods contaminated with pre-formed toxin. The most common symptoms are nausea, vomiting, retching, abdominal cramping, and prostration, also similar to the *B. cereus* emetic syndrome.

Foods that are frequently incriminated in staphylococcal food poisoning are bakery products such as cream-filled pastries, cream pies, and chocolate eclairs, milk and milk based puddings. However, meat and meat products, poultry and egg products, salads such as egg, tuna and chicken, potato, and macaroni have also been named. Foods that require considerable handling during preparation, and those that are allowed to cool slowly from high temperatures of cooking and baking, such as cakes and puddings, are frequently involved in staphylococcal food poisoning. Staphylococci exist in air, dust, sewage, water, milk, and food, and on food equipment, environmental surfaces, humans, and animals. Humans and animals are the primary reservoirs. Staphylococci are present in the nasal passages and throats and on the hair and skin of 50% or more of healthy individuals. Although food handlers are usually the main source of food contamination in food poisoning outbreaks, equipment and environmental surfaces can also be sources of contamination with *S. aureus*. Humans contract food poisoning by ingesting pre-formed enterotoxins produced in food by some strains of *S. aureus*, usually because the food has not been kept consistently hot enough (60°C/140°F, or above) or cold enough (7.2°C/45°F, or below).

Clostridium perfringens

Sources at the CDC, state that perfringens food poisoning is one of the most commonly reported foodborne illnesses in the USA, around 10 000 actual cases occur annually. At least 10–20 outbreaks have been reported annually in the USA in the past two decades, some involving tens of hundreds of patients. It is probable that many outbreaks go unreported because the implicated foods or patient feces are not tested routinely for *Clostridium perfringens* or its toxin.

Food poisoning due to *C. perfringens* is characterized by intense abdominal cramps and diarrhea which begin typically 12–24 hours after consumption of contaminated foods. Examination of foodstuffs implicated (and patients' feces) will show large numbers ($>10^8$) of *C. perfringens* capable of producing the food poisoning toxin. Toxin can also be detected in the feces. The illness lasts no more than 24 hours but less severe symptoms may persist in some individuals for 1 or 2 weeks. A few deaths have been reported as a result of dehydration and other complications.

In most instances, the primary cause of poisoning by *C. perfringens* is inadequate temperature maintenance of prepared foods. Small numbers of the organisms, often present after cooking, multiply to food poisoning levels during cool down and storage of prepared foods. Meats, meat products and gravy are the foods most frequently implicated. Institutions such as school cafeterias, hospitals, nursing homes, prisons, etc., where large quantities of food are prepared several hours before serving, are particularly at risk. The young and elderly are the most frequent victims of perfringens poisoning (Box 8.5).

Escherichia coli O157

Escherichia coli O157:H7 is an important and potentially dangerous cause of foodborne illness. An estimated 73 000 cases of infection and 61 deaths occur in the USA each year. The illness is characterized by severe cramping (abdominal pain) and diarrhea which is initially watery but becomes grossly bloody (hemorrhagic

Box 8.5 Gastroenteritis associated with corned beef served at St Patrick's Day meals – 1993 (*MMWR* March 4, 1994/43(08); 137–138,143–144)

On March 18, 1993, the Cleveland City Health Department (CCHD) received telephone calls from 15 persons who became ill after eating corned beef purchased from one delicatessen. After a local newspaper article publicized this problem, 156 persons contacted CCHD to report onset of illness within 48 hours of eating food from the delicatessen on March 16 or March 17. Of the 156 persons reporting illness, 144 (92%) reported having eaten corned beef, 20 (13%) pickles, 12 (8%) potato salad, and 11 (7%), roast beef.

In anticipation of a large demand for corned beef on St Patrick's Day (March 17), the delicatessen had purchased 1400 pounds of raw, salt-cured product.

Beginning March 12, portions of the corned beef were boiled for 3 hours at the delicatessen, allowed to cool at room temperature, and refrigerated. On March 16 and 17, the portions were removed from the refrigerator, held in a warmer at 120°F (48.8°C), and sliced and served. Corned beef sandwiches also were made for catering to several groups on March 17; these sandwiches were held at room temperature from 11 am until they were eaten throughout the afternoon.

Cultures of two of three samples of leftover corned beef obtained from the delicatessen yielded greater than or equal to 10^5 colonies of *C. perfringens* per gram. Read on to complete the exercise.

❓Describe the pathogenesis and virulence factors associated with this organism.
❓What symptoms would the patients have displayed?
❓What is the incubation period for illness with this organism (state a range)?
❓Name one simple measure that could have prevented the outbreak.

colitis). Occasionally vomiting occurs. Fever is either low-grade or absent. The illness is usually self-limited and lasts for an average of 8 days. The infective dose can be as few as 10 organisms. Some victims, particularly the very young and the elderly, risk developing serious complications such as hemolytic uremic syndrome (HUS), characterized by renal failure and lysis of red blood cells leading to hemolytic anemia. From 0 to 15% of hemorrhagic colitis victims may develop HUS. The disease can lead to permanent loss of kidney function. Other complications include a syndrome of fever, neurologic damage, and a fall in thrombocytes (platelets), known as thrombotic thrombocytopenic purpura (TTP). This illness can have a mortality rate in the elderly as high as 50%.

Undercooked or raw hamburger (ground beef) has been implicated in many of the documented outbreaks, however *E. coli* O157:H7 outbreaks have implicated alfalfa sprouts, unpasteurized fruit juices, dry-cured salami, lettuce, game meat, and cheese curds. Raw milk was the vehicle in a school outbreak in Canada. A novel source of *E. coli* O157:H7 infection has been the petting farm or zoo, where children are encouraged to play with young farm animals and have then reportedly put their unwashed hands into their mouths. The largest *E. coli* O157:H7 outbreaks worldwide and the sources implicated are illustrated in Table 8.3.

Most illness has been associated with eating undercooked, contaminated ground beef. Person-to-person contact in families and childcare centers is also an important mode of transmission. Infection can also occur after drinking raw milk and after swimming in or drinking sewage-contaminated water. Consumers can prevent *E. coli* O157:H7 infection by thoroughly cooking ground beef, avoiding unpasteurized milk, and washing hands carefully. As the organism lives in the intestines of healthy cattle, preventive measures on cattle farms, in abattoirs, and during meat processing are recommended. No other organism has had as much impact on the beef industry and on the federal agencies that regulate food safety (Box 8.6).

Table 8.3 Largest *E. coli* O157:H7 outbreaks worldwide and the sources implicated

Year	Place	No. of people sick	Contamination source
1989	Montana, USA	243	Undercooked ground beef
1996	Sakai, Japan	5727	Poorly washed white radish sprouts
1996	Scotland, UK	496	Undercooked ground beef
2000	Walkerton, Canada	>2000	Contaminated drinking water
2002	Pennsylvania, USA	51	Petting infected dairy animals

Box 8.6 Hudson Foods recalls beef burgers nationwide (Food Safety and Inspection Service, United States Department of Agriculture, Washington, DC 20250-3700. Consumer Education and Information Release No. 0272.97)

Washington, August 12, 1997 – The Hudson Foods Company, a Rogers, Ark., meat processing firm, is voluntarily recalling about 20 000 pounds of frozen ground beef patties distributed nationwide, because the product may be contaminated with a bacteria, the US Department of Agriculture's Food Safety and Inspection Service announced today.

USDA learned of the problem from the Colorado Department of Public Health and Environment after it received reports of illness from several Colorado consumers who had eaten the Hudson product in early July. Laboratory tests showed the same strain among many of those who became ill, some of whom had eaten the Hudson product.

One elderly patient was critically ill with focal neurological symptoms, falling platelets, and renal failure. Read the rest of the chapter and attempt these questions:

- ❓ Name the organism that may have caused the outbreak.
- ❓ Detail the pathogenesis of illness caused by the organism, relating it to the patient's illness.
- ❓ How did the organism contaminate the beef product?
- ❓ At the consumer end what measure can render the product safe for eating?

Shigella spp.

There are four species of *Shigella: dysenteriae, flexneri, boydii* and *sonnei*. *Shigella sonnei* accounts for over two-thirds of the shigellosis in the USA. *Shigella flexneri* accounts for almost all of the rest. Other types of *Shigella* are rare in the USA, although they are important causes of disease in the developing world and of travellers' diarrhea. See Chapter 21 for a more detailed description of the shigellae.

S. sonnei is the commonest cause of gastroenteritis, an estimated 300 000 cases of shigellosis occur annually in the USA. The number attributable to food is unknown, but given the low infectious dose it is probably substantial. Humans and other primates are the only reservoirs for *S. sonnei*, and transmission occurs through the fecal–oral route. As few as 10–100 organisms can cause disease; infection is transmitted person-to-person where hygienic conditions are compromised. In the USA, *S. sonnei* primarily infects young children and is a common cause of diarrheal outbreaks in childcare centers. Although reported infrequently, foodborne outbreaks of shigellosis have been associated with raw produce, including green onions, iceberg lettuce, and uncooked baby maize. Patients typically describe loose stools, with abdominal pain and fever.

Reports of outbreaks from restaurants indicate that salads (potato, tuna, shrimp, macaroni, and chicken), raw vegetables, milk and dairy products, and poultry are all implicated. Contamination of these foods is usually through the fecal–oral route. Fecally contaminated water and unsanitary handling by food handlers are the most common causes of contamination.

Box 8.7 Summary exercise

Twenty-five guests attended a wedding reception on a hot summer afternoon. Wild rice, soft cheeses, chicken, salad greens, and mayonnaise were amongst the ingredients used for the menu. The catering was provided by a well known gourmet food company. Between 12 and 18 hours later, 12 of the guests attended the emergency department with abdominal pain and profuse diarrhea tinged with blood.

❓Name all the organisms that could be associated with the each of the foods mentioned.

❓Now look at the incubation period and rule out the ones that may not apply.

❓Match the patients' symptoms with all the organisms that could be implicated in this incident.

❓Why do you think this outbreak occurred and what could have been done to prevent it?

Worldwide, isolates of *Shigella* spp. have been found to be resistant to many antimicrobial agents, including ampicillin and trimethoprim-sulfamethoxazole, which are commonly used to treat shigellosis. Reports from CDC indicate that antimicrobial resistance among the shigellae have increased substantially in the USA: resistance to ampicillin increased from 32% to 67%, resistance to trimethoprim-sulfamethoxazole increased from 7% to 35%, and resistance to both agents increased from 6% to 19%. A history of international travel was the strongest risk factor for *Shigella* infection resistant to trimethoprim-sulfamethoxazole (see Chapter 21).

Now attempt the exercise in Box 8.7.

Sometimes you can ingest a toxin orally via food and suffer the effects of food poisoning at other sites in the body, read Box 8.8 for examples of these.

Box 8.8 Botulism, scrombotoxin and shellfish poisoning: ingested via the oral route; effects felt elsewhere

Foodborne botulism occurs when a person ingests pre-formed toxin produced by *Clostridium botulinum*. Symptoms begin within 6 hours to 2 weeks (most commonly between 12 and 36 hours) after eating toxin-containing food. Symptoms of botulism include double vision, blurred vision, drooping eyelids, slurred speech, difficulty swallowing, dry mouth, muscle weakness that always descends through the body: first shoulders are affected, then upper arms, lower arms, thighs, calves, etc. Paralysis of breathing muscles can cause a person to stop breathing and die, unless assistance with breathing (mechanical ventilation) is provided. Botulism is not spread from one person to another. Foodborne botulism can occur in all age groups. A supply of antitoxin against botulism is maintained by CDC. The antitoxin is effective in reducing the severity of symptoms if administered early in the course of the disease. Most patients eventually recover after weeks to months of supportive care.

Scrombotoxin poisoning is caused by the ingestion of scromboid foods that contain high levels of histamine. Certain fish such as tuna and mahi mahi are rich in an amino acid called histidine. Bacterial spoilage of such foods causes histidine to be broken down into histamine, a substance that acts on blood vessels. Initial symptoms may include a tingling or burning sensation in the mouth, a rash on the upper body, and a drop in blood pressure. Frequently, headaches and itching of the skin are encountered. The symptoms may progress to nausea, vomiting, and diarrhea and may require hospitalization, particularly in the case of elderly or impaired patients. Fishery products that have been implicated in scrombotoxin poisoning include the tunas (e.g. skipjack and yellowfin), mahi mahi, bluefish, sardines, mackerel, amberjack, and abalone.

Shellfish poisoning is caused by a group of toxins elaborated by planktonic algae upon which the shellfish feed. The toxins are accumulated and sometimes metabolized by the shellfish. There are four types of shellfish poisoning named after the major symptoms they produce: Paralytic Shellfish Poisoning (PSP); Diarrheic Shellfish Poisoning (DSP); Neurotoxic Shellfish Poisoning (NSP); Amnesic Shellfish Poisoning (ASP).

Viral diarrheas

Human caliciviruses, i.e. the noroviruses (formerly known as "Norwalk-like" viruses) and the sapoviruses (formerly known as "Sapporo-like viruses"), are the most common cause of viral diarrhea in the USA. Data from the Center for Disease Research & Policy (CIDRAP), University of Minnesota, suggests that they have been estimated to cause 23 million cases per year in the USA. An estimated 181 000 cases of this type of food poisoning occur annually.

Antibodies to these viruses are detectable in young children from 3 to 4 years old, and seropositivity is greater than 50% by the age of 50 years. Transmission of noroviruses occurs all year round but mainly peaks in winter in temperate countries, such as the USA. In one study by CDC, using PCR assays, during 2000–2004, 81% (181/226) of suspected viral diarrhea outbreaks was associated with human caliciviruses (noroviruses). Norovirus outbreaks are particularly common in enclosed areas, where there is a "captive population" that can transmit the virus to each other, e.g. cruise ships, nursing/retirement homes, hospitals, schools/daycare centers, military/recreational camps, and also swimming pools (as this nonenveloped virus can resist low levels of chlorine for some time). Viral transmission can be via food, water (or other drinks) and person-to-person (due to vomiting-inhalation or fecal–oral transmission). For an illustration of the multiple routes of transmission of norovirus read Box 8.9. Norovirus is also a common cause of "traveler's diarrhea."

In children, rotavirus is the most common cause of viral diarrhea, accounting for about 25% of cases hospitalized for gastroenteritis. In the community (non-hospital-based) setting, one study found that viruses were responsible for most cases of diarrhea where an organism was identified, but an organism was only

---

Box 8.9 The multiple transmission routes of norovirus ("winter-vomiting disease")

Part 1: The football game (from Becker et al. *New England Journal of Medicine* 2000;343:1223–1227)

During a college football game in Florida, many players on a North Carolina team developed diarrhea and vomiting. The next day, similar symptoms developed in some members of the opposing team. Investigations showed that a lunch box eaten the day before the game by some members of the North Carolina team was the most likely source of the norovirus ("Norwalk-like virus") infection. However, the opposing team members had not eaten this lunchbox, and shared no food and had no other contact with the North Carolina team members after the game. How had the virus been transmitted? It became apparent that some members of the infected North Carolina team were playing whilst wearing uniforms contaminated with vomit and feces, and the opposing team members had probably contracted the disease via aerosol and fecal–oral transmission of the virus.

Part 2: The concert hall (from Evans et al. *Epidemiology and Infection* 2002;129:355–360)

An outbreak of more than 300 cases of norovirus occurred over a 5-day period in people who had attended a concert hall. The index case was found to have vomited in the auditorium on the carpeted floor, into a waste bin, and in a nearby male toilet, the night before. Gastroenteritis symptoms occurred in children who attended the lunchtime concert the next day, who sat at the same level of the auditorium as the index case. These children came from different schools, but only the children who attended the concert became ill. Investigations revealed that the vomit had been cleaned up in the noncarpeted areas after the auditorium had cleared the night before, but not using a chlorine-based solution. Also, the carpet was cleaned only the next day using an ordinary vacuum cleaner, but not until after the lunchtime concert. It was likely that the outbreak occurred when the children touched contaminated surfaces with their hands in the auditorium then contaminated food which they ate, or touched their mouths directly. Alternatively, they could have inhaled virus aerosolized by the action of walking feet over the still contaminated carpeted areas.

Table 8.4 Viruses causing diarrhea: a ready reckoner

Organism	Pathogenesis	Incubation period (h)	Vomiting	Diarrhea	Abdominal pain	Fever	Mode of transmission
Human caliciviruses (e.g. norovirus "winter-vomiting disease")	Precise mechanisms of diarrhea and vomiting unknown, but may involve transient malabsorption of fat due to decreased activity of enzymes in intestinal mucosa	12–24	Frequent, can be projectile	Moderate, nonbloody	Cramps	Often present, low grade	Fecal–oral; waterborne; foodborne (especially shellfish); person-to-person, via contaminated hands, toys, and other fomites. Common cause of point source diarrhea outbreaks in enclosed areas, mainly in adults
Rotavirus	Incompletely understood and complex, thought to involve malabsorption due to mucosal damage, decreased disaccharidase activity, a viral enterotoxin and excess fluid secretion by the enteric nervous system	1–3 days	Present	Profuse and watery, nonbloody	Cramps	Present but low grade	Mode of transmission as for noroviruses, but less commonly transmitted via food; often causing outbreaks in children in hospitals and nurseries and among the elderly in nursing homes
Enteric adenoviruses (subgenus F, serotypes 40 and 41)	Similar to rotavirus, infection of intestinal enterocytes lead to villus* damage and atrophy, malabsorption and fluid loss	5–10 days	Common	Watery	Common	Low grade	Mode of transmission as for noroviruses, mainly causing outbreaks in children, but not usually via food
Astroviruses	Poorly understood, but thought to involve small intestinal villus* shortening, decreased disaccharidase activity inducing an osmotic diarrhea – similar to rotavirus	3–4 days	Common	Moderate, nonbloody	Occasional	Frequent low grade	Mode of transmission as for noroviruses, but less commonly transmitted through food, more often causing outbreaks in children in schools

* These are mucosal folds in the upper small intestine and are primarily responsible for nutrient absorption and secretion of enzymes that break down complex sugars – the disaccharidases

identified in about 20% of all cases (a 6-month prospective cohort study of 604 healthy children, 6–35 months old). The prevalence of the identified viruses causing diarrhea in these children were: enteric adenoviruses (5.7%), rotavirus (5.2%), astrovirus (3.5%), sapovirus (similar to norovirus also in the calicivirus family – 3.0%), and norovirus (1.9%). See Table 8.4 for a ready reckoner of viruses causing diarrhea.

Norovirus and rotavirus testing is common in most diagnostic laboratories as these are the most common diarrhea-causing viruses in hospitalized patients. Enteric adenovirus and astrovirus testing is less commonly performed, often in specific studies only. Therefore, from the above data on the hospital and community prevalence of diarrhea-causing viruses, it suggests that norovirus and rotavirus infections tend to cause more serious diarrhea and illness than enteric adenoviruses and astrovirus.

The incubation of the most common diarrhea-causing viruses can be as short as 1–2 days for norovirus and rotavirus, 3–4 days for astroviruses, and as long as 5 days for enteric adenoviruses. The symptoms are generally clinically indistinguishable between the viruses, being a combination of nausea, vomiting (more common in norovirus infections, particularly in children – hence "winter vomiting disease"), loose watery stool occurring more than five times a day in children or three times a day in adults, with or without fever. It is important to note that definitions of diarrhea may vary and can be very broad (e.g. "a change in stool habits with stools that are more frequent than usual or stools that are more watery than usual," for "diarrhea"), or very narrow (e.g. "vomiting in >50% of patients, mean incubation period of 24–48 hours, mean duration of illness 12–60 hrs, no bacterial pathogen," for "norovirus gastroenteritis"), depending on the purposes of a particular study.

Pathophysiology of diarrheas

Bacterial diarrheas

Salmonella

Microbiology
The taxonomy of the genus *Salmonella* is very confusing: to make it both simple and accurate let us call all salmonellae *Salmonella enterica* and differentiate them by the serovar/serotype, i.e. (Agona as above). Please note that the serovar is not italicized, is written with the first letter in uppercase, and for convenience the species name "*enterica*" is omitted as in S. Agona. The commonest salmonella implicated in eggs are S. Enteritidis and S. Typhimurium.

Salmonellae are Gram negative, rod shaped, non-spore-forming organisms, most serovars are motile (Figure 8.1). Salmonellae are capable of withstanding dry and desiccated environments and cold temperatures; this has lead to outbreaks linked to desiccated coconut, oatmeal cereals, and ice and ice creams. There are over 2000 serovars of salmonella that are implicated in foodborne disease; many are given names of the geographic location where they were first isolated, i.e. S. London, S. Panama, etc.

Pathogenesis and virulence
Once in the lumen of the small intestine salmonellae penetrate the epithelium, multiply, and enter the blood within 24–72 hours. As few as 15–20 bacteria can produce symptoms of infection.

Humans get salmonella gastroenteritis when contaminated food is ingested. Person-to-person spread of salmonellae also occurs. To cause disease, salmonellae need to colonize the lower ileum and colon, invade and proliferate within the intestinal epithelial cells, and elicit a local inflammatory response. The mechanism by which salmonellae invade the epithelium is only partially understood and may be mediated by binding to specific receptors on the epithelial cell surface. The local inflammatory response is attributed to release of various proinflammatory cytokines, including: IL-1, IL-6, IL-8, and TNF. This results in breakdown of the epithelial lining of the gut and local ulceration. The intestinal inflammatory reaction contributes to symptoms of inflammation such as fever, chills, abdominal pain, leukocytosis, and diarrhea. Diarrhea occurs due to secretion of fluid and electrolytes by the small and large intestines and is thought to be due to

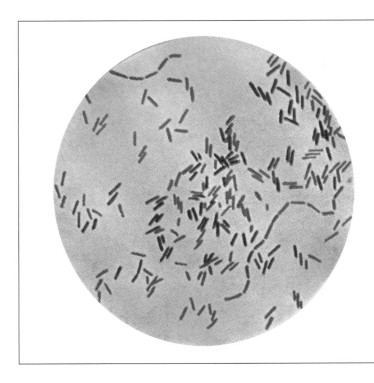

Figure 8.1 Gram stain of *Salmonella* spp. showing Gram negative rods

activation of mucosal adenylate cyclase; the resultant increase in cyclic AMP induces secretion. Activation of adenylate cyclase is thought to be due to secretion of prostaglandins and a local inflammatory response rather than to a specific enterotoxin.

Infants, the elderly, hospitalized and immunosuppressed individuals are the most susceptible to disease and suffer the most severe symptoms. The acute symptoms of *Salmonella* gastroenteritis include sudden onset of nausea with vomiting and abdominal pain; the diarrhea is often bloody and with mucus. The disease is rarely fatal but may be associated with complications such as reactive arthritis.

An effective salmonella vaccine is available for poultry stocks and in some countries like the UK, eggs are branded with the red lion mark to indicate this. The majority of outbreaks currently in the UK are associated with the use of imported eggs from nonvaccinated stock.

Campylobacter jejuni

Microbiology
Globally, *C. jejuni* subsp. *jejuni* accounts for more than 80% of all *Campylobacter* enteritis. They are Gram negative curved rod shaped organisms with a characteristic sea-gull appearance (Figure 8.2). They display darting motility in wet mount preparation under phase contrast or dark field illumination because of their polar flagella. As in all invasive diarrheas, fecal leukocytes are readily seen in stained preparations.

Pathogenesis and virulence
The pathogenesis of *C. jejuni* is not fully understood. *C. jejuni* is an invasive pathogen; most of the invasive tissue injury occurs in the small and large intestines, the lesions show an acute inflammatory response accompanied by hemorrhage. The lesions seen in campylobacter colitis are similar to those seen in ulcerative colitis. The presence of blood and fecal leukocytes in the stool is a common finding. Some *C. jejuni* isolates elaborate very low levels of cytotoxins similar to Shiga toxin. Strains from developing countries show presence of an enterotoxin which may explain why infection by *C. jejuni* has been associated with watery diarrhea.

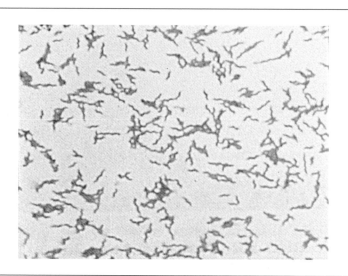

Figure 8.2 Gram stain of *Campylobacter jejuni* showing Gram negative rods in the characteristic "sea-gull" shape

Most commonly it presents as acute enteritis with bloody diarrhea, malaise, fever, cramping abdominal pain, and nausea, but rarely any vomiting. The illness has an incubation period of 1–7 days with acute onset of abdominal cramps and diarrhea. It is a self-limiting illness and subsides in a week, with some patients having longer episodes of diarrhea. Complications following campylobacter gastroenteritis include Guillain–Barré syndrome (an acute inflammatory or demyelinating neuropathy due to molecular or antigenic mimicry with neural tissue), reactive arthritis, and chronic infection in immuno-deficient patients.

Bacillus cereus

Microbiology

Bacillus cereus is an aerobic, spore forming, Gram positive rod with a ubiquitous distribution in the environment (Figure 8.3). Spores of *B. cereus* have been found in a wide variety of cereals, pulses, vegetables, spices, and pasteurized fresh and powdered milk.

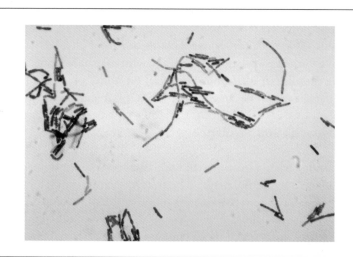

Figure 8.3 Gram stain of *Bacillus cereus* showing Gram positive (purple) rods (some may appear pink because they are over-decolorized or damaged). Provided by Dr William A. Clark. Courtesy of the Centers for Disease Control and Prevention; from CDC website: http://phil.cdc.gov/phil/details.asp

Pathogenesis and virulence

B. cereus spores are frequently present in uncooked rice; being heat resistant they survive cooking. If large vats of cooked rice are subsequently held at room temperature, for long periods of time, spores germinate and vegetative forms multiply. They produce a heat-stable toxin that can survive brief heating, such as stir frying. The emetic form of the infection is caused by this preformed heat-stable enterotoxin. The mechanism and site of action of this toxin are unknown. The toxin is thought to act directly on the vomiting center of the brain. The long-incubation form of illness is mediated by a heat-labile enterotoxin which activates intestinal adenylate cyclase and causes intestinal fluid secretion.

Staphylococcus aureus

Microbiology

Strains of *Staphylococcus aureus* that produce food poisoning are indistinguishable from other staphylococci in that they all appear as Gram positive cocci in clusters on Gram stain and display similar cultural characteristics as all other strains of *S. aureus* (see Chapter 7).

Pathogenesis and virulence

S. aureus that is capable of producing enterotoxin usually produce one or more of five distinct antigenic types of enterotoxin labeled A, B, C, D, E. They are water soluble, low molecular weight proteins that are heat stable (resist boiling for 30 minutes). Their mode of action is unknown but they each cause a neurologic effect (by acting on the vomiting center in the brain), and an enteric effect (diarrhea). All are exotoxins produced by chromosomal genes.

Clostridium perfringens

Microbiology

Clostridium perfringens is an anaerobic, Gram positive bacterium widely found in soil and the intestinal tract of vertebrates (Figure 8.4). It is responsible for three clinical syndromes, including gas gangrene (see Chapter 7), enteritis necroticans or pig-bel (very rare in the USA), and food poisoning.

Pathogenesis and virulence

At least 12 toxins are produced by *C. perfringens*, including four lethal toxins: hemolysin, protease, neuraminidase, and enterotoxin. The ability of individual strains to produce the four lethal toxins forms the

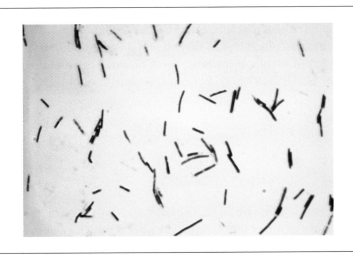

Figure 8.4 Gram stain of *Clostridium perfringens* showing Gram positive (purple) rods. Provided by Don Stalons. Courtesy of the Centers for Disease Control and Prevention; from CDC website: http://phil.cdc.gov/phil/details.asp

basis for a classification scheme that divides the species into five types, A to E. Enterotoxin is produced by Type A strains, and is the primary mediator of *C. perfringens* food poisoning. Upon ingestion, *C. perfringens* comes in contact with the acidic conditions of the stomach or bile salts in the intestines; this initiates and stimulates sporulation of the organism. During the sporulation process, bacteria produce the enterotoxin, which is then released into the intestine when the mother cell lyses. Enterotoxin binds to receptors on the surface of intestinal epithelial cells inducing intestinal tissue damage resulting in an inflammatory diarrhea.

Escherichia coli O157

Microbiology

Escherichia coli is a Gram negative rod belonging to the family Enterobacteriacae. *E. coli* are part of the normal intestinal flora of all animals, including humans. The serotype designated *E. coli* O157:H7 (and lately a few other serotypes as well) is a virulent diarrhea causing organism also known as enterohemorrhagic *E. coli* (EHEC).

Pathogenesis and virulence

This serotype of *E. coli* produces large amounts of two potent enterocytotoxins or verotoxins (VT 1 and 2); because they are remarkably similar to the shiga toxins produced by *Shigella dysenteriae*, they are sometimes referred to as shiga like toxins (SLT 1 and 2). These toxins adhere to the intestinal epithelium and inhibit protein synthesis. The verotoxin is a potent toxin of the A–B type, i.e. it has one A and five B subunits. B subunits bind to the cell and inject the A subunit. By cleaving a specific adenine residue from the 28S ribosomal RNA in the 60S ribosome, the toxin inhibits protein synthesis, causing cell death and intestinal damage.

Shigella species

The shigellae causing gastroenteritis will be dealt with in more detail in Chapter 21; here we mention them because they can contaminate food and cause foodborne illness.

Microbiology

Shigella are Gram negative, nonmotile, non-spore-forming rod shaped bacteria. *Shigella* rarely occurs in animals; it is principally a disease of humans, sometimes of primates such as monkeys and chimpanzees. The organism is frequently found in water polluted with human feces.

Pathogenesis and virulence

The disease is caused when virulent *Shigella* organisms attach to, penetrate and damage epithelial cells of the intestinal mucosa. After invasion, they multiply intracellularly, and spread to contiguous epithileal cells resulting in tissue destruction. Figure 8.5 is the sigmoidoscopic view of the red and inflamed mucosa of the rectum in a patient with shigella dysentery. Some strains such S. *dysenteriae* type 1 produce an enterotoxin called Shiga toxin (very much like the verotoxin of *E. coli* O157:H7). For more information on the pathogenesis of shigellae see Chapter 21.

Viral diarrheas

Human caliciviruses

Virology

The human calicivirus family contains two members, the noroviruses and sapoviruses. Both are structurally similar, being small (26–34 nm), nonenveloped, single-stranded RNA viruses (Figure 8.6). There are animal caliciviruses, e.g. in marine mammals, pigs, cats and rabbits, some of which can be cultured, unlike their

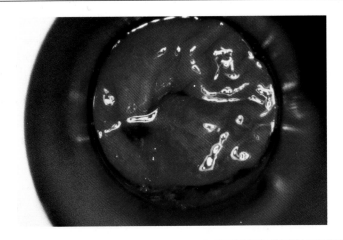

Figure 8.5 Interior mucosal surface of the rectum from a sigmoidoscopic view in a patient who presented with shigella dysentery. Note inflamed and engorged mucosa. Courtesy of the Centers for Disease Control and Prevention; from CDC website: http://phil.cdc.gov/phil/details.asp

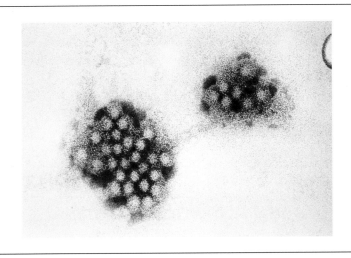

Figure 8.6 An electron micrograph of norovirus, with 27–32 nm size viral particles. Courtesy of the Centers for Disease Control and Prevention; from CDC website: http://phil.cdc.gov/phil/details.asp

human calicivirus counterparts. The name "calici" comes from the Latin for chalice or "cup-like" as the virus has "cup-like" indentations on its surface under electron microscopy.

Pathogenesis and virulence

Most work has been performed on noroviruses. This has been difficult due to a lack of an animal model. Experiments in human volunteers have shown histological changes in the jejunum and ileum with sparing of the stomach and rectum. After 24 hours, shortened microvilli and widened intracellular spaces can be identified that persist for up to 2 weeks after infection. During acute illness, no enterotoxin has been detected, though a variable amount of intestinal fluid is produced. Also, adenylate cyclase levels have been shown to be normal in jejunal biopsies taken during acute infection, so the exact mechanism of the virus-induced diarrhea and vomiting is unclear.

Rotavirus

Virology

Rotavirus is a nonenveloped, double-stranded, 11-segmented RNA virus, of icosahedral symmetry and about 70–80 nm in diameter (Figure 8.7). It is the most common cause of diarrhea and dehydrating gastroenteritis in all socioeconomic groups in all regions worldwide, with a mortality of 6%, primarily in

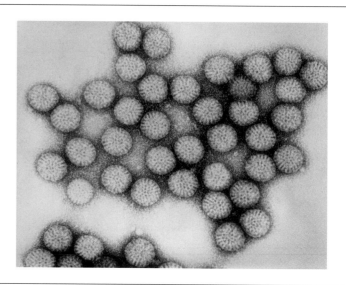

Figure 8.7 Transmission electron micrograph of rotavirus particles showing the distinctive wheel like rim of radiating capsomeres. Courtesy of the Centers for Disease Control and Prevention; from CDC website: http://phil.cdc.gov/phil/details.asp

children in developing countries. The name "rota" comes from the Latin for "wheel" due to the "wheel-like" appearance of the intact virus under electron microscopy. Being nonenveloped, double shelled viruses, rotaviruses are relatively stable in the environment.

Pathogenesis and virulence

The pathogenesis of rotavirus infection is complex and not completely understood. Viral replication appears to be limited to the small intestinal villous epithelium, as can be seen upon histological examination of duodenal biopsies from children with severe rotavirus gastroenteritis. Light microscopy demonstrates shortened, blunted villi with cuboidal epithelium and crypt hypertrophy. The severity of the intestinal mucosal damage seems to correlate with the diarrheal severity, suggesting that malabsorption may also contribute to the diarrhea later on in the disease. Other mechanisms of diarrhea include the inhibition of the glucose co-transport mechanism, reducing the amount of water reabsorbed from the intestine, the possible roles of a viral protein (nonstructural protein 4 – NSP4) acting as an extracellular viral enterotoxin on the enteric nervous system resulting in excessive secretion of fluid. Therefore, generally, there seem to be other mechanisms responsible for rotavirus diarrhea besides the simple destruction of the intestinal epithelium.

Enteric adenoviruses (serotypes 40 and 41)

Virology

Adenoviruses are nonenveloped, double-stranded DNA viruses with icosahedral symmetry, about 70 nm in diameter (Figure 8.8). The virus was first isolated from adenoid tissue, from where its name originates. There are multiple serotypes that are grouped into several subgenera (A–F), and serotypes 40 and 41 that mainly cause diarrhea are in subgenus F.

Pathogenesis and virulence

Adenoviruses can infect cells in three different ways: a lytic infection, which results in cell death and the production of 10 000 to 1 million progeny per cell; a latent or chronic infection, usually in lymphoid cells (e.g. tonsils, adenoids), where the virus only produces a few progeny, with little cell death and asymptomatic infection; and oncogenic transformation, where viral DNA is integrated into the host cell DNA, without the production of viral progeny. Oncogenic transformation has only been described in animals, not in humans, so far. Enteric adenoviruses cause diarrhea mainly in infants, by a similar mechanism to that of rotavirus, with intestinal villous atrophy, epithelial damage, and malabsorption.

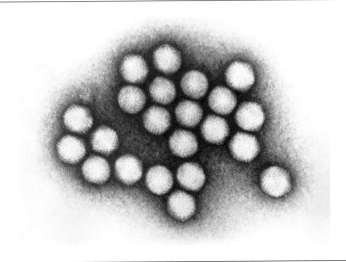

Figure 8.8 Transmission electron micrograph of adenovirus. Courtesy of the Centers for Disease Control and Prevention; from CDC website: http://phil.cdc.gov/phil/details.asp

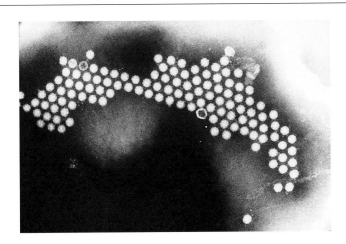

Figure 8.9 Transmission electron micrograph of astrovirus; note the typical star-like morphology. Reprinted from H.P. Lambert and W.E. Farrar (1982) *Slide Atlas of Infectious Diseases*, Gower Medical Publishing Ltd. Reproduced with permission of Elsevier

Astrovirus

Virology

Astroviruses are small (28–30 nm), nonenveloped, single-stranded, positive-sense RNA viruses, displaying cubic symmetry. The name derives from its five- to six-pointed "star-shape" appearance under electron microscopy (Figure 8.9). It causes diarrhea in both adults and children and there are at least eight different serotypes (HastV-1 to HastV-8), which are distributed worldwide.

Pathogenesis and virulence

This is poorly understood, but the diarrhea seems to be induced by mechanisms very similar to that of rotavirus, including small intestinal villous shortening and reduced disaccharidase activity resulting in an osmotic diarrhea.

Parasitic diarrheas

Parasitic agents known to cause diarrhea are:

- *Giardia lamblia*
- *Cryptosporidium* spp.

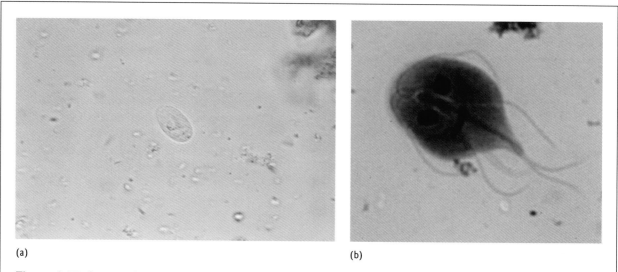

(a)   (b)

Figure 8.10 Cyst and trophozoite forms of *Giardia lamblia*. (a) Cyst (iodine stained). (b) Trophozoite (Giemsa stained). Courtesy of the Centers for Disease Control and Prevention; from CDC website: http://www.dpd.cdc.gov/dpdx/HTML/

- *Cyclospora*
- *Entamoeba histolytica*
- *Isospora belli*
- *Balantidium coli*.

Giardiasis

Giardiasis is caused by *Giardia lamblia* (intestinalis; Figure 8.10) a single celled protozoan parasite (see Chapter 2 for a description of the parasite). It is the most frequent cause of nonbacterial diarrhea in North America; the organism is implicated in 25% of the cases of gastrointestinal disease and may be carried asymptomatically. The overall incidence of infection in the USA is estimated at 2% of the population. Giardiasis is more prevalent in children than in adults. This disease afflicts many homosexual men, both HIV positive and HIV negative individuals. This is presumed to be due to sexual transmission. The disease is also common in child daycare centers and elderly care homes, probably because these individuals are more likely to need assistance with diapers and may be incontinent.

When a groundwater source is located close enough to nearby surface water, such as a river, lake or shallow well, it receives direct surface water recharge. Groundwater source is at risk of contamination from pathogens such as *G. lamblia* and cryptosporidia, if there has been excess rainfall and local flooding occurs and particularly when animal dung is washed into surface waters.

A person becomes infected by ingesting water or food containing *G. lamblia* cysts. The cyst then develops into a trophozoite in the duodenum (see Chapter 2). The trophozoites adhere to the surface of the duodenum and jejunum. In time the organism causes shortening and thickening of the villus surfaces. Diarrhea occurs as a result of sugar (lactose, i.e. milk sugar) intolerance; bloating and flatulence is also common. Chronic infections can lead to malabsorption and fatty diarrhea (steatorrhea). Infection is best prevented by boiling all drinking water while on extended outdoor adventures. Chlorination will not kill the cysts. Proper maintainance of the filtration systems at water plants is also essential. Antiparasitic agents such as metronidazole and their derivatives are the mainstay of treatment (see Further reading).

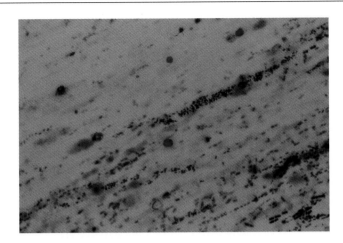

Figure 8.11 *Cryptosporidium* oocysts acid fast stain. Courtesy of the Department of Clinical Microbiology, UCLH, London

Cryptosporidiosis

Cryptosporidiosis is caused by *Cryptosporidium parvum*, an intracellular protozoan parasite (Figure 8.11). *Cryptosporidium* sp. infects many herd animals (cows, goats, sheep among domesticated animals, and deer and elk among wild animals). Direct human surveys indicate prevalence is about 2% in the North American population. Serological surveys indicate that 80% of the population has been exposed to *C. parvum*.

Human infection results from ingestion of the oocyst (see Chapter 2), usually from contaminated water. It is a frequent cause of watery diarrhea in daycare centers and among male homosexuals. Immunodeficient individuals, especially AIDS patients, may have the disease for life, with intractable, severe, watery diarrhea contributing to death. Invasion of the pulmonary system may also be fatal. How it causes disease is not completely understood; it is known that the parasite affects intestinal ion transport and causes inflammatory damage of the microvilli resulting in malabsorption. The cysts are resistant to most chemical disinfectants including chlorine. Boiling drinking water is recommended if contamination has occurred. Read about an interesting waterborne outbreak in Box 8.10.

Infection with *Cyclospora cayetanensis*, *Isospora belli*, *Balantidium coli*, and *Microsporida* (*Enterocytozoon bieneusi*) is seen less often than *C. parvum* but the symptoms are clinically indistinguishable. Like *C. parvum*, infection in most is self-limiting whereas immunocompromised patients may have protracted symptoms. Read Chapter 21 for more information on travel related diarrheas.

Amebiasis

Amebiasis is caused by the unicellular protozoan parasite, *Entamoeba histolytica* (Figure 8.12). The infection is common in the tropics and also in crowded situations of poor hygiene in temperate-zone urban environments. Many infections may go undiagnosed as patients often fail to report symptoms. It is a frequent occurrence among homosexual men.

The parasite occurs in two forms: the motile, ameboid, trophozoite form, and the cyst form (see Chapter 2). The active or trophozoite stage exists only in the host and in fresh feces; cysts survive outside the host in water and soil and on foods left exposed to warmth and moisture. The cyst form is the infective stage of the parasite. When swallowed, cysts cause infection by excysting (to the trophozoite stage) in the digestive tract. Amebiasis is transmitted by fecal contamination of drinking water and foods, but also by direct contact with dirty hands or objects as well as by sexual contact. Symptoms only result from invasion of the colon by

Box 8.10 Cryptosporidiosis – Los Angeles County (report from *MMWR* May 25, 1990/39(20);343–345)

From July 13 through August 14, 1988, 44 persons in five separate swimming groups developed a gastrointestinal illness after using a swimming pool in Los Angeles County. The outbreak began several days after an unintentional human defecation occurred in the pool during the first week of July. A case was defined as any person with watery diarrhea or diarrhea plus cramping and/or fever during July or August.

Cryptosporidium was identified in stool specimens by modified acid-fast staining from seven of 11 patients tested. Results of other laboratory examinations, including bacterial culturing for salmonella, shigella and campylobacter and testing for ova and parasites, were negative. Assessment for viral agents was not performed.

The pool implicated in this outbreak was a 100 000-gallon pool at a school in Los Angeles County. Inspection of the pool during the outbreak period confirmed adequate chlorine levels (2 ppm) but detected a 30% diminished filtration flow rate and established that one of three diatomaceous earth (DE) filters was inoperative.

Editorial note: The investigation revealed that cryptosporidium may be acquired through recreational water contact. Resistance of cryptosporidium to chlorination, an inadequately maintained filtration system, and repeated and prolonged exposure may have contributed to the size and extent of this outbreak. Continued pool use and possible ongoing contamination by infected persons, many of whom continued to swim despite their illness, could also have sustained transmission.

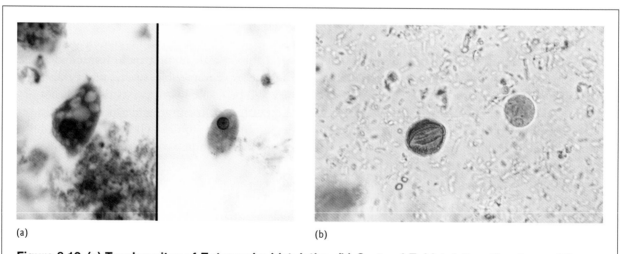

(a)   (b)

Figure 8.12 (a) Trophozoites of *Entamoeba histolytica*. (b) Cysts of *E. histolytica*. Courtesy of the Centers for Disease Control and Prevention; from CDC website: http://www.dpd.cdc.gov/dpdx/HTML/

trophozoites. The amebae secrete enzymes such as proteases, hyaluronidase, and mucopolysaccharidases that facilitate penetration of the mucosa causing ulceration and resulting in the classic symptoms of dysentery. Trophozoites can gain access to other organs via the bloodstream; amebic liver abscess is the most common form of extraintestinal amebic disease. Metronidazole and their derivatives are good amebicidal agents. See Further reading for treatment recommendations.

The principal diagnostic tests for the common causes of diarrheal disease are summarized in Table 8.5. Diagnosis of fecal pathogens is a complex and painstaking exercise. Human feces contains 10^{11} bacterial cells

Table 8.5 Diagnosis of infectious diarrhea

Bacteria	Principal diagnostic test
Salmonellae	Culture of organism in feces and food with serological identification of specific type
Campylobacter spp.	Culture of organism in feces and food
Bacillus cereus	Culture of strains of the same serotype from the suspect food and feces or tests for toxin in food (emetic toxin) and feces (diarrheagenic toxin)
Staphylococcus aureus	Culture of toxin producing strains or detection of toxin in food
Clostridium perfringens	Culture of toxin producing organism in large numbers or detection of toxin in food and feces
Escherichia coli O157	Culture of same type of verotoxin-producing *E. coli* from feces and food. Presence of verotoxin directly from feces
Shigella spp.	Culture of organism in feces
Viruses	
Noroviruses, rotavirus, enteric adenoviruses, astroviruses	All these common diarrhea-causing viruses cannot be routinely cultured and diagnosis relies on electron microscopy (particularly for rotavirus), or antigen assays on the stool samples (again for rotavirus), or PCR assays
Parasites	
Giardia lamblia	Detection of *G. lamblia* trophozoites or cysts in the feces by microscopy.
Cryptosporidium parvum and *Cyclospora* sp.	Differentiated by acid-fast staining of oocysts shed in feces or in biopsy. Fluorescent antibody stains also available for *C. parvum*
Entamoeba histolytica	Stains (including fluorescent antibody) for detection of cysts under the microscope. Motile trophozoite can be seen in fresh feces. Serological tests for extraintestinal infections
Isospora belli and *Balantidium coli*	Characteristic morphology of cysts in feces on microscopy

per gram. Up to 1000 species are represented, including enteric rods (mainly *E. coli*), streptococci, clostridia, and lactobacilli. To find a pathogen, let alone a pathogenic *E. coli*, is like finding a needle in a haystack. Culture methods use a battery of media, enrichment cultures to select out potential pathogens followed by biochemical and serological identification. Many toxins may be difficult to detect in stool and need to be identified from contaminated food. Toxin detection in feces and food is usually done in specialized reference laboratories.

Principles of management of diarrheal disease

The main treatment for bacterial diarrheal disease is to replace fluids and electrolytes, i.e. rehydrate the patient. If vomiting is not an issue encourage the patient to drink small quantities of a suitable oral rehydration solution and often. Children, in particular, may need close observation. Intravenous administration may be the only option if the patient has severe vomiting.

Antibiotics are rarely needed for foodborne illness and in some cases such as in patients with *E. coli* 0157, antibiotics can increase the risk of complications. For guidelines regarding management of diarrhea in children, see Further reading.

Box 8.11 Rotavirus vaccines

Currently there are two rotavirus vaccines on the international market: RotaTeq produced by Merck and Rotarix produced by GlaxoSmithKline (GSK). Both are live-attenuated, oral vaccines intended to be given to infants together with their other childhood immunizations. Only RotaTeq is approved by the US FDA and is the only rotavirus vaccine officially available in the USA. Rotarix is licensed in more than 30 other countries, including those of the European Union, as well as Panama and Brazil. The two vaccines differ in composition. RotaTeq is pentavalent, containing five human-bovine re-assorted viruses. The bovine strain used, WC3, is already naturally attenuated for humans as it comes from cows, but it is poorly cross-protective. Hence, it contains five different re-assorted viruses, each one expressing a different human rotavirus surface protein, to protect against the most common human rotavirus serotypes. As it is mainly a bovine rotavirus, it replicates poorly in the human gut so a larger dose is required to produce immunity. It is less frequently shed in the stool than human rotavirus, and three oral doses are required, each at least 1 month apart. Rotarix uses a different approach and is based on the most common human rotavirus strain that has been attenuated by serial passage. It is given in two oral doses, 1 month apart. This vaccine replicates well in the human gut and is shed by more than 50% of vaccinees after the first dose. Like the natural human rotavirus infection, this vaccine provides cross-protection against most other human rotavirus serotypes. Although trials are still ongoing in populations of more developing countries, so far RotaTeq and Rotarix seem to be highly protective and relatively safe, particularly with respect to "intussusception" – an abnormal telescoping of the bowel within itself that can lead to fatal bowel obstruction. It was this particular complication that led to the withdrawal of the previously licensed rotavirus vaccine in the USA (RotaShield from Wyeth-Ayerst Pharmaceuticals, withdrawn in 1999 – see Further reading).

Generally, viral diarrhea in immunocompetent patients is a self-limiting disease. For babies and young children, careful monitoring of rehydration is required as their lower circulating volume can be more quickly depleted than adults. This is probably best performed in hospital where intravenous rehydration is usually required, as oral fluid intake may be difficult and unreliable. For older children (teenagers) and adults, oral rehydration at home is more acceptable. In developing countries, the shortage of readily available, clean drinking water still makes viral (and other) diarrheal diseases a significant killer of young children. The diarrheal disease may also persist longer with the resulting dehydration being more severe in immunocompromised and elderly patients. There is no specific antiviral therapy for viral diarrhea. A vaccine against rotavirus has been recently licensed and a second rotavirus vaccine will probably be licensed shortly (Box 8.11).

By contrast, parasitic diarrheas require treatment with specific antiparasitic agents. Commonly used antiparasitic agents are metronidazole, tinidazole, iodoquinol, paromomycin, or diloxanide furoate (not commercially available in the USA). For additional information, see the recommendations in The Medical Letter (http://www.dpd.cdc.gov/dpdx/HTML/PDF_Files/2004%20Parasitic.pdf; see Further reading).

Further reading

Glass RI, Parashar UD. The promise of new rotavirus vaccines. *N Engl J Med* 2006;354(1):75–77

Parashar UD, Alexander JP, Glass RI; Advisory Committee on Immunization Practices (ACIP), Centers for Disease Control and Prevention (CDC). Prevention of rotavirus gastroenteritis among infants and children. Recommendations of the Advisory Committee on Immunization Practices (ACIP). *MMWR Recomm Rep* 2006;55(RR-12):1–13

Useful websites

CDC. www.cdc.gov/mmwr/preview/mmwrhtml/rr5216a1.htm

This is the latest CDC report and includes recommendations, for pediatricians in the USA, to manage acute diarrhea in children

CDC. A–Z Index of Parasitic. Management of parasitic diarrheas.
  http://www.cdc.gov/ncidod/dpd/parasites/index.htm

Guidelines from the Infectious Diseases Society of America. Practice Guidelines for the Management of Infectious Diarrhea. *Clin Infect Dis* 2001;32:331–351.
  http://www.journals.uchicago.edu/CID/journal/issues/v32n3/001387/001387.html

Drugs for parasitic infections http://www.dpd.cdc.gov/dpdx/HTML/PDF_Files/2004%20Parasitic.pdf

Useful overviews of viral diarrheas

http://digestive.niddk.nih.gov/ddiseases/pubs/viralgastroenteritis/

http://www.ibms.org/pdf/bs_articles_2005/viral_diarrhea.pdf

http://web.uct.ac.za/depts/virology/teaching/notes/gastroenteritis.htm

Chapter 9
Cardiac and respiratory tract infections

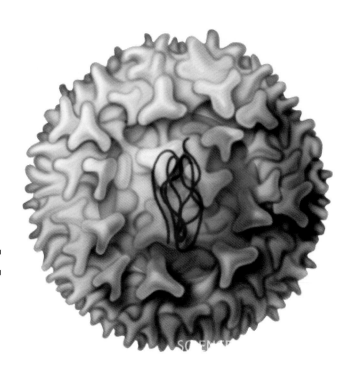

N. Shetty, J.W. Tang, J. Andrews

Infections of the cardiovascular system
Infective endocarditis
Myocarditis
Pericarditis
Infections of the respiratory system
Infections of the upper respiratory tract
Otitis media and sinusitis
Viral infections of the upper and lower respiratory tract
Upper respiratory tract viral infections: the common cold

Viral infections of the middle and lower respiratory tract
Bronchitis and bronchiectasis
Community acquired pneumonia (CAP)
Empyema
Microbiology, pathogenesis and virulence
Diagnosis
Treatment
Prevention

Infections of the cardiovascular and respiratory systems are some of the most common infections seen in primary care and in hospital emergency departments. They are often serious and carry a significant risk of death and debilitation. Many of the infections present insidiously and are mistaken for mild respiratory or systemic viral infections; however they can be rapidly fatal if left untreated. We discuss these infections under two broad section headings:

Infections of the cardiovascular system:
   Infective endocarditis
   Myocarditis
   Pericarditis.
Infections of the respiratory system:
   Infections of the upper respiratory tract
   Otitis media and sinusitis
   Croup and bronchiolitis
   Bronchitis and bronchiectasis
   Community acquired pneumonia

Empyema
Influenza is discussed in Chapter 20 and SARS in Chapter 24
Pulmonary tuberculosis is discussed in Chapter 16
Pneumonia in the immunocompromised patient is discussed in Chapter 13
Hospital acquired pneumonia is discussed in Chapter 14.

Infections of the cardiovascular system

See Box 9.1.

Infective endocarditis

Infective endocarditis (IE) is caused by microorganisms adhering to and multiplying on the innermost aspect of the chamber of the heart and its valves (the endocardium). Infections often involve an abnormal heart valve such as one previously damaged by rheumatic fever, atherosclerotic plaques, or a prosthetic (artificial) valve. Less frequently, infection occurs at the site of congenital cardiac abnormalities such as a septal defect or an arteriovenous shunt. It is very important to remember that infection can occur on a normal heart valve.

The annual incidence is estimated to be 16/million of the population in the USA. It can occur at any age although 50- to 60-year-old patients are more commonly affected with a male to female ratio of 2 : 1. The mortality rate can be up to 40% and this high rate has not decreased in the last 50 years. Some important predisposing factors are summarized in Box 9.2.

Box 9.1 At the heart of the matter

A 64-year-old retired school teacher presented to her primary care physician with several week's history of low grade fever and extreme tiredness. Her past medical history included open heart surgery for a coronary artery bypass graft 4 years ago. She has had longstanding dental problems and has had to see her dentist regularly for dental treatments. On listening to her chest, her physician noted abnormal heart sounds (cardiac murmur) that were not present last year on a routine check-up. He referred her to hospital for specialist advice and further investigations.

At hospital she was noted to have a temperature of 38.0°C. Among other investigations three sets of blood cultures were taken. These became positive after 24 hours of incubation; a Gram stain was performed on the blood culture broth (see figure right). She was also noted to have traces of blood in her urine on microscopic examination (microscopic hematuria).

Read on to find the answers to these questions:

- Based on the Gram stain what is the organism likely to be?

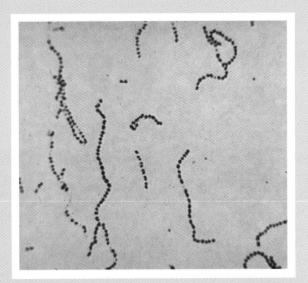

- Given the history and examination findings where do you think the organism has lodged in the body?
- Why is the visit to the dentist a significant factor?
- What common predisposing conditions make an individual susceptible to this infection?

Box 9.2 Important predisposing factors for infective endocarditis

- Congenital heart disease
- Previous rheumatic heart disease
- Atherosclerotic aortic valve disease
- Prosthetic valve heart surgery

- Severe mitral valve prolapse
- Intravenous drug use
- Infections of intravascular devices

Pathophysiology

Ulceration on the endothelial surface of any of the heart valves may be caused by turbulent blood flow around areas of previous damage. This promotes bacterial adherence by at least two possible mechanisms:

1 Direct contact between blood and damaged tissue results in production of a small clot or vegetation made up of fibrin and platelets. When transient bacteremia occurs, as it does (for example) during vigorous brushing of teeth that are diseased and bleed readily, or during dental treatments, organisms (most commonly the "viridans" streptococci) enter the bloodstream and bind avidly to the clot. Monocytes are attracted to clot and become activated producing cytokines, resulting in progressive enlargement of "infected vegetations" (Figure 9.1).

2 In addition, local inflammation induces endothelial cells to express transmembrane proteins that bind fibronectin. Pathogens such as *Staphylococcus aureus* carry fibronectin on their surface and facilitate build up of *S. aureus* on endothelial surfaces. Similarly, clot build up can lead to vegetations on an artificial or prosthetic heart valve (Figure 9.2).

Other than the mouth, transient bacteremia may occur from the urinary tract, intravenous drug misuse, or colonized intravascular catheters. Infective vegetations are most likely to develop on damaged endothelium of the aortic or mitral valves, this accounts for about 85% of cases. Enlarging vegetations may break down and travel in the bloodstream (embolize) to other parts of the body such as the brain, lung, or spleen (Figure 9.3). Immune complexes (antigen + antibody + complement) may also form in distal sites such as the skin and subcutaneous tissue and kidney.

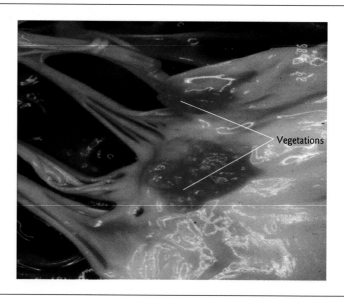

Figure 9.1 Native aortic valve with bacterial vegetations

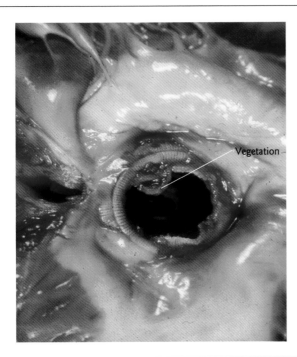

Vegetation

Figure 9.2 Prosthetic valve endocarditis

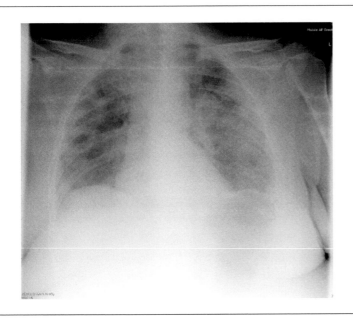

Figure 9.3 Infected emboli in both lung fields. University College Hospital, London is gratefully acknowledged for the use of this image

Clinical presentation

In patients with IE the onset of symptoms can often be insidious and include tiredness, malaise, anorexia, and/or weight loss. Fever, which is often low grade and intermittent, is present in 90% of patients. Most patients will have a new or changed cardiac murmur and some patients may have evidence of cardiac failure. When endocarditis is secondary to more virulent organisms such as *S. aureus*, infection may progress quite rapidly and signs of acute sepsis may predominate. An enlarged spleen is noted in a quarter of patients. Organisms causing IE circulate in the bloodstream causing a transient or intermittent bacteremia.

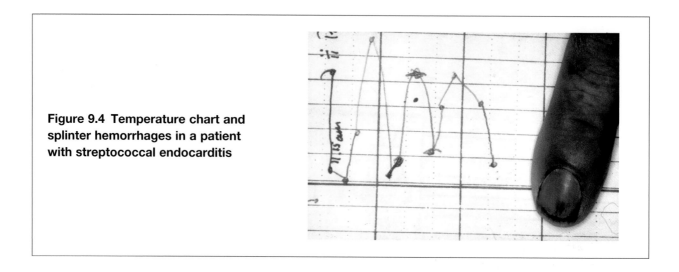

Figure 9.4 Temperature chart and splinter hemorrhages in a patient with streptococcal endocarditis

Patients may present with signs secondary to infected emboli and immune complex deposition. These are described as stigmata of IE as many are classically associated with IE. Inflammation of the small blood vessels and microemboli can manifest as splinter hemorrhages under the nail bed (Figure 9.4).

If embolization occurs in the brain the patient may present with signs of a stroke. Microemboli (**Roth's spots**) can occur in the retina of the eye, these can by visualized using an ophthalmoscope where retinal hemorrhages with white centers can be seen. If immune complex deposition occurs in the skin and subcutaneous tissues, classical stigmata include painless, red (erythematous) or hemorrhagic macules or nodules in the palms or soles, called **Janeway lesions** and **Osler's nodes** characterized by painful, red, raised lesions on the finger pulps. Immune complex related disease, e.g. glomerulonephritis, may also be found. Anemia is often present due to microscopic bleeding characteristic of many of the stigmata.

Microbiology

The microorganisms associated with IE and their isolation rates in cases of IE are described in Table 9.1.

Table 9.1 Microorganisms implicated in infective endocarditis

Causative organisms	Percentage of cases
"viridans streptococci"	54
Staphylococcus aureus	19
Enterococcus spp.	9
Other streptococci	5
Staphylococcus epidermidis	5
Anaerobic streptococci	1
HACEK* bacteria	4
Other bacteria	3
Blood culture negative	Up to 20

* HACEK: *Haemophilus, Actinobacillus, Cardiobacterium, Eikenella, Kingella.*

"viridans" streptococci

These organisms form part of the commensal flora of the oropharynx. They cause IE by gaining access to the bloodstream through dental manipulation or because of pre-existing dental disease. The viridans streptococci comprise several different species including *Streptococcus mutans*, *S. sanguis*, *S. salivarius*, *S. mitior*, *S. mitis*, and *S. milleri*. Viridans streptococci are Gram positive cocci found in chains causing α–hemolysis around colonies on blood agar (see Figure 4.6c).

Enterococcus spp.

Enterococcus faecalis and *E. faecium* are the most common enterococci isolated from patients with IE. They are also Gram positive organisms found in pairs and short chains. On blood agar they produce α, β, or nonhemolytic colonies. As well as endocarditis, enterococci are associated with urinary tract and wound infections.

Staphylococcus aureus

For a full description of the organism and its virulence factors see Chapter 7. *S. aureus* has become a more common cause of IE in recent years and is the leading cause in patients with associated intravenous drug use.

Staphylococcus epidermidis

S. epidermidis are one of a group collectively known as coagulase negative staphylococci (CoNS). They form part of normal skin flora. Coagulase negative staphylococci were once dismissed as contaminants in blood cultures but they are now recognized as important pathogens if conditions favor multiplication. As well as IE, CoNS are associated with urinary tract and prosthetic implant or device infections. CoNS secrete a sticky substance called glycocalyx, sometimes referred to as "slime" or biofilm. Biofilms tend to coat foreign body surfaces, including prosthetic heart valves. Organisms trapped within biofilms are protected from the action of antimicrobial agents and attack from host defence mechanisms. Consequently they are notoriously difficult to treat and often necessitate removal of the prosthetic device.

HACEK group

The HACEK group of organisms are slow growing Gram negative rods that form part of the body's normal mouth and gut flora. The name comes from the first letter of each of the following organisms *Haemophilus* spp., *Actinobacillus actinomycetemcomitans*, *Cardiobacterium hominis*, *Eikenella* spp., and *Kingella* spp.

Blood culture negative endocarditis

In up to 20% of cases of IE blood cultures may be negative. This may be because of previous antibiotic therapy or infection with organisms that are difficult to culture in the laboratory such as fastidious streptococci, a HACEK organism, or *Coxiella burnetii*.

Diagnosis

Blood cultures remain the most important investigation and ideally at least two sets of blood cultures (aerobic and anaerobic) should be collected before the start of therapy. These should be set up for aerobic and anaerobic culture and any organism found should be identified to species level and full sensitivities to a range of antimicrobials determined. Other important investigations include echocardiography, chest X-ray, measurement of inflammatory markers, and urine microscopy. Echocardiography can be used both to demonstrate the presence of vegetations and any complications such as abscess formation or valvular damage. Serological testing can be useful for the diagnosis of IE due to *C. burnetii*.

Treatment

Ideally antimicrobials should not be commenced until blood cultures have been taken. The best guess treatment or empirical treatment is usually a β lactam agent such as penicillin or flucloxacillin/nafcillin and gentamicin first, then changed according to organism and sensitivity pattern. Typical regimens include benzylpenicillin and gentamicin for viridans streptococci, or flucloxacillin/nafcillin/vancomycin and gentamicin for staphylococci. Therapy is usually continued for 2–6 weeks. Surgical management may be required to deal with nonfunctioning or malfunctioning valves as a consequence of endocarditis, especially in cases caused by *S. aureus* or if infection is unresponsive to antimicrobial therapy (see Further reading).

Prevention

Infective endocarditis may be prevented by administering antibiotic prophylaxis treatment to patients with damaged valves before they undergo procedures which would give rise to significant bacteremia, e.g. infected dental work or urogenital surgery (see Further reading).

Myocarditis

Prevalence and etiology

Myocarditis or inflammation of the myocardium (heart muscle) may result from infectious or noninfectious causes. With infection, many different agents (viral, bacterial, parasitic, or fungal) may produce myocarditis, but it is most commonly associated with viral infections. The viruses that have been associated with myocarditis are mainly those that cause an accompanying systemic infection, such as measles, mumps, rubella, chickenpox, parvovirus B19, adenovirus, hepatitis A and B, cytomegalovirus (CMV), and even influenza. However, the viral species most commonly associated with myocarditis are enteroviruses. The enteroviruses consist of several different groups of viruses: coxsackievirus A (serotypes 1–24), coxsackievirus B (serotypes 1–6), echoviruses (serotypes 1–34), polioviruses (serotypes 1–3), and other un-named enteroviruses (serotypes 68–71). Although there are reports of myocarditis caused by most of these different species of enteroviruses, coxsackieviruses A and B are the most commonly reported to cause myocarditis, particularly in young children. Such infections can be very severe – some cases requiring heart transplantation, or they may even be fatal. In the USA and Europe, most cases of myocarditis are associated with a relatively small number of viral agents: coxsackievirus B, adenoviruses, and possibly parvovirus B19. As myocarditis often arises as a complication of a systemic infection with these viruses, the incubation period has little meaning here as the patient may have been infected for some time before the myocarditis becomes clinically manifest.

See Table 9.2 for etiological agents causing myocarditis.

Pathogenesis

The pathogenesis of viral myocarditis is poorly understood, but is thought to be due to either direct viral damage to the heart muscle cells (myocytes) or damage to the blood vessels that supply the myocytes, leading to myocardial ischemia (reduced blood supply) that leads to cell dysfunction and death.

Clinical presentation

Clinically, patients with myocarditis may exhibit a wide range of manifestations, from being asymptomatic to having rapidly progressive, fatal disease. Often, the presentation is of a young person who develops unexplained heart failure or arrhythmias, with or without other signs of systemic illness. These other systemic symptoms may include fever, general malaise, joint and/or muscle pains, respiratory symptoms (e.g. a "flu-like" illness), and/or chest pains. The presentation of viral myocarditis may mimic a heart attack (acute myocardial infarction), or even present with sudden death. Laboratory serum markers of myocarditis may be similar to those of a heart attack with elevated specific cardiac enzymes, and similar changes (ST elevation and T wave inversion) on the electrocardiogram (EKG).

Table 9.2 Reported causes of viral myocarditis and pericarditis, in relative order of frequency

Myocarditis	Pericarditis
Coxsackieviruses (A and B)	Coxsackieviruses (A and B)
Other enteroviruses	Other enteroviruses
Adenovirus	Adenovirus
Mumps	Mumps
Measles	Influenza (A and B)
Influenza (A and B)	Lassa fever
Rabies	Herpesviruses (VZV, CMV, EBV, HSV)
Rubella	Hepatitis B virus
Vectorborne diseases (dengue, chikungunya, yellow fever)	HIV
Hemorrhagic fevers (Junin, Machupo, Lassa)	
Herpesviruses (VZV, CMV, EBV, HSV)	
Hepatitis viruses (B and C)	
RSV	
Parvovirus B19	
HIV	

Investigations

Virological investigations are unsatisfactory and in most cases, can only provide circumstantial evidence of viral involvement. Hence, the incidence of viral myocarditis is probably greatly underdiagnosed and unreported. The strongest connection between a virus and myocarditis would be from a myocardial (heart) biopsy where the virus is then grown from this tissue directly. However this type of biopsy is rarely performed (it has some associated risk), and where it has been done the virus has only been grown from immunocompromised patients and neonates (babies less than 1 month old). The demonstration of a concomitant systemic viral infection, e.g. with enterovirus, adenovirus, or parvovirus B19, may go some way to associating the myocarditis with this particular viral infection, but the link may still be circumstantial. Such systemic viral infections can be diagnosed using routine laboratory methods appropriate to that specific virus, such as serology, or PCR testing on blood, stool and throat swabs together with viral culture, e.g. for enterovirus and adenovirus in stool and throat swabs. If no other infectious or noninfectious cause for the myocarditis is found, then this systemic viral infection may be assumed to be the cause of the myocarditis, using a process of elimination.

Treatment

The mainstay of therapy is bed rest, as exercise has been found to worsen the cardiac dysfunction in myocarditis patients. Non-steroidal anti-inflammatory drugs (NSAIDs), many of which are common analgesics, e.g. ibuprofen and aspirin, have been successful for symptom relief, as has the antigout agent, colchicine. However, with regular NSAIDs use, a tablet to control the gastric acid needs to be taken to prevent gastrointestinal bleeding (NSAIDs can reduce the body's natural protection against the stomach acid). Steroids alone may have detrimental effects on such patients due to their inhibition of the host antiviral immune responses. Some cardiac drugs may be helpful in treating the effects of the myocarditis, such as the associated heart failure and arrythmias. There is a specific antiviral agent, called pleconaril, which can be given to patients whose myocarditis is specifically associated with an enterovirus species infection, but this drug is still undergoing clinical trials and has not yet received full licensing approval (at the time of writing). Intravenous immunoglobulin (pooled sera from blood donations containing various antibodies) has been used and may be of benefit in some cases. Other immuno-modulating agents have also been tried, but none have proven consistently effective in all cases. Cardiac transplantation may be required in severe cases of myocarditis that do not adequately recover from the acute phase of the viral myocarditis, despite the use of circulatory support devices. Long-term prognosis is usually good.

Prevention

Existing viral vaccines may have already played a role in preventing many cases of viral myocarditis, as many of the systemic viral infections listed above are vaccine preventable (i.e. measles, mumps, rubella, chickenpox, hepatitis A and B, influenza). However, there are no vaccines yet licensed for general use against enteroviruses, adenoviruses, or parvovirus B19, so these viruses may well continue to be the most common cause of viral myocarditis.

Pericarditis

The pericardium is a thin, approximately 1 mm thick membrane of dense collagen forming a sac, and lying in contact with the heart. Within it there is normally 15–50 mL of clear fluid that may act to lubricate the heart's movements. Damage to this pericardium, by infectious or noninfectious means, results in fluid, fibrin and various cells being exuded or secreted from this membrane into this sac. This may constrict the heart to various degrees, compromising its contractile function ('tamponade'). After recovery, the pericardium may return to its former state or may become thickened with scar tissue that may lead to long-term cardiac dysfunction due to constriction or adhesions.

Prevalence and etiology

Pericarditis or inflammation of the pericardium may arise from both infectious and noninfectious causes. Identifying the cause is difficult and the proportion of so-called "idiopathic" ("of unknown cause") cases of pericarditis may be as high as 40–90% in some reported studies. There are no distinguishing features between infectious and noninfectious pericarditis cases. It is likely that viral infections again account for the majority of infectious pericarditis since myocarditis frequently coexists with the pericarditis ("myopericarditis"), for which viruses are the most frequent cause. Hence, the coxsackieviruses are likely to be the most common viruses associated with pericarditis for reasons already discussed earlier. A form of acute benign pericarditis has been historically referred to as "Bornholm disease" or "epidemic pleurodynia" (roughly meaning "epidemic chest pain") after outbreaks were described in Bornholm, an island off the coast of Denmark, over 100 years ago. These epidemics were subsequently found to be caused by coxsackievirus B species. Other important causes of pericarditis include bacteria such as *S. aureus* and *Mycobacterium tuberculosis*, as well as HIV and its related opportunistic infections, including the atypical *Mycobacteria* spp. Similar to myocarditis, as pericarditis often arises as a complication of a systemic infection with these pathogens, the incubation period has little meaning here as the patient may have been infected for some time before the pericarditis becomes clinically manifest. See Table 9.2 for the viral etiology of myocarditis.

Clinical presentation

Depending on the causal agent, infection-related pericarditis may present in different ways. Viral pericarditis may typically present with chest pain, mimicking a heart attack with 'retrosternal' (behind the breast bone) chest pain radiating to the shoulder and neck. It differs from a true heart attack in that fever is often present, and there may be a recent or current "flu-like" illness with malaise, joint and muscle pains, and sometimes respiratory symptoms such as a cough or sore throat. Also, different from a true heart attack, the patient may be able to exacerbate the symptoms by breathing, swallowing, or lying supine. Bacterial pericarditis usually develops as part of a severe septicemia when the patient is already severely ill and the pericardial sac may be filled with pus, causing tamponade. Tuberculous pericarditis has a more insidious onset, with the patient complaining of vague chest pains, weight loss, night sweats, cough, and shortness of breath. HIV-infected patients may have asymptomatic pericarditis due to opportunistic infections that may become more manifest as the patient progresses to end stage AIDS, in the absence of antiretroviral treatment. Clinical investigations such as an EKG and echocardiography are useful for diagnosing pericarditis, as well as assessing the heart function. The EKG may show characteristic changes indicative of pericarditis (which can also mimic those for an acute myocardial infarction), and the echocardiogram can demonstrate a pericardial effusion (fluid collecting around the heart in the pericardial sac), and detect signs and the degree of tamponade.

Pathogenesis

Cardiotropic viruses, such as enteroviruses, infecting the myo- and pericardium, may produce inflammation and cause exudation of fibrinous fluid into the pericardial sac. Infection with other agents may result in a similar inflammatory reaction, leading to an accumulation of fluid in the sac and possible constriction of the beating myocardium (heart). This reduces the cardiac filling and therefore its output, which may lead to mild, moderate or severe heart failure, depending on the extent and duration of the inflammatory reaction.

Investigations

As many different infectious pathogens have been associated with pericarditis, it may be difficult to find a definitive causal agent in any particular patient with pericarditis. In most young adults presenting with chest pain, the pericarditis is likely to be idiopathic or viral in cause. A stool sample and throat swab may be taken for viral culture or PCR testing for enteroviruses or adenoviruses. Yet, this is only circumstantial evidence for the cause of the pericarditis as these viruses may also be grown from such samples from the same patient at other times when he/she is well. Even pericardial tissue and/or fluid may fail to culture live viruses, though nowadays with PCR testing available, the viral RNA or DNA may be more easily detected from these tissues. Bacterial and tuberculous pericardial infections may lead to purulent pericardial effusions and life-threatening tamponade. Such effusions can be drained with a procedure called 'pericardiocentesis' where a needle is inserted into the pericardial space to remove some of the fluid. This has a dual purpose in such severe cases of pericardial effusion, of removing fluid for diagnostic testing, as well as relieving the tamponade on the heart.

Treatment

The medical (nonsurgical) treatment for the most common form of viral pericarditis is similar to viral myocarditis, as described above. In addition to this, bacterial or tuberculous pericarditis with pericardial effusions may require more invasive, surgical procedures to permanently remove and prevent the recurrence of fluid surrounding the heart.

Prevention

For viral pericarditis, the preventative measures are similar to those described above for viral myocarditis, and the disease is often self-limiting. Prompt diagnosis and treatment of bacterial or tuberculous infections with appropriate antibiotics will reduce the risk of pericarditis and pericardial effusion as a complication of generalized bacterial sepsis. Steroids are also sometimes used in conjunction with antituberculous drugs to reduce inflammation, scarring, and constriction in tuberculous pericarditis. However, steroids are probably detrimental in any form of viral myopericarditis, and empirical therapy with antituberculous drugs and steroids should only be started when a viral cause has been excluded as far as possible.

Infections of the respiratory system

Infections of the upper respiratory tract

Upper respiratory tract infections are some of the most common infections in man and include **pharyngitis** (sore throat), epiglottitis (infection around the vocal chords), laryngitis (infection of the upper airway or voice box), and the common cold.

Pharyngitis is an infective process of the pharynx and surrounding structures, which most often has a viral aetiology. Common bacterial organisms known to cause pharyngitis are shown in Box 9.3. The most important bacterial cause is *Streptococcus pyogenes* (Group A beta hemolytic streptococcus, GAS). **Laryngitis** is predominately secondary to viral causes and epiglottis is almost always caused by *Haemophilus influenzae* type b (Hib) infection.

It is important to diagnose acute streptococcal infection, as untreated throat infections may lead to serious sequelae such as rheumatic fever or acute glomerulonephritis. These sequelae can usually be prevented by appropriate antibiotic treatment (see Further reading). Streptococcal pharyngitis or "strep. throat" is more common in the winter months and may present with significant pharyngeal redness (erythema) and swelling (edema) (Figure 9.5). Petechiae (bleeding spots in the skin) may be found and enlarged cervical lymph nodes are a common finding. Most patients have a raised temperature on examination.

Box 9.3 Bacterial causes of acute pharyngitis

- *Streptococcus pyogenes*
- Groups C and G beta-hemolytic streptococci
- *Corynebacterium* sp. including *Corynebacterium diphtheriae*
- *Haemophilus influenzae*

- *Neisseria meningitidis*
- *Neisseria gonorrhoeae*
- *Arcanobacterium haemolyticum*
- *Legionella pneumophila*

Figure 9.5 Child with streptococcal pharyngitis or "strep throat." Note inflammed pharynx. Courtesy of the Centers for Disease Control and Prevention; from CDC website: http://phil.cdc.gov/phil/details.asp

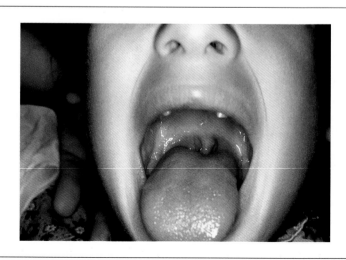

Following infection with a strain of *S. pyogenes* producing erythrogenic toxin some patients may develop scarlet fever. After a prodromal illness of about 48 hours the patient develops a characteristic erythematous rash on the body and/or face sparing the area around the mouth (circumoral pallor). A "strawberry tongue" (see Fig. 7.7) due to loss of tongue papillae may be present and skin affected by rash that desquamates after about a week. Without antibiotic treatment the illness will usually resolve but rheumatic fever could follow.

Corynebacterium diphtheriae is now an uncommon cause of pharyngitis in developed countries since the introduction of widespread vaccination. In recent years diphtheria has re-emerged as an important threat to health in many parts of the world. In patients with an appropriate travel history, who have not been vaccinated, it therefore remains an important clinical and public health problem. *C. diphtheriae* usually causes a severe pharyngitis with pseudomembrane formation and is associated with serious systemic toxicity (see Chapter 25).

Acute epiglottitis can result in swelling and inflammation that may threaten the airway. *Haemophilus influenzae* type b was the most common cause until vaccination became widely available. Infection with *S. pyogenes* causes some cases. It presents usually in children with sore throat, high fever, and drooling. Sometimes stridor (labored breathing) is present. Oral examination should be avoided as it may precipitate acute respiratory obstruction.

Bordetella pertussis and *B. parapertussis* cause **whooping cough**, which is a tracheo-bronchitis, characterized by recurrent paroxysms of coughing.

The pathogenesis of pertussis is not well understood. The bacteria attach to the respiratory tract and release a toxin that causes inflammation and paralyzes the cilia, this prevents the removal of respiratory secretions. The disease is transmitted to susceptible individuals via aerosolized droplets from a cough or sneeze, or by direct contact with a patient's respiratory secretions. The incubation period is commonly 7–10 days. Infection progresses through three stages:

The catarrhal stage is characterized by a runny nose, sneezing, low-grade fever, and a mild, occasional, nonproductive cough similar to that of a common cold or minor viral infection. The cough gradually becomes more severe. The disease is most infectious during this period, which lasts 1–2 weeks.

The paroxysmal stage is when pertussis is usually suspected; the patient has bursts, or paroxysms, of rapid coughs, related to the difficulty of expelling thick mucus from the tracheobronchial tree. The paroxysms continue without inspiration until the coughing ends and the high-pitched inspiratory whoop occurs. The episode is often followed by vomiting, exhaustion, and possibly cyanosis.

The paroxysmal stage generally lasts from 1 to 6 weeks but can persist for up to 10 weeks. During the first 2 weeks of this stage, the attacks become more frequent particularly at night.

The convalescent stage is characterized by gradual recovery. The coughs become less paroxysmal and may disappear in 2–3 weeks.

Whooping cough is a vaccine preventable illness, however because of waning herd immunity the disease is making a comeback (Box 9.4).

Otitis media and sinusitis

Infection in the middle ear (otitis media) is usually secondary to occlusion from inflammation. Young children are at particular risk of infection as the Eustachian tube is shorter and more horizontal. The main infecting organisms include *Streptococcus pneumoniae*, *H. influenzae*, and *Moraxella catarhalis*. Otitis media usually presents with fever and local pain although young children may find it difficult to localize the pain. Infection may be complicated by eardrum perforation, development of glue ear, or rarely acute mastoiditis. Auroscope reveals fluid behind an inflamed tympanic membrane (Figure 9.6) or a purulent discharge associated with perforation.

Infection of the sinuses with bacteria from the nasopharynx follows impaired drainage of sinus secretions often as a result of a prior upper respiratory tract infection. The infecting organisms are the same as for otitis media. Patients present with fever and pain, which is generally worse on movement.

Box 9.4 School-associated pertussis outbreak in Yavapai County, Arizona: September 2002–February 2003 (report from *MMWR* March 19, 2004/53(10);216–219)

On September 21, 2002, a pertussis case (confirmed by isolation of *Bordetella pertussis*) was reported to the Yavapai County Health Department (YCHD). The patient was a child aged 13 years in the 8th grade at a middle school in Yavapai County; the child had attended school during the illness. Subsequent investigation identified five additional persons (two students in the same classroom, two 8th-grade teachers, and one parent of an ill student) with prolonged cough illnesses. Healthcare providers were told to consider pertussis in persons of any age with acute cough illnesses and consider obtaining nasopharyngeal specimens for *B. pertussis* culture.

A total of 485 pertussis cases were reported from six communities in the county, a rate of 580.5 per 100 000 population.

Editorial: A substantial number of cases among older children and adolescents (i.e. persons aged 10–19 years) initially caught the infection. This spread to the community, with cases occurring among infants aged <1 year. In the USA, cases in older children and adolescents are reported most commonly in the fall, when students return to school. Because of waning immunity, older children and adolescents can become susceptible to pertussis 5–15 years after the last dose of DTaP vaccine (diphtheria, tetanus toxoid, and acellular pertussis).

Although infants with pertussis can become severely ill and die, no pertussis-associated hospitalizations or deaths were reported during this outbreak. By contrast, older persons with pertussis often have a mild illness. As a result, older persons might not visit a healthcare provider until several weeks after cough onset, when recovery of the fastidious *B. pertussis* bacterium is unlikely and diagnosis might not be confirmed. Early recognition, treatment, and chemoprophylaxis can help prevent transmission to others; because of its severity in young unvaccinated infants, preventing pertussis in this population is of greatest importance.

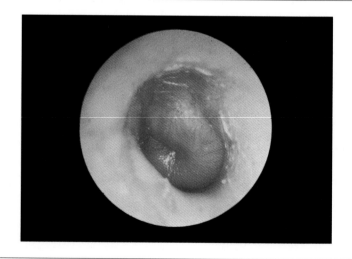

Figure 9.6 Acute otitis media (red, bulging tympanic membrane) as seen on auroscope. Reprinted from H.P. Lambert and W.E. Farrar (1982) *Slide Atlas of Infectious Diseases*, Gower Medical Publishing Ltd. Reproduced with permission of Elsevier

Viral infections of the upper and lower respiratory tract

Viral infections probably account for most of the mild "colds" and "flus" that we all experience each year. There are many viruses that contribute to these mild illnesses so it is common to get a "cold" or "flu" several times a year. In fact, different viruses become common at different times of the year, so this seasonality of the common cold or "flu-like illness" can be predicted on a population level for certain viruses, such as influenza, respiratory syncytial virus (RSV), and parainfluenza viruses. Newly discovered viruses such as human metapneumovirus (hMPV) and new coronaviruses (e.g. NL63-CoV) and human bocavirus (HBoV) may also contribute to the burden of URTIs, and further research is ongoing to quantify their contributions.

Viral infections of the respiratory tract can be divided loosely (with a lot of overlap) into upper (naso-pharynx), middle (larynx-trachea-bronchi), and lower (bronchiole-alveolar) respiratory tract infections. Generally the severity of illness is greater the further down the respiratory tract that the infection progresses. Each virus may move up and down the respiratory tract with the action of cilia, inhalation, coughing or sneezing to assist viral transport, so that any of the respiratory viruses may be found to be causing disease in any part of the respiratory tract.

Upper respiratory tract viral infections: the common cold

These are the mildest and most common forms of respiratory viral infections. The majority of them are self-limiting, and depending on the symptoms experienced, the infected individual may manage to continue working, with or without the aid of some over-the-counter symptom relief medication, or they may feel that a day off work may help speed up their recovery, with the added bonus of reducing the risk of transmitting the illness to others in the workplace. Common colds still account for a significant number of days off work and can have an important impact on a nation's economy (see Box 9.5).

Pathogenesis

The symptoms of the common cold (cough, sneeze, sore throat, rhinorrhea or runny nose, headache, malaise, etc.) appear to arise from a combination of local and systemic cytokine released by the host immune system in response to viral infection, replication, and damage to the respiratory epithelial cells in the upper respiratory tract (URT). Coughing and sneezing are thought to be due to a combination of cytokine stimulation and specific nerve reflexes supplying the facial and respiratory muscles (see Further reading). In addition nose-blowing may force infected mucus into sinuses and the Eustachain tube giving the "bunged up" or "stuffy nose" feeling commonly found with URTIs. However, such infected mucus may then give rise to infection in these localized areas, giving rise to sinusitis and otitis media (the middle ear – connects to the mouth via the Eustachian tube). These infections can be serious, especially if due to bacteria which are inadequately treated. Severe infections of the central nervous system can result from such localized infections (see Chapter 10).

Box 9.5 The economic burden of the common cold

One study has estimated that each common cold illness in an adult leads to an average of 8.7 lost work hours (consisting of 2.8 hours of absenteeism, 5.9 hours of on-the-job loss), 1.2 work hours lost to attending their children (<13 years old) with common colds. The total cost was approximated to $US 25 billion, with $US 16.6 billion of this from on-the-job productivity losses, $US 8 billion due to absenteeism, and $US 230 million due to caregiver absenteeism. Absenteeism was defined as being the total number of work hours missed due to staying at home, arriving late or leaving early from work, going to the pharmacy, grocery store or doctor for medications. On-the-job productivity loss was defined by asking employees to complete a Work Productivity and Activity Impairment (WPAI) questionnaire that compared their performances whilst healthy and then with a cold on a scale of 1–10. Any difference between the two scores was then assigned to the effect of the common cold infection on the employee (see Further reading).

Table 9.3 Typical viral causes of upper, middle and lower respiratory tract infections, in relative order of frequency, though they may all overlap to a certain extent

Upper respiratory tract infections	Middle and lower respiratory tract infections
Rhinoviruses	Parainfluenza viruses (types 1–3)
Coronaviruses (OC43, 229E)	Adenoviruses
Influenza A and B	Influenza A and B
Adenoviruses	RSV
Parainfluenza viruses (types 1–3)	Rhinoviruses
RSV	Coronaviruses (OC43, 229E)
Measles	Measles
VZV	VZV

RSV, respiratory syncytial virus; VZV, varicella zoster virus.

Etiological agents

Rhinoviruses and coronaviruses OC43, 229E (i.e. the non-severe acute respiratory syndrome associated coronaviruses, the non-SARS coronaviruses) account for about two-thirds of all viral causes for the common cold. The rest are caused by a mixture of adeno-, parainfluenza (PIF), respiratory syncitial virus (RSV), and influenza viruses. See Table 9.3 for the etiological agents commonly implicated in viral respiratory tract disease.

The incubation period for these viruses ranges from 0.5–1 day for rhinoviruses to up to 5–7 days for adeno- and influenza viruses. Peak clinical symptoms usually occur after 2–3 days of illness, and most people recover by 7–10 days, though some may still suffer from the symptoms for up to 3 weeks.

Clinical presentation

Rhinoviruses and the non-SARS coronaviruses tend to remain in the URT and cause self-limiting disease, with symptoms of cough, sneezing, rhinorrhea or blocked nose, and rarely, fever. Fever is commoner in children who are generally more likely to become febrile after infection by any of the respiratory viruses. Other symptoms associated with the common cold include sore throat and hoarse voice, headache, lethargy, and poor or loss of appetite. Although secondary bacterial infections are uncommon in adults, children may develop bacterial infections leading to acute otitis media, which can occur in up to 20% of children with URT viral infections. Sinusitis may also be a complication in up to 0.5–2% of common cold. Other complications include triggering an asthma attack, the exacerbation (resulting in increased breathlessness) of asthma or chronic obstructive pulmonary disease (COPD) – a condition often found in chronic smokers.

Investigations

These are similar for virtually all the respiratory viruses. The best clinical sample to take for diagnosing a viral URTI is a nasopharyngeal aspirate (NPA) for direct viral antigen, RNA or DNA detection, and viral culture. A throat or nasal swab can also be taken, but the diagnostic yield is usually lower than with an NPA. An acute then convalescent (taken 10–14 days later) blood serum sample can be also taken for specific viral antibody testing. Virological testing includes specific immunofluorescence (IF) to detect the presence of viral antigen, the polymerase chain reaction (PCR) to detect the specific viral RNA or DNA, viral culture to grow the whole virus, or antibody testing on paired acute and convalescent sera to demonstrate a rising antibody titer indicating a recent infection with a specific virus.

Generally, viral culture is a catch-all technique, but different respiratory viruses grow better on different cell lines, and in different incubation conditions, so these need to be chosen to suit the suspected viruses concerned. Direct antigen detection and PCR require reagents specific for the virus to be detected, so they are not catch-all techniques. However, multiple viruses can be tested for by developing multiple specific IF and PCR reagents to cover all the typical respiratory viruses. There are many commercially available kits that will detect most respiratory viruses. Paired antibody titers are useful if the other tests prove negative and the patient gives a good clinical history of a respiratory tract infection. The patient may present during convalescence (recovery) sometime after the acute illness, for a retrospective diagnosis. Antibodies take about 10–14 days to develop and mature, so the two serum samples are required for this test: an acute one taken around the time of illness, and a convalescent one taken 10–14 days later. These two sera can be tested together by a variety of techniques, to determine the relative antibody concentrations in them. The sera are tested neat, then at successively higher dilutions, until antibody can no longer be detected in them. If there is a fourfold rise (or difference) in titer (i.e. dilution ratio) between them, then it indicates a recent infection with the virus concerned.

Treatment and prevention

There is no licensed specific antiviral agent or vaccine for the noninfluenza common cold viruses (rhinoviruses, non-SARS coronaviruses, RSV, parainfluenza virus, adenoviruses). For influenza, specific antiviral drugs exist, as well as an annually updated influenza vaccine (see below). For the other respiratory viruses, the treatment is symptomatic and the illness is self-limiting in normally healthy individuals. Caution must be taken not to treat such individuals indiscriminately with antibiotics. These drugs are antibacterial and are ineffective against viruses, but may contribute to the community levels of antibiotic-resistant bacteria that are now being found in the community at an increasing (and worrying) rate. Clinical acumen and close liaison with the local hospitals's diagnostic virology laboratory may allow for rapid testing and diagnosis of viral infections and avoid such unnecessary antibiotic use. In the immunocompromised, viral infections and the associated symptoms may persist and even become more severe if the infection descends into the lower respiratory tract (LRT). In such situations, high-dose intravenous antibiotics may then be required to treat any secondary bacterial infections.

Viral infections of the middle and lower respiratory tract

Croup (pronounced "croop") is a manifestation of laryngo-tracheo-bronchitis, which is the inflammation of the middle to lower part of the respiratory tract. This clinical symptom is most commonly seen in children. The middle section of the respiratory tract (larynx and trachea) is quite narrow and constricted by cartilaginous rings. Inflammation in this area can cause considerable swelling and narrowing of this airway, producing the "croupy" symptoms. Croup can also involve the upper large bronchi, hence the name "laryngo-tracheo-bronchitis," as it involves the larynx, the trachea, and the large bronchi as the viral infection descends to the LRT.

Lower down, viral infections may infect and damage the terminal bronchioles, the alveoli, and the lung tissue itself. This latter condition becomes the realm of viral pneumonia and can be caused by other viruses besides the typical respiratory viruses (e.g. measles and chickenpox).

Clinical presentation

Symptoms of croup most commonly present in children. Affected children may initially develop a sore throat and hoarse voice due to inflammation of the pharynx and larynx, respectively, then progress to more croup-like symptoms. This is often characterized by a barking cough (often described as like that of a seal), with grunting and wheezing sounds and difficulty breathing. Similarly, the presentation of bronchiolitis can be quite characteristic. It may first present as a common cold with URT symptoms of cough, sneezing, rhinorrhea with fever, before worsening over the next 24–48 hours with the appearance of wheezing, more rapid, shallow breathing movements ("tachypnea"), and visible in-drawing or "retraction" of the skin between the child's ribs and around the clavicles (collar-bones) with each breath. The heart rate is also often increased ("tachycardia"). Visible flaring of the nostrils may also be seen with gradual signs of exhaustion and poor sleeping. Children with bronchiolitis more commonly have fever and in some cases may stop breathing completely (called "apnea") before the other symptoms become obvious. The condition may deteriorate rapidly as the child becomes too tired to breathe and may become oxygen-deprived or "cyanotic," where the lips, fingernails, and skin turn visibly blue, as the oxygen levels in the circulating blood drops. In addition the child becomes dehydrated and may have difficulty eating and drinking, vomiting up any feed as it struggles to breathe. Eventually, the child may need intensive care support to raise the oxygen levels circulating in its blood.

Viral infections causing bronchiolitis result in the blockage of the small diameter respiratory bronchioles with inflammatory and dead cells and debris. This blockage produces a ball-and-valve effect such that inhaled air can enter the lung but air cannot be exhaled easily past this blockage. The typical appearance of a child with bronchiolitis, therefore, is of a hyperinflated "barrel-shaped" chest, with visible retraction of the skin into the spaces between the ribs and around the clavicles as the child tries desperately to exhale the trapped air, creating the paradoxical negative pressure effect to cause the visible skin retraction.

Etiological agents

Parainfluenza viruses are typically the cause of croup in children. There are four types of PIF, but type 4 is rare and most of the serious infections arise from type 3. Influenza types A and B can also cause croup. There is an influenza type C, but like PIF type 4, it is rare and not often tested for routinely in patients presenting with respiratory illness. Respiratory syncytial virus (RSV) is the typical causal agent for childhood bronchiolitis. Quite why RSV targets specifically the bronchioles (lower end of the respiratory tract, just before the alveoli) in children is still being investigated. However, RSV is responsible for much of the severe, life-threatening respiratory illness in children.

Adenoviruses are also commonly isolated from children with respiratory infections, and can cause URTIs as well as LRTIs. They can also cause more systemic disease such as hepatitis, cystitis (bladder infection), kerato-conjunctivitis (eye infections), myocarditis, and meningo-encephalitis (infection of the brain and its covering membrane). However, these latter complications are not often seen in otherwise healthy children.

All respiratory viruses as well as others such as measles and varicella zoster virus (VZV that causes chickenpox) have the potential to cause disease in both the upper and lower respiratory tract. A significant contribution to the mortality from such viral infections comes from secondary bacterial infections that can cause a more serious pneumonia, subsequent to the initial viral infection. See Table 9.3 for etiological agents implicated in viral respiratory tract disease.

Bronchitis and bronchiectasis

Bronchitis is a lower respiratory tract infection with cough and sputum production but no radiographic changes on the chest X-ray. Infection may be with *S. pneumoniae*, *H. influenzae*, *Mycoplasma pneumoniae* or one of the common respiratory viruses. Bronchiectasis is defined as abnormal dilatation of the bronchi and has a variety of etiologies, including genetic and infective factors. *Bordetella pertussis* and *Mycobacterium tuberculosis* are the principal bacteria that cause bronchiectasis. Cystic fibrosis (CF) is currently the most important cause of bronchiectasis in the western world, and patients with CF bronchiectasis are prone to early respiratory infection with pathogens such as *S. aureus* and *H. influenzae* and later infection with mucoid *Pseudomonas aeruginosa* or *Burkholderia cepacia*.

Community acquired pneumonia (CAP)

See Box 9.6.

Pneumonia is infection of the terminal air sacs ("alveoli") and tissue of the lung. Since the alveoli are the main air-exchange surface for replenishing the blood oxygen levels, infection and damage to the alveoli in viral and/or bacterial pneumonias can be severe and life-threatening. Pneumonia can present with fever, malaise, tachypnea (increased respiratory rate), and tachycardia (increased heart-rate). In more serious, end-stage cases, a patient can present with shock (due to a large drop in blood pressure as the circulation fails resulting in multi-organ failure), with few or no breath sounds (apnea), due to overwhelming exhaustion and in some cases, viral or secondary bacterial sepsis.

Community acquired pneumonia (CAP) is defined as pneumonia (infection of the lung parenchyma seen on chest X-ray) whose onset occurs either prior to or immediately after admission to hospital. CAP is the sixth most common cause of death worldwide and the leading cause of infectious death in the USA. As many as 4 million patients are diagnosed with CAP each year in the USA and about 20% of those require hospitalization. It may be a primary disease occurring in an otherwise healthy patient or it may be secondary to a predisposing factor such as chronic lung disease, diabetes mellitus, or malignancy. There are many organisms associated with CAP (Box 9.7), with *S. pneumoniae* being the most important in all age groups apart from the under 2 year olds. Respiratory syncytial virus (RSV) is the most common cause in this age group. No causative agent is found in up to 40% of patients with CAP.

Patients with acute pneumonia usually have a cough (often productive of purulent sputum but can be nonproductive). Hemoptysis (blood in the sputum) and chest pain may be present. Chest signs heard on auscultation can be variable but usually include coarse breath sounds. Atypical pneumonia refers to the clinical presentation of pneumonia with the so called "atypical organisms" (Box 9.7). In such cases infection

Box 9.6 Fever, cough, and sputum

A 37-year-old train driver presented to the emergency department of his hospital with sudden onset of chest pain and fever. He had also noticed a bad cough producing sputum that was green-brown in color. His breathing was difficult and he was short of breath on exertion. On examination he had a fever of 38°C and coarse breath sounds on auscultation of his chest. His white cell count was raised at 30×10^9/L. Blood cultures and a sputum sample were sent and a chest X-ray was performed. A Gram stain of the positive blood cultures showed Gram positive cocci in pairs. The chest X-ray (see right) demonstrated a homogenous opacity in the right upper lobe. Read the rest of the chapter before you attempt these questions.

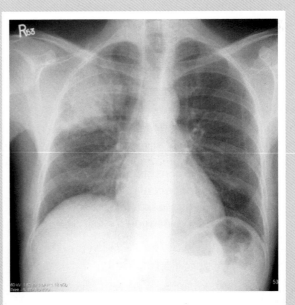

University College Hospital, London is gratefully acknowledged for use of this image

❓From what clinical illness is the patient suffering?
❓What is the most likely organism implicated?
❓What other illnesses does this organism commonly cause?
❓Could this illness have been prevented?

Box 9.7 Common causes of community acquired pneumonia

- *Streptococcus pneumoniae*
  - Penicillin-sensitive *S. pneumoniae*
  - Penicillin-resistant *S. pneumoniae*
- *Haemophilus influenzae*
  - Ampicillin-sensitive *H. influenzae*
  - Ampicillin-resistant *H. influenzae*
- *Moraxella catarrhalis* (all strains penicillin resistant)
- *Staphylococcus aureus*
- "The atypicals"
  - *Legionella pneumophila*
  - *Mycoplasma pneumoniae*
  - *Chlamydia pneumoniae* and *Chlamydia psittaci*
- Primary viral pneumonia

is associated with nonrespiratory symptoms such as myalgia, headache, confusion, or abdominal pain, and the chest X-ray does not show the typical lobar consolidation or homogenous shadowing over a lung field. The most important consequence of acute pneumonia is impairment of respiratory function and needs to be assessed urgently by studying respiratory rate and oxygen saturation of blood.

Three main patterns of acute pneumonia on chest X-ray are recognized; lobar, bronchopneumonia, and interstitial. Lobar pneumonia is pulmonary consolidation demarcated by border of lung segment or lobe (Figure 9.7). It is particularly associated with *S. pneumoniae* infection and can also be seen in infections with *S. aureus* and *L. pneumophila*. Sputum production is often marked. Bronchopneumonia is seen as patchy consolidation around the larger airways caused by the above organisms and also *H. influenzae* (Figure 9.8). Interstitial pneumonia is demonstrated by fine areas of shadowing in the lung fields and there is usually no sputum production at presentation. It is usually seen in mycoplasma, legionella, and viral pneumonia (Figure 9.9). Aspiration pneumonia can follow aspiration of oral or gastric contents and the bacteria associated with this are the oral streptococci or anaerobes. For an overview of community acquired pneumonia and all its variations see Figure 9.10.

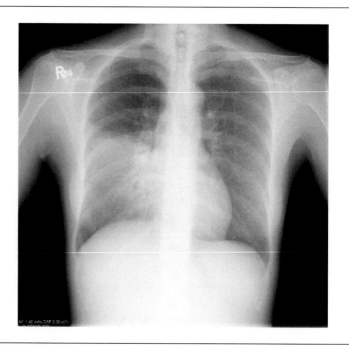

Figure 9.7 Lobar consolidation typical of pneumococcal pneumonia. University College Hospital, London is gratefully acknowledged for use of this image

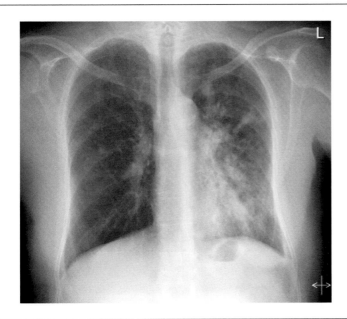

Figure 9.8 Bronchopneumonia – patchy consolidation around the airways. University College Hospital, London is gratefully acknowledged for use of this image

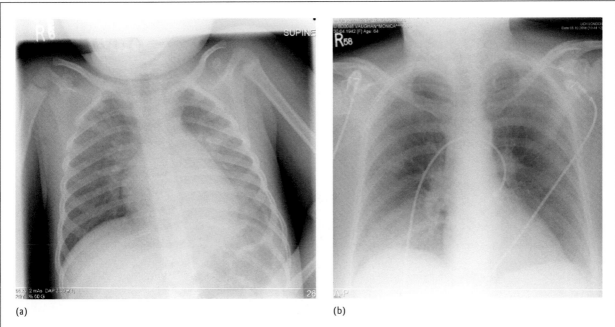

(a)   (b)

Figure 9.9 Interstitial pneumonia showing diffuse shadowing in both lung fields. (a) *Mycoplasma* pneumonia. (b) *Legionella* pneumonia. University College Hospital, London is gratefully acknowledged for use of these images

Empyema

An empyema is an accumulation of purulent fluid in the pleural space (Figure 9.11). It is caused by either direct extension from underlying pneumonia or trauma or hematogenous spread from another focus. The common bacteria associated with empyema include *S. aureus*, *S. pneumoniae*, the Enterobacteriaceae, and anaerobic bacteria. Patients present most often with ongoing fever, chest pain, and cough.

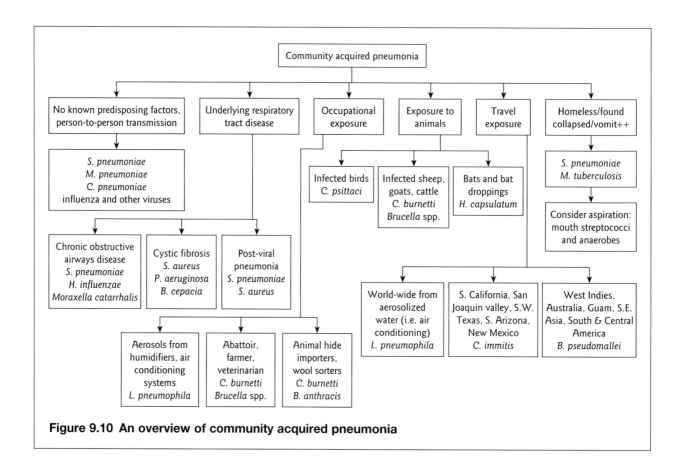

Figure 9.10 An overview of community acquired pneumonia

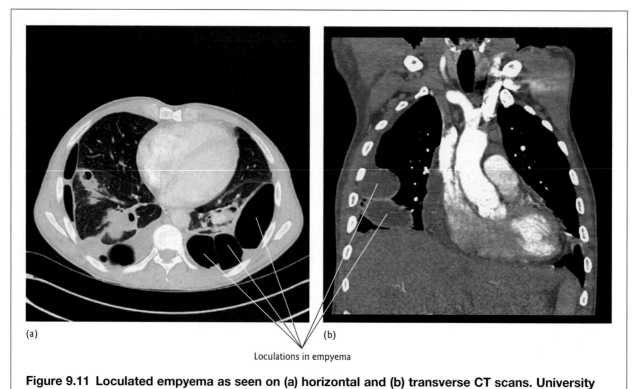

(a)   (b)

Loculations in empyema

Figure 9.11 Loculated empyema as seen on (a) horizontal and (b) transverse CT scans. University College Hospital, London is gratefully acknowledged for use of these images

Microbiology, pathogenesis, and virulence

Host defence in the lower respiratory tract

Many of the organisms above are part of the normal flora of the upper respiratory tract. However, the lower part of the respiratory tract is virtually sterile despite the large numbers of microorganisms present in the upper airway and in inspired air. A variety of host defence mechanisms exist to maintain this sterile environment and one or more of these may be overcome leading to the development of lower respiratory tract infection including pneumonia. Important physical host defences include the cough reflex that guards the lower respiratory tract from respiratory secretions. The mucociliary escalator is another mechanism. Cilia (tiny hairs in the mucosa of the respiratory tract) bind microorganisms that are inhaled and waft them upwards and out; this greatly reduces the number of organisms entering the lower respiratory tract. Cigarette smoking, narcotics and alcohol consumption can reduce the efficiency of this important defense mechanism. Recent respiratory viral infection also affects the function of the mucociliary barrier.

There are also nonspecific cellular and humoral factors produced in the lung including immunoglobulin A, complement, neutrophils, and macrophages that are able to destroy many potential respiratory pathogens by binding, engulfing, or directly killing them. Opsonization by antibody and complement aids the phagocytic process by neutrophils and macrophages. The recruitment of macrophages from the reticuloendothelial system, especially the spleen, is particularly important for destroying capsulated organisms such as *S. pneumoniae* and *H. influenzae*, and therefore patients without a functioning spleen are particularly susceptible to these organisms. There are also specific immune responses such as specific antibody production and production of recruitment factors for neutrophils and lymphocytes that serve to kill potential pathogens.

Streptococcus pyogenes and *Staphylococcus aureus*

The microbiology and virulence determinants of these organisms have been discussed in full in Chapter 7.

Streptococcus pneumoniae

Microbiology

S. pneumoniae is a Gram positive diplococcus (Figure 9.12) that appears α-hemolytic (partial lysis of red blood cells) on blood agar (Figure 9.13). Mature colonies can have a depressed center causing the so-called "draughtsman" appearance. The cocci are elongated along their long axis and many possess a polysaccharide

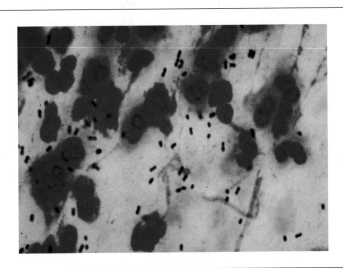

Figure 9.12 Gram stain of a sputum sample showing neutrophils and Gram positive diplococci of *Streptococcus pneumoniae*

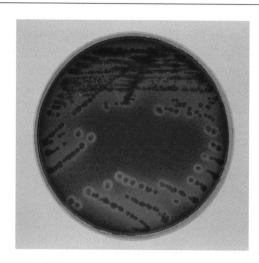

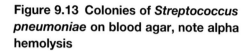
Figure 9.13 Colonies of *Streptococcus pneumoniae* on blood agar, note alpha hemolysis

capsule. Humans are the only host of *S. pneumoniae* and they can be found as normal flora in the upper respiratory tract. Transmission is via the respiratory route in droplet nuclei. As well as respiratory infections, *S. pneumoniae* can cause septicemia and meningitis. The overuse of beta-lactam and macrolide antibiotics has caused a gradual increase in the resistance of *S. pneumoniae* to these antibiotics.

Virulence mechanisms

The polysaccharide capsule, of which there are over 80 known serotypes, is the major virulence factor since it interferes with phagocytosis by neutrophils. The organism is also able to produce a variety of toxins including IgA protease, an enzyme able to digest mucosal IgA, pneumolysin, neuraminidase, and hyaluronidase. Pneumolysin is particularly interesting as it is able to inhibit the mucociliary escalator and it also directly damages the delicate cilia cells that form part of the physical barrier. Adhesins such as pneumococcal surface protein A are also important in the pathogenesis of disease.

Haemophilus influenzae

Microbiology

This small Gram negative cocco-bacillus requires growth factors, known as X and V factors (Figure 9.14), present in blood to grow on solid media. Noncapsulate forms are found in the upper respiratory tract mucosa and cause otitis media (middle ear infection), sinusitis, and chest infections, particularly in patients with obstructive airways disease (chronic bronchitis). The majority of invasive infections occur in preschool children and are caused by strains carrying the polysaccharide capsule type b. Invasive infections include meningitis, facial cellulitis, osteomyelitis, and septicemia, as well as acute epiglottis. Blood cultures are often positive in invasive disease. *H. influenzae* produces beta-lactamase capable of destroying penicillin and amoxicillin.

Virulence mechanisms

H. influenzae expresses an antiphagocytic polysaccharide capsule of which there are six types (a–f). Most invasive disease is associated with type b. It also expresses a lipopolysaccharide that damages cilia and an IgA protease. Pili are present on the outer surface of the organism that can aid adherence of the bacteria to components of mucus in respiratory secretions. The organism can also directly inhibit neutrophil migration.

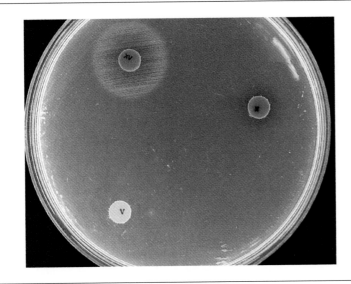

Figure 9.14 Growth of *Haemophilus influenzae* colonies around XV disc only demonstrating reliance on both factors for growth

Moraxella catarrhalis

This Gram negative cocco-bacillus which grows easily on blood agar is usually a commensal of the upper respiratory tract. It is associated with acute sinusitis and occasionally lower respiratory tract infections. It produces a beta-lactamase enzyme rendering it resistant to penicillin and amoxicillin.

Bordetella pertussis

Microbiology

Bordetella organisms are small, Gram negative coccobacilli; they are strict aerobes and require enriched growth media for culture

Virulence mechanisms

B. pertussis expresses fimbriae that aid adhesion to receptors on respiratory cilia and produces a number of exotoxins including pertussis toxin and tracheal cytotoxin. Pertussis toxin acts via adenyl cyclase and ultimately inhibits neutrophil function. Tracheal cytotoxin and a released dermonecrotic toxin cause local damage. The lipopolysaccharide component of the Gram negative cell wall initiates cytokine release and contributes to shock and circulatory collapse.

Legionella pneumophila

Microbiology

There are many members of the *Legionella* genus but over two-thirds of infection is caused by *L. pneumophila* serogroup 1. *L. pneumophila* is a fastidious aerobic Gram negative bacillus, normally found in a wide variety of aquatic environments. Patients are infected after exposure to warm (25–42°C), contaminated water, e.g. showers, air conditioning, humidifiers, and sprays (Box 9.8). Infections are more common in the summer months, unlike most other respiratory infections that are more common in the winter. Infection with *L. pneumophila* can cause a spectrum of disease from a mild viral like illness to a severe pneumonia with high mortality (referred to as legionnaires' disease). As discussed previously the presentation may be atypical with gastrointestinal symptoms or confusion. Person-to-person transmission does not occur. Diabetes, history of heart disease, or smoking are known to be risk factors for legionnaires' disease.

Box 9.8 Legionnaires' disease associated with a whirlpool spa display: Virginia, September–October, 1996 (report from *MMWR* January 31, 1997/46(04);83–86)

On October 15, 1996, a district health department in southwestern Virginia contacted the Office of Epidemiology, VDH, about a hospital (hospital A) report that 15 patients had been admitted during October 12–13 with unexplained pneumonia. On October 23, the district health department was informed about three area residents with legionellosis (with *Legionella pneumophila* serogroup 1 antigen detected in urine); one was a patient at hospital A.

To identify potential exposures associated with legionnaires' disease, case-patients were asked about their activities during the 2 weeks before the onset of their illness.

A history of having visited a large home-improvement center during the 2 weeks before onset of illness was reported by 14 (93%) of the 15 cases, compared with 12 (27%) of 45 controls. Ten (77%) case-patients reported spending time in the area surrounding the spas during their visits to the store, compared with three (25%) of the 12 controls. No other activity, including drinking from the store's water fountains or visiting the 14 other locations in the community, was associated with illness.

Samples were collected and cultured for the presence of legionella from water sources in the home-improvement center, including a whirlpool spa basin, spa filters, a greenhouse sprinkler system, a decorative fish pond and fountain, potable water fountains, urinals, and hot and cold water taps in the store's restrooms. *Legionella pneumophila* serogroup 1 was isolated from the filter of the spa; the isolate was an exact match, by monoclonal antibody subtyping and primed polymerase chain reaction, to the sputum isolates cultured from two of the cases

Editorial note: Approximately 10 000–15 000 cases of legionnaires' disease occur each year in the USA; most occur sporadically. Investigations of outbreaks have documented aerosol transmission of legionella from contaminated cooling towers and evaporative condensers, showers, decorative fountains, humidifiers, respiratory therapy equipment, and whirlpool spas.

Following the investigation, VDH recommended that whirlpool spas being used as displays should be regularly inspected and maintained with biocides and that filters be regularly changed or decontaminated. In response to a recent outbreak of legionnaires' disease on a cruise ship, CDC has developed guidelines for the maintenance of whirlpool spas on cruise ships.

Legionellae are difficult to culture and require special media such as buffered charcoal yeast extract (BCYE). Antigen can be detected directly in clinical samples such as urine. Serological methods are also widely used. The organism is susceptible to erythromycin and rifampin.

Virulence determinants

The organism has a major outer protein that inhibits the acidification of the phagolysosome that, together with other factors, resist intracellular killing. It also produces a potent exoproteinase that has hemolytic and cytotoxic effects.

Mycoplasma pneumoniae

Microbiology

M. pneumoniae is a bacterium with no rigid cell wall and limited metabolic capabilities. It grows slowly on special media and under a plate microscope the colonies give a pitted appearance The lack of cell wall prevents staining with Gram stain. *M. pneumoniae* respiratory infection occurs sporadically and in epidemics every 4 years and is more common in children and young adults. As well as respiratory infections, *M. pneumoniae* rarely causes encephalitis. As the organism is relatively difficult to isolate, infection may be diagnosed retrospectively by testing for antibody production, a fourfold increase between acute and convalescent antibody titer is indicative of current infection. Most isolates are sensitive to erythromycin, tetracyclines, or quinolones.

Virulence determinants
The organism adheres to mucosal epithelium (via P1 receptors on its surface) and interferes with ciliary function.

Chlamydia pneumoniae and *Chlamydia psittaci*

Microbiology
The chlamydiae are a group of small Gram negative bacteria that require an intracellular environment for growth. There are three medically important species: *C. trachomatis*, *C. pneumoniae*, and *C. psittaci*. *C. pneumoniae* is associated with an atypical pneumonia. *C. psittaci* is the cause of an uncommon infection, psittacosis, acquired from contact with birds such as parrots. *C. trachomatis* rarely causes primary community aquired pneumonia. Although culture of these organisms is possible, serological diagnosis is more common. Chlamydial infection is treated with erythromycin or tetracycline.

Viral causes of pneumonia
Viral causes of severe pneumonia in adults and children can include influenza, as well as measles and chickenpox (VZV) pneumonitis.

More common in children, RSV and PIF type 3 can cause a similar picture. In immunocompromised patients, all of these pathogens as well as others, such as adenovirus, may cause systemic, multi-organ failure due to severe pneumonia.

Rarely and usually more clinically severe, pure viral pneumonias can be caused by more virulent agents, such as the severe acute respiratory syndrome-associated coronavirus (SARS-CoV), as well as in the more recent human H5N1 influenza cases (see Chapters 20 and 24).

Virulence
The pathogenesis of middle and lower respiratory tract infections is generally due to direct viral damage to the respiratory tract epithelial cells. The host immune response stimulates cytokine production and triggers nerve reflexes that give rise to the symptoms typically seen with these respiratory infections, but can also contribute to the severe respiratory failure seen in some viral pneumonias, such as those seen in the 2003 SARS outbreaks and the more recent cases of human H5N1 influenza infections (see Chapters 20 and 24).

Generally true viral pneumonias are relatively rare and more often cases of viral-associated pneumonia turn out to be secondary bacterial infections (e.g. with *S. pneumoniae* or *S. aureus*). As previously described cilia are small hair-like structures that line the respiratory tract that move potentially infected mucus and cell debris up from the lungs to the mouth where they are then swallowed and destroyed by the stomach acid. They are commonly damaged by respiratory viral infections and this can lead to secondary bacterial infections that take advantage of the virally-damaged cilial ladder to sit within the damage lung tissue and replicate, entering the bloodstream and causing bacterial sepsis, shock, and multi-organ failure, if appropriate antibiotic treatment is not initiated early and aggressively.

Less common causes of community acquired pneumonia

Coxiella burnetii
C. burnetii causes a zoonotic infection of humans called Q fever and is distributed globally. Infection usually occurs by inhalation of these organisms from air that contains airborne barnyard dust contaminated by dried

placental material, birth fluids, and excreta of infected herd animals. Patients present with high fevers (up to 104–105°F), severe headache, general malaise, myalgia, confusion, sore throat, chills, sweats, nonproductive cough, and pneumonia. A majority of patients have altered liver function and some will develop overt hepatitis.

Patients who have had acute Q fever may develop the chronic form several years later; endocarditis in a previously damaged valve is a recognized complication of chronic infection.

Burkholderia cepacia

B. cepacia is the name for a group of Gram negative bacteria found in soil and water. They do not pose an infection risk to individuals with a normal immune system. They are, however, an important cause of pneumonia in patients with cystic fibrosis; an inherited condition where patients suffer from excessively sticky mucus especially in the bronchi and lungs. The sticky mucus provides an ideal environment for bacterial growth with organisms such as *S. aureus*, *P. aeruginosa*, and *B. cepacia*. *B. cepacia* is readily spread between susceptible persons and by contact with contaminated environments.

Burkholderia pseudomallei

Generally considered a saprophyte (grows on and uses dead or decaying organic matter as an energy source), this Gram negative organism causes the infectious disease melioidosis that is mostly restricted to Southeast Asia, northern Australia, South and Central America, and the West Indies. It causes serious invasive diseases like septicemia and pneumonia in susceptible individuals. Although the epidemiology of melioidosis is not yet fully understood, it is thought that infections are contracted by contact with the organism from contaminated groundwater (e.g. in rice paddies) through puncture wounds, cuts, or abrasions in the skin.

Coccidioides immitis

Coccidioidomycosis, a fungal disease caused by *Coccidioides immitis*, is endemic in certain parts of Arizona, California, Nevada, New Mexico, Texas, Utah, and Northern Mexico. Infection is caused by inhalation of airborne, infective arthroconidia (fungal spores) from the soil; this is one stage in the organism's lifecycle. In the host, these conidia convert into endosporulating spherules, the organism's other morphologic form (Figure 9.15). The disease is not transmitted from person to person. Approximately 60% of persons infected with *C. immitis* remain asymptomatic. Symptomatic coccidioidomycosis has a wide clinical spectrum, ranging from mild influenza-like illness to serious pneumonia, to widespread dissemination (Box 9.9).

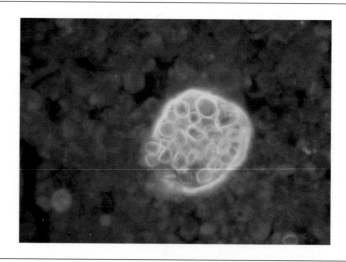

Figure 9.15 Spherule of *Coccidioides immitis*. Provided by Mercy Hospital, Toledo, OH/Brian J. Harrington. Courtesy of the Centers for Disease Control and Prevention; from CDC website: http://phil.cdc.gov/phil/details.asp

Box 9.9 Coccidioidomycosis in California (report from *MMWR* January 22, 1993/42(02);21–24)

In August 1992, a 13-year-old black male from Georgia developed symptoms that included hoarseness, noisy breathing, and difficulty in breathing 2 months after visiting southern California, Nevada, and northern Mexico. During initial evaluation, a laryngeal mass was detected; a laryngeal papilloma (tumor) was suspected. Treatment with steroids and bronchodilaters resulted in symptomatic improvement. In October 1992, a subsequent laryngoscopy detected diffuse granular tissue on the larynx. Histopathologic examination of the biopsy revealed spherules of *Coccidioides immitis* and culture of the biopsy specimen grew *C. immitis*. The patient was treated with an intravenous antifungal agent and, after 5 days was discharged on an oral antifungal agent.

Histoplasma capsulatum

Histoplasmosis is a fungal infection that can affect many organ systems in the body. It is a dimorphic fungus, i.e. it exists in the host as a yeast (Figure 9.16) but grows as a fluffy mold under laboratory conditions (Figure 9.17). It usually causes a short-term, treatable lung infection; however, disseminated histoplasmosis

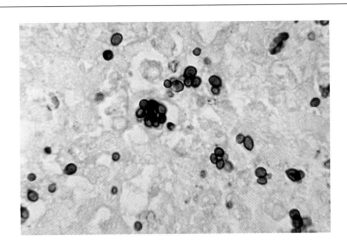

Figure 9.16 *Histoplasma capsulatum* as seen in lung tissue; note budding yeast cells. Provided by Dr Libero Ajello. Courtesy of the Centers for Disease Control and Prevention; from CDC website: http://phil.cdc.gov/phil/details.asp

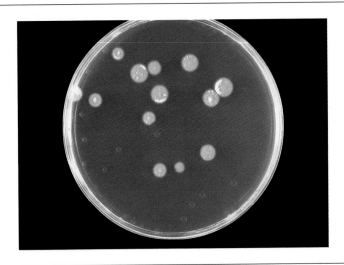

Figure 9.17 Culture of *Histoplasma capsulatum*; note mold form when grown in the laboratory at 20°C. Provided by Dr William Kaplan. Courtesy of the Centers for Disease Control and Prevention; from CDC website: http://phil.cdc.gov/phil/details.asp

can be fatal. The fungus grows naturally in soil in some areas of the USA, mostly in the midwestern and southeastern states and along the Ohio and Mississippi River valleys. It thrives in soil that is enriched with bat or bird droppings. *H. capsulatum* produces spores that can survive in the environment for a long time and infection is acquired by inhalation of spores from soil that is disturbed. The disease is not spread from person to person. In the USA infection with *H. capsulatum* is common, but the disease is rare. As many as 80% of persons living in endemic areas in the USA, have a positive skin test, indicating that they have been exposed to the organism at some time. However, most of these people do not have a history of active disease. To prevent histoplasmosis people are advised to take care to avoid exposure to dust from soil that might be contaminated with bat or bird droppings, and to avoid disturbing accumulations of bat or bird droppings.

Diagnosis

Throat cultures are the mainstay of diagnosis for *S. pyogenes* and *C. diphtheriae* pharyngitis. Blood cultures may be positive in acute epiglottitis due to *H. influenzae*.

For cases of pneumonia, history, examination and investigations should focus on two main issues: the degree of respiratory compromise and clues to the causal microorganism. Since a wide range of pathogens need to be considered, the number of likely candidates should be reduced as much as possible. Accurate information on the age of the patient, co-morbidity, recent travel, occupation, pets, and contact with patients with similar symptoms should be sought.

Sputum can be obtained from the respiratory tract with ease when a patient has a productive cough but the value is often limited by contamination by the flora of the oral and upper respiratory cavity. The upper respiratory tract may be bypassed using techniques such as bronchoalveolar lavage (BAL: a long telescopic device is inserted down the trachea into the bronchi and the lung, specifically designed to examine the LRT) or protected brush specimens but they are invasive and used only in the sicker patients or those failing to respond to empirical treatment. Sputum can be subject to direct Gram stain or acid–alcohol fast stains for *M. tuberculosis* and then set up for culture. Blood cultures should always be sent from febrile patients and are most useful in diagnosing *S. pneumoniae* and other bacterial infections. Specific antigen tests are available for testing urine from patients with suspected pneumococcal or *Legionella pneumophila* serogroup 1 infections. Paired serology (antibody estimations done 1 week apart) is used to diagnose atypical pneumonia as the "atypical" organisms are difficult to culture; however this is often retrospective and not therefore helpful in the acute situation and does not influence initial management.

Q fever is also diagnosed by serologic testing to detect the presence of antibodies to *C. burnetii* antigens. Other useful methods are the indirect immunofluorescence assay (IFA) and DNA detection methods.

The diagnostic techniques used for viral infections of the lower respiratory tract infections (LRTI) are the same as for the upper respiratory tract infection (URTIs), however, LRTIs require a deeper clinical specimen for a more accurate, specific diagnosis. These may include a bronchoscopically collected sample, such as a bronchoalveolar lavage (BAL) or biopsy from the LRT. If the patient has been intubated on the intensive care unit (ICU) to support respiration, an endotracheal aspirate (ETA) may also be obtained – this is more of a middle respiratory tract specimen.

C. immitis and *H. capsulatum* are cultured from sputum samples or bronchial washings using appropriate fungal media. In the laboratory they develop into the highly infectious mold form and may pose a hazard to laboratory workers if arthroconidia or spores from cultures are inadvertently aerosolized. When clinical laboratories handle these organisms, laboratory activities should be performed at biosafety level 3.

Chest X-rays are a fundamental part of the evaluation of lower respiratory tract infections and provide evidence of the distribution and extent of disease more reliably than signs elicited by auscultation. Chest X-ray may also show complications of acute pneumonia such as cavitation or empyema formation.

Treatment

Treatment guidelines are being constantly updated. We refer you to American Thoracic Society (ATS) and Infectious Disease Society of America (IDSA) documents (see Further reading).

Prevention

There is a 23-valent capsular polysaccharide vaccine available that provides immunity against the most common serotypes causing pneumococcal disease. It is offered to at risk patients including those without functioning spleens, those over 65, and patients with cardiovascular or respiratory disease. The vaccine is not effective in the under 2 year olds or in the immunocompromised. A conjugate vaccine is available against seven of the capsular types most often implicated and is given to children as part of routine vaccination in the USA. It has recently been introduced in the UK for vaccination of 2- to 4-month-old babies. Invasive *H. influenzae* disease has vastly decreased in communities where the new protein conjugated vaccine has been introduced to the routine vaccination schedule. An acellular vaccine against *B. pertussis* forms part of the universal childhood vaccination schedule of many countries.

Infection with *Legionella* species can be avoided by maintenance of air conditioning systems including regular hyperchlorination treatment and ensuring that hot water supplies are above 45°C to prevent bacterial multiplication.

There is an annually updated vaccine against the influenza virus whose composition is recommended by the WHO (see Chapter 20 for more details).

Test yourself

Case study 9.1

A 67-year-old previously healthy man was admitted with intermittent fever, weight loss, microscopic hematuria (blood in the urine), and anemia. He was a painter/decorator by profession and had never suffered serious illness before. His only complaint was the numerous cuts and scratches he sustained as a result of his building and decorating work. He came to hospital because he began to notice left sided limb weakness. On examination, he was febrile, anemic, but otherwise well. In the photographs below you can see small bleeding points under his nail bed and lesions in his palm and in the pulp of his finger.

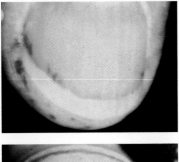
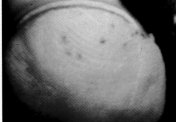
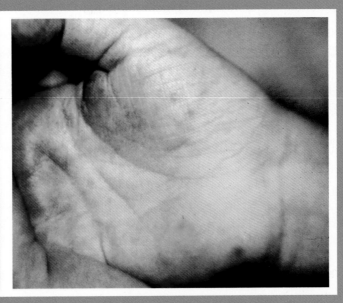

Test yourself

❓1. What are the lesions in the photographs on the previous page called?
❓2. What is your tentative diagnosis?
❓3. What is the pathogenesis of these lesions in the context of this infection?
❓4. What is the commonest organism/group of organisms causing this condition?

Case study 9.2

An 86-year-old lady was admitted with a 3-day history of fever, cough, and right-sided chest pain. On examination she was confused, had labored breathing and a fever of 38.2°C. Blood and sputum cultures were taken and the patient was started on antibiotics.

Her sputum Gram stain result is shown in a figure below and also her chest X-ray (note right lower lobe consolidation).

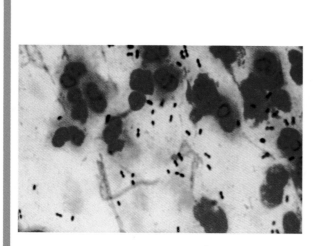 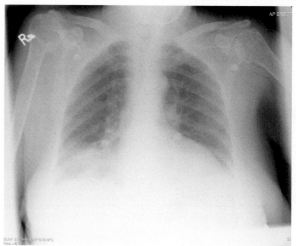

University College Hospital, London is gratefully acknowledged for use of this image

❓1. What is the likely identity of the organism depicted in the Gram stain?
❓2. What is the major virulence determinant of this organism?
❓3. What special patient groups are particularly susceptible to overwhelming infection with this organism?
❓4. How is resistance to penicillin mediated by this organism?

Case study 9.3

An 8-month-old girl presents with a 3-week history of a cough. She initially had a runny nose and her mother thought she had a viral infection. However, the cough appears to be worsening, particularly at night. It often comes in spasms and she frequently vomits after coughing. The mother, who is a teacher, also has a mild cough and has taken the past 2 weeks off work, both to nurse the child and because she was feeling unwell herself.

On examination, the child appears mildly dehydrated but not distressed. Her chest is clear and her abdominal examination is normal.

Test yourself

1. What additional information would you like to ask the mother?
2. What is the possible infectious cause of this girl's cough?
3. What are the major virulence determinants of this organism?
4. Why is this infection making a come-back particularly in young adults and adolescents?

Case study 9.4
A young man developed headache, shivering, muscle pains, and marked lassitude, followed by vague abdominal symptoms and later a distressing cough. No respiratory distress was evident on initial examination and there were signs on clinical examination of the chest. He had just completed a summer job working in a garden center operating the sprinkler system. He deteriorated rapidly requiring intensive care.

1. What is the probable causative organism in this case?
2. What important piece of information suggests that this organism is the most likely cause?
3. How could the diagnosis be confirmed in the laboratory?
4. How could the infection be prevented?

Case study 9.5
A shop assistant working in a pet shop received a large shipment of budgerigars and helped unload them into the shop. He later developed an influenza-type illness with severe headache and muscle pains, persistent dry cough and breathlessness. His spleen was palpable.

1. What is the probable causative organism?
2. How did the shop assistant acquire the infection?
3. How could the diagnosis be confirmed?
4. Is the infection spread from one person to another?

Further reading
American Thoracic Society Guidelines for the Management of Adults with Community acquired Pneumonia: Diagnosis, Assessment of Severity, Antimicrobial Therapy, and Prevention. *Am J Respir Crit Care Med* 2001;163:1730–1754

Bayer AS, Bolger AF, Taubert KA, et al. Diagnosis and management of infective endocarditis and its complications. *Circulation* 1998; 98:2936–2948

Bramley TJ, Lerner D, Sames M. Productivity losses related to the common cold. *J Occup Environ Med* 2002;44(9):822–829

Dajani AS, Taubert KA, Wilson W, et al. Prevention of bacterial endocarditis. Recommendations by the American Heart Association. *JAMA* 1997;277:1794–1801

Ellis CR, Di Salvo T. Myocarditis: basic and clinical aspects. *Cardiol Rev* 2007;15(4):170–177

Infectious Disease Society of America. Practice Guidelines for the Diagnosis and Management of Group A Streptococcal Pharyngitis. *Clin Infect Dis* 2002;35:113–125

Infectious Disease Society of America. Update of Practice Guidelines for the Management of Community acquired Pneumonia in Immunocompetent Adults. *Clin Infect Dis* 2003;37:1405–1433

Tingle LE, Molina D, Calvert CW. Acute pericarditis. *Am Fam Physician* 2007;76(10):1509–1514

Wilson WR, Karchmer AW, Bisno AL, et al. Antibiotic treatment of adults with infective endocarditis due to viridans streptococci, enterococci, other streptococci, staphylococci, and HACEK microorganisms. *JAMA* 1995;274:1706–1713

Useful websites

Myocarditis

http://www.mayoclinic.com/health/myocarditis/DS00521

http://www.medicinenet.com/myocarditis/article.htm

Pericarditis

http://www.mayoclinic.com/health/pericarditis/DS00505/DSECTION=2

http://www.medicinenet.com/pericarditis/article.htm

Pneumonia disease information

http://www.cdc.gov/ncidod/diseases/submenus/sub_pneumonia.htm

http://www.immunitytoday.com/resvirin.html

http://www.medscape.com/viewarticle/498439

http://www.merck.com/mmhe/sec23/ch273/ch273i.html

Chapter 10
Infections of the central nervous system

N. Shetty, J.W. Tang

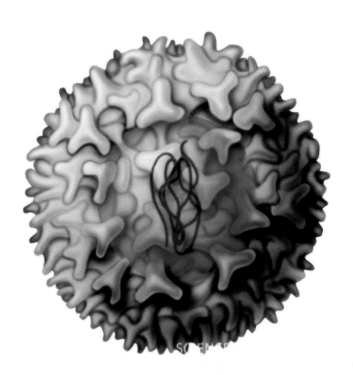

The brain and its coverings
Meningitis
    Public health impact of meningitis
    Clinical presentation
Encephalitis
    Public health impact of rabies
    Clinical presentation
    Prevention

Brain abscess
Pathogenesis and virulence
    Microbiology of bacterial meningitis
    Viral meningitis and encephalitis
    Rabies encephalitis

Infections of the brain and its coverings have been the source of intense media interest and evoke strong emotions in the public psyche (Figure 10.1). This is not without reason, as some forms of bacterial meningitis can be rapidly fatal.

The brain and its coverings

Before we study the infectious processes that commonly involve the brain and its coverings we must first know what they are. The organs of the central nervous system (CNS) comprise the brain and spinal cord; they are covered by three connective tissue layers collectively called the meninges (Figure 10.2). From inside out they are called the pia mater (closest to the brain and spinal cord), the arachnoid (in the middle), and the dura mater (outermost layer). The meninges protect the brain from injury and infection. The brain floats in a protective cushion of cerebrospinal fluid (CSF), which flows within the subarachnoid space, beneath the arachnoid membrane, on top of the pia mater. It also surrounds the spinal cord and fills open spaces (ventricles) inside the brain. The amount of CSF that circulates around the brain normally stays the same, constantly equilibrated by the body; CSF helps to maintain a constant pressure inside the skull, known as intracranial pressure (ICP).

At the cellular level we need to be familiar with the concept of the blood–brain barrier (BBB) including the blood–CSF barrier, as this is central to understanding the pathogenesis and management of CNS

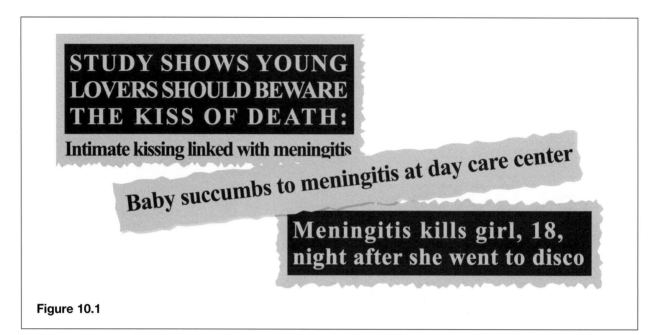

Figure 10.1

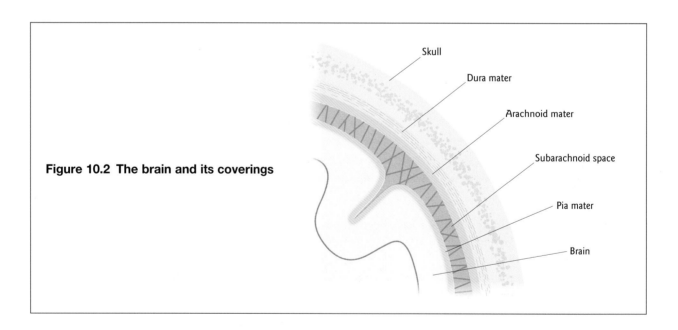

Figure 10.2 The brain and its coverings

Skull

Dura mater

Arachnoid mater

Subarachnoid space

Pia mater

Brain

infections. The BBB (Figure 10.3) is created by the tight apposition of endothelial cells lining blood vessels in the brain; this forms a barrier between the blood vessel and the surrounding brain substance (consisting of astrocytes and microglia for example). A thin basement membrane, comprising laminin, fibronectin, and other proteins, surrounds the endothelial cells and provides both mechanical support and a barrier function. A similar barrier exists between blood and CSF at the arachnoid membrane and in the ventricles. Blood-borne immune cells of the immune system, such as lymphocytes, monocytes and neutrophils, cannot penetrate this barrier. The BBB is crucial for preventing infiltration of pathogens and restricting antibody-mediated immune responses in the CNS. In addition, some, but not all, antimicrobial agents penetrate the BBB; others only penetrate the barrier if the meninges are inflamed, when the junctions between the endothelial cells become more permeable. On rare occasions, pathogens (e.g. bacteria, viruses,

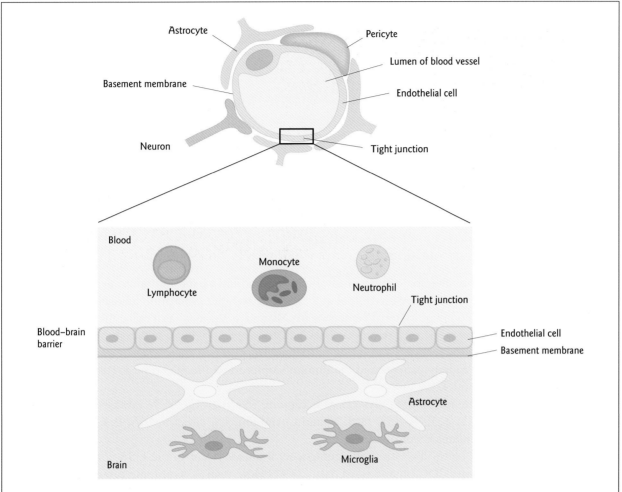

Figure 10.3 The blood–brain barrier. Modified from Expert Reviews in Molecular Medicine © 2003 Cambridge University Press, reproduced with permission

fungi, and protozoa) and cells involved in the immune response breach the endothelial barrier and enter the brain or the meninges resulting in the typical inflammatory changes seen in the CSF as a result of infection.

The three major categories of CNS infections listed below are the most common; we will limit our discussion to these:

- Meningitis
- Encephalitis
- Brain abscess.

Meningitis

Meningitis is the inflammation of the meninges and occurs commonly as a result of infection. The infectious causes of meningitis are tabulated in Table 10.1.

Causes of neonatal meningitis will be discussed in Chapter 12.

Tuberculous meningitis caused by the bacterium *Mycobacterium tuberculosis* will be discussed elsewhere (see Chapter 16).

Table 10.1 Some of the commonest causes of meningitis worldwide

Bacteria	Viruses	Fungi	Protozoa
The three most important causes: **Neisseria meningitidis** **Streptococcus pneumoniae** **Haemophilus influenzae**	*Enteroviruses*: Echoviruses Coxsackie viruses A and B poliovirus *Herpes viruses*: Herpes simplex virus 1 and 2 *Paramyxovirus*: As a complication of mumps	*Cryptococcus neoformans*	*Amebae* (rare) *Naegleria* *Acanthameba*

Causes of neonatal meningitis will be discussed in Chapter 12.

Public health impact of meningitis

Bacterial meningitis is responsible for significant morbidity (severe illness) and mortality (death) throughout the world. The attack rate in the USA is reported at 3 cases per 100 000 population annually. As indicated in Table 10.1, the three most common bacterial pathogens are *Neisseria meningitidis* (also called the meningococcus), *Streptococcus pneumoniae* (also called the pneumococcus), and *Haemophilus influenzae* type b (referred to as Hib). *Listeria monocytogenes* is a relatively rare cause of meningitis; maternal infection can result in serious infection of the newborn. Elderly patients and the immunocompromised may also be at risk. It will be discussed in detail in Chapter 12.

Based on antigenic differences in the polysaccharide capsule, 13 serogroups of *N. meningitidis* have been identified (A, B, C, D, X, Y, Z, E, W-135, H, I, K, and L) and four (*N. meningitidis* A, B, C, and W135) are recognized to cause epidemics worldwide.

Each year, an estimated 1400–2800 cases of meningococcal disease occur in the USA, a rate of 0.5–1.1/100 000 population (CDC, unpublished data, 2004). More than 98% of these cases of meningococcal disease are sporadic, i.e. they are not normally associated with outbreaks. Serogroups B, C, and Y are the major causes of meningococcal disease in the USA, each being responsible for approximately one-third of cases. The proportion of cases caused by each serogroup varies by age group. Among infants aged <1 year, >50% of cases are caused by serogroup B, for which no vaccine is licensed at present. Of all the cases of meningococcal disease among persons aged >11 years, 75% are caused by serogroups (C, Y, or W-135), which are included in vaccines now available in the USA (CDC, 2004). The proportion of meningococcal cases caused by serogroup Y increased from 2% during 1989–1991 to 37% during 1997–2002 (CDC, 2004). Even though the infection can occur at any age, in general, there are two clear epidemiological peaks for meningococcal disease: the under 1 year old and the 15–17 year old.

Multiple studies have been conducted in the USA and the UK concerning the risk for meningococcal disease among college students. The risk for meningococcal disease among US college students was higher for those who resided in dormitories than for those residing in other types of accommodations. Among the approximately 600 000 college freshmen living in dormitories, rates were higher (5.1/100 000) than among any age group in the population other than children aged under 2 years old. In the UK, rates of meningococcal disease were higher among university students than among nonstudents of similar age. Therefore there is good epidemiological evidence showing that meningococcal meningitis is a disease associated with overcrowding and living in closed and intimate communities: military bases, daycare facilities, nurseries, and student dorms are well known settings. In the event of an outbreak, throat swabs taken for bacterial culture from healthy individuals who are close contacts of patients (surveillance cultures) have shown a marked increase in the carriage rate of the organism in the upper airways.

S. pneumoniae is the most common cause of bacteremia, pneumonia, meningitis, and middle ear infection in young children. Each year in the USA, *S. pneumoniae* causes approximately 700 cases of meningitis,

17 000 cases of bacteremia or other invasive disease in children under the age of five. The public health problem related to meningitis caused by *S. pneumoniae* is driven by the emergence of resistant strains; rates as high as 40–60% are reported from some regions in Spain and South Africa. In the USA 20–35% of strains show intermediate or high level resistance to penicillin. During 2005–2006 a new pneumococcal childhood vaccine was introduced in the USA and the UK for all infants and toddlers younger than 24 months as part of their primary immunization schedule. It is also given to children aged 24–59 months at highest risk of infection, such as those with sickle cell anemia, HIV infection, chronic lung or heart disease.

Before the availability of the Hib conjugate vaccine in the USA and other industrialized countries, more than one-half of Hib cases presented as meningitis. The remainder presented as cellulitis, arthritis, or sepsis. In developing countries, Hib is still a leading cause of bacterial pneumonia and deaths in children. During 1980–1990, the incidence in the US was 40–100/100 000 in children younger than 5 years old. Due to routine use of the Hib conjugate vaccine since 1990, the incidence of invasive Hib disease has decreased to 1.3/100 000 children. Hib meningitis can be fatal in 3–6% of cases and up to 20% of surviving patients have permanent hearing loss or other long-term sequelae.

In recent years important developments in immunization have had a dramatic impact on the spectrum of disease caused by the "big three" (i.e. *N. meningitidis*, *S. pneumoniae*, and *H. influenzae* type b). As discussed, childhood vaccination against Hib has been the single most important development that has brought about this change: the widespread use of childhood Hib vaccination has decreased the incidence of Hib meningitis in children in many countries by more than 90%. As a result there is a shift in the age group to older children and young adults presenting with bacterial meningitis.

The second breakthrough came in the form of a successful vaccine against meningococcus group C (the MenC vaccine); in the UK the MenC conjugate vaccine was made available for everybody up to the age of 18 years, and to all first year university students from November 1999. This has since been extended to include everybody less than 25 years of age. The results of this mass vaccination program were soon evident. Meningococcal serogroup C disease has virtually disappeared in the UK (Figure 10.4). However, in the UK as in the USA, serogroup B meningococcal disease is still a public health problem. Unfortunately, there is no vaccine against meningococcus Group B yet, because of poor immunogenicity induced by the serogroup B antigens. One consequence of this is that serogroup B disease may become the predominant cause of meningitis in populations immunized against the other serogroups.

In the absence of an effective serogroup B vaccine and in keeping with national prevalence data, a new meningococcal conjugate vaccine (MCV4), against serogroups A,C,Y,W135 was introduced in the USA in 2005. The vaccine was recommended for all children at age 11–12 years as well as for unvaccinated adolescents at high school entry (age 15 years) and all college freshmen living in dormitories. The vaccine is expected to be efficacious in young children, confer long-term protection, and provide herd immunity by reducing nasopharyngeal carriage and transmission. Other risk groups needing this vaccine include pilgrims to the Hajj in Mecca, Saudi Arabia (where outbreaks of serogroup W135 have been reported); patients with

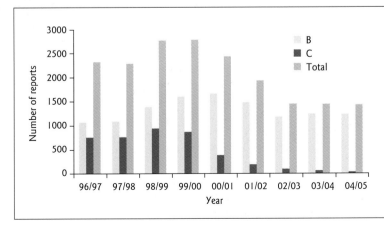

Figure 10.4 Meningococcal disease by serogroup, England and Wales, 2004

poor or absent splenic function, and travelers to areas where serogroup A is prevalent (the "meningitis belt", see Chapter 21).

Viral meningitis (also known as aseptic meningitis) has a reported incidence rate of 10.9 cases per 100 000 person-years in the USA. This is probably a gross underestimate as many cases present with mild disease (associated with just a headache and general malaise); they rarely present to a hospital, may be treated with over the counter medication, and therefore may go undiagnosed. If appropriate diagnostic methods are performed, a specific viral agent is identified in 55–70% of cases of viral meningitis. In previous studies, enteroviruses accounted for 90% of cases and herpes simplex virus (HSV) for 0.5–3% of cases. However, a more recent 5-year study from Finland (see Further reading), using modern molecular detection techniques, revealed that enteroviruses were responsible for only 26% of cases, with 17% being caused by HSV type 2 (HSV-2) and 8% by varicella-zoster (chickenpox) virus out of 95 adult patients with aseptic meningitis. Usually, HSV-2 is a more common cause of viral meningitis than HSV-1, and first-time attacks are often associated with primary genital HSV-2 infection, though subsequent attacks through reactivation of this virus may occur without any reactivation of the genital lesions. As a consequence of this epidemiology, viral meningitis in children will be mostly caused by enteroviruses.

Other causes of viral meningitis include the mumps virus especially in unimmunized populations, occurring in 30% of all patients with mumps. It affects males between two and five times more often than females.

The public health aspects of cryptococcal meningitis will be discussed in Chapter 13.

Naegleria and *Acanthameba* spp. are ubiquitous, free-living amebae, that cause primary amebic meningitis or encephalitis. These infections are very rare and difficult to diagnose. Most *Naegleria fowleri* infections have been reported in children and young adults who have had recent exposure to swimming or diving in warm fresh water. *N. fowleri* is a thermophilic organism that survives well in temperatures of 45°C; they thrive in waterways contaminated by thermal discharges from power plants, heated swimming pools, and hot springs. Most cases of primary amebic meningitis (PAM) occur during the summer months when freshwater sources are warm. When water temperatures decrease, *N. fowleri* encyst and enter a dormant stage, which allows them to survive until the next summer. A short discussion on primary amebic meningitis illustrated by a case report is described in Box 10.1.

Box 10.1 Primary amebic meningoencephalitis – Georgia, 2002 (report from *MMWR* October 10, 2003/52(40);962–964)

In early September 2002, the Georgia Division of Public Health and CDC were notified about a fatal case of primary amebic meningoencephalitis (PAM) caused by *Naegleria fowleri* in a boy aged 11 years who had recently swum in a local river. In response to this case, the district health department recommended that local community authorities advise persons to avoid swimming in this river during periods of high temperature and low water depth.

No organisms were observed on a Gram stained smear of cerebrospinal fluid (CSF); CSF antigen-detection tests were negative for bacterial pathogens. CSF red blood cell count was 1550/mm³ (normal: 0/mm³), white blood cell count was 13 650/mm³ (normal: 0–5/mm³), glucose was <5 mg/dL (normal: 40–70 mg/dL), and protein was 679 mg/dL (normal: 12–60 mg/dL). Follow-up lumbar puncture later the same day revealed motile amebae in a centrifuged CSF specimen. *N. fowleri* was isolated from two of three river water samples tested and from a control sample taken from a local lake.

Learning points: PAM is a rare but nearly always fatal infection caused by *N. fowleri*, a thermophilic, free-living ameba that inhabits freshwater ponds, lakes, and rivers, minimally chlorinated pools, and hot springs throughout the world. Only three survivors of PAM have been documented. Successful therapy is related to early diagnosis and administration of intravenous and intrathecal amphotericin B with intensive supportive care.

Acanthameba keratitis occurs in patients who sustain minor corneal abrasions; this is usually associated with wearing contact lenses. Amebae can be introduced into the eye by swimming while wearing contact lenses or using contaminated contact lens solutions, especially homemade solutions.

Clinical presentation

Many organisms that cause meningitis gain entry by colonizing the upper airways and are spread by airborne transmission. In many cases there may even be a short history of a prodromal upper respiratory tract infection. The organism evades local innate defence mechanisms and gains entry into the bloodstream and eventually lodges in the brain or meninges. Organisms can also gain entry by contiguous spread from a sinusitis, otitis media, or trauma to the face and skull. Once inside the CNS, the relative impermeability of the blood–brain barrier to antibodies, complement components, and white blood cells (WBCs) allows the bacterial infection to proceed unchecked.

Inflammatory changes in the meninges account for the classic clinical symptoms of headache, neck stiffness, and photophobia (discomfort when looking directly at bright light). Though theoretically meningitis is divided into acute (<7 days' since onset) and chronic (>7 days' since onset) presentations, these categories are often blurred and are of little clinical significance. Meningococcal meningitis is often accompanied by a petechial (bleeding under the skin), nonblanching skin rash. This may be so severe as to cause gangrene of the digits (Figure 10.5a and b). This is evidence of meningococcal septicemia. Approximately a third of sufferers develop endotoxic shock and disseminated intravascular coagulation. Acute bacterial meningitis is a life-threatening condition (see "Pathogenesis and virulence", p. 283) and prompts immediate investigation and appropriate management. If treatment is delayed patients may be left with residual neurological impairment including deafness.

By contrast, viral meningitis has a less severe presentation and is rarely associated with sequelae. In the case of enterovirus meningitis, there may be a short history of a flu-like upper respiratory tract infection, prior to meningitis symptoms, and there may or may not be a typical enterovirus maculo-papulo-vesicular rash. Many patients present with a nondescript rash which is nonblanching (Figure 10.6). With HSV meningitis, which is often associated with primary HSV infection (usually HSV-2), there may be vesicular lesions in the genital area or occasionally around the mouth. Cases of recurrent HSV meningitis (also referred to as Mollaret's meningitis or syndrome) have been described, which may not present with any accompanying skin manifestations (see Further reading).

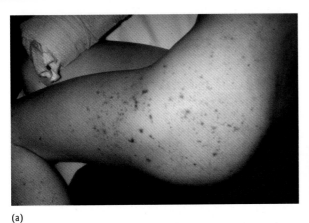
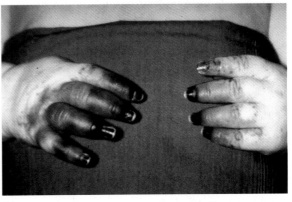

(a)   (b)

Figure 10.5 (a) Classic petechial rash associated with meningococcal disease. (b) Severe meningococcal disease associated with gangrene of the digits

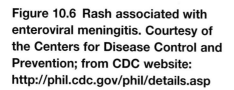

Figure 10.6 Rash associated with enteroviral meningitis. Courtesy of the Centers for Disease Control and Prevention; from CDC website: http://phil.cdc.gov/phil/details.asp

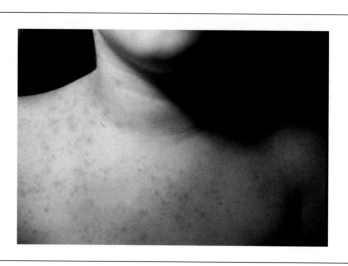

Table 10.2 Characteristic CSF changes in meningitis

Condition	Appearance	Cells (per mm³)	Gram stain or antigen tests or culture for bacteria	Protein (mg/dL)	Glucose (mg/dL)
Normal	Clear	0–7 lymphocytes★	Negative results	12–40	40–80 (should be interpreted as approx. 50% of blood glucose)
Bacterial meningitis	Clear or turbid	100–2000 polymorphs	Positive results	50–300	0–5
Viral meningitis or partially antibiotic treated bacterial meningitis	Clear or slightly turbid	15–500 lymphocytes (polymorphs may predominate in the acute stage)	Negative results	50–100	Normal
Tuberculous meningitis	Clear or slightly turbid; fibrin web may develop	30–500 lymphocytes plus polymorphs	Negative results (scanty by auramine stained smear)	100–600	0–5

★ In a neonate, up to 30 cells/mm³, mainly polymorphs, may be considered normal

Diagnosis of meningitis includes submission of blood cultures or CSF for Gram stain and culture (most pathogens) or for detection of antigens (*C. neoformans*) and for nucleic acid amplification tests by PCR (bacteria and viruses). A combined biochemical and microbiological analysis of CSF is an important rapid tool to differentiate the various causes of meningitis (Table 10.2).

Encephalitis

Encephalitis is best described as inflammation of the brain due to an infection. The commonest cause of encephalitis is usually viral in origin. Viruses gain access to the CNS through the blood or by traveling within nerve cells (neurons).

Encephalitis manifests either as:

- **Primary encephalitis.** This occurs when the first exposure to a virus results in the virus directly affecting the brain and spinal cord. Spinal cord infection is also called myelitis.

or

- **Secondary encephalitis.** This form occurs when a virus first infects another part of the body, lies latent for a while and secondarily affects the CNS when reactivated.

There are approximately 20 000 cases of encephalitis in the USA each year, and the most common cause of acute viral encephalitis is the herpes simplex virus. Other viruses causing encephalitis are arthropod borne viruses (arboviruses, see below), transmitted by mosquitoes, ticks or other insects; and rabies virus – transmitted by certain animal bites or contact with their saliva (Box 10.2).

Box 10.2 Human rabies – Tennessee, 2002 (report from *MMWR* September 20, 2002/51(37);828–829)

On August 24, a boy aged 13 years residing in Franklin County, Tennessee was seen at the local hospital emergency department (ED) with a 3-day history of headache, neck pain, right arm numbness and weakness, and a temperature of 100°F (37.8°C); he also complained of diplopia (double vision). He was discharged home with a diagnosis of "muscle strain." On August 25, he again sought medical care at the local hospital ED. Symptoms at this time included fever of 102.0°F (39.0°C), right arm weakness, slurred speech, diplopia, nuchal (neck) rigidity, and dysphagia (difficulty in swallowing). Laboratory results from the CSF revealed a WBC count of 220/mL (normal: 0–7/mL) with 80% lymphocytes, a protein concentration of 96 mg/dL (normal: 5–40 mg/dL), and a glucose concentration of 57 mg/dL (normal: 40–80 mg/dL). A CT scan of the head revealed no focal lesions. On August 26, the patient had difficulty breathing because of decreased mental status and hypersalivation. He was intubated, mechanically ventilated, and sedated because of agitation. Rabies was suspected on the basis of focal neurologic symptoms and hypersalivation. The patient's mental status deteriorated rapidly, and by the next morning, he was unresponsive and no longer required sedation. On August 31, the patient was pronounced brain dead, support was withdrawn, and the patient died.

Samples of serum, CSF and saliva that were sent to CDC on August 29 showed rabies virus-specific antibody. The nuchal skin biopsy and saliva from August 29 were positive for rabies virus RNA by reverse transcription polymerase chain reaction. The virus was identified by genetic sequence analysis as a variant associated with silver-haired and eastern pipistrelle bats.

The patient's family had several pets, including cats, dogs, and horses, none of which had been ill. The parents reported that the patient had found a bat on the ground during the day at a nearby lake on approximately July 1 and brought it home. No other family members handled the bat, which was released the same day. The family was unaware of any animal bite or that bats might be rabid and can transmit rabies virus to humans. Four household members and one other family member received postexposure prophylaxis (PEP) for rabies because of possible exposure to the virus through contact with the patient's saliva. In addition, 18 healthcare workers who had contact with the patient received PEP.

Editorial note: The public should be informed that bats carry the rabies virus. CDC strongly advises that persons should avoid direct contact with bats, other wildlife, and stray or ill domestic animals; however, if direct contact with bats has occurred, exposed persons should see their healthcare provider, and the exposure should be reported to local public health officials.

Box 10.3 Lyme disease

Lyme* disease is caused by a spirochaete, *Borrelia burgdorferi* (left above) and is transmitted to humans by the bite of infected blacklegged ticks (*Ixodes scapularis*, left below). When a young tick feeds on an infected animal, the tick sucks the bacterium into its body along with the blood meal.

The bacterium lives in the gut of the tick; as it feeds again, it can transmit the bacterium to its new host. Usually the new host is another small rodent, but sometimes the new host is a human. The first sign of infection is usually a circular to oval rash called erythema migrans (right).

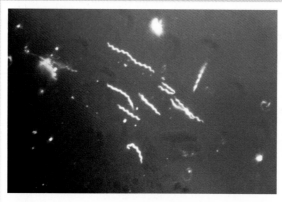

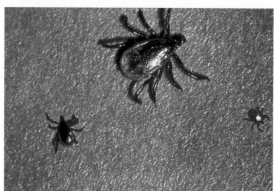

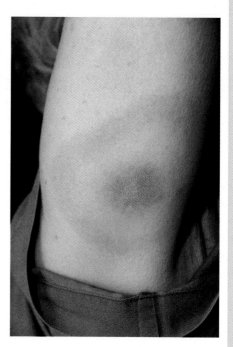

Courtesy of the Centers for Disease Control and Prevention; and CDC website: http://phil.cdc. gov/phil/details.asp. Image of spirochaetes provided by Robert D.Gilmore, CDC

Systemic symptoms of fatigue, chills, fever, headache, muscle and joint aches, and swollen lymph nodes are common. Meningitis or encephalitis may follow if left untreated. Late stage manifestations of the disease include arthritis and other neurological complaints. Prevent Lyme disease by applying an insect repellent when walking in the woods, especially in the months of May through July. Check clothing for ticks, remove ticks attached to your body with tweezers. See Further reading for a full account of treatment and prevention methods.

* Named after Lyme, Connecticut after a cluster of cases occurred there.

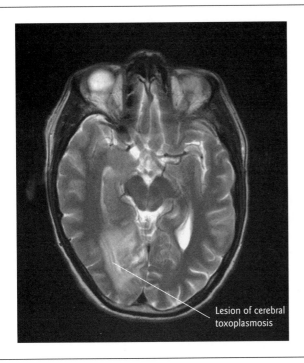

Figure 10.7 Encephalitis due to cerebral toxoplasmosis: MRI of brain

Lesion of cerebral toxoplasmosis

In rare instances, secondary encephalitis occurs after common childhood viral infections, such as measles, mumps, rubella (German measles), chickenpox, or infectious mononucleosis. In these cases encephalitis may occur as a result of a heightened immune response to the virus rather than the virus itself. They will be discussed in greater detail in Chapter 15.

Encephalitis can also be a feature of other infections such as Lyme disease (Box 10.3), caused by the bacterium *Borrelia burgdorferi*, and toxoplasmosis (caused by the parasite *Toxoplasma gondii*). In Figure 10.7 you can see the inflammatory changes in the occipital lobe of the brain caused by cerebral toxoplasmosis. Toxoplasmosis will be discussed in Chapter 13.

Patients with encephalitis complain of headache, irritability, or lethargy. Most cases are mild and recovery is spontaneous. More severe disease may manifest with seizures, nausea and vomiting, sudden fever, and altered levels of consciousness.

Nowadays, the most common method of diagnosis involves analyzing CSF or blood for viral nucleic acid by amplification tests. Viral culture and antigen (viral protein) detection techniques can also be used, for confirmation. Other nonmicrobiological tests include looking for electroencephalographic (EEG) changes, magnetic resonance imaging (MRI) of the brain, and brain biopsy.

See Further reading for the various treatment options available for encephalitis.

Public health impact of rabies

Rabies virus causes an acute encephalitis in all warm-blooded hosts, including humans, and the outcome is almost always fatal. Although all species of mammals are susceptible to rabies virus infection, only a few species are important as reservoirs for the disease. In the USA, several distinct rabies virus variants have been identified in terrestrial mammals, including raccoons, skunks, foxes, and coyotes. In addition to these terrestrial reservoirs, several species of insectivorous bats are also reservoirs for rabies.

Overall, rates of human rabies cases in the USA remain low, averaging three cases per year during the previous 10 years. Since 1990, a total of 26 (74%) of the 35 human rabies deaths in the USA have been associated with bat-variant rabies viruses. This is in marked contrast with human rabies cases in Asia, Africa, and South America where canine-variant rabies predominates. In the USA, human fatalities associated with rabies occur in people who fail to seek medical assistance, usually because they were unaware of their exposure. Modern day prophylaxis has proven nearly 100% successful.

Clinical presentation

Typically patients may present initially with nonspecific flu-like symptoms – malaise, fever, or headache. There may be discomfort or paresthesia (abnormal sensations) at the site of the bite. In the later stages, often within days of onset, there is progression with signs and symptoms of altered mental status, including anxiety, confusion, agitation, progressing to delirium, abnormal behavior, hallucinations, and insomnia. The difficulty in swallowing can cause spasms at the sight and sound of water which is characteristic of some forms of clinical rabies. The location and severity of the bite can influence the speed with which clinical signs develop. If the bite is severe and close to the head or face rather than in the lower limbs the chances of rapid progression to CNS signs are greater. Once clinical rabies has set in the outcome is nearly always fatal. Treatment is typically supportive. Disease prevention is entirely prophylactic and includes both passive antibody (immune globulin) and vaccine. Nonlethal exceptions are extremely rare. To date only six documented cases of human survival from clinical rabies have been reported and each included a history of either pre- or postexposure prophylaxis (see below).

Prevention

There is no antiviral treatment for rabies after symptoms of the disease appear. However, there is a safe and extremely effective new rabies vaccine regimen that provides immunity to rabies when administered after an exposure (postexposure prophylaxis) or for protection before an exposure occurs (preexposure prophylaxis). Although rabies among humans is rare in the USA, every year an estimated 18 000 people receive rabies preexposure prophylaxis and an additional 40 000 receive postexposure prophylaxis.

Preexposure vaccination is recommended for persons in high-risk groups, such as veterinarians, animal handlers, and certain laboratory workers.

For the latest information on the recommended postexposure prophylaxis see Further reading.

Brain abscess

Abscesses may form anywhere in the body and the brain is no exception. Brain abscesses usually occur secondary to a focus of infection outside of the CNS. An abscess usually begins as a diffuse inflammation of brain matter and progresses to form a focal lesion visualized, using a variety of imaging techniques (CT scan, MRI etc), as an encapsulated, well demarcated lesion (Figure 10.8).

Nasopharyngeal infections such as otitis media, mastoiditis, and sinusitis are common predisposing factors and account for about 40% of brain abscesses. Organisms that enter the bloodstream and lodge in the brain from sites remote to the CNS contribute to about 30% of brain abscesses. Previously, lung abscesses were traditionally cited as being principal sources. This pattern is changing; dental abscesses are increasingly the primary focus. Many patients also have a history of alcohol dependence and poor nutrition. Direct inoculation into the brain as a result of trauma (fractures of the skull and face) or surgery accounts for 10% of cases.

The microbiology of brain abscesses reflects the oral–nasopharyngeal flora seen in infections at these sites (Figure 10.9). The organisms most often implicated are a combination of aerobic Gram positive cocci (i.e. *Streptococcus milleri*, *Staphylococcus aureus*, and other alpha and beta hemolytic streptococci) and anaerobic Gram positive and negative organisms (i.e. *Bacteroides* species, *Fusobacterium* spp., anaerobic streptococci). See Chapter 7 for the pathogenesis of abscess formation related to these organisms. An abscess whether in skin, bone, joint, heart valve, or brain evolves in pretty much the same way.

In patients who are immunocompromised (see Chapter 13) as a result of HIV, organ transplantation or malignancy, the spectrum expands to include protozoan parasites such as *Toxoplasma gondii*, fungi such as *Aspergillus* and *Candida* species and *Nocardia* spp. (a branching Gram positive bacterium).

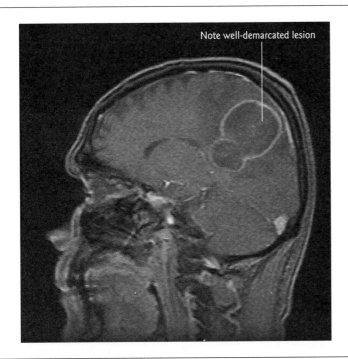

Note well-demarcated lesion

Figure 10.8 Brain abscess in the occipito-parietal lobe secondary to a dental abscess (MRI)

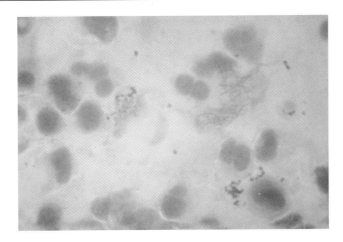

Figure 10.9 Pus from a brain abscess stained by Gram stain. Note numerous polymorphs, Gram positive cocci and slender, filamentous Gram negative rods. The abscess was caused by a mixture of organisms including *Bacteroides* spp., a *Fusobacterium* sp., and a *Streptococcus* sp. Provided by Dr V.R. Dowell. Courtesy of the Centers for Disease Control and Prevention; from CDC website: http://phil.cdc.gov/phil/details.asp

Patients manifest with a variety of symptoms that include fever, headaches, focal seizures, and altered mental status.

Diagnosis is confirmed on magnetic resonance imaging (MRI) or CT scans and diagnostic aspiration of the pus for microbiological smear and culture analysis.

For up to date management guidelines for all of the CNS infections see Further reading.

Pathogenesis and virulence

Microbiology of bacterial meningitis

Neisseria meningitidis is a Gram negative diplococcus that may be found within polymorphonuclear leukocytes. About 20% of the population carry this bacterium in the oropharynx (Figure 10.10). The

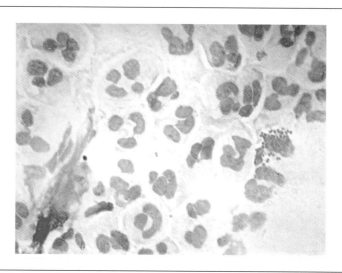

Figure 10.10 Gram stain smear of CSF showing *N. meningitidis*. Note Gram negative (pink) bean shaped intracellular diplococci

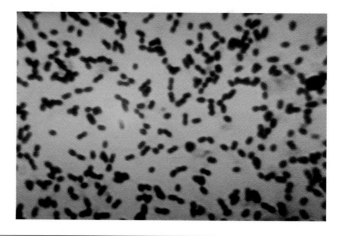

Figure 10.11 Numerous Gram positive diplococci with a few fragments of degenerating polymorphonuclear leukocytes. Some diplococci show a clear unstained halo. Reprinted from H.P. Lambert and W.E. Farrar (1982) *Slide Atlas of Infectious Diseases*, Gower Medical Publishing Ltd. Reproduced with permission of Elsevier

organism is surrounded by a polysaccharide capsule. There are 13 antigenic "serogroups," depending on the antigenic differences in the polysaccharide capsule.

S. pneumoniae is a Gram positive diplococcus characterized by a large polysaccharide capsule that remains unstained on Gram stain, giving the impression of a halo around the organism (Figure 10.11). The capsule of *S. pneumoniae* is also antigenic in nature – to date there are over 90 different types. A pneumococcal vaccine, currently available, cannot obviously include all the different antigenic types. Those that are currently available include the most prevalent types that cause severe invasive disease.

H. influenzae is a Gram negative pleomorphic (different shapes: coccoid, bacillary, or cocco-bacillary) capsulated organism (Figure 10.12). There are six serological types of *H. influenzae*: types a, b, c, d, e, and f. Like other capsulated organisms these separate types are based on the antigenic structure of the capsular polysaccharide. The invasive strain is that which is surrounded by a type B capsule, hence the name *H. influenzae* type b (or Hib).

Virulence mechanisms

In recent years there have been important advances in understanding the mechanisms by which bacteria cause the many devastating consequences of meningitis and septicemia. Some of this has already been referred to in Chapter 3 (see Systemic Inflammatory Response Syndrome or SIRS). Bacterial cell wall

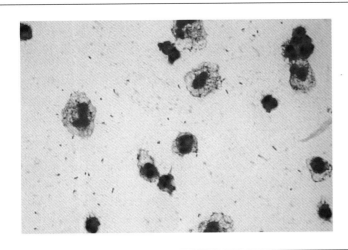

Figure 10.12 Gram stain smear of CSF showing *H. influenzae*. Note Gram negative (pink) pleomorphic organisms and numerous polymorphs. www.yamagiku.co.jp/ pathology/case/ case100.htm

components (i.e. peptidoglycan and lipopolysaccharide) mediate a complex cascade of events that involves complement and certain key cytokines. TNF-α and IL-1 are the most prominent among the cytokines that mediate this inflammatory cascade. Other chemokines such as IL-6, IL-8, nitric oxide, prostaglandins (PGE$_2$), and platelet activation factor (PAF), are presumed to amplify the inflammatory response.

The net result is that the blood–brain barrier becomes more permeable, there is increased intracerebral pressure because of swelling of the brain, and toxic metabolic end products of bacterial metabolism accumulate in the brain and CSF. This accounts for the characteristic biochemical and cellular changes that are described in Table 10.2. In addition exudates (purulent material seen in Figure 10.13) extend throughout the CSF, particularly in the base of the brain, damaging cranial nerves (damage to the VIII cranial nerve results in deafness), obstructing CSF flow (causes hydrocephalus), and inducing inflammation of and injury to the small blood vessels (decreasing the blood supply to the brain). If untreated, the end result is gross neuronal injury.

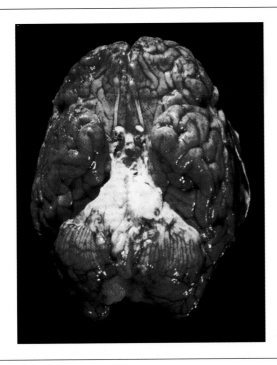

Figure 10.13 Exudate covering the base of the brain as a result of pneumococcal meningitis. Courtesy of the Centers for Disease Control and Prevention; from CDC website: http://phil.cdc.gov/phil/details.asp

Encapsulated pathogens are still the major causes of meningitis due to the production of diverse capsular types (e.g. pneumococcus) or to the capsule being nonimmunogenic (e.g. *N. meningitidis* group B). A poorly immunogenic capsule is due to the molecular structure of the polysaccharide subunits within the capsule; they are so similar to sugars found on host cells that an immune response is not mounted against them. Polysaccharide capsules also interfere with the processes of phagocytosis and complement-mediated bacterial killing. The importance of the capsule in the virulence of some organisms has been demonstrated at the molecular level. The molecular mechanisms of activity of capsular polysaccharide still remain to be defined. It is known that sialyl sugar groups on capsular polysaccharides of some organisms may prevent the activation of the complement pathway by these organisms. Antibodies to capsular polysaccharide usually confer protective immunity through opsonization (coated with antibody and/or complement) of bacteria promoting phagocytosis.

The pneumococcus also produces a toxin, pneumolysin, that interferes with the immune response. At high concentrations this membrane damaging toxin lyses all eukaryotic cells. Pneumolysin inhibits the respiratory burst of phagocytes and also inhibits random migration and chemotaxis by these cells. The toxin inhibits antibody production by lymphocytes and blocks mitogen induced proliferation of B cells. *In vivo* the toxin induces a large inflammatory response and this may be due to its ability to stimulate the production of inflammatory cytokines (IL-1β and TNF-α) and to activate the classical complement pathway. Activation of the classical complement pathway is due, at least in part, to the ability of the toxin to bind to the Fc portion of IgG.

Important predisposing factors for overwhelming pneumococcal/meningococcal and Hib infections are sickle cell disease (a blood disorder in Afro-Caribbean ethnic groups) and other conditions which result in the absence of a functioning spleen. The spleen serves two major functions in protecting the individual against serious bacterial infections, especially those due to the capsulated organisms mentioned above. It is a phagocytic filter that removes bacteria from the bloodstream and it is an antibody producing organ. Although the liver appears to remove the majority of well opsonized bacteria from the bloodstream, the spleen plays an important role through its ability to sequester bacteria that are not as well opsonized and, thus, is of vital importance in the nonimmune host. The spleen may also be critical in the production of opsonizing antibodies, which are important for the rapid and efficient removal of these bacteria from the bloodstream.

Viral meningitis and encephalitis

Enteroviruses are small RNA viruses that include echoviruses, coxsackie viruses A and B, and polioviruses. Certain enterovirus types, i.e. 70 and 71, are associated with meningoencephalitis as well as meningitis. Coxsackievirus B subgroups cause over 60% of meningitis seen in children less than 3 months old (Figure 10.14).

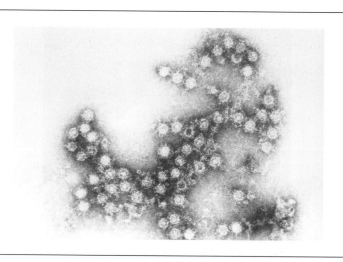

Figure 10.14 An immune electron micrograph of a Coxsackie virus – a cause of viral meningitis. Courtesy of the Centers for Disease Control and Prevention; from CDC website: http://phil.cdc.gov/phil/details.asp

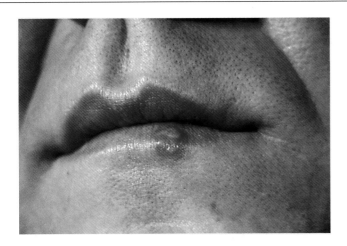

Figure 10.15 A "cold sore" caused by herpes simplex virus. Provided by Dr Herrmann. Courtesy of the Centers for Disease Control and Prevention; from CDC website: http://phil.cdc.gov/phil/details.asp

Herpes simplex virus type 1 (HSV-1) is usually associated with the "cold sore" infections of the lips, mouth, and face and is transmitted by contact with infected saliva (Figure 10.15).

Herpes simplex virus 2 (HSV-2) is sexually transmitted. Symptoms include genital and oral ulcers. Cross-infection of HSV-1 and -2 may occur from oral–genital contact. Herpes viruses are DNA viruses.

The **mumps virus** is an RNA virus that typically causes painful swelling of parotid glands. This is preceded by primary replication of the virus in epithelial cells of the upper respiratory tract and local lymph nodes, followed by viremia. A proportion of mumps cases (mainly adults) develop complications: meningitis and encephalitis (also orchitis, pancreatitis, myocarditis, and nephritis).

The **enteroviruses** enter the human host by the oral–fecal or respiratory routes, the latter route is also responsible for entry of the mumps virus. Most other viruses gain access to the CNS along the nerve roots. This includes the herpes viruses (HSV-1, HSV-2, and varicella zoster virus). The herpes viruses are known for their latency in neural ganglia. HSV-1 remains the most common cause of sporadic encephalitis, while HSV-2 commonly causes meningitis. HSV-2 DNA has also been the most common finding in many reported cases of recurrent viral meningitis. HSV-2 genital infection often precedes meningitis; sexual contact with actively infected individuals is one of the known risk factors. For this reason this type of meningitis is rare in children, unless mother–fetus transmission occurs, when significant systemic sequelae including death may occur.

Replication of viruses in neuronal cells leads to inflammation of the brain and characteristic CSF changes: early polymorphonuclear reaction in the first 24–48 hours, followed later by increasing numbers of monocytes and lymphocytes. Hence, in the early stages of viral meningitis, the CSF picture may be mistaken for bacterial meningitis.

Arboviruses are a large group of enveloped RNA viruses that are transmitted by mosquitoes and ticks and are the most common cause of epidemic encephalitis. Organisms that transmit disease from one animal host to another are called vectors. Mosquitoes are vectors for the transmission of several viruses that can cause encephalitis, they transmit from small animals – usually rodents and birds – to humans. In fact, with many of these arbovirus infections, man is a "dead-end" host, though it is possible for uninfected mosquitoes to feed on an infected human and become infected. Sometimes, however, the viral load in humans may be too low for the mosquitoes to become infected (see Chapter 24: West Nile virus).

However, if a mosquito feeds on an infected bird, the mosquito becomes a lifelong carrier of the virus. The mosquito transmits the infection to the next bird it feeds on, which in turn passes it on to more mosquitoes. Usually, this transmission pattern is maintained without serious impact on mosquito or bird or, indeed, man. However, this balance can be upset by a number of environmental or ecological disasters, involving weather or other climate changes and encroachment of human populations into the natural habitats of birds. Under these conditions, humans and other animals may be affected.

In the USA, the following types of mosquito-borne encephalitis occur:

Eastern equine encephalitis is a rare infection that mainly affects horses; on average less than 10 human cases are reported per year. Eastern equine encephalitis outbreaks occur most commonly in the eastern USA.

Western equine encephalitis, like eastern equine encephalitis, this infection affects horses and, rarely, humans. Most reports of western equine encephalitis come from the central and western plains of the USA.

St. Louis encephalitis: The mosquito vector of St Louis encephalitis breeds in stagnant water, including polluted pools, roadside ditches and containers such as birdbaths, flowerpots, and discarded tires. About 130 cases are reported each year in the USA, although severe outbreaks have affected up to 3000 people in one year.

La Crosse encephalitis is named for La Crosse, Wisconsin, where the virus was first isolated. Unlike other forms of viral encephalitis, this virus is passed to mosquitoes from chipmunks and squirrels.

West Nile encephalitis cases first appeared in the USA in 1999. The virus and the disease it causes will be discussed in greater detail in a separate chapter (see Chapter 24) dealing with emerging viral infections.

Rabies encephalitis

Virology

The rabies virus is an RNA virus that belongs to the Rhabdoviridae family. Viruses in this group possess characteristic bullet shaped morphology (Figure 10.16). The virus particle is surrounded by an envelope and 10-nm glycoprotein spikes called peplomers.

Pathogenesis

Transmission of rabies virus to humans usually occurs through the bite or lick of an infected animal, when virus containing saliva is inoculated into an uninfected individual. Various other routes of transmission have been documented and include contamination of mucous membranes (i.e. eyes, nose, mouth), aerosol transmission, and corneal transplantations.

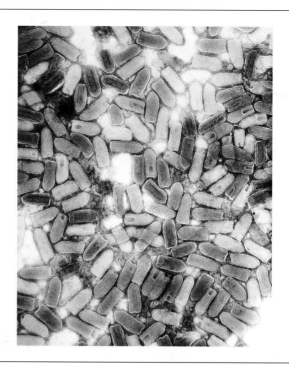

Figure 10.16 An electron micrograph of the rhabdovirus virion; note the characteristic bullet shape. Courtesy of the Centers for Disease Control and Prevention; from CDC website: http://phil.cdc.gov/phil/details.asp

Following primary infection the virus enters an eclipse or latent phase in which it cannot be easily detected within the host. This phase may last for several days or months. Virus can enter directly into peripheral nerves at the site of infection or replicate locally in non-neural tissue (i.e. muscle cells). Subsequent uptake of virus into peripheral nerves is important for progression of disease.

After uptake into peripheral nerves, rabies virus is transported to the CNS via sensory and motor nerves at the initial site of infection. The incubation period, i.e. the time from exposure to onset of clinical signs of disease, may vary from a few days to several years, but is typically 1–3 months. Dissemination of virus within the CNS is rapid, amplification of infection within the CNS occurs through cycles of viral replication and cell-to-cell transfer of progeny virus. During this period of cerebral infection, the classic behavioral changes associated with rabies develop.

The virus causes both encephalitis and myelitis. Rabies infection frequently causes cytoplasmic eosinophilic inclusion bodies (Negri bodies) in neuronal cells, especially pyramidal cells of the hippocampus and Purkinje cells of the cerebellum. These inclusions have been identified as areas of active viral replication by the identification of rabies viral antigen and are useful for markers for diagnosis of rabies in human and animal brain tissue.

Test yourself

Case study 10.1

A 5-month-old baby presents to the emergency department with a 12-hour history of vomiting, incessant crying, and irritability. The parents have elected not to vaccinate the child.

On examination she is listless, has a fever, cries when her head is moved, the fontanelles (soft spot on top of a baby's head) are full; there is a small conjunctival hemorrhage in one eye. The chest and abdomen are clear; there is a suggestion of a rash over the shoulder.

Specimen	Appearance	Cells (per mm³)	Gram stain or antigen tests or culture for bacteria	Protein mg/dL	Glucose (mg/dL)
Normal CSF	Clear	0–5 lymphocytes★	Negative results	12–60	40–70 (should be interpreted as approx. 50% of blood glucose)
Patient's CSF	Clear	500 polymorphs	Few polymorphs, very scant? Gram negative coccoid bacteria, some are more rod shaped	80	10; Blood glucose = 80

❓1. Interpret the CSF results above; suggest a possible organism causing the infection. Justify your answer from: (a) patient details and (b) CSF findings.

❓2. How could the infection have been prevented?

Case study 10.2

A 19-year-old freshman student, living in dormitory accommodation, took to his bed early one Friday evening, complaining of a flu-like illness and headache. The next morning he was found cold and unresponsive with a widespread nonblanching rash. He was taken to the emergency department where a

Test yourself

lumbar puncture was done after a CT scan. The whole freshman year had received a meningococcal vaccine prior to starting their course. Below are the results of his CSF examination and the Gram stain picture.

Specimen	Appearance	Cells (per mm³)	Gram stain or antigen tests or culture for bacteria	Protein mg/dL	Glucose (mg/dL)
Normal CSF	Clear	0–5 lymphocytes	Negative results	12–60	40–70 (should be interpreted as approx. 50% of blood glucose)
Patient's CSF	Clear	10 000 red blood cells*, 800 polymorphs	Few polymorphs, occasional Gram negative diplococci some appear intracellular	75	8; Blood glucose = 120

* Normal blood has a ratio of approximately 1 white cell for 500 red cells.

1. What do you think is the cause of his infection?
2. What are the predisposing factors in this patient's history that make him at risk for this infection?
3. Why was he not protected by the vaccine?
4. How would you manage the other residents in his "dorm"?

Case study 10.3

A 70-year-old man presents to the outpatient clinic with a 3-week history of general malaise. More specifically, over the last week he has noticed a throbbing headache and has lost his appetite. He feels that the left side of this body is weak and he has no energy. He has vomited on two occasions. He smokes ten cigarettes a day, and consumes 8–10 units of alcohol per day. He lives on his own at home and usually manages to cope well. On examination, he has a temperature of 38.5°C and a pulse rate of 90 beats/min, and his blood pressure is 140/90 mm Hg. A Gram stain is made of a sample of his CSF fluid.

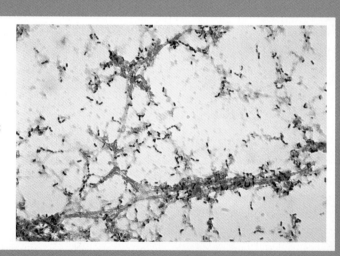

Provided by Dr Mike Miller. Courtesy of the Centers for Disease Control and Prevention; from CDC website: http://phil.cdc.gov/phil/details.asp

Test yourself

❓1. Interpret the Gram stain. What is the cause of his infection?
❓2. What other serious infection does this organism cause?
❓3. What important changes are associated with this organism that would impact antimicrobial therapy?
❓4. Is there any way you could protect him from recurrent infection?
❓5. If this patient was a young African-American what specific risk factor would you look for?

Case study 10.4
A 4-year-old child was taken to the emergency department by her parents with a 1-day history of fever and irritability. On examination the child had neck stiffness and a temperature of 37.5°C. The remainder of the clinical examination revealed no abnormalities except for a faint blanching rash (see below).

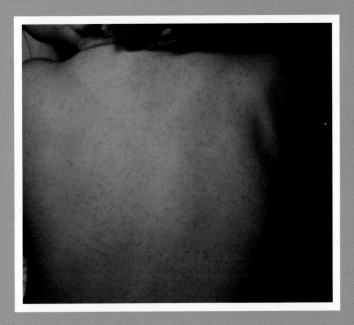

A lumbar puncture was performed. Analysis of the CSF showed the following

Specimen	Appearance	Cells (per mm³)	Gram stain or antigen tests or culture for bacteria	Protein mg/dL	Glucose (mg/dL)
Normal CSF	Clear	0–5 lymphocytes	Negative results	12–60	40–70 (should be interpreted as approx. 50% of blood glucose)
Patient's CSF	Clear	89 predominantly lymphocytes	Negative	60	50; Blood glucose = 120

❓1. Based on the CSF results and the appearance of the rash what is the most likely diagnosis? Justify your answer.

Test yourself

?2. Name the agents most commonly implicated in this type of infection.

?3. Of the agents you have enumerated one is unlikely because of the age of the child, which one is it?

?4. Will the patient have any residual neurological sequelae following her acute illness?

Case study 10.5

A 40-year-old man presented to the emergency department with a history of fever, headache, and altered mental status after a single seizure. His past medical notes indicated a longstanding history of chronic sinusitis and poor teeth; he had seen his dentist 2 weeks earlier for a dental extraction. Below is an MRI image, showing a lesion in the frontal lobe.

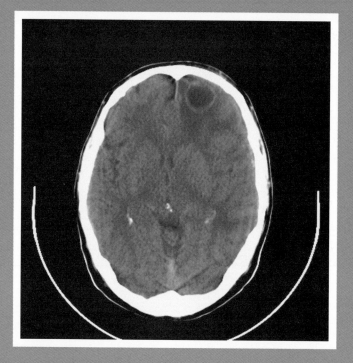

?1. What do you think is being visualized in this scan?

?2. Name two predisposing factors in this patient's story that could have contributed to this infection.

?3. Name at least three groups of organisms (at genus level) that are commonly implicated in this type of infection.

Further reading

Guidelines from the Infectious Diseases Society of America. Practice Guidelines for the Management of Bacterial Meningitis. *Clin Infect Dis* 2004;39:1267–1284. http://www.journals.uchicago.edu/CID/journal/issues/v39n9/34796/34796.htm

Guidelines from the Infectious Diseases Society of America. Practice Guidelines for the Treatment of Lyme Disease. *Clin Infect Dis* 2000;31:1–14. http://www.journals.uchicago.edu/CID/journal/issues/v31nS1/000342/000342.htm

Kupila L, Vuorinen T, Vainionpaa R, Hukkanen V, Marttila RJ, Kotilainen P. Etiology of aseptic meningitis and encephalitis in an adult population. *Neurology* 2006;10;66(1):75–80

Mandell GL, Bennett JE, Dolin R (eds). *Principles and Practice of Infectious Diseases*, 6th edn. Philadelphia: Churchill Livingstone, 2005, chaps 79, 80, 83, 84

Tyler KL. Herpes simplex virus infections of the central nervous system: encephalitis and meningitis, including Mollaret's. *Herpes* 2004;11(suppl 2):57A–64A

Useful websites

CDC. Learn About Lyme Disease. www.cdc.gov/ncidod/dvbid/lyme/

CDC. Traveler's Health: Yellow Book. Meningococcal Disease. http://wwwn.cdc.gov/travel/yellowBookCh4-Menin.aspx

Read this website for a for a full discussion on Lyme disease

Prevention and control of rabies

http://www.cdc.gov/mmwr/preview/mmwrhtml/00056176.htm

http://www.cdc.gov/ncidod/dvrd/rabies/Prevention&Control/preventi.htm

Chapter 11
Infections of the genitourinary system

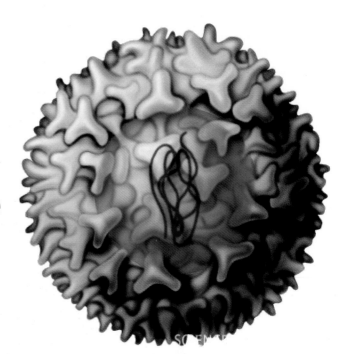

N. Shetty, R. Smith

Sexually transmitted diseases
  The public health impact of sexually transmitted
    diseases
  Feel free to talk: the first step to diagnosing an STD
  Clinical presentation of sexually transmitted diseases
  Diagnosis of genital tract infections
  Management of STDs
  Microbiology, pathogenesis, and virulence

Urinary tract infections
  Predisposing factors
  Bacterial pathogenesis
  Classification of UTIs
  Clinical presentation
  Diagnosis
  Management

Infections of the genitourinary tract are among the most difficult to manage because of social and cultural taboos, the threat of ostracism, and the fear of blame. Interestingly, many early public health posters issued by the Departments of Health in the UK and USA during the Second Word War (circa 1940–1942) clearly imply "beware of women carrying venereal disease" (Figure 11.1). The global AIDS epidemic saw a sharp about turn in this kind of thinking. Taking the view that apportioning blame was neither constructive nor helpful but taking responsibility was, the UN issued a worldwide call to all men, across global and cultural divides, to embrace the campaign known as "Men can make a difference" (Box 11.1).

In the following section we will examine common infections related to the genitourinary system: their epidemiology, clinical presentation, management, prevention, and control.

Infections of the genitourinary tract can be broadly divided into:

- Infections that are sexually transmitted (e.g. gonorrhea, chlamydia, syphilis, herpes, and warts), and
- Urinary tract infections.

Infections due to HIV and hepatitis B virus, though sexually transmitted, are not included here. Due to their global and public health importance they merit their own chapters – Chapters 18 and 19 respectively.

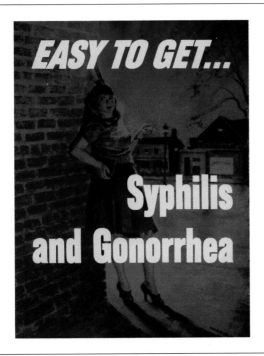

Figure 11.1 Public health poster warning against "Venereal Disease". Charles Casa, 1940

Box 11.1

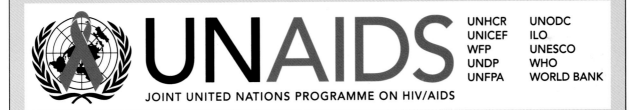

How do men make a difference, let us count the ways. Drawing on UN studies across geographic and cultural boundaries we know that:

- The sex partners of men outnumber those of women, making men more common vectors of transmission.

- Men more often than women determine whether safe sex is practised.
- Men, especially under the influence of alcohol, are more likely to use violence to coerce women into having sex.
- Men are less likely than women to be health conscious.

Sexually transmitted diseases

By virtue of their name, sexually transmitted infections are transmitted by sexual contact and their rise is a reflection of cultural changes in sexual behavior, particularly the increasing likelihood of multiple sexual partners. The main risk factors for acquiring a sexually transmitted infection (STI) are young age, unmarried status, high numbers of reported sexual partners, concurrent sexual partners, and unprotected sexual intercourse. An additional factor in the spread of sexually transmitted diseases (STDs) is the often asymptomatic nature of the infection. The asymptomatic nature of early HIV infection is well known, but other infections may also go unnoticed. Chlamydial infection is asymptomatic in approximately 70% of women and up to 50% of men. Gonococcal infection is asymptomatic in up to 50% of women. This contributes to the silent transmission of infections between sexually active people. While many STDs are easily treatable, some bring with them irreversible sequelae. The most serious of these sequelae affect women. Chlamydial infection in women can lead to pelvic inflammatory disease and tubal scarring causing infertility or the risk of ectopic pregnancy. Untreated syphilis infection, although rare, can cause progressively destructive lesions of the cardiovascular and central nervous systems. There is also evidence that the presence of a STI increases the chance of contracting HIV infection.

Lactobacilli predominate in the healthy vagina where they are able to metabolize glycogen to lactic acid. The resultant acid pH of the adult vagina is protective against many infectious microorganisms. Organisms that cause STIs do not survive well outside the body. For transmission to occur there must be direct contact between mucosal surfaces in order to transfer the organisms unharmed. Indirect contact between mucosal surfaces via the fingers can very occasionally transfer viable organisms.

The public health impact of sexually transmitted diseases

Sexually transmitted diseases remain a major public health challenge in the USA. Despite tremendous advances and economic investment in the prevention, diagnosis and management of STDs, the CDC estimates that 19 million new infections occur each year, almost half of them among young people from 15 to 24 years old. The three notifiable STDs in the USA are chlamydia, gonorrhea, and syphilis. They represent only a small proportion of the true national burden of STDs. Many cases of notifiable STDs go undiagnosed, and some highly prevalent viral infections, such as human papillomavirus and genital herpes, are not reported at all.

Chlamydia remains the most commonly reported infectious disease in the USA. In 2004, 929 462 chlamydia diagnoses were reported to the CDC, up from 877 478 in 2003. Even so, most chlamydia cases go undiagnosed. It is estimated that there are approximately 2.8 million new cases of chlamydia in the USA each year. The national rate of reported chlamydia in 2004 was 319.6 cases per 100 000 population, an increase of 5.9% from 2003. The increases in reported cases and rates likely reflect the continued expansion of screening efforts and increased use of more sensitive diagnostic tests, rather than an actual increase in new infections. CDC data shows that young women are the most likely to acquire chlamydia (Figure 11.2).

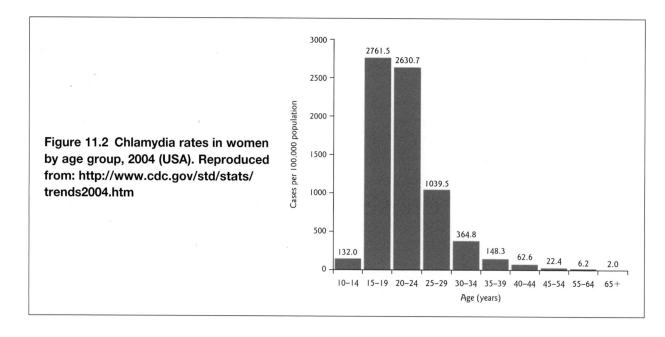

Figure 11.2 Chlamydia rates in women by age group, 2004 (USA). Reproduced from: http://www.cdc.gov/std/stats/trends2004.htm

The chlamydia case rate per 100 000 population for females in 2004 was 3.3 times higher than for males (485.0 vs. 147.1). However, much of this difference reflects the fact that women are far more likely to be screened than men. Females ages 15–19 years had the highest chlamydia rate (2761.5), followed by females ages 20–24 years (2630.7). African-American women have disproportionately higher rates of chlamydia. In 2004, the rate of reported chlamydia among black females (1722.3) was more than 7.5 times that of white females (226.6). All rates are per 100 000 population.

Lymphogranuloma venereum (LGV), an infection caused by certain types of chlamydia (see below), is prevalent in parts of Africa, Asia, and South America but has been rare in Western Europe for many years. Since 2003 there have been a series of outbreaks of LGV in European cities among men who have sex with men (MSM). All current European outbreaks are of the L2 genotype. Most cases have been in white HIV-positive males, reporting multiple sexual contacts and associated with high levels of concurrent sexually transmitted infections such as gonorrhea and syphilis. It does not appear to have spread outside this specific population. In 2004, 27 cases of LGV were reported to the CDC. Studies are underway to identify LGV throughout the USA through genotypic confirmation

From CDC surveillance data it is evident that **gonorrhea** is the second most commonly reported infectious disease in the USA, with 330 132 cases reported in 2004. African-Americans remain the group most heavily affected by gonorrhea. The reported 2004 rate per 100 000 population for blacks (629.6) was 19 times greater than for whites (33.3). American Indians/Alaska natives had the second highest gonorrhea rate in 2004 (117.7, up 14.8% from 2003), followed by Hispanics (71.3, up 2.3% from 2003), whites (33.3, up 2.1% from 2003), and Asians/Pacific Islanders (21.4, down 3.2% from 2003). Ethnic minorities in the USA have higher rates of reported gonorrhea and other STDs, this is, in part, a reflection of poor access to quality healthcare and a higher background prevalence of disease in these populations.

Syphilis cases in the USA decreased throughout the 1990s, and in 2000 they reached an all-time low. However, between 2003 and 2004 alone, the national syphilis rate increased 8%, and the total numbers of reported cases in the USA increased from 7177 to 7980. Overall, increases in syphilis rates between 2000 and 2004 were observed only among men (2.7/100 000 population in 2004); the rate among females did not decrease, remaining at 0.8. More detailed investigation by the CDC showed that syphilis in the group MSM was responsible for the overall increases in the national syphilis rate observed since 2000. Additionally, CDC estimates that MSM comprised 64% of syphilis cases in 2004, up from 5% in 1999. Syphilis remains a public health problem in metropolitan areas with large populations of MSM. For the third consecutive year, San Francisco had the highest rate of any US city in 2004 (45.9/100 000).

Feel free to talk: the first step to diagnosing an STD

People with STDs are often asymptomatic or may not recognize symptoms that are present. Many may be too ashamed or afraid to confront the reality that they have acquired an STD. While sexual health clinics are well equipped to manage these patients, they are often seen by health services such as family practice, obstetrics and gynaecology or urology clinics where the presence of an STI may not be considered. A thorough sexual history is essential in order to make an informed risk assessment and gauge the likelihood of infection being present (Box 11.2). Important information includes symptoms, details of last sexual

---

Box 11.2 Golden rules for taking a sexual history (reproduced with permission from the Department of Genito-urinary Medicine, University College London)

- Assume **NOTHING**
- Demonstrate that you've heard it all before

- **Try not to** look shocked or surprised if you haven't!
- Do not appear judgmental

contact, details of previous partners (number of partners, casual versus long-term and partners' symptoms), the use of barrier contraception (condom or diaphragm), the nature of the sexual contact (oral, vaginal, anal), previous STI history, and other high-risk behavior such as drug taking or heavy alcohol use. The presenting symptoms and the nature of the sexual contact will guide examination and diagnostic sampling, for instance, the need for throat or rectal swabs in addition to routine genital specimens.

A person harboring one STI is at increased risk of being coinfected with a second or even third STI and, therefore, a full sexual screen is advisable for any patient at risk of having a STI. Laboratory processing of clinical swabs will detect most common pathogens, but serology testing on a venous blood sample is usually necessary to confirm the presence of syphilis, HIV, and hepatitis B infection.

Once a patient has been assessed and initial investigations performed, treatment needs to be given promptly to reduce the risk of complications and to minimize further transmission of the infection. A syndromic approach is normally taken: treatment is determined by the symptoms and initial microscopy findings and not delayed until full laboratory results are available.

The patient is advised to avoid sexual contact until treatment and partner tracing are completed. This will prevent further transmission to others and also prevent reinfection from an untreated, infected partner. Tracing of current and recent partners is a crucial part of management in order to break the chain of transmission, to detect asymptomatic cases, and to promote safer sexual practice. However, patient and contact confidentiality should not be breached.

The patient should be reviewed after treatment to ensure that symptoms have resolved and that contact tracing of partners has been completed. A "test of cure," repeat testing to confirm clearance, is advised for some infections.

Clinical presentation of sexually transmitted diseases

STDs can present with a number of different clinical symptoms and signs. The main presenting features are:

- Urethritis
- Cervicitis (and pelvic inflammatory disease)
- Vulvovaginitis
- Genital lesions:
  - Genital herpes
  - Genital warts
  - Syphilis
  - Lymphogranuloma venereum
  - Chancroid
  - Donovanosis (granuloma inguinale)
- Genital infestations
  - Pubic lice
  - Scabies.

Urethritis

Urethritis, or inflammation of the urethra, is the most common presentation in men attending sexual health clinics in the USA. It is characterized by a discharge and/or dysuria (pain when passing urine), and/or urethral pruritis (itching), but it can be asymptomatic. The discharge may only become apparent after "milking" or massaging the urethra on examination.

Complications include ascending infection causing epididymo-orchitis and prostatitis.

Up to 4% of cases of urethritis progress to sexually acquired reactive arthritis (SARA) or Reiter's syndrome, an immune-mediated arthritis, conjunctivitis, and mucocutaneous lesions in association with urethritis. *Chlamydia trachomatis* is the organism most commonly associated with the syndrome.

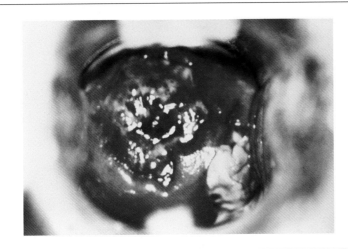

Figure 11.3 Cervicitis – erosive inflammation of the uterine cervix. Image donated by Dr G.L. Ridgway

The most common causes of urethritis in general, are *C. trachomatis* and *Neisseria gonorrheae*: gonococcal urethritis accounts for 20–30% of all urethritis cases. Nongonococcal urethritis (NGU) is caused by *C. trachomatis* in 30–50% of cases, and *Ureaplasma urealyticum* or *Mycoplasma genitalium* in 10–20% of cases. Other causes include *Trichomonas vaginalis*, *Candida* species, herpes simplex virus, urinary tract infection; Group A streptococcus, presence of a foreign body, and allergic reaction. In 20–30% of cases no organism is detected.

Cervicitis and pelvic inflammatory disease

Cervicitis is inflammation of the uterine cervix (Figure 11.3). The condition is often asymptomatic (particularly chlamydial cervicitis) but presenting symptoms can include mucopurulent discharge, intermenstrual bleeding, dyspareunia (pain during intercourse), and dysuria.

Pelvic inflammatory disease (PID) is the clinical syndrome that results when infection ascends from the cervix to infect the endometrium, fallopian tubes, and contiguous pelvic structures causing: endometritis, salpingitis, tubo-ovarian abscess, or perihepatitis (Fitz–Hugh–Curtis syndrome). Symptoms of PID include lower abdominal pain and signs of systemic infection such as fever and rigors.

Progressive inflammation leads to scarring and blockage of the fallopian tubes and uterus resulting in infertility, the risk of ectopic pregnancy, and chronic pelvic pain. Thirteen percent of women will become infertile following a single episode of PID; this increases to 25–30% after a second episode and 50–75% after three or more episodes of PID.

It is thought that much PID is asymptomatic: 60% of patients with evidence of old PID on laparoscopy do not recall any symptoms yet have enough scarring to cause infertility. This highlights the importance of screening asymptomatic women.

By far the most common causes of cervicitis and PID are *Chlamydia trachomatis* and *Neisseria gonorrheae*, which preferentially infect the columnar epithelium of the cervix and ascend upwards into the endometrium, rather than infecting the squamous epithelium of the vagina.

Vulvovaginitis

The adult vaginal epithelium is inhabited largely by lactobacilli (>10^5/ml of vaginal material), which maintain the normal vaginal pH between 3.8 and 4.4 and may play a role in defence against infection. A number of other organisms may inhabit the vagina in small numbers: *Gardnerella vaginalis* is carried in 30–90%, *Candida* species are carried by 15–20%, and even *Staphylococcus aureus* is carried by up to 5%.

The prepubescent vaginal epithelium is inhabited mainly by anaerobes, particularly *Bacteroides* species.

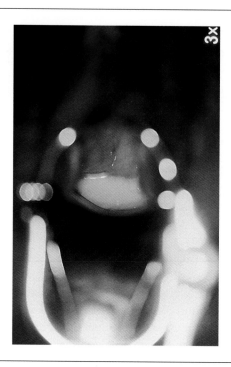

Figure 11.4 Vulvovaginitis. Image donated by Dr G.L. Ridgway

Some degree of vaginal discharge is normal, the quality and quantity being influenced by hormonal changes, pregnancy, and age. What is normal discharge for one patient may be deemed excessive by another patient and, generally, the individual patient is the best judge of what is normal or abnormal for her.

Vulvovaginitis (Figure 11.4) is characterized by a combination of increased vaginal discharge, irritation, erythema, dysuria, odor, and lower vaginal tenderness. The causes of adult vulvovaginitis include *Candida* species, bacterial vaginosis, *Trichomonas vaginalis*, *Neisseria gonorrheae*, and *Chlamydia trachomatis*. Men carry *T. vaginalis* asymptomatically; however they need to be treated if the female partner has been diagnosed with it.

Candida albicans is the organism present in the majority of cases of vulvovaginal candidiasis. Episodes may be associated with pregnancy and after treatment with broad-spectrum antibiotics. The patient complains of a white curdy discharge – like "cottage cheese" with vulvar redness and itching. *Candida* is not transmitted sexually and is included here to complete the spectrum of organism implicated in vulvovaginitis.

Bacterial vaginosis (BV) is a specific condition characterized by a thin grayish discharge with a "fishy" odor; BV is occasionally accompanied by inflammation, irritation, and dysuria. The cause of BV is thought to be

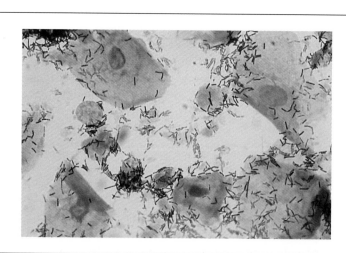

Figure 11.5 Normal vaginal flora. Note the preponderance of Gram positive lactobacilli. Image donated by Dr G.L. Ridgway

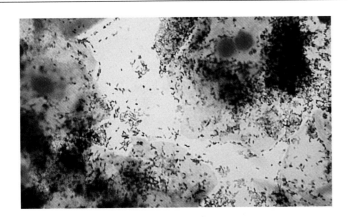

Figure 11.6 Presence of clue cells in bacterial vaginosis. Note vaginal epithelial cells studded with tiny coccobacilli. Image donated by Dr G.L. Ridgway

polymicrobial overgrowth and an ecologic shift in the flora of the vagina. Figure 11.5 is a Gram stain of normal vaginal flora showing a preponderance of Gram positive lactobacilli. In BV almost no lactobacilli are seen on smear examination. A number of organisms have been implicated in BV: *Gardnerella vaginalis* is associated with >90% of BV cases, but can also be present in up to 70% of asymptomatic women. *Mobiluncus* species is also associated with >95% of cases, but in only 6% of asymptomatic controls. Although both organisms can be found in the partners of BV cases, they are not usually regarded as sexually transmitted infections, more as an overgrowth of anaerobic bacteria due to disruption of the normal vaginal flora by environmental factors such as perfumed bubble bath, washing powder, new sexual partner, condoms, and vaginal douching. Culture for BV organisms is not routinely performed; instead Amsel's diagnostic criteria are used – three out of four of the criteria must be present to diagnose BV.

Amsel's diagnostic criteria:

1 Homogeneous gray discharge.
2 Vaginal pH >4.5 (present in 90% of BV cases).
3 Addition of 10% potassium hydroxide solution to the discharge intensifies the fishy odor – the "whiff test" (present in 70% of cases).
4 The wet preparation reveals "clue cells" (Figure 11.6) – vaginal epithelial cells studded with tiny coccobacilli (present in 90% of cases).

Although generally benign, there is an association between BV during pregnancy and premature rupture of membranes and premature labor (*G. vaginalis* possesses phospholipase A_2 activity which initiates labor).

Genital lesions

The causes of the most common genital lesions is shown in Table 11.1.

General features

The most common causes of genital lesions seen in the USA are human herpes simplex virus (HSV), papillomavirus (HPV), and syphilis. It is important to determine whether there are multiple lesions, how long the lesion has been present, whether it is painful or painless, and whether the condition has occurred before.

HSV and syphilis are the most common causes of genital ulcer disease. HSV ulcers are usually multiple, invariably painful, and tend to recur in the same site. By contrast, the ulcer associated with primary syphilis, the syphilitic chancre, is solitary and painless. An accurate travel history is also important if lymphogranuloma venereum, chancroid, or donovanosis is suspected. It is important to remember that intravaginal and rectal lesions will not be visible and thorough examination is necessary.

Table 11.1 Causes of common genital lesions

Ulcers	Papules	Crusted
Herpes simplex virus (HSV)	Warts (HPV)	HSV
Syphilis	Molluscum contagiosum	Scabies
Chancroid	Syphilis	
Lymphogranuloma venereum (LGV)		**Miscellaneous**
Granuloma inguinale (donovanosis)	**Vesicles**	Linear tracks of scabies
Candidiasis	HSV	Crab louse excreta and eggs
Gonorrhea	Scabies	
Trichomonas		

Genital herpes

Genital herpes is caused by herpes simplex virus (HSV). HSV has two types: HSV1 and HSV2. Transmission occurs when virus from actively shedding lesions comes into contact with the mucous membranes of a nonimmune partner. While both types can cause both oro-facial and genital lesions, HSV2 is the main cause of genital lesions and HSV1 is the main cause of oro-facial lesions. Like all herpesviruses, HSV exhibits latency and remains in the body for life. After primary infection, HSV remains latent in the local sensory ganglia with the potential to reactivate causing recurrent episodes of infection.

Primary genital infection (when a patient has acquired the infection for the first time) usually presents with a crop of painful vesicles, which develop into ulcers and eventually crust and heal (Figure 11.7a and b). Other local symptoms include pain on dysuria, discharge, and lymphadenopathy. Twenty percent of cases have symptoms and recognizable lesions on the external genitalia, 60% have symptoms but no visible lesions (often cervical, urethral or anal lesions), and 20% are asymptomatic. The viremia that accompanies the primary infection can cause systemic symptoms such as fever, headache, malaise, and myalgias. Complications

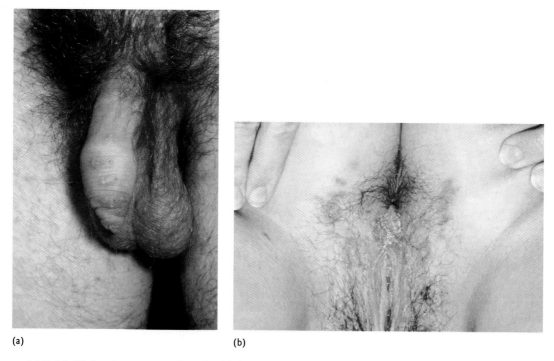

(a)   (b)

Figure 11.7 Multiple ulcers associated with herpes simplex virus. (a) Penile lesions. (b) Perineal lesions

include viral meningitis, hepatitis, and pneumonitis, and an association with high mortality in immunosuppressed and pregnant cases.

HSV2 genital infection is associated with a 90% recurrence rate within the first year following primary infection. HSV1 genital infection has a 55% recurrence rate. Recurrence is localized to a defined site, usually the site of initial inoculation. The lesions are smaller, symptoms are milder, and duration shorter. There is usually a gradual decrease in recurrence rates over time, but some patients are plagued by regular, painful recurrences.

Herpes infection in pregnancy has a risk of severe, disseminated infection and transplacental spread leading to spontaneous abortion. Women with primary lesions during vaginal delivery are at greater risk of transmitting HSV to the neonate as compared to those with recurrent lesions. This is because maternal antibody will not have had time to develop or cross the placenta. Women with recurrent herpes have a much lower risk (<5%) of transmitting infection to the neonate. Severe disseminated herpes in the neonate manifests with jaundice, hepatosplenomegaly (enlarged liver and spleen), thrombocytopenia (low platelets), a widespread vesicular rash, and a high mortality.

Genital warts

Genital warts (condylomata acuminata) are caused by human papillomavirus (HPV). HPV has numerous different types, all of which cause warts; certain types are associated with a particular type of wart or region of the body. Types 6 and 11 most commonly cause genital warts. Warts are generally benign tumors of the skin with virus-induced proliferation of both keratinized (skin) and nonkeratinized (mucous membranes) squamous epithelium (Figure 11.8). Like the herpesviruses, HPV can remain latent within tissues and recurrent episodes can be seen. Besides the unsightly nature of warts, complications are rare. There is, however, an association between some genital HPV types and the development of cervical cancer. Approximately 93% of cervical cancers contain HPV DNA, usually of types 16 and 18, but a number of other types, including 31, 33, 35 and 45, are also implicated.

In June 2006, the first vaccine developed to prevent cervical cancer and other diseases in females caused by certain types of HPV was licensed. The vaccine protects against four HPV types (6, 11, 16, 18), which are responsible for 70% of cervical cancers and 90% of genital warts. It is recommended for use in females

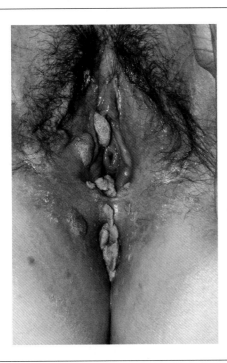

Figure 11.8 Human papillomavirus causing vulvo-vaginal warts

aged 9–26 years. However, this vaccine will not replace other prevention strategies since it will not work for all genital HPV types. Ideally, the vaccine should be administered before onset of sexual activity. However, females who are sexually active may also benefit. Females who have already been infected with one or more HPV type would still get protection from the vaccine types they have not acquired. Few young women are infected with all four HPV types in the vaccine. Currently, there is no test available for clinical use to determine whether a female has had any or all of the four HPV types in the vaccine.

Syphilis

One of the important clinical conditions to consider when a patient presents with a genital lesion is the complex and often systemic disease called syphilis. The panoply of clinical disease associated with syphilis will therefore be discussed here.

Treponema pallidum, the organism that causes syphilis can be acquired by sexual contact, *in utero* transplacental transmission, or contaminated blood transfusion. Syphilis is a chronic infection with distinct clinical stages separated by periods of latency during which the patient is entirely asymptomatic, making detection of cases more difficult. The patient is most infectious in the early stages of the disease (primary and secondary stages), gradually becoming less infectious so that transmission of infection is unlikely beyond 4 years post-acquisition.

The widespread dissemination of *T. pallidum* throughout the body leads to numerous clinical manifestations, which have earned syphilis its name as "the great imitator."

Clinically, syphilis is divided into the following stages: incubation, primary, secondary, latent, and late. Intrauterine transmission leads to congenital syphilis.

Incubation stage

T. pallidum penetrates intact mucous membranes or abraded skin to enter the lymphatics and bloodstream to disseminate throughout the body. A very low dose is sufficient to cause infection but clinical lesions will not appear until a concentration of 10^7 organisms/g of tissue is reached, hence the incubation period will depend on the inoculating dose. The median incubation period is 3 weeks, but can vary from 3–90 days.

Primary syphilis

A chancre forms at the site of inoculation. Classically, the chancre is a solitary, painless, clean ulcer with raised, firm edges, a smooth base, and no exudates (Figure 11.9). The ulcer carries a high number of spirochaetes and is highly infectious. Atypical lesions can occur in up to 60%, and can often go unnoticed. Local lymph nodes are enlarged and accompany the primary lesion. The chancre will heal in 1–12 weeks but the enlarged lymph nodes (lymphadenopathy) remain for longer.

Secondary syphilis

This stage begins 2–8 weeks after appearance of the primary chancre and reflects the uncontrolled multiplication and dissemination of spirochaetes throughout the body until a sufficient host response develops. Manifestations are numerous with any region of the body affected.

The most common manifestation is a widespread rash, which can affect the whole body including the palms and soles. The rash can be macular, maculopapular, or pustular (Figure 11.10a and b). In moist areas the papules enlarge, coalesce, and erode to produce large painless and highly infectious plaques termed condyloma lata, or mucous patches when occurring on mucous membranes (Figure 11.11). Systemic symptoms such as fever, malaise, pharyngitis, weight loss, arthralgias, and lymphadenopathy commonly accompany the rash. Other manifestations are listed in Table 11.2.

Latent syphilis

The patient is asymptomatic during this stage. Latent syphilis can be divided into "early" latent syphilis – the first 4 years after infection during which time relapse is possible and the patient remains infectious – and "late" latent syphilis where relapse and transmission become less likely.

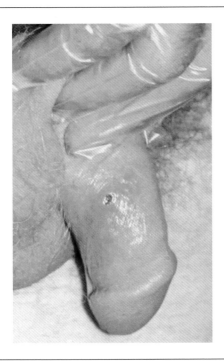

Figure 11.9 Syphilitic primary chancre on the shaft of the penis

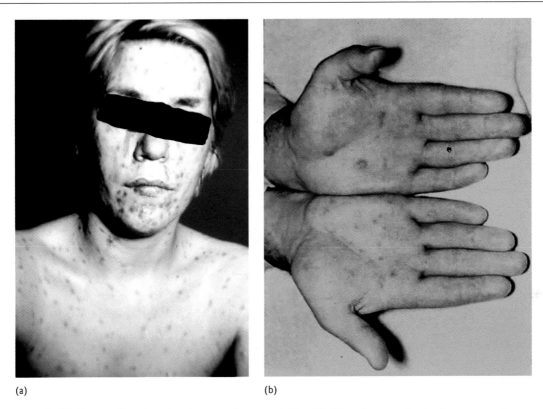

(a) (b)

Figure 11.10 (a) Generalized rash of secondary syphilis. (b) Maculo-papular lesions on palms

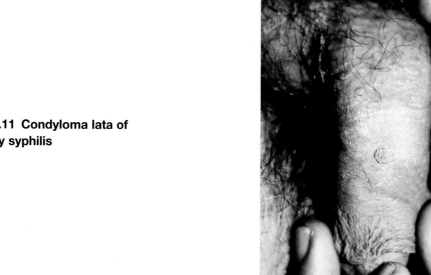

Figure 11.11 Condyloma lata of secondary syphilis

Table 11.2 The many manifestations of secondary syphilis

Central nervous system (involved in 40% of cases)	Headache Meningitis Cranial nerve involvement Visual disturbance Hearing loss Tinnitus (CSF protein and lymphocyte count are raised in 8–40%)
Ocular (involved in 5–10% of cases)	Anterior uveitis
Liver	Hepatitis
Renal	Glomerulonephritis Nephritic syndrome
Gastrointestinal	Ulceration of the GI tract
Musculoskeletal	Arthritis Synovitis Osteitis Periosteitis

Late syphilis

There is gradual, progressive inflammation of the inner (intima) layer of small blood vessels leading to endarteritis obliterans (narrowing of the lumen of the blood vessel). This can affect any organ in the body, most classically the nervous, cardiovascular and musculoskeletal systems:

- **Cardiovascular syphilis:** endarteritis obliterans of the ascending aorta and the coronary arteries are most commonly seen, giving rise to aneurysms, aortic regurgitation, and coronary artery stenosis. Symptoms

Table 11.3 Manifestations of neurosyphilis

Meningovascular syphilis (endarteritis obliterans of meninges, brain, and spinal cord)	Basal meningitis, headache, seizures, stroke, cervical myelopathy, cranial nerve lesions	5–10 years post-acquisition
Parenchymatous syphilis (atrophy of nerve cells)	General paresis (cerebral atrophy): dementia, seizures, tremors	15–20 years post-acquisition
	Tabes dorsalis (posterior spinal column atrophy): autonomic neuropathy, ataxia, sensory loss, lightning pains, sphincter disturbance, cranial nerve lesions, Argyll–Robertson pupils	25–30 years post-acquisition

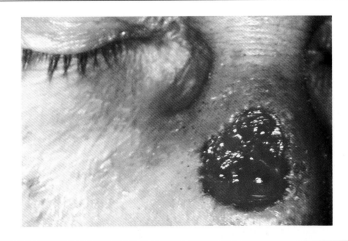

Figure 11.12 Gumma of the nose – a lesion in late syphilis. Provided by J. Pledger. Courtesy of the Centers for Disease Control and Prevention; from CDC website: http://phil.cdc.gov/phil/details.asp

develop in 10% of untreated cases, although >80% of untreated cases have evidence of cardiovascular syphilis on post-mortem.

- **Neurosyphilis:** used to be known as general paralysis of the insane, occurs in 6–8% of untreated cases. The numerous manifestations are shown in Table 11.3.
- **Gummatous syphilis:** occurs in 15% of untreated cases. Large, granulomatous lesions ("gummata") develop, mainly in the skin, mucous membranes, and skeletal system, although viscera can also be involved (Figure 11.12). The lesions are locally destructive leading to soft-tissue deformity, fractures, and organ failure (e.g. liver cirrhosis).
- **Congenital syphilis:** screening for syphilis is part of the routine antenatal screening program and congenital syphilis is now a rare event where antenatal care is provided. Transmission *in utero* can occur with any stage of untreated infection, but is more likely in early infection. Transmission across the placenta is rare before 4 months' gestation. The consequences depend on the severity of the infection, ranging from late miscarriage, stillbirth and neonatal death to neonatal disease or latent infection.

In a child born with neonatal disease, there are often no abnormal findings at birth. The earliest signs are rhinitis (syphilitic snuffles) and a diffuse, maculopapular rash. Visceral organ infection causes significant morbidity and mortality with liver failure, pneumonia, and pulmonary haemorrhage being the major killers. In surviving children, bone infection affects musculoskeletal development causing the classical syphilitic facies (saddle nose and frontal bossing, Figure 11.13) and sabre shins (Figure 11.14). After 6–12 months, the untreated child enters the latent phase. Between the ages of 5 and 30 years neurosyphilis and interstitial keratitis (inflammation of the cornea, Figure 11.15) can occur. Cardiovascular syphilis is rarely seen.

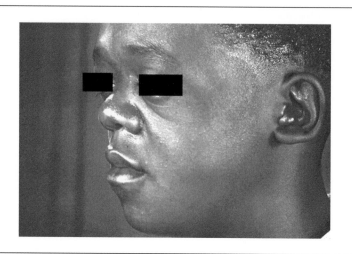

Figure 11.13 Saddle nose deformity of congenital syphilis. Courtesy of the Centers for Disease Control and Prevention; from CDC website: http://phil.cdc.gov/phil/details.asp

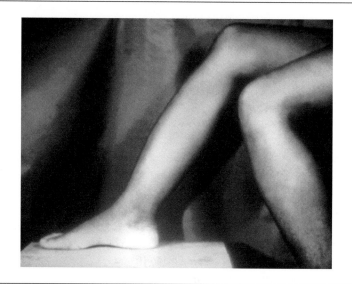

Figure 11.14 Sabre shins in congenital syphilis. Provided by Susan Lindsley. Courtesy of the Centers for Disease Control and Prevention; from CDC website: http://phil.cdc.gov/phil/details.asp

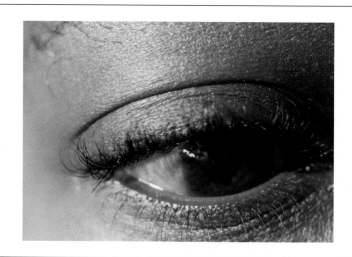

Figure 11.15 Keratitis associated with congenital syphilis. Provided by Susan Lindsley. Courtesy of the Centers for Disease Control and Prevention; from CDC website: http://phil.cdc.gov/phil/details.asp

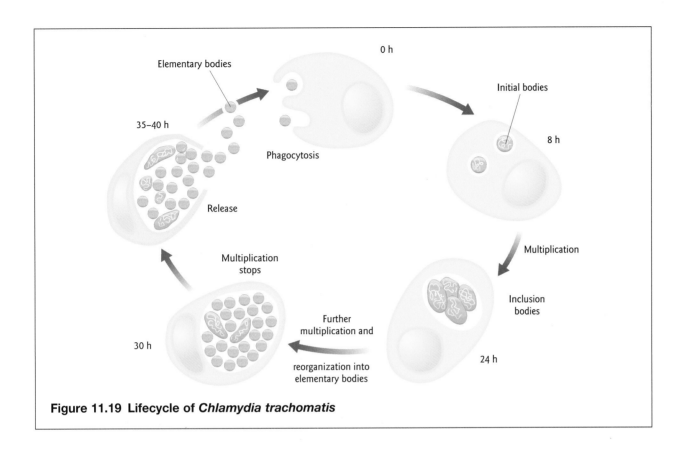

Figure 11.19 Lifecycle of *Chlamydia trachomatis*

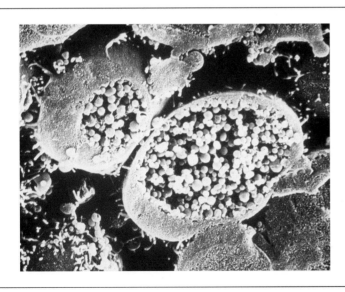

Figure 11.20 Chlamydia: inclusions containing numerous elementary bodies. www.chlamydiae.com

Virulence mechanisms

The pathogenesis of chlamydial infection is only partially understood. LGV strains gain entrance through breaks in the skin or infect squamous epithelial cells of the mucous membranes of the genital tract or rectum. They are carried by lymphatic drainage to the regional lymph nodes where they multiply within mononuclear phagocytes. Histologically, there is granuloma formation with abscess development that may become necrotic or coalesce into large focal abscesses.

Genital strains infect the squamo-columnar epithelial cells of the endocervix in women and the conjunctiva, urethra, and rectum in men and women. The initial response to infection is primarily a polymorph response. Lipopolysaccharide is thought to be the predominant antigen responsible for inducing proinflammatory cytokines. The polymorph response is later replaced by lymphocytes, macrophages, plasma cells, and eosinophils, and lymphoid follicles form as the acute inflammatory response subsides. There is thinning of the overlying epithelium and cells may become necrotic as disease progresses. As infection resolves, fibrosis and scarring occur. Initial infection is thought to leave little residual damage but recurrent infection produces a rapid and intense response with inevitable tissue damage and scarring.

Cell culture sensitivity varies between 70% and 90% depending on the expertise of the laboratory.

Neisseria gonorrheae

Microbiology

Neisseria gonorrheae (the gonococcus) is a small, nonmotile Gram negative diplococcus (Figure 11.21). The organism has fastidious growth requirements and is cultured in the laboratory using enriched media. Rapid nucleic acid amplification tests are also available.

Virulence mechanisms

Attachment to mucosal epithelium is followed by penetration between and through epithelial cells to the submucosal tissues. The acute neutrophil response leads to breakdown and sloughing of the epithelium, submucosal micro-abscesses, and formation of pus.

Neisseria gonorrheae has a number of virulence factors that aid its role as an intracellular pathogen. The organism is able to turn on and off the expression of some of these factors, allowing it to switch between a low virulence infector of mucous membranes to a highly pathogenic organism capable of disseminated infection when conditions are right.

Pili aid attachment to mucosal surfaces, entry into mucosal epithelial cells, and resistance to killing by neutrophils. The most remarkable feature of *N. gonorrheae* is its ability to evade the host's immune system through variation of its surface antigens, primarily the pili proteins. *N. gonorrheae* has a repertoire of up to 1 million antigenic variations of its surface (pili) proteins. Recombination between different variants of the same gene is the most common mechanism of antigenic variation. Similarly, phase shifting can occur in which repeated sequences in the pili genes are added or cleaved, changing the likelihood that the gene will be expressed. Both mechanisms add variation into the local bacterial population on the order of 1/100 to 1/10 000. This small amount of variation sufficiently ensures that, as the host mounts an antibody response to the original pili protein, a new variation will go undetected and become the dominant form in the population.

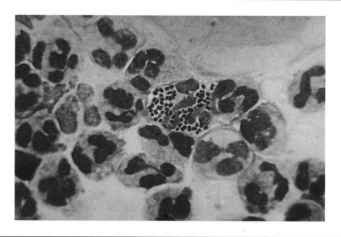

Figure 11.21 Urethral discharge showing numerous polymorphs and Gram negative diplococci typical of *Neisseria gonorrheae*. Gram stain (1000×)

Outer membrane porin proteins (PorA and PorB) promote invasion of epithelial cells, and strains carrying certain porins (PorA) are more likely to cause bloodstream infection.

A range of other proteins like the membrane proteins (Opa) increase adherence between gonococci and to a variety of eukaryotic cells, another reduces the bactericidal effect of serum by stimulating the production of blocking antibodies, while other outer membrane proteins have iron-scavenging roles. The organism can also produce IgA protease that cleaves locally formed antibody. Cell wall constituents, lipopolysaccharide (LPS) and peptidoglycan stimulate the inflammatory response.

Traditionally, gonorrhea has been treated with penicillin-based antibiotics but as resistance to penicillin increased, tetracycline and then ciprofloxacin became the treatment of choice. This has been followed by a rapid increase in both tetracycline and ciprofloxacin resistance. *N. gonorrheae* is an excellent example of an organism which can adapt rapidly to an antibiotic environment.

The organism has three mechanisms conferring resistance to penicillins:

1 Destruction of the antibiotic: β-lactamase-producing strains are now commonplace and confer high level resistance to penicillin that cannot be overcome by high dose penicillin.
2 Mutation of the antibiotic target: chromosomal mutation (PenA) alters the penicillin binding protein PBP2 to gradually reduce its affinity for penicillin.
3 Efflux of the antibiotic: The *mtr* determinant is a chromosomal mutation encoding an efflux pump for penicillin.

The organism can also carry chromosomal mutations conferring resistance to ciprofloxacin and a plasmid containing the tetM determinant that confers resistance to tetracycline.

Trichomonas vaginalis

Microbiology

Trichomonas vaginalis is a flagellated protozoan and is a common parasite in both men and women (see Chapter 1). Transmission is usually sexual although there have been instances where the parasite has been transmitted via fomites such as towels and bathing suits. Microscopy of a fresh wet preparation of discharge will show motile flagellated protozoa. Acridine orange and Giemsa stain (Figure 11.22) can also be used to highlight the protozoa on microscopy.

Virulence mechanisms

T. vaginalis infection is superficial and penetration through the vaginal or urethral epithelium is not seen. Specific virulence factors and the immune response are poorly understood. Low level inflammation and microulceration of the genital epithelium, with neutrophil infiltration, is thought to be stimulated by direct contact with protozoal surface proteins.

Candida albicans

Microbiology

Candida species are yeast-like fungi that can form true hyphae (strands) and pseudohyphae. The pseudohyphae are so called because they can give rise to yeast cells by apical or lateral budding. They stain Gram positive on Gram stain (Figure 11.22b).

Virulence mechanisms

Virulence factors of the *Candida* species have not been well characterized. The main contenders are surface molecules that permit adherence of the organism to a variety of surfaces: e.g. human epithelial cells, extracellular matrix, and prosthetic devices; acid proteases and the ability to convert to an invasive hyphal

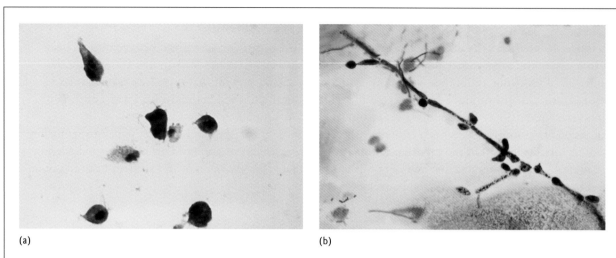

(a)   (b)

Figure 11.22 (a) *Trichomonas vaginalis.* **Giemsa stain. Courtesy of the Centers for Disease Control and Prevention; from CDC website: http://phil.cdc.gov/phil/details.asp. (b) Gram stain of** *Candida albicans* **showing pseudo hyphae and budding cells. Provided by Dr Stuart Brown. Courtesy of the Centers for Disease Control and Prevention; from CDC website: http://phil.cdc.gov/phil/details.asp**

form. As with most fungal infections, host defects also play a significant role in the development of candidal infections. Immunosuppressed patients are at greater risk of developing candidal infections.

Treponema pallidum

Microbiology
Spirochaetes do not stain with Gram stain, so darkfield or immunofluorescent microscopy must be used. On microscopy, spirochaetes are seen as slender, corkscrew-shaped rods (Figure 11.23). They have several flagella, attached at either end of the cell, that wrap around the cell body. This gives the organism its characteristic spiral shape and wave-like motility.

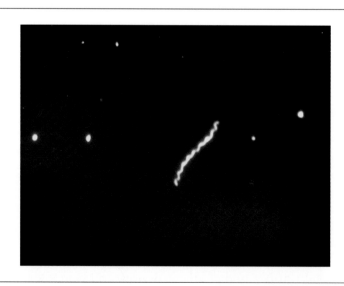

Figure 11.23 Photomicrograph of a *Treponema pallidum* **bacterium using darkfield microscopy (400×). Provided by Schwartz. Courtesy of the Centers for Disease Control and Prevention; from CDC website: http://phil.cdc.gov/phil/details.asp**

Virulence mechanisms

The virulence factors of *T. pallidum* are unknown. The organism has an outer membrane that is rich in lipid but contains relatively little protein and it has been suggested that the immune system does not initially recognize *T. pallidum*, and so it manages to go unnoticed until it has multiplied to a level that finally stimulates the host response. By this time, *T. pallidum* has spread throughout the body and the host response is never strong enough to eradicate the organism completely. A chronic process is set up, whereby a delicate balance between immune system and organism is achieved and maintained unless the immune system is damaged in some way that allows *T. pallidum* to gain control.

The primary chancre is a direct result of the host's cellular response to the increasing numbers of spirochaetes at the entry site. Histologically, polymorphs and macrophages can be seen ingesting treponemes and there is infiltration of plasma cells and histiocytes. Concentric endothelial and fibroblastic proliferative thickening of the small blood vessels leading to narrowing of the arteries (endarteritis obliterans) is seen.

Secondary syphilis occurs when there are the greatest numbers of organisms throughout the body and the battle between the cellular immune system and infection is at its most intense. Immune complexes containing *T. pallidum*, immunoglobulin, and complement can be found in those who develop glomerulonephritis and evidence of endarteritis obliterans is widespread.

Latency occurs when balance is achieved. The majority of cases will remain in the latent stage and will not progress to late disease unless the immune system is impaired and endarteritis obliterans allowed to progress unchecked.

The release of microbial components from dying treponemes, as a result of treatment, can cause the Jarisch–Herxheimer reaction: the abrupt onset of fever, flu-like symptoms, hyperventilation, and vasodilatation following the first treatment injection. The reaction is usually self-limiting. Although, the reaction is most commonly seen during treatment of secondary syphilis, it can occur at any stage of disease.

Herpes simplex virus (HSV)

HSV is an enveloped virus that is visible by electron microscopy (Figure 11.24). It can also be cultured on a suitable cell line and detected by nucleic acid amplification tests.

The pathogenesis of HSV is related to its ability to replicate in the basal and intermediate layers of the epithelium of skin and mucous membrane leading to cell lysis and inflammation. HSV is able to escape the immune response and persists indefinitely in a latent state in certain tissues like the sensory nerve ganglia. Reactivation occurs via replication in the ganglion and peripheral spread through sensory

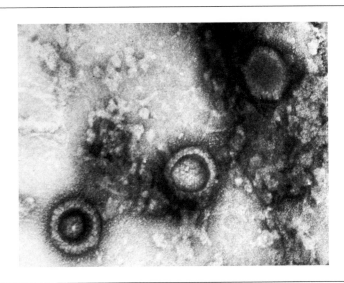

Figure 11.24 Electron photomicrograph of herpesvirus. Provided by Dr John Hierholzer. Courtesy of the Centers for Disease Control and Prevention; from CDC website: http://phil.cdc.gov/phil/details.asp

nerves. Triggers include sunlight, fever, local trauma, trigeminal nerve manipulation, menstruation, and emotional stress.

Human papillomavirus (HPV)

Papillomaviruses have icosahedral symmetry and are nonenveloped. It is believed that the HPV virus enters the body after slight trauma to the epithelium. The virus needs mature epithelial cells for replication.

One of the key events of HPV-induced carcinogenesis (transformation of a normal cell to a malignant cell) is the integration of the HPV genome into a host chromosome(Figure 11.25). Integration follows a more specific pattern with respect to the HPV genome. Expression of the viral E6 and E7 genes is consistently maintained, whereas other portions of the viral DNA are deleted or their expression is disturbed. Loss of expression of the HPV E2 transcriptional repressor is also significant, as it may result in deregulated HPV E6 and E7 expression. Cells that express E6/E7 from integrated HPV sequences have a selective growth advantage over cells with nonintegrated HPV genomes. Additional cofactors, such as cigarette smoking, may be required as a carcinogen to advance HPV-infected cells toward neoplastic (cancer) progression.

Haemophilus ducreyi

Microbiology

Haemophilus ducreyi is a Gram negative cocco-bacillus. Culture of the organism is difficult and requires enriched media.

Virulence mechanisms

H. ducreyi produces a potent cyto-lethal distending toxin. This toxin probably contributes to both the generation and the slow healing of ulcers. Chancroid facilitates HIV transmission. The two main co-receptors essential for HIV entry into a cell are CCR5 and CXCR4 (see Chapter 18). Macrophages in lesions of chancroid have significantly increased expression of CCR5 and CXCR4 compared with peripheral blood cells, and CD4 T cells have significant upregulation of CCR5. Together with the disruption of mucosal and

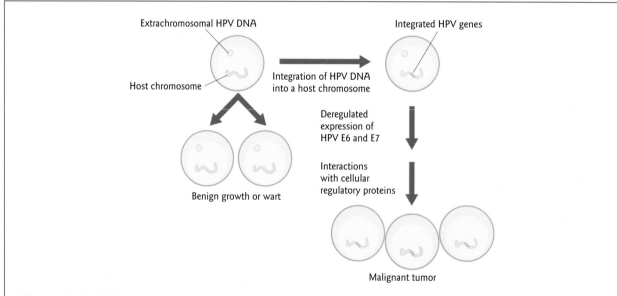

Figure 11.25 Malignant transformation of cells infected by HPV. From Beutner KR et al. Human papillomavirus and human disease. *American Journal of Medicine* **1997;102(5A):9–15**

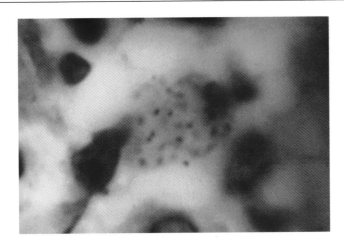

Figure 11.26 Donovan bodies or cellular inclusions of Gram negative rods confirming the diagnosis of Donovanosis. Provided by Susan Lindsley. Courtesy of the Centers for Disease Control and Prevention; from CDC website: http://phil.cdc.gov/phil/details.asp

skin barriers, the presence of cells with upregulated HIV-1 co-receptors in lesions infected with *H. ducreyi* provides an environment that facilitates the acquisition of HIV-1 infection.

Calymmatobacterium granulomatis

Microbiology
Calymmatobacterium granulomatis is a Gram negative bacillus. There are no culture techniques available for *C. granulomatis*. Diagnosis depends upon histological examination of biopsy material demonstrating characteristic "Donovan bodies," encapsulated Gram negative rods within macrophage vacuoles (Figure 11.26).

Virulence mechanisms
The organism appears to have a special tropism for dermal macrophages, in which it seems able to avoid damage by lysosomal enzymes and toxic oxygen metabolites. The response to infection is characterized by vigorous granulomatous inflammation that damages the skin and subcutaneous tissues. Extension of the infection is predominantly a local process of spreading ulceration. The frequent inguinal lesions are probably seeded by lymphatic spread. Lesions in women tend to be more extensive and may progress rapidly during pregnancy.

Urinary tract infections
Urinary tract infections (UTIs) are among the most common of all bacterial infections. Up to 60% of women will experience at least one UTI at some point in their lifetime.

UTI accounts for over 6 million patient visits to physicians per year in the USA. Approximately one fifth of those visits are to emergency departments.

Predisposing factors

UTIs are usually caused by bacteria that inhabit the gastrointestinal tract. These organisms can also colonize the perineal and lower urethral areas and if organisms ascend the urinary tract from the lower urethra they can give rise to infection. Very rarely, infection can reach the urinary tract via the bloodstream, usually presenting with renal abscesses. Table 11.4 shows the common causal agents of UTI.

The host has a number of defence mechanisms to prevent infection of the urinary tract. Table 11.5 shows the main mechanisms involved and the groups at risk of impaired defence. The main risk factors for

Table 11.4 Common causes of urinary tract infections

Ascending route (% of total UTIs)	Hematogenous route
E. coli (75%) *Proteus mirabilis* (5%) Other Enterobacteriaceae (5%) *Enterococcus* spp. (5%) *Staphylococcus saprophyticus* (5%, but 30% of UTIs in young women)	*Staphylococcus aureus* *Candida albicans* *Mycobacterium tuberculosis*

Table 11.5 Factors that protect against and those that contribute to urinary tract infections

Defence	Protective mechanism	Predisposing factors to infection
Urethral anatomy	The long male urethra reduces the likelihood of bacteria ascending Position of male urethra away from anus and perineum reduces colonization	**Women:** short urethra, close proximity to highly colonized vulva and perineum, sexual activity forces bacteria into the urethra ("honeymoon cystitis")
Urinary tract mucosa	Cytokine production and neutrophil secretion prevent adherence	**Stones, scarring, catheters:** act as nidus for bacteria to adhere in the urinary tract **Surgical instrumentation, catheterization:** bacteria bypass the lower urinary tract mucosa, allowing immediate access to the bladder
Urinary pH and osmolality	Inhibit bacterial growth	**Women:** osmolar tension is less than in men; it is reduced further in **pregnancy**
Urinary substances	IgA and prostatic fluid inhibit bacterial growth	**Diabetes:** glucosuria (glucose in urine) levels promote bacterial growth
Normal micturition: flushing mechanism and complete bladder emptying	Eliminates bacteria from urethra and prevents stagnation of urine	**Pregnancy, obstruction, neurological abnormality, catheterization, elderly men (enlarged prostate):** all associated with incomplete bladder emptying and stagnation
Competent vesicoureteric valves	Prevents backflow of urine from bladder to kidney	**Congenital abnormality:** can cause reflux nephropathy
Low urethral colonization	Normal vaginal pH reduces colonization of the vulval and periurethral areas. Urinary flow	**Women:** altered vaginal flora; sexual activity can force bacteria into the urethra **Elderly:** fecal incontinence
Bowel carriage	Healthy bowel flora (lactobacilli, etc.) reduce presence of uropathogenic bacteria	Disturbed colonic flora

developing a UTI are: female sex, structural or neurological abnormalities of the urinary tract, increasing age, and catheterization. The prevalence of UTIs changes with age, reflecting the presence of risk factors in different age groups (Table 11.6).

Bacterial pathogenesis

While many species of bacteria are capable of causing urinary tract infection, *E. coli* is the predominant organism implicated and only a few serogroups of *E. coli* cause UTIs, the so-called uropathogenic strains.

Table 11.6 The age-related risk of acquiring UTI

Age	Point prevalence data	Reason
Neonate	1% males > females	Congenital abnormality such as urethral valves or stenosis
School children	1–2% in girls 0.03% in boys	30–50% will have vesicoureteric reflux
Young adults	1–3% in women 0.1% in men	Sexual activity, altered vaginal flora
Older adults	20% in women 10% in men	Bladder prolapse, prostatic hypertrophy, calculi, catheterization, fecal incontinence

All these strains contain adhesins that enhance adherence to uroepithelium. The main adhesin is P fimbria, a filamentous protein on the surface of *E. coli* that attaches to globoseries receptors present on uroepithelium. Uropathogenic strains of *E.coli* may also possess other virulence factors including K capsular antigen, which protects against phagocytosis; hemolysin, which promotes tissue invasion, and aerobactin, an iron-scavenging mechanism.

Other urinary pathogens also have virulence mechanisms: *Staphylococcus saprophyticus* is much less pathogenic than *Staphylococcus aureus* but, due to its powerful adherence to uroepithelium, it has found itself a niche as the major cause of UTIs in young, sexually active women, by comparison *S. aureus* rarely causes UTIs. Urease production is strongly associated with a pyelonephritogenic strain of *Proteus* sp.

Classification of UTIs

Urinary tract infections can be classified in a number of different ways: which can have an impact on clinical presentation, diagnosis, and management.

Anatomical localization

Lower urinary tract infection of the urethra or bladder presents with different symptoms and signs and tends to be less severe than upper urinary tract infections of the renal pelvis or parenchyma.

Uncomplicated versus complicated

Infections affecting a structurally and neurologically normal urinary tract are classed as uncomplicated urinary tract infections. Infections affecting a urinary tract with structural or neurological abnormalities are termed complicated infections and are more difficult to eradicate, prone to complications, and to recurrent infection.

Patient group affected

- UTIs in young children suggest structural problems and can lead to scarring of the immature renal tract if not managed rigorously. Bacterial invasion of the bladder with overt UTI is more likely to occur if urinary stasis or low flow conditions exist. Some causes of these conditions are infrequent or incomplete voiding, reflux, or other urinary tract abnormalities. Even in the absence of urinary tract abnormalities, cystitis causes reflux of urine back into the ureters, and it may worsen pre-existing reflux. Reflux may cause development of pyelonephritis. Chronic or recurrent pyelonephritis results in renal damage and scarring that may progress to chronic renal failure if it continues or is severe. Approximately 5–10% of children with symptomatic UTI and fever develop renal scarring. These children should be treated promptly and all of them referred to a specialist urology clinic. This is done by imaging the renal tract 3–6 weeks after the infection as part of outpatient follow-up, except in cases in which urinary tract obstruction is suspected.

- Pregnant women are at an increased risk of pyelonephritis, which can cause intra-uterine growth retardation, premature labor, and all its associated complications. They should be screened for the presence of bacteriuria and treated even if asymptomatic. When treating pregnant women care should be exercised to prescribe those antibiotics that are safe in pregnancy (see Chapter 5).
- Young men should not be at risk of acquiring a UTI; diagnosis of UTI in this group warrants further investigation to look for an underlying structural or neurological abnormality.
- UTIs in the elderly are common; patients who were previously self-caring may suddenly become confused and presentation of typical signs and symptoms may therefore be masked. In men older than 50 years, the incidence of UTI rises dramatically because of enlargement of the prostate, prostatism, and subsequent instrumentation of the urinary tract.
- UTIs in diabetics and those with underlying renal abnormalities are at high risk of complications and must be treated promptly.
- Catheter-associated UTI is a particular problem; almost all patients with an indwelling catheter will develop infection, and the risk of infection increases with duration of catheterization. It is the most common hospital acquired infection, a major cause of hospital acquired Gram negative bacteremia, and is often caused by more unusual pathogens and resistant organisms. The management must include removal of the offending catheter.

Clinical presentation

Symptoms of lower urinary tract infection include dysuria, frequency, urgency, suprapubic pain, and hematuria. There may be an associated low grade fever, but the patient is not usually systemically unwell. Overt fever, rigors, systemic toxicity, and loin pain are suggestive of pyelonephritis. Presentation at the extremes of age is less clear-cut: young children present with nonspecific fever, abdominal pain, vomiting, poor feeding, or failure to thrive. In the elderly, new onset urinary incontinence and confusion are common presentations.

Diagnosis

Bladder urine is sterile. Urine samples are prone to contamination from lower urethral and periurethral flora. A mid-stream urine (MSU) specimen is the sample of choice for UTI diagnosis. The initial urine stream will flush these bacteria away, so that the mid-stream sample should be a true reflection of what is happening higher up in the urinary tract. To avoid contamination, the periurethral area should be cleaned and then wiped with sterile saline; the first portion of urine should be discarded and the mid-stream collected in a sterile container. The patient is rarely instructed thoroughly and, therefore, contaminated MSU specimens are common.

Obtaining a MSU from a child is almost impossible, yet a positive diagnosis in this age group warrants thorough investigation for structural abnormalities, so it important get the right specimen. A suprapubic aspirate of urine directly from the bladder is the most reliable specimen. Bag urine samples are useful only when they yield a negative result and, therefore, exclude infection; positive results are impossible to interpret, as the rate of contamination is unacceptably high.

The sample must be transported to the laboratory as quickly as possible: any bacteria, including contaminants, will multiply in the urine leading to an unreliable result if culture is delayed. Moreover,

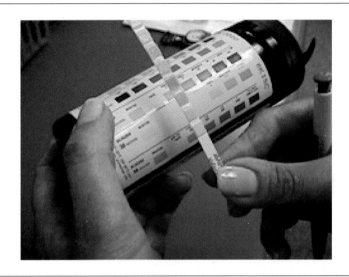

Figure 11.27 Examination of urine by dipstick. From www.brooksidepress. org/ . . . /Lab/UrineDipstick.htm

WBCs, RBCs, and casts degrade in urine, so that microscopy performed on a sample that is more than 12 hours old will be invalid. The collected sample can be analysed using urinalysis, microscopy, and culture.

Urinalysis sticks (dipsticks) are being used increasingly in the diagnosis of UTIs (Figure 11.27). Dipsticks are immersed in the urine sample; they record a change in color of embedded substrates on the paper strip. They measure protein, leukocyte esterase (produced by WBCs), and nitrites (produced by bacteria which utilize nitrates). The negative predictive value of dipstick is 95–99%, meaning that if the dipstick test is negative for all three measures, there is a 95–99% chance that infection is not present. The positive predictive value is only 40%, so a positive result does not confirm infection. Dipsticks are a useful rapid screening test and many laboratories now use them as an initial test and will only perform further investigations on urines with a positive result.

Microscopy of an unstained sample of urine is performed to visualize WBCs, RBCs, casts, and epithelial cells. A count of 10–50 WBC/mm^3 of urine is considered the upper limit of normal, a higher number is highly suggestive of infection. The presence of WBC casts is suggestive of pyelonephritis, RBCs are suggestive of an inflammatory process, and high numbers of epithelial cells are indicative of contamination. Organisms are not examined by microscopy, as it is impossible to differentiate between contaminating organisms and those causing infection.

Some degree of contamination is expected, so urine **culture** requires quantification of bacteria in order to differentiate between contamination and infection. Studies have shown that a growth of $>10^5$ bacteria/ml of urine is a good predictor of infection, whereas contaminating organisms are usually present in much lower concentrations. 1 μl of urine is spread onto agar (or a dip slide is used) and the presence of >100 colonies of a single bacterial species after overnight incubation correlates to $>10^5$ organisms/ml of urine (Figure 11.28).

Lower counts may be obtained if the patient is already on antibiotics, if there is frequent bladder voiding (bacteria do not have time to reach high concentration), and in suprapubic urine samples (where the presence of any bacteria is concerning).

Slow-growing or fastidious organisms such as *S. saprophyticus* and *Candida albicans* can also give lower counts. *M. tuberculosis* will not grow at all on routine culture plates and is a well recognized cause of "sterile pyuria." If no obvious cause for pyuria (WBCs or "pus" cells in urine) is found, large amounts of urine (three entire early morning urine samples) should be submitted for mycobacterial culture.

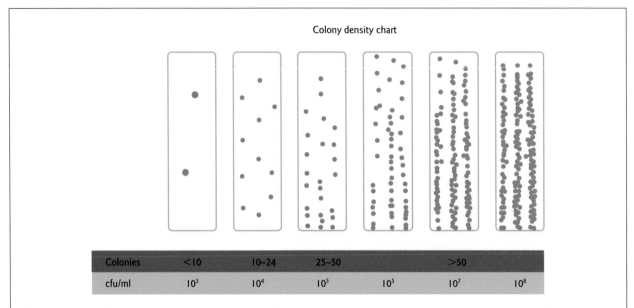

Figure 11.28 Quantitative urine cultures using a dip slide. From http://www.novamed.co.il/distreak%20advertisement.htm

Management

The patient with an uncomplicated presumed lower UTI or simple cystitis who has symptoms of less than 48 hours' duration may be treated with an oral agent for a total of 3 days.

Common antibiotics used in the treatment of uncomplicated UTIs include oral therapy with an antibiotic effective against Gram negative aerobic coliform bacteria, such as *E coli*. The Infectious Disease Society of America recommends the use of co-trimoxazole (Bactrim) as first-line therapy in patients without an allergy and in areas where resistance is not high (>15%).

Reserving the use of fluoroquinolones such as ciprofloxacin for complicated infections or cases with documented drug resistance may help decrease the incidence of bacterial resistance to drugs in the fluoroquinolone class. These drugs must be avoided in pregnancy. Other options are nitrofurantoin macrocrystals (e.g. Macrodantin) and co-amoxiclav (e.g. Augmentin).

Complicated UTIs, pyelonephritis, or UTIs in high-risk groups such as children require prompt, effective treatment before laboratory results are ready. The choice of empirical antibiotic needs to cover all the likely organisms present, reflect local antibiotic resistance patterns, and have good penetration into the urinary tract. These antibiotics tend to be more broad spectrum and common choices include ciprofloxacin, co-amoxiclav, third generation cephalosporins, and aminoglycosides. Intravenous treatment is warranted in cases of pyelonephritis and other severe infections, and may be necessary for more resistant organisms where no oral options are available.

Catheter-associated infection warrants removal of the catheter, as no amount of antibiotics will eradicate bacteria from the catheter plastic. Urine samples from indwelling catheters are often positive for microorganisms, caregivers need to be educated to resist treating such organisms with antibiotics. Asymptomatic patients are carefully watched and symptomatic patients need catheter removal as the mainstay of treatment.

Long-term suppressive antibiotic treatment may be attempted in those with recurrent UTIs, but break-through infections may occur with resistant organisms and the choice of suppressive agent becomes increasingly restricted over time.

Case study 11.1

An 18-year-old woman presents with a 2-week history of white vaginal discharge with odor. She also reports vulvar itching and has been scratching. Last sexual intercourse was 2 days ago with a regular male partner of 5 months. He has no symptoms. They do not use condoms and she has stopped using the pill. She reports no other sexual partners in the past 3 months but two partners within the past 12 months.

Microscopy (Gram stain) of vaginal discharge shows the following:

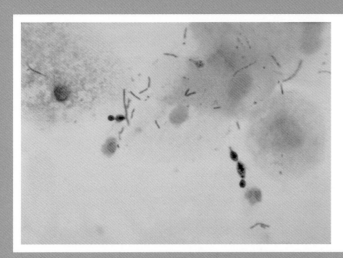

Provided by Dr Stuart Brown; Courtesy of the Centers for Disease Control and Prevention; from CDC website: http://phil.cdc.gov/phil/details.asp

1. What is the probable cause of her symptoms?
2. What may have predisposed her to getting this infection?

Case study 11.2

A 22-year-old woman presents with a 1-week history of yellowish discharge with an offensive odor. She reports vulvo-vaginal soreness and superficial (vulval) dyspareunia (pain during sex). Last sexual intercourse was 2 days ago with a regular male partner of 12 months. They do not use condoms as she is taking the combined oral contraceptive pill.

She reports unprotected vaginal intercourse with a casual male partner whilst on holiday in Thailand 2 weeks ago. She has had no other sexual partners in the past 3 months.

The vaginal pH is 7. The discharge is frothy and watery; microscopy reveals an organism (shown below) that has a typical flagellating motility.

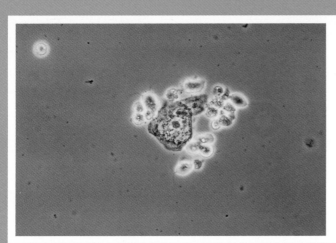

Courtesy of the Centers for Disease Control and Prevention; from CDC website: http://phil.cdc.gov/phil/details.asp

Test yourself

1. What is the probable cause of her symptoms?
2. In addition to treating her what else would you do?

Case study 11.3

A 38-year-old married woman comes in for a routine cervical smear test (Pap's smear to screen for cervical cancer). She incidentally mentions that she has noticed an increased vaginal discharge. There is no odor. Last sexual intercourse was 5 weeks ago with her regular male partner of 15 years. They do not use condoms as she has had a laparoscopic sterilization. There are no other sexual partners. The vaginal pH is 4.5. Discharge is creamy and odorless. Below you can see the microscopy result (Gram stain) of a high vaginal swab taken at the clinic.

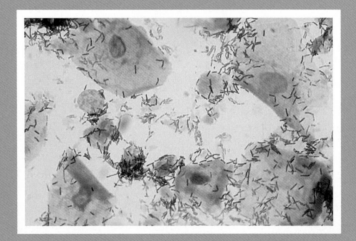

1. What is your interpretation of the smear?
2. How will you address the patient's concerns?

Case study 11.4

A 22-year-old female presents with a 48-hour history of severe vulval pain, dysuria, and vaginal discharge. She has flu-like symptoms and has noticed tender glands all over. She has recently started having sex with a new male partner who is 38 and who has had many previous partners. Her previous sexual relationship finished 9 months ago. Neither she nor her partner has any previous history of genital or oral ulceration.

Examination shows small tender nodes in several areas, especially in the groin. There are multiple small ulcers 1–2 mm in diameter on the labia minora and vulva. Internal examination cannot be performed because of pain.

Test yourself

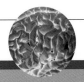

Microscopy (transmission electron micrograph) reveals the following:

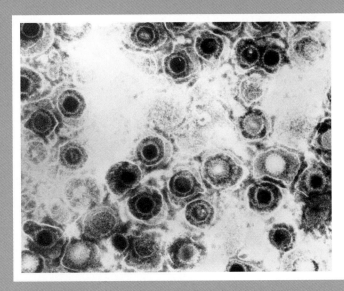

Provided by Dr. Erskine Palmer; Courtesy of the Centers for Disease Control and Prevention. From CDC website: http://phil.cdc.gov/phil/details.asp

1. Suggest a causative agent that fits best with her story.
2. Describe what stage of the natural history of infection with this agent is depicted.
3. How would you answer questions the patient puts to you about the source of her infection, the danger of spreading it to other parts of her own body or to others, and what preventive measures she should consider?

Case study 11.5
A 33-year-old man presents to the sexual health clinic complaining of a urethral discharge. He gives a history of several casual, unprotected sexual contacts with a sex worker while on business trips to New York over the last few months. You notice that he appears to have conjunctivitis. When questioned he says his newborn baby daughter has developed a red and purulent eye infection and he fears he may have got it from her. This is his and his partner's first child.

1. Having taken a detailed sexual history, what further questions would you ask about any other possible symptoms?
2. What is the most likely organism implicated in his illness, do you think he was infected by his baby daughter? If not what do you think was the chain of transmission?
3. What is this the likely pathogenesis of his eye ailment; what is the condition called?
4. What investigation would you perform to detect the infecting organism?
5. What are your concerns about his baby daughter, particularly as regards mode of acquisition, pathogenesis, complications, and treatment options?
6. His partner has had no symptoms, would you: (a) investigate her; (b) if so what specimen would you request; (c) what test would you order and for what organisms/organisms?
7. Would you treat his partner? Note that she is reluctant to take any medication as she is keen to continue breast feeding.

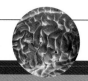

Test yourself

Case study 11.6

A 22-year-old male presents to the sexual health clinic with his male partner. Both have had several previous male partners and have had casual anal and oral sex while on holiday in Mexico. He complains of pus discharging from the urethra accompanied by dysuria. He has a fever and also complains of pain in his left knee joint.

Microscopy of the pus showed the following organism on Gram stain:

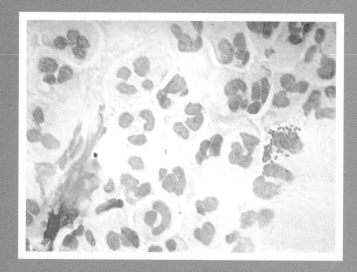

1. Interpret the Gram stain and suggest a causative organism.
2. How does the organism cause disease?
3. What are the current concerns about this organism in terms of treatment?
4. What are the complications associated with urethritis with this organism?

Case study 11.7

A 19-year-old male presents with a 2-week history of flu-like symptoms and a generalized rash which appeared the day before his visit to the clinic. He has had a new, regular male partner for 6 weeks. He saw his family doctor who prescribed amoxicillin. He is on no other medication. He has not been abroad for 4 years; his partner travels extensively. On examination he has a red throat and a generalized nonitchy maculopapular rash photographed on the following page.

Test yourself

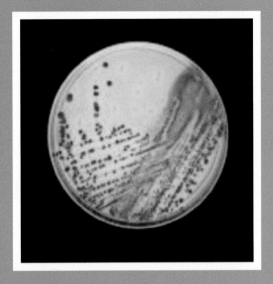

1. Interpreting the quantitative culture result above, do you think this is a significant count, suggestive of a UTI?
2. What is the basis of your interpretation?
3. What important biochemical characteristic of *E. coli* is demonstrated in this culture plate (hint: see Chapter 4)?
4. What are your concerns when treating a child with a UTI? What are the important principles of management of this child?

Further reading

Emond RTD, Rowland HAK, Welsby PD. *Colour Atlas of Infectious Diseases*. St Louis, MO: Mosby, 1994

Gorbach SL, Bartlett JG, Zorab Z, Blacklow NR. *Infectious Diseases*, 3rd edition. New York: Lippincott Williams & Wilkins, 2003

Useful websites

Guidelines from the Infectious Diseases Society of America. Guidelines for Antimicrobial Treatment of Uncomplicated Acute Bacterial Cystitis and Acute Pyelonephritis in Women. http://www.journals.uchicago.edu/IDSA/guide/p745.pdf

Treatment Guidelines for Sexually Transmitted Infections in the USA. http://www.cdc.gov//treatment/

Part 3
Infections in special groups

Chapter 12

Obstetric, congenital and neonatal infections

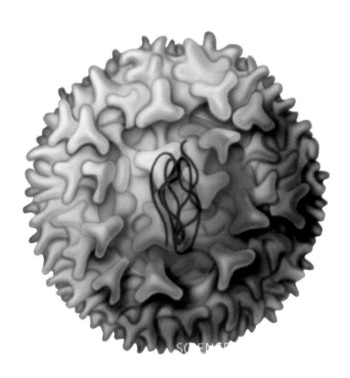

N. Shetty, J.W. Tang, J. Andrews

Obstetric infections (infections during pregnancy and childbirth)
  Postpartum (puerperal) sepsis
  Pyelonephritis in pregnancy
Congenital infections and neonatal infections
Congenital infections: bacterial
  Listeriosis
  Syphilis
Congenital infections: viral
  Rubella, varicella zoster, and parvovirus B19
    infections
  Cytomegalovirus (CMV)

Congenital infections: parasitic
  Toxoplasmosis
Neonatal/perinatal infections
Neonatal/perinatal infections: bacterial
  Early onset sepsis
  Late onset sepsis
Neonatal/perinatal infections: viral
  Bloodborne viruses: human immunodeficiency virus
    (HIV), hepatitis B (HBV), hepatitis C (HCV)
  Herpes simplex viruses 1 and 2 (HSV-1, HSV-2)
  Enteroviruses
  Emerging infections, pregnancy, neonatal infections

This chapter discusses infections that may cause disease in up to three populations of patients: the mother, the fetus, and the neonate. When discussing each infection and the causative agents consideration must be given to the possible effects on each group.

Obstetric infections (infections during pregnancy and childbirth)

In the developed world today pregnancy carries few risks and childbirth is a relatively safe procedure with an increasing number of women opting to give birth in the comfort of their own homes without an attendant obstetrician. There is also a more relaxed approach to many former sterile "operating theatre-like" routines in the labor room: healthcare staff do not wear masks and gowns and several support people like the husband and other members of the immediate family are allowed into the delivery suite.

In addition, the antibiotic era has accounted for much of the relaxed attitude we have today to safe pregnancy and delivery. Routine prophylaxis is widely accepted for caesarean sections, which account for 20–25% of deliveries in the USA. Many antibiotics are now licensed for use in pregnancy and any pregnant woman presenting with an obvious infection will automatically receive an antibiotic. Antibiotics are also indicated for pregnant women with ruptured membranes for a prolonged length of time and for any woman in labor with a raised temperature. However, until relatively recently in developed countries, and still in many developing countries, puerperal (postpartum) sepsis was and is a killer. In the USA, in the 1890s, 20 000 women a year died in childbirth. In 2000, there were 396 maternal deaths related to complications of pregnancy, childbirth, and the postpartum period, a rate of 9.8 per 100 000 live births.

Postpartum (puerperal) sepsis

Globally, in years gone by, the most common and the most feared infecting organism was the Group A beta hemolytic streptococcus (*S. pyogenes*, see Chapter 7). Normally found on the skin, in the nose and throat, and in the vagina, as well as in skin lesions, the streptococcus was introduced into the genital tract during examinations and deliveries performed by midwives who did not wash their hands. The virulence of this agent is dreaded even today though it is far less common, possibly due to improved socioeconomic conditions, the basic principles of good hygiene, and the use of antibiotics. Staphylococci, *E. coli*, other bowel flora, as well as anaerobes, were less likely culprits, but have assumed greater importance in recent years, as has the Group B streptococcus.

Immediately postnatally, the placental site is a large open wound – easily invaded by ascending bacteria. For thousands of years, it was recognized that postpartum women were at risk of a fever that could be fatal. Puerperal infection is suspected when the mother's temperature rises to ≥38°C (≥100.4°F) on any two successive days after the first 24 hours after delivery. Certain conditions predispose normal vaginal bacteria (such as anaerobic streptococci and staphylococci) to migrate to the uterine cavity and cause infection of the raw uterine bed; they include anemia, prolonged rupture of the membranes, prolonged labor, operative or traumatic delivery, repeated examination, retention of placental fragments within the uterus, and postpartum hemorrhage. The most commonly implicated organisms are *E. coli*, and other gut associated Gram negative organisms, and anaerobes such as anaerobic cocci, *Bacteroides* spp., and less commonly *Clostridium* spp. The pathogenesis is similar to gas gangrene and anaerobic infections described in Chapter 7.

Patients manifest with pain and tenderness over the uterus. This is accompanied by chills, headache, malaise, an increased pulse rate, and a raised white blood cell count. Vaginal discharge just postpartum is called lochia; this may be profuse and foul smelling. In extreme cases endotoxemia and endotoxic shock may follow and may be fatal.

Less serious infections in this period are bladder (cystitis) and kidney (pyelonephritis) infections. Other causes of fever are pelvic thrombophlebitis (inflammation of the pelvic veins) and breast infection (mastitis); these tend to occur after the third day postpartum. Breast abscesses are rare and are treated with incision, drainage, and antibiotics aimed at *Staphylococcus aureus*. Breastfeeding need not be stopped if the breast infection improves.

Pyelonephritis in pregnancy

Pregnant women are at an increased risk of pyelonephritis, which can cause intrauterine growth retardation, premature labor, and all its associated complications. The infection may begin as asymptomatic bacteriuria during pregnancy. Bacteria have a greater to tendency to ascend into the upper renal tract in pregnancy, due in part to the pressure of the fetus on the bladder and in part due to lax sphincter tone associated with hormonal changes in pregnancy. All pregnant women are screened for the presence of bacteriuria and treated even if asymptomatic. When treating pregnant and breast feeding women, care should be exercised to prescribe those antibiotics that are safe for the fetus/newborn (see Chapter 5).

Congenital infections and neonatal infections

The placenta provides nutrients from the mother, via the placental blood supply, to the fetus. The placenta also has a protective role as a barrier against microorganisms reaching the fetus. Should organisms cross the placenta infection of the fetus may occur. Organisms infecting the mother can lead to transplacental infection, this in turn can cause congenital infection with serious consequences to the fetus such as growth retardation, anatomical malformations, and fetal loss. *Toxoplasma gondii*, *Treponema pallidum*, rubella virus, and cytomegalovirus, (CMV) are examples of organisms that cause congenital infection.

Definitions of terms: For definitions of the terms congenital, perinatal and neonatal infections see Box 12.1.

Early onset neonatal infection may be contracted during the process of birth, by direct contact with maternal blood or genital secretions. The manifestations of such infections tend to be less severe than congenital infection and include presentations such as meningitis, pneumonia, or conjunctivitis. Prolonged rupture of membranes (over 18 hours prior to delivery) predisposes to fetal and neonatal infection. Infections can also be transmitted to the neonate after birth, known as late onset neonatal infection. Late onset neonatal infection can occur via person to person spread, via breast milk, or via the environment. Read the case illustrated in Box 12.2 and read on to figure what might be the problem.

Different microorganisms can cause infection at various stages in pregnancy, labor and after birth. Table 12.1 outlines the most important with their route(s) of acquisition.

Box 12.1 Definitions of terms (source World Health Organization (WHO))

- **Congenital** infection is an infection of the fetus acquired *in utero* either via maternal bloodstream or across the placenta
- **Perinatal** infection is an infection that is acquired any time after 22 completed weeks (154 days) of gestation to seven completed days after birth
- **Neonatal** infection is an infection that occurs any time from birth to 28 completed days after birth

- **Early onset neonatal infection** occurs from birth to seven completed days after birth
- **Late onset neonatal infection** occurs from after seven completed days after birth to 28 completed days after birth.

There is clearly some overlap between perinatal and early onset neonatal periods

---

Box 12.2 A baby born at term is not quite right

A 2-day-old female baby is seen on the postnatal ward after the mother has noticed her baby is unable to suck and seems to have some difficulty with her breathing. The pediatric doctor examines the baby and notices she has a high breathing rate, crackles in her chest, and a temperature of 38°C. The baby has no rash or evidence of an enlarged liver or spleen (hepatosplenomegaly).

❓1. What other important information would you like to know from the mother?
❓2. What investigations should this baby undergo?
❓3. Name two important bacteria that commonly cause sepsis in the neonatal period.

Table 12.1 Important microorganisms associated with congenital and neonatal infections

Infection and route of acquisition	Organisms
Congenital	
Bacterial	*Listeria monocytogenes* *Treponema pallidum*
Viral	Rubella Parvovirus Cytomegalovirus (CMV) Varicella zoster virus (VZV)
Protozoal	*Toxoplasma gondii*
Neonatal: early onset via an infected/colonized birth canal	
Bacteria	Group B streptococcus *Escherichia coli* *Listeria monocytogenes* *Chlamydia trachomatis* *Neisseria gonorrhoeae*
Viruses	Hepatitis B virus Herpes simplex virus Hepatitis C Enterovirus HIV
Neonatal: late onset	
Via healthcare workers	Group B streptococcus *Staphylococcus aureus*
Via breast milk	*Staphylococcus aureus*
Via the environment	Gram negative bacteria
Via intravenous catheters	Coagulase negative staphylococci *Candida* species

Congenital infections: bacterial

Listeriosis

The CDC estimates that 2500 people become seriously ill with listeriosis each year in the USA. Of these, one in five dies from the disease. Listeriosis can be particularly dangerous for pregnant women and their unborn babies. Foodborne illness caused by *Listeria* spp. in pregnant women can result in premature delivery, miscarriage, fetal death, and severe illness or death of a newborn from the infection. Data from the CDC puts the incidence of infection from *L. monocytogenes* from 0.5 to 0.3 cases per 100 000 people per year (Box 12.3).

L. monocytogenes is found in soil or in foodstuffs where contamination by animal feces has occurred. Cross-contamination of food products may occur. Infection follows consumption of contaminated food, e.g. soft cheeses other unpasteurized dairy products, undercooked poultry, and prepared meats such as paté.

Box 12.3 Outbreak of listeriosis – Northeastern United States, 2002 (report from *MMWR* October 25, 2002/51(42);950–951)

A multistate outbreak of *Listeria monocytogenes* infections with 46 culture-confirmed cases, seven deaths, and three stillbirths or miscarriages in eight states has been linked to eating sliceable turkey deli meat. Cases have been reported from Pennsylvania (14 cases), New York (11 in New York City and seven in other locations), New Jersey (five), Delaware (four), Maryland (two), Connecticut (one), Massachusetts (one), and Michigan (one). Outbreak isolates share a relatively uncommon pulsed-field gel electrophoresis (PFGE) pattern. One intact food product and 25 environmental samples from a poultry processing plant have yielded *L. monocytogenes*. The isolate from the food product had a PFGE pattern different from the outbreak strain; however, two environmental isolates from floor drains shared a PFGE pattern indistinguishable from that of outbreak patient isolates, suggesting that the plant might be the source of the outbreak.

Clinical presentation

L. monocytogenes usually causes a mild, self-limiting infectious mononucleosis-like syndrome. Rarely acute meningitis or encephalitis (with a high mortality) can develop in patients with reduced cell-mediated immunity. Maternal listeriosis may be associated with bacteremia and minimal associated symptoms or signs. Transplacental infection can lead to dire consequences such as intrauterine death, premature labor, or neonatal sepsis. Listeriosis can also manifest in the early neonatal period if infection has been acquired via a contaminated birth canal. Neonatal listeriosis manifests most usually as neonatal meningitis presenting within the first week of life.

Diagnosis

Diagnosis of maternal infection is usually via blood cultures. Diagnosis of neonatal infection is via placental and surface swab cultures as well as blood and cerebrospinal fluid culture. *L. monocytogenes* grows readily on simple media, exhibiting a narrow zone of hemolysis on blood agar. It can be selected for by incubating at low temperatures or by using selective media. Further identification is by biochemical or serological testing.

Treatment and prevention

L. monocytogenes is susceptible to ampicillin/amoxicillin but resistant to the cephalosporins and penicillin.

Pregnant women are advised to avoid any meat and dairy products that are unpasteurized to reduce their possible exposure to *L. monocytogenes* containing items. Listeriosis can also be prevented by good food hygiene, effective refrigeration, and adequate re-heating of pre-prepared food. Women who work with animals are also advised to avoid contact with aborted animal fetuses.

Microbiology and virulence

L. monocytogenes is a Gram positive rod-like ubiquitous organism that displays tumbling motility under the microscope particularly at low temperatures such as 4°C. See Figure 12.1 for a typical Gram stain of *L. monocytogenes*.

Virulence mechanisms

Host susceptibility plays a major role in the presentation of clinical disease upon exposure to *L. monocytogenes*. Normally, the cellular immune system eliminates infection before it spreads. Thus, most listeriosis patients

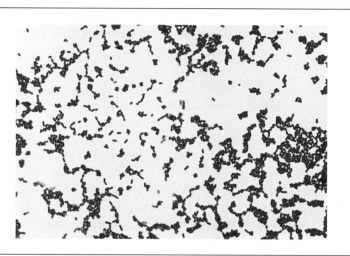

Figure 12.1 Gram stain of *Listeria monocytogenes.* Courtesy of Department of Microbiology, University College Hospitals London

have a physiological or pathological defect that affects T-cell-mediated immunity. An invasin secreted by the pathogenic bacteria enables the listeriae to penetrate host cells of the epithelial lining. *L. monocytogenes* multiplies not only extracellularly but also intracellularly, within macrophages after phagocytosis, or within parenchymal cells which are entered by induced phagocytosis. Unlike other bacterial pathogens, *Listeria* are able to penetrate the endothelial layer of the placenta and thereby infect the fetus.

After engulfment, the bacterium may escape from the phagosome before phagolysosome fusion occurs; this is mediated by the toxin, listeriolysin O (LLO), which also acts as a hemolysin. This toxin is one of the so-called SH-activated hemolysins, which are produced by a number of other Gram positive bacteria, such as group A streptococci (streptolysin O), pneumococci (pneumolysin), and *Clostridium perfringens.* The hemolysin gene is located on the chromosome within a cluster of other virulence genes which are all regulated by a common promoter. Survival of the bacterium within the phagolysosome may be aided by its ability to produce catalase and superoxide dismutase which neutralize the effects of the phagocytic oxidative burst.

Additional genetic determinants are necessary for further steps in the intracellular lifecycle of *L. monocytogenes.* An important gene product, Act A (encoded by *act*A), promotes the polymerization of actin, a component of the host cell cytoskeleton. Within the host cell environment, surrounded by a sheet of actin filaments, the bacteria reside and multiply. The growing actin sheet functions as a propulsive force and mediates direct cell-to-cell spread of *Listeria* in an infected tissue. Other, less well characterized, hemolysins and phopholipases may also contribute to virulence of the organism.

Syphilis

According to the CDC, health officials in the USA reported over 32 000 cases of syphilis in 2002, including 6862 cases of primary and secondary syphilis. In 2002, half of all primary and secondary syphilis cases were reported from 16 counties and one city (San Francisco); and most primary and secondary syphilis cases occurred in persons 20–39 years of age. The incidence of infectious syphilis was highest in women 20–24 years of age and in men 35–39 years of age. Reported cases of congenital syphilis in newborns decreased from 2001 to 2002, with 492 new cases reported in 2001 compared to 412 cases in 2002.

Between 2001 and 2002, the number of reported syphilis cases increased 12.4%. Rates in women continued to decrease, and overall, the rate in men was 3.5 times that in women. This, in conjunction with reports of syphilis outbreaks in men who have sex with men (MSM), suggests that rates of syphilis in MSM are increasing (see also Chapter 11).

Clinical features

Women who acquire the infection just before or during pregnancy may transmit the infection to the fetus across the placenta to cause congenital disease. Congenital syphilis is more likely if maternal infection occurs after the fourth month of gestation rather than early in pregnancy. Early congenital syphilis presents in the first 2 years of life with signs of secondary syphilis such as fever, skin rash (see Figure 11.10), skeletal abnormalities (see Figures 11.13 and 11.14), low platelets or an enlarged liver and spleen. Persistent rhinitis (syphilis snuffles) is common. Later (beyond 2 years) manifestations of congenital syphilis include deafness, atrophy of the optic nerve, and abnormalities of the incisor teeth called Hutchinson's teeth.

Diagnosis

Although acquisition of *T. pallidum* just prior or during pregnancy is rare (maternal incidence approximately 1 in 10 000), it is important to screen all women in early pregnancy with the aim of preventing the serious sequelae of congenital syphilis. All women in the USA are offered routine testing for presence of antibodies against treponemal species at their first antenatal appointment towards the end of their first trimester. Any women who are found to have positive treponemal serology are offered further testing and, if necessary, treatment with a course of long-acting penicillin. It is important to note that most serological tests used have cross-reactivity with other treponemal illnesses such as yaws and pinta.

Management

Treatment with penicillin during pregnancy prevents most cases of congenital syphilis. Neonates who present with any features of congenital syphilis can be screened using an IgM test against treponemal antigens and dark ground microscopy of any skin or mucosal lesions. If they test positive with serology, or *T. pallidum* are demonstrated by microscopy, neonates should be given intravenous or intramuscular penicillin for at least 10 days.

For detailed information on *Treponema pallidum*, the causative organism in syphilis read Chapter 11.

Congenital infections: viral

Several viruses may cause congenital infection and damage to the fetus if the mother is infected with any of them for the first time ("primary infection") during her pregnancy. The clinical illnesses and natural histories of three of these infections in children – rubella, varicella zoster virus (VZV), and parvovirus B19 – are described in the chapter on childhood rash illnesses (see Chapter 15). A fourth viral infection, cytomegalovirus (CMV), will be described separately, here.

Rubella, varicella zoster, and parvovirus B19 infections

Clinical features

Generally primary infection in adults with rubella, varicella zoster virus, and parvovirus B19 will be more symptomatic in adults, when complications of acute infection are also more common.

For acute primary rubella and parvovirus B19 infection in adults, the symptom of arthralgia (painful joints) may be very prominent, whereas in children this particular symptom may be very mild or absent. There is no specific antiviral therapy for either of these infections. Occasionally, infections with either of these viruses in adults (and occasionally in children) may result in a persistent arthritis, for which long term analgesia may be required. Normally, this persistent arthritis is nondestructive and self-limiting, though it can be very debilitating. Similarly, adult chickenpox infection can be very severe – even life-threatening – due to the most common complication of VZV pneumonitis that is seen more often in adults than children. For this reason, aciclovir treatment is usually given to adults with chickenpox, even during pregnancy if life-threatening VZV pneumonitis develops.

Other than this, the other aspects of primary infection with these viruses (incubation period, transmissibility, and laboratory diagnosis) are similar to those described in Chapter 15 for children.

Pathogenesis, prenatal diagnosis, and management options

The value of prenatal diagnosis (i.e. diagnosing an infection of the fetus whilst it is still in the womb, "*in utero*", before delivery) depends on the ability to apply potentially life-saving interventions. For rubella, VZV, and parvovirus B19 infections during pregnancy, the management options are very closely related to the gestational age at which the mother is infected. This, in turn, depends on the mechanism by which the infecting virus damages the fetus. This is not the case with congenital CMV infections, however, which are dealt with separately, below.

Rubella

Congenital rubella infection is relatively rare nowadays due to the widespread use and coverage of the live-attenuated, combined MMR (Measles, Mumps and Rubella) vaccine. Also, rubella IgG testing (indicating immunity if positive) is now routine during all antenatal checks, as long as the mother attends and such facilities are available to her.

Pathogenesis

In susceptible (rubella IgG negative) mothers, once infected, the rubella virus replicates and circulates in the maternal bloodstream, eventually reaching the placenta. In the placenta, the virus replicates and enters the fetal side of the placental circulation, spreading throughout the fetal organs. During the first trimester, this occurs relatively free of any immune restriction, as the fetal immune response is too immature to react at this time. The virus infects and destroys cells in the developing fetal heart, brain, eyes, ears, liver, spleen, and bone marrow. Hence, during the first and early part of the second trimester (1–16 weeks of pregnancy), maternal rubella infection infects and damages the fetus in 80–90% of cases of maternal primary rubella infections, resulting in "congenital rubella syndrome" (CRS). The affected fetus can be born with any number of abnormalities, including a characteristic petechial rash (appearing like pinpoint bruising), cataracts (see Figure 12.2), microphthalmia ("small eyes"), microcephaly ("small head"), heart defects (e.g. "hole in the heart" requiring surgical correction), enlarged liver and spleen ("hepato-splenomegaly", reversible), and

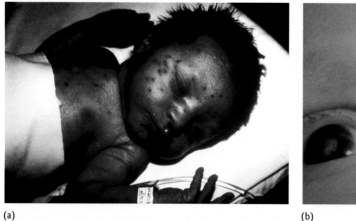
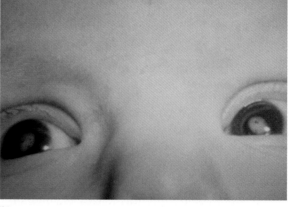

(a)   (b)

Figure 12.2 Congenital rubella syndrome. Note characteristic petechial or purpuric (similar to bruising) skin rash in the newborn (a) and bilateral cataracts (b). Courtesy of the Centers for Disease Control and Prevention; from CDC website: http://phil.cdc.gov/phil/details.asp

varying degrees of nerve ("sensorineural") deafness (irreversible). In addition, congenital rubella infection can result in spontaneous abortion, intrauterine death, or stillbirth. Since the severity and timing of occurrence of the abnormalities in CRS are so well documented, prenatal diagnosis may be less commonly offered, as the probability of rubella fetal infection and damage is >80%. In addition, many such abnormalities can be detected on ultrasound scanning.

Prenatal diagnosis

This can still be performed by carrying out rubella IgM and PCR testing (see Chapter 15 and Further reading) on fetal blood (obtained by "cordocentesis"). Testing of amniotic fluid (which is actually fetal urine and surrounds the fetus in the amniotic sac), obtained by "amniocentesis," may also be performed. Obtaining either of these samples requires a needle to be inserted into the mother's womb under ultrasound scan guidance. Cordocentesis (fetal blood sampling via the intrauterine umbilical cord) carries a slightly higher risk of fetal loss (1–2%), but can be usefully performed slightly earlier (at 18–20 weeks' gestation) than amniocentesis. Amniocentesis, which is safer (risk of fetal loss <1%), can only be usefully performed after maturation of the fetal kidneys after 21 weeks' gestation. However, rubella virus is not normally shed in the urine so amniotic fluid testing to rubella is usually less sensitive and may give false negative results. There is also an additional delay in the performance of either procedure. It is necessary to wait until 4–6 weeks after maternal rubella infection before sampling fetal fluids. This is to avoid any false positive result obtained from the sampling needle as it passes through maternal blood vessels that may still be carrying the maternal rubella virus. This delay makes prenatal diagnosis of congenital rubella in the first trimester even more difficult. If termination is chosen, normally it is not practical to wait until the 20–22 week of gestation, as the fetus is quite large by then, requiring a medical ("induced") rather than a surgical ("suction") termination of pregnancy, which is more unpleasant for many women. Fetal blood can be tested by serology (testing for rubella IgM) and rubella RNA by PCR, which may be more sensitive for first trimester fetal infections, as fetal antibodies are generally only produced after 22 weeks' gestation. Ultrasound scanning may detect the more gross morphological abnormalities in CRS.

Management options

With true, early, first trimester maternal primary rubella infections, termination is often recommended due to the extremely high rate of fetal infection and damage (>80–90% before 11 weeks' gestation). Where prenatal diagnosis becomes useful is if the mother becomes rubella infected during the end of the first and early in the second trimesters (weeks 11–16 of pregnancy). Between 16 and 20 weeks of pregnancy, about 40–50% of mothers with primary rubella infection may pass the virus onto their fetuses. Not all of these rubella-infected fetuses will be damaged by the virus. Fetal damage at this stage generally only involves fetal deafness of variable severity (one-sided, two-sided, total or partial sensorineural deafness), due to rubella virus destruction of the hearing "hair" cells in the inner ear. This occurs in about 15–20% of fetuses whose mothers have had primary rubella infection at this stage of pregnancy, i.e. probably less than half of the 40–50% of fetuses who are infected with rubella from their mothers end up damaged.

Hence, it is important to note that although prenatal diagnosis may *confirm* fetal viral infection, it cannot confirm whether that fetus will actually be damaged by the virus. Unfortunately, this is the question of interest to the parents and this sort of uncertainty can be very difficult for both them and their doctors.

There is no specific antiviral treatment for rubella virus infection and no postexposure prophylaxis that can be offered to rubella-susceptible pregnant women who are exposed. Unfortunately, rubella in children and even adults can be very mild and pregnant women may not be aware that they have been exposed, or even infected themselves and that they may be shedding the virus which may infect others (pregnant mothers-to-be often meet in antenatal clinics and exercise classes). Maternal susceptibility to rubella infection may arise in countries where routine childhood (or adult catch-up) MMR immunization is absent, where coverage is poor, or where there is an individual vaccine failure (in about 5% of all vaccines), for which there is no universal explanation.

Varicella zoster virus (VZV)

Unlike rubella infection, which is otherwise mild and relatively inconsequential for nonpregnant women, chickenpox (primary VZV infection) in pregnancy may also be clinically severe for the mother, as well as for the fetus. In adults the risk of complications from chickenpox (e.g. VZV pneumonitis – a viral pneumonia) are already higher than in children. During pregnancy, the growing fetus compresses the maternal lungs from the bottom upwards, reducing her lung capacity and making it more difficult for her to cough and clear infected phlegm. Especially in smokers, this reduced lung capacity may increase the risk of pneumonia, either viral (VZV) or from secondary bacterial infections. Treatment with aciclovir to save the mother in severe VZV infections during pregnancy is not so uncommon and so far has not been associated with fetal damage.

The new live-attenuated VZV vaccine can be offered to VZV-susceptible, nonpregnant women who are planning for pregnancy. This will give them protection against VZV if they are exposed during pregnancy. However, they need to wait at least 4 weeks after the vaccine before getting pregnant. As with all live-attenuated vaccines (containing live but weakened, replicating virus), it is contraindicated *during* pregnancy. The USA has already initiated universal VZV vaccination for all healthy children before school entry, starting at 1–2 years of age. A booster dose of VZV vaccine may be required during adolescence and young adulthood. It is probably wise for any young woman planning pregnancy to check her existing VZV IgG levels as part of this preparation. Universal antenatal screening for VZV IgG is not yet practiced, since at present most (>80–90%) women in most countries of child-bearing age are likely to be VZV IgG positive, usually through natural childhood chickenpox infections. However, in some tropical countries like Singapore, the overall VZV IgG positivity rate is surprisingly low at around 40%. It is, however, unclear exactly how the universal VZV immunization program in the USA (and elsewhere where it is in use) may change this in the future. The longer term duration of immunity induced by the VZV vaccine, and its impact on the natural epidemiology of VZV, is still uncertain (see Further reading).

Pathogenesis

Circulating VZV from maternal primary infection eventually reaches the placenta and crosses into the fetal circulation. Damage to the fetus from congenital VZV infection is thought to arise from direct fetal skin and nerve damage from the virus reactivating from latency from fetal nerve ganglia (i.e. fetal shingles) after an initial primary VZV viremia (see Chapter 15). As with congenital rubella syndrome (CRS), congenital varicella syndrome (CVS) defects primarily occur during the first 20 weeks of gestation, i.e. during fetal organogenesis. The virus replicates by lytic destruction of infected fetal cells resulting in a number of abnormalities, particularly skin lesions and contractures, shortened and deformed limbs resulting from VZV-damaged nerves being unable to provide growth factors for their normal development. Congenital varicella syndrome (CVS) therefore is characterized by intrauterine growth retardation (IUGR – i.e. a small baby), skin scarring, brain abnormalities (cortical atrophy, seizures), microcephaly ("small head"), microphthalmia ("small eyes"), eye abnormalities ("optic atrophy," "chorioretinitis"), shortened and deformed limbs, gut, kidney and bladder abnormalities.

Prenatal diagnosis

The overall risk of congenital varicella syndrome (CVS) is low, about 1–2% if the mother develops chickenpox within the first 20 weeks of pregnancy. Maternal shingles (VZV reactivation in the mother, in the presence of VZV IgG antibodies) poses very little or no risk to the fetus at any stage of pregnancy. In such a situation, prenatal diagnosis is not routinely offered, as the risk of the procedure (cordocentesis rather than amniocentesis, as VZV is present in blood, not urine) is about as great as the risk of having an affected fetus. So, with maternal chickenpox infection, even in the first 20 weeks of pregnancy, about 99% of the fetuses will be born normal. Ultrasound scanning may also detect abnormal limb formation in CVS.

Management options

Where a VZV-susceptible mother has had a close contact with a case of chickenpox (see Box 12.4 for definitions of close contact), there are several options for postexposure prophylactic intervention to reduce

Box 12.4 Contact between pregnant women and infected individuals: how close is close?

When in public places such as shopping malls, restaurants, the movie theatre, sports venues, sitting in the bus, train or plane, visiting friends and relatives, etc., it is very difficult to know whether a person sitting nearby may have an infectious disease that may harm the developing fetus. Unfortunately, in hospitals and other healthcare settings, pregnant women come into contact with other pregnant women and their children, e.g. in antenatal clinic and ultrasound scan waiting areas. Not infrequently, a midwife or physician receives a call from a pregnant woman saying that she attended the clinic the previous day and that she (or one of her accompanying children) has now come out in spots or a rash of some kind. Waiting areas vary in size and sometimes can be very busy with anything between 10 and 100 people waiting to be seen. So, how do you determine if another pregnant woman has had a "significant contact" with the woman with a rash?

Using the most common scenario involving chickenpox, this rash illness is known to be infectious for up to 2 days before the typical vesicular rash appears. Therefore, the movements of the woman (or child) with the rash needs to be traced during the time they were in the antenatal waiting area (with all the other pregnant women). Both of the other viral rash illnesses, rubella and PVB19, are generally less transmissible than chickenpox which is transmitted by the airborne route, but "contact tracing" will also have to be performed for these infections – just in case. In addition, the natural history of the individual viral infections also matters. For example, PVB19 is generally no longer infectious by the time the rash appears, since this is an immune-mediated rash and indicates the appearance of PVB19 neutralizing antibodies. For both rubella and chickenpox, they are infectious for a few days before and for a few days after the appearance of the rash. In the scenario presented, the following guidelines for "significant contact" for chickenpox have been suggested:

1 **Living in the same household as the person with "active" chickenpox.*** "Active" means that new lesions are still appearing and that they are not all dried and crusted. Sharing the same living space is possibly the most intense form of contact, and for chickenpox, it is quite common for all other nonimmune household members (usually young children) to become infected from each other.

2 **Face-to-face contact (i.e. at conversational distance, <1 m apart) with the person with "active" chickenpox* for at least 5 minutes.** Since VZV is airborne, conversational distance is sufficiently close for each person to inhale each other's exhaled air. Exhaled air will carry VZV from the infected person to the other, uninfected person who will inhale it during the course of the conversation.

Such unsuspecting contacts usually occur during the 2 days before the chickenpox rash appears in the "index" case (the one who has the infection first), as after this time, the risk becomes obvious once that person develops the characteristic rash. In this situation the person who subsequently contracts and develops the disease (the "secondary" case) would have had little or no warning about the infectious nature of the index case, though there are usually other signs of infection – a so-called infectious "prodrome," usually consisting of fever, cough, sore throat, headache, etc. With rubella and PVB19, the rashes are less obvious and the clinical symptoms of disease milder, so that even the index case may not be aware that he/she is ill at all.

This does not exclude other forms of contact being significant in some circumstances, e.g. sitting in a waiting room for 2 hours, sharing the same air as an index case, who may be on the other side of the room, or sharing a six-bedded bay in a hospital ward where a patient with chickenpox pneumonitis (viral pneumonia), lying opposite, may be coughing or using an oxygen mask.

* Immunocompromised patients (e.g. with AIDS, on chemotherapy for cancer, or with inherited immunodeficiencies) with shingles are considered as infectious as someone with chickenpox. In addition, a person with facial shingles is also considered to be as high a risk as someone with chickenpox.

the risk of the mother developing severe chickenpox, and therefore reducing the VZV risk to the fetus. If a VZV-susceptible (VZV IgG antibody negative) mother within the first 20 weeks of pregnancy presents to a physician with a recent (within 8–10 days) contact with chickenpox (or direct contact with exposed shingles lesions), then a dose of VZV IgG can be given to her. This preparation, VZV immunoglobulin or "VZIG," is produced from the pooling of VZV IgG-containing sera from blood donors, after purification and screening for bloodborne viruses (HIV, hepatitis B, and C). This dose of high concentration, ready-made VZV IgG antibodies will neutralize some, but not all, of the virus currently incubating within the mother. Even after receiving VZIG, the mother may still experience a mild form of chickenpox, with a few spots (usually <50). However, the VZV viral load is usually sufficiently reduced to make any damage to the fetus extremely unlikely. Some mothers may prefer not to take such donor blood products. In these situations, some may choose to do nothing, i.e. take the 1% risk of CVS, if within the first 20 weeks of pregnancy. Others may accept the theoretical (yet still unproven) risk to their fetus from aciclovir used in the first 20 weeks of pregnancy, and take prophylactic aciclovir postexposure, to reduce the VZV levels in their body to protect their fetus. Beyond 20 weeks' gestation, maternal chickenpox poses little risk to the fetus – until the final week before delivery. Maternal shingles has not been associated with CVS so far, presumably because maternal VZV IgG is already present, limiting any maternal viremia and therefore fetal VZV infection.

Maternal chickenpox in the final week before delivery and within the first 7 days after childbirth, poses an additional risk to the newborn. Since the mother had no VZV IgG during pregnancy, and the immune system of the newborn (neonate) is still not yet fully developed (not until after 22 weeks, normally), it will be completely unprotected against VZV infection. Neonatal varicella can be fatal in up to 30% of cases if untreated. Neonates born to mothers who experienced chickenpox either 7 days before, or after delivery should be given VZIG, as well as intravenous aciclovir treatment to prevent the onset of severe neonatal varicella infection. They should be monitored in hospital for at least 2 weeks. Neonates who lack maternal VZV antibodies should be monitored and treated aggressively if they develop VZV infection and disease during their first 28 days of life, as VZV can cause life-threatening illness in such young babies.

Maternal antibody transfer to the fetus normally occurs after the 28th week of gestation. However, some premature babies are now being born and surviving from 24 weeks' gestation. These babies will not have received any maternal VZV IgG, even if the mother is already immune with circulating VZV IgG. Such babies should be given VZIG and aciclovir treatment if there is any contact with chickenpox, either from their mother or anyone else. In fact, for premature babies of <28 weeks' gestational age, they cannot be assumed to be immune to any viral infection (rubella, chickenpox – VZV, parvovirus B19, measles, etc.), since no maternal antibodies would have been transferred at this age.

Parvovirus B19

Maternal parvovirus B19 (PVB19) infection may potentially be more common than either maternal rubella or varicella zoster infections. This is because, whilst most women of child-bearing age are rubella and VZV immune (>80% rubella and VZV IgG positive), previous infection and subsequent immunity to PVB19 is less common (around 50–60% PVB19 IgG positive by adulthood). Although systemic primary PVB19 infection may be more symptomatic in adults (with joint pains – arthralgia), it can also be very mildly symptomatic and may be just dismissed as a "cold" or the "flu." Unlike rubella and VZV, there is no vaccine currently available for PVB19 infection, and as with rubella, there is no specific antiviral drug for treating PVB19 infection.

Pathogenesis

Circulating maternal PVB19 can reach very high levels in primary infection (10^{10}–10^{12} viruses per ml). There is about a 30–40% chance of PVB19 being transmitted to the fetus, with an overall rate of untreated fetal loss of about 5–10%. Again, most fatalities occur when fetal infection occurs within the first 20 weeks of pregnancy. The mechanism of fetal loss involves the destruction of oxygen-carrying fetal precursor red blood cells by the virus. These cells have a receptor (the "P" antigen) specific for PVB19, which enters these cells and destroys them during viral replication. The very high circulating PVB19 load in primary infection can lead to rapid destruction of these red cells. To compensate, the fetal heart goes into overdrive to try to pump the remaining oxygen-carrying fetal red blood cells around its body faster, to distribute the limited amount of oxygen. The result is a type of "high-output" heart failure and the fetal organs and tissues start to swell. Also, the red cell producing ("erythropoietic") fetal tissues (liver and bone marrow) attempt to produce more red cells to replace those destroyed, but these have a short half-life and may not be fully functional. The fetal liver enlarges and partially obstructs the fetal blood flow, leading to a build up of back pressure, resulting in "ascites" or fluid accumulation and swelling of fetal body tissues. This process of gradual fetal swelling is called "fetal hydrops" and usually becomes manifest about 3–8 weeks after maternal PVB19 infection, though it may appear as late as 12–18 weeks later. Ultrasound scanning may show this fetal ascites, with generalized swelling under the skin including the scalp, fluid in the membranes surrounding the heart and lungs, as well as an enlarged amniotic sac and liver. Other manifestations of fetal hydrops include a petechial skin rash (perhaps similar to that shown for congenital rubella), intrauterine death, spontaneous abortion, and stillbirth.

The risk of fetal hydrops is greatest when maternal PVB19 occurs between 12 and 18 weeks' gestation. Fetal hydrops in the first trimester has been described but may be due to the action of PVB19 directly on the heart muscle, rather than the red cell precursors, as they would not be fully functional at this time. Congenital PVB19 infection does not cause morphological fetal abnormalities in the same way as CRS and CVS, though a few reports have described possible eye, facial and limb defects associated with congenital PVB19 infection. If fetal blood transfusion can be performed (possible in an increasing number of specialist centers), the fetal hydrops is reversible and the baby usually suffers no further long term sequelae. However, occasionally, a persistent PVB19-induced pure red anemia can be present in newborns, resulting in a variable period of blood transfusion dependency.

Prenatal diagnosis

The most reliable way to detect fetal PVB19 infection is to sample fetal blood, but again sampling needs to wait for at least 4–6 weeks after maternal PVB19 infection so as not to give false positive results. The fetal PVB19 IgM antibody response is probably unreliable before 22 weeks' gestational age, so PCR testing for PVB19 DNA is preferred prior to this age. Detailed ultrasound scanning may also reveal early signs of fetal hydrops or other signs of fetal anemia. Nowadays, modern methods can give fairly accurate information about fetal blood flow, e.g. fetal middle cerebral artery bloodflow velocity Doppler, which can determine whether the fetal blood is less viscose (due to a decreased fetal red blood cell count), as well as an increased cardiac output in response to the anemia and an attempt to pump the remaining red cells around the body, faster. Ultrasound scanning can also detect fetal ascites, and the swelling of other fetal organs, e.g. in the lungs ("pleural" effusion) and the heart ("pericardial" effusion). Hence, following confirmed maternal PVB19 infection, fetal ultrasound monitoring should continue weekly for at least 12 weeks, may be even up to 18 weeks.

Management options

Some cases of fetal hydrops may resolve spontaneously without the need for any further intervention. This conservative management (a "wait-and-see") approach has been reported to have some success – even from some very severely affected cases, as seen on ultrasound. This may result from maternal anti-PVB19 antibodies crossing the placenta after 28 weeks and neutralizing any fetal PVB19, allowing a restoration of fetal red cell counts and normalization of the fetal circulation. However, it is not possible at present to determine which PVB19-infected fetuses will have such a good outcome, without intervention. Another option is intrauterine blood transfusion (via the intrauterine umbilical cord). This has produced good results in specialist centers where this is possible, even though this has some associated procedural risk to the fetus. What seems fairly certain, however, is that once the PVB19-induced anemia and infection have resolved, the fetuses do not suffer any other abnormality or long term complications.

Cytomegalovirus (CMV)

Cytomegalovirus (CMV) infection is usually acquired, asymptomatically, during childhood. Unlike rubella and PVB19 infections that are transmitted by short range respiratory droplets, or VZV transmitted by the airborne route, CMV is usually transmitted by direct contact – probably by saliva from parents to children. Since many primary CMV infections are asymptomatic, the incubation period is not always easy to determine, but is generally accepted to be about 3 weeks at the most. Symptomatic infection more often occurs in teenagers and adults, where the clinical presentation mimics glandular fever (acute Epstein–Barr virus infection) with fever, sore throat, swollen glands (lymphadenopathy), and occasionally a faint, generalized maculopapular rash. Usually, the clinical disease has no serious complications in normal, healthy immunocompetent individuals. The virus is shed in the saliva and urine during primary infection and can be shed intermittently throughout life during CMV reactivation. After primary infection, CMV remains latent in a type of circulating white cell (monocytes), with occasional reactivations throughout life. In immunocompromised individuals (e.g. those on chemotherapy for cancer, with advanced AIDS or other acquired or inherited immunodeficiency), CMV reactivation can cause severe, life-threatening disease.

For maternal infection, the diagnosis of primary CMV infection is usually made using a combination of viral culture (usually from urine), serology for CMV IgG (going from negative to positive) or IgM (a single strong positive result), and CMV DNA PCR testing (to detect CMV DNA in blood, cerebrospinal fluid surrounding the brain, biopsy tissues, etc.). Unlike rubella, VZV, and PVB19, where major fetal damage occurs only with maternal viral infections present within the first 20 weeks of pregnancy, CMV can cause fetal damage throughout pregnancy. However, there is data to show that again, CMV causes the most damage during fetal organogenesis during the first 20 weeks of gestation.

Currently, there is no licenced CMV vaccine, though there are some very toxic anti-CMV antiviral drugs available. Now, CMV is the most common cause of congenital infection in the developed world, affecting 0.5–1.3% of all live births.

Pathogenesis

Maternal primary CMV infection results in a systemic viremia that includes the placenta. CMV enters maternal white blood cells where they replicate, and some are carried across the placenta into the fetal circulation. Fetal CMV viremia results, which is relatively uninhibited in the absence of a mature fetal immune response or maternal anti-CMV antibodies. Fetal damage occurs through several mechanisms, including "apoptosis" (virus-induced cell death) of fetal brain cell, fetal cell chromosomal damage, downregulation of growth factors in fetal lungs, and disruption of fetal blood vessels leading to heart abnormalities. Maternal immune responses may limit some of this damage.

Unlike rubella that interferes with the development of fetal organs, CMV allows fetal organs to form normally, but then damages them making them dysfunctional. Thus, whilst the damage from rubella is limited to the first 20 weeks of gestation during fetal organogenesis, CMV can continue to damage organs up to, and even after birth. Even after birth, in up to 15% of otherwise apparently healthy CMV-infected neonates, CMV continues to damage mainly the hearing "hair" cells, causing variable degrees of irreversible sensorineural ("nerve") deafness, as well as inducing more subtle effects, such as mental retardation and learning difficulties. Hence, at birth a CMV-infected baby may be of low birth weight, have a petechial skin rash, "thrombocytopenia" (i.e. low platelets – blood cells that assist clotting), enlarged liver and spleen, suffer from inflammation of the liver ("hepatitis" and "jaundice" – a yellowing of the skin and eyes), the lungs ("pneumonitis"), the heart ("myocarditis"), the brain ("encephalitis"), with damage to the eyes ("chorioretinitis", cataracts, blindness), and ears (sensorineural deafness). Often these abnormalities are not severe enough to kill the neonate, but may make life more difficult for both the baby and the parents. Some of these abnormalities will be difficult or impossible to detect on ultrasound scanning (e.g. sensorineural deafness and mental retardation).

Prenatal diagnosis

It must be again emphasized that an infected fetus may not necessarily mean a damaged fetus – especially with CMV, when sometimes the only damage may be a variable degree of deafness or mental retardation that cannot be diagnosed using ultrasound. With confirmed maternal primary CMV infection, about 40% of these mothers will transmit the CMV to their fetuses, and overall, about 7–10% of babies born to such mothers will have some CMV-induced damage identifiable at birth. So, if we take 100 such CMV-infected mothers, about 40 will infect their fetuses, resulting in three or four babies (7–10% of 40) who will be born with some identifiable CMV-related damage. However, of the remaining asymptomatic, apparently normal 36–37 CMV-infected babies, another four or five (10–15% of 36–37) of these will then go on to develop CMV-related sensorineural deafness or mental retardation. Hence in this example, out of 100 CMV-infected mothers, between about seven and nine babies will be CMV-affected. Reactivated CMV infection during pregnancy has also been shown to cause fetal damage that can be just as severe as that caused by primary CMV infection, but this is much less frequent (0.24–2.2% as compared with 7–10%).

Prenatal diagnosis for possible congenital CMV infection relies mainly on amniocentesis (amniotic fluid sampling) for CMV culture and PCR, and cordocentesis (fetal blood sampling) for CMV IgM and PCR. Both are useful in confirming fetal CMV infection. However, again sampling should take place about 4–6 weeks after maternal infection to avoid false positive results. In addition, sampling for both fetal blood and amniotic fluid should be performed after 21 weeks' gestational age to avoid false negative results from an immature fetal immune response, or immature fetal kidneys that have yet to excrete CMV positive urine as amniotic fluid, respectively. More recently, there have been some studies showing that the probability of fetal damage can be related to the CMV load in the amniotic fluid, though this is not universally accepted yet, and CMV assays may vary considerably between different testing laboratories.

Management options

It is very difficult to advise the parents on the likely outcomes and best course of action for their child for a number of reasons: (i) the abnormalities caused by congenital CMV infection are generally less severe than those of CRS; (ii) the majority of CMV-infected fetuses will be normal (at least, above the background rate of fetal abnormalities from other causes); (iii) the severity of CMV-induced fetal damage can be very variable and may not be easily detected on ultrasound; and (iv) CMV-induced damage may continue evolving even after birth. For a very small group of severely damaged CMV-infected fetuses, clinical trials with an antiviral drug against CMV (ganciclovir) have shown that intravenous treatment with this drug for CMV-infected fetuses for their first 6 weeks of life can limit any further, evolving CMV damage (consisting mainly of sensorineural deafness). However, such treatment does not reverse any damage already done by the virus and there are also serious side-effects from the ganciclovir. In addition, treatment requires a lengthy hospital stay for intravenous therapy, although there is a now a new, oral form of this drug available (valganciclovir) that may eventually allow long term treatment, as an outpatient. In addition, long term sequelae of congenital CMV infection may still be detected as long as 2 years after birth, so it remains to be seen whether such treated babies benefit significantly later in life and whether the CMV disease is truly halted.

Congenital infections: parasitic

Toxoplasmosis

Toxoplasmosis is not a nationally reportable disease in the USA, and no reliable data are available at the national level about the number of cases diagnosed each year. Since the 1960s, rates of infection with *Toxoplasma gondii* in the USA appear to be declining. The most reliable estimate of *T. gondii* seroprevalence in the USA is derived from the third National Health and Nutrition Examination Survey, which was conducted during 1988–1994. Of 5988 women of childbearing age (i.e. age 12–49 years), 14% were seropositive (CDC, unpublished data, 1994). No recent US studies of a large population of pregnant women have been conducted to determine the incidence of new infections during pregnancy.

Two prospective studies in the 1970s both reported rates of congenital toxoplasmosis of approximately 10 per 10 000 live births. More recent data regarding the rate of congenital toxoplasmosis are available from the New England Regional Newborn Screening Program. During 1986–1992, of 635 000 infants who underwent serological testing, 52 were infected, representing an infection rate of approximately 1 per 10 000 live births. If these rates (i.e. 1 per 10 000 and 10 per 10 000) were extrapolated to the approximately 4 million live births in the USA each year, an estimated 400–4000 infants would be born each year with congenital toxoplasmosis.

Clinical features

Human infection is acquired most commonly by ingestion of tissue cysts in raw, poorly cooked or cured meat or via ingestion of oocysts derived from cat feces contaminating soil or inadequately washed vegetables. A report conducted by USDA's Economic Research Service concluded that one half of the toxoplasmosis cases in the USA are caused by eating contaminated meat. Pork has been implicated by some authorities as the meat most commonly associated with foodborne toxoplasmosis. Tachyzoites of *T. gondii* (see lifecycle under "Microbiology and virulence" below) are also able to cross the placenta, infect the placenta, and in a second step infect the fetus.

Most immunocompetent individuals develop few if any symptoms and infection persists for life without any signs of disease. Maternal infection often occurs with no or mild symptoms only. Maternal infection may lead between 4 and 8 weeks later to placental infection followed by fetal infection with potential for congenital damage. The incidence and severity of congenital toxoplasmosis depends on when in pregnancy the women acquires the infection. Transplacental infection occurs in about one-third of affected pregnancies. Later maternal infection (in the third trimester) is more likely to result in fetal infection as the placental blood flow is of higher volume, but risk of severe damage is less because the fetus is more developed. Fetal infection may however lead to abortion or stillbirth. Severe congenital damage is associated with infection in early gestation, less than 16 weeks.

The most extreme form of congenital toxoplasmosis is the classic triad of chorioretinitis (lesions on the retina), hydrocephalus, and intracranial calcification, but this is fortunately rare. More common clinical manifestations of congenital toxoplasmosis include encephalitis, cerebral palsy, epilepsy, jaundice, enlarged liver and spleen (hepatosplenomegaly), thrombocytopenia, and rash. Many congenitally infected neonates show no signs of infection at birth but develop chorioretinitis later in life.

Diagnosis

In many countries screening for antibodies to *T. gondii* is not routinely performed on antenatal women at their booking visit. However if there are concerns about possible acquisition during pregnancy then serological tests to detect presence of IgM and seroconversion from no antibody against *T. gondii* to an IgG positive response during pregnancy is the mainstay of maternal diagnosis. Congenital toxoplasmosis is most commonly diagnosed by serological tests on both maternal and neonatal blood. Serology on amniotic fluid or fetal blood from cordocentesis can be useful for diagnosing congenital infection. *T. gondii* can be cultured at a reference laboratory but culture methods are slow. Rapid molecular techniques such as PCR have recently been introduced for testing blood and amniotic fluid. Ultrasound can be used to search for features of congenital toxoplasmosis in the fetus *in utero* and in neonates following birth.

Management and prevention

Antiprotozoal treatment consists of simultaneous administration of sulfadiazine and pyrimethamine and is directed against the active tachyzoite form. Spiramycin is a macrolide antimicrobial that concentrates in the placenta, reducing placental infection by 60%. It does not pass through the placental barrier and is therefore only used to prevent vertical transmission from mother to fetus. Complete eradication of the dormant cyst form (the bradyzoite form) is not achievable.

In congenital toxoplasmosis, the drug therapy may be intended to treat the mother, the fetus, or the newborn. If fetal infection is diagnosed, the risk of serious congenital disease (especially in early pregnancy) may outweigh any consideration of potential teratogenic effects of antifolate antimicobials such as sulfadiazine or pyrimethamine. The maternal regimen should be switched to sulfadiazine plus pyrimethamine. All infected newborns should have sulfadiazine plus pyrimethamine for at least 6 months, usually 12. Termination of pregnancy is commonly offered to women who seroconvert in the first 8 weeks of pregnancy and to those infected in the first 22 weeks of pregnancy when fetal infection is confirmed.

Primary prevention of congenital toxoplasmosis is via health education for all women in the immediate preconception period and during pregnancy (especially for women known to be seronegative for *T. gondii*). Women should be advised to avoid any potential *T. gondii* cyst contact such as consumption or handling of undercooked meats or the changing of cat litter or gardening unless wearing gloves.

Microbiology and virulence

T. gondii is a protozoal organism with a complex lifecycle (Figure 12.3). The sexual cycle occurs in the gut epithelium of the definitive host (members of the cat family) and leads to excretion of oocysts in their feces.

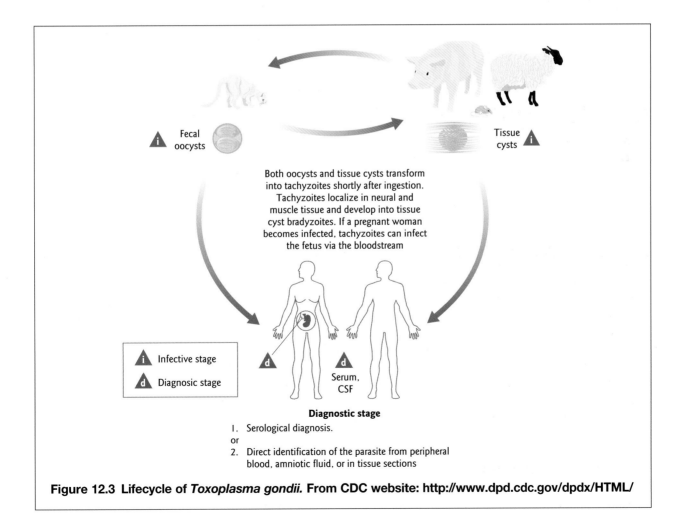

Figure 12.3 Lifecycle of *Toxoplasma gondii*. From CDC website: http://www.dpd.cdc.gov/dpdx/HTML/

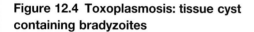

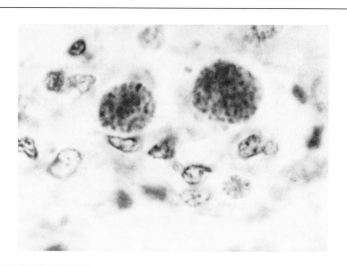

Figure 12.4 Toxoplasmosis: tissue cyst containing bradyzoites

The asexual cycle occurs in secondary hosts (birds and most mammals including man) when ingestion of the oocyst is followed by release of the active forms, the *T. gondii* tachyzoites. The tachyzoites then disseminate by blood, lymphatic system and by active cell invasion. Multiplication of tachyzoites occurs in all nucleated cells, infected cells rupture and 8–32 tachyzoites are produced which can infect new cells. The immune response controls infection but some surviving parasites persist as bradyzoites within tissue cysts (Figure 12.4). Predation of secondary hosts (birds and rodents) completes the lifecycle as tissue cysts release their contents into gut lumen of cat and the active tachyzoites invade the intestinal epithelium.

Neonatal/perinatal infections

Neonatal sepsis is usually considered under two separate categories: early onset and late onset sepsis. Early onset sepsis is defined as sepsis that manifests in the first week of life and late onset is that which occurs after the first week of life. This is important because early onset sepsis is associated with organisms that are acquired during passage through the maternal birth canal, while late onset sepsis is associated with person to person transmission and therefore represents hospital or environmentally acquired organisms.

Neonatal/perinatal infections: bacterial

Early onset sepsis

Neonatal sepsis occurs at an estimated rate of 1–2 cases per 1000 live births in the USA. Blood cultures may be positive in up to 20% of infants in neonatal intensive care units (NICUs). The organisms that cause early onset (first week of life) sepsis include group B beta hemolytic *Streptococcus* (GBS) and *Escherichia coli*, which together may account for 70–80% of blood and cerebrospinal fluid cultures. Although less common, enterococci, *Listeria monocytogenes*, and species of Gram negative enteric bacilli other than *E. coli* are known to cause disease in neonates

Group B streptococcal sepsis

Asymptomatic colonization of the female genitourinary tract with GBS occurs in 17–25% of the population. However, GBS accounts for significant obstetric infections including urinary tract infection and endometritis (infection of the endometrium, the lining of the uterus). GBS is also the most important causative organism

Box 12.5 Important risk factors for early onset GBS disease

Maternal

- Previous delivery of an infant with GBS disease
- GBS bacteruria during pregnancy

Labor

- Clinically evident amnionitis (infection of the amniotic fluid surrounding the fetus)

- Prolonged interval between rupture of membranes and delivery (>18 hours)

Neonate

- Preterm birth (birth before 37 weeks' gestation)

---

of neonatal sepsis. In the USA more than 300 deaths occur annually as a result of GBS sepsis in the first 90 days of life. Early neonatal GBS infection is acquired through vertical transmission of GBS from mother to neonate during labor or delivery. Early GBS sepsis accounts for about 80% of GBS disease in the newborn and presents a variety of symptoms and signs.

Clinical features
Box 12.5 outlines the important risk factors for early onset GBS infection, although it can occur without any of these being present.

A GBS infected neonate may have a fever, feed or handle poorly, or develop difficulty with his/her breathing. There may be signs of a pneumonia or meningitis on examination or non-specific features of sepsis such as a bulging fontanelle, a skin rash, hepatosplenomegaly, or low blood sugar.

Diagnosis
An infection screen including blood, urine, and surface swab cultures should be sent as soon as infection is suspected. A lumbar puncture with urgent microscopy and culture of cerebrospinal fluid may be indicated. Group B streptococci grow readily on simple agar and demonstrate beta hemolysis. Antigen detection tests are available and can be applied to body fluids for rapid diagnosis. Full blood count, inflammatory marker measurement, and chest X-ray are also required.

Management and prevention
Urgent intravenous antimicrobials should be commenced after obtaining appropriate cultures; high dose benzylpenicillin and gentamicin are the usual empirical choices.

Studies in the 1980s demonstrated that treatment of mothers intrapartum or infants immediately postpartum with penicillin or ampicillin could reduce the incidence of early onset GBS infections in infants. In addition, it was noted that women who are at high risk of delivering infants who develop early onset GBS infections could be identified either by detection of GBS carriers through collection of recto-vaginal cultures at 35–37 weeks of gestation (the screening-based approach) or by recognition of certain obstetrical risk factors, such as having a threatened premature delivery or prolonged rupture of the membranes (the risk-based approach; see Box 12.5).

In 1996, the Centers for Disease Control and Prevention (CDC), in collaboration with the American College of Obstetricians and Gynecologists and the American Academy of Pediatrics, developed GBS prevention guidelines that advocated intrapartum antibiotics for women who are at high risk for delivering an infant with GBS disease. Using a GBS screening-based approach, it is estimated that an 80% reduction of early onset neonatal GBS infections would be possible, while an estimated 40% reduction would be possible using the risk-based prophylaxis approach. Most obstetric centers will use a combination of both these strategies.

Microbiology and virulence

Group B streptococci (GBS), also known as *Streptococci agalactiae*, are Gram positive cocci that demonstrate beta hemolysis on blood agar and test positive with Lancefield group B antisera.

The polysaccharide antiphagocytic capsule is the main pathogenicity determinant of GBS and babies of mothers with antibody to the four capsular types (Ia, Ib, II, and III) are protected from infection. Group B streptococci also produce enzymes capable of local inflammation and invasion.

Escherichia coli sepsis

E. coli bacteria have been discussed at length in the previous chapters on gastrointestinal and urinary tract infections (see Chapters 8 and 11). The clinical manifestation of *E. coli* sepsis in a neonate is similar to that caused by GBS.

Diagnosis and management

E. coli are readily cultured from blood, CSF, urine, and surface swabs on various types of agar. They are further identified by biochemical tests such as indole and urease. As some strains produce β-lactamases and aminoglycoside degrading enzymes treatment should be guided by sensitivity tests.

Microbiology and virulence

These, mainly lactose fermenting, Gram negative organisms are normal flora of the gastrointestinal tract. They may be present on and around the perineal area. *E. coli* is the commonest cause of urinary tract infections in pregnancy, can cause a chorioamnioitis (infection of the placenta and amniotic fluid surrounding the fetus) by ascending the genital tract, and is associated with early neonatal meningitis.

E. coli have lipopolysaccharide (LPS) molecules that are responsible for resistance to the bactericidal actitivity of complement. The lipid A core stimulates host macrophages to produce interleukin 1 and tumor necrosis factor responsible for fever and shock associated with *E. coli* sepsis. K1 is an extracellular capsular polysaccharide produced by some *E. coli* organisms; this is the most common type associated with neonatal meningitis. Fimbrae are bacterial organelles that allow attachment to host cells and are important in promoting colonization. *E. coli* organisms associated with meningitis and obstetric infections express P type fimbrae.

Ophthalmia neonatorum

Neonates who are born via a contaminated birth canal may present early (within 5 days) with a purulent conjunctivitis known as ophthalmia neonatorum (Figure 12.5). Ophthalmia neonatorum can be caused by *Neisseria gonorrheae* or by *Chlamydia trachomatis*, the two most common sexually transmitted infections (see also Chapter 11).

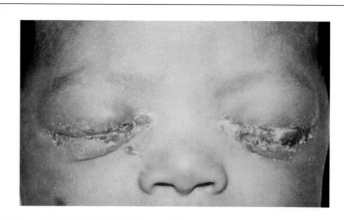

**Figure 12.5 Ophthalmia neonatorum.
Courtesy Department of Microbiology,
University College Hospitals, London**

Neisseria gonorrheae

The diagnosis is suspected by microscopy of eye swabs that demonstrate characteristic intracellular Gram diplococci. The diagnosis is confirmed with the growth of *N. gonorrheae* on chocolate agar and further biochemical and serological tests. Systemic benzylpenicillin or a third generation cephalosporin is used to treat this condition. The mother and all sexual contacts should be counseled, screened, and treated for *N. gonorrheae* if found. Dual infection with *N. gonorrheae* and *C. trachomatis* is common.

Microbiology and virulence

N. gonorrheae are Gram negative intracellular diplococci that are almost exclusively sexually transmitted. The organism is able to adhere to the genitourinary epithelium via pili and antigenic variation of these pili means that recovery from infection provides no immunity. The organism invades the epithelial layer and provokes a local acute inflammatory response.

Chlamydia trachomatis

C. trachomatis is the commonest agent causing sexually transmitted disease. In the USA the prevalence of *C. trachomatis* infection in antenatal women is between 8% and 10% and there is recent evidence that this figure is on the rise. Up to 70% of infected antenatal women may be asymptomatic. Neonates acquire infection via transit through the birth canal. Approximately 30% of neonates born to mothers infected with *C. trachomatis* will develop a mucopurulent unilateral or bilateral severe conjunctivitis that presents on average 6–10 days following birth, chlamydial ophthalmia neonatorum (Figure 12.5). Between 10% and 20% of colonized neonates may develop *C. trachomatis* pneumonitis that presents as difficulty in breathing and recurrent cough between 3 weeks and 3 months of life.

Diagnosis and management

C. trachomatis conjunctivitis and pneumonitis can be most easily diagnosed by molecular techniques such as polymerase chain reaction (PCR) performed on eye swabs or respiratory secretions. The organism can be cultured using cell cultures but this is usually only available in a reference laboratory setting. Erythromycin administered systemically is the antimicrobial of choice for chlamydial pneumonitis and conjunctivitis.

Microbiology and virulence

C. trachomatis is a nonmotile obligate intracellular bacterium with a two phase lifecycle. Unable to synthesize its own adenosine triphosphate (ATP), the chlamydia organism requires an exogenous (host) source. The infectious form of the organism is referred to as the elementary body (EB) which attaches to and enters the host cell. After entering the host cell, the EBs begin a second lifecycle as metabolically active reticulate bodies (RBs). The RBs use host-derived ATP to replicate by binary fission. Up to several hundred progeny are produced within a large cytoplasmic inclusion. These newly replicated RBs reorganize into the infectious EBs and are released by the host cell – thus completing the lifecycle (see Figures 11.19 and 11.20). The major outer membrane protein participates in attachment to mucosal cells and a large cysteine rich protein may also be associated with virulence.

Late onset sepsis

See Table 12.1 for the organisms implicated in neonatal late onset sepsis. Late GBS neonatal sepsis (occurring after 1 week) is associated with lower mortality, often presents as acute meningitis, and may result from hospital or community acquired infection. Several other organisms such as *Staphylococcus aureus* and *Candida* spp. are common causes of sepsis in the neonatal unit; their severity is related to the unique vulnerability of the neonate, in particular the preterm neonate. Immaturity of the neonatal immune system, particularly in the preterm neonate, is the single most important factor that predisposes to sepsis. Management of sepsis depends on the organism implicated and the severity of infection.

Neonatal/perinatal infections: viral

The congenital viral infections (rubella, varicella zoster, parvovirus B19, and cytomegalovirus) are so named as they usually infect the developing fetus by crossing the placenta during maternal infection. The neonatal or perinatal viral infections that will be discussed in this chapter (HIV, hepatitis B and C, herpes simplex virus, enteroviruses) usually infect the baby as it progress from the uterus through the vagina, around the time of delivery.

Varicella zoster virus (VZV) can cause both congenital infection ("congenital varicella syndrome"), during the first 20 weeks of pregnancy, as well as severe neonatal varicella infection and disease. Perinatally, VZV infects the baby during delivery if the mother develops chickenpox during the week before birth (when she is still viremic), or during the week after birth. This has been covered above in the section "Varicella zoster virus (VZV)."

Bloodborne viruses: human immunodeficiency virus (HIV), hepatitis B (HBV), hepatitis C (HCV)

Due to their more "peripheral" route of transmission, more effective interventions are available to protect the baby from neonatal/perinatal viral infections than from the congenital viral infections. The bloodborne viruses HIV, hepatitis B (HBV) and C (HCV) are generally acquired from the mother who is infected with these viruses, which are circulating in her blood (see also Chapters 18 and 19). Although HIV, HBV, and HCV rarely infect the fetus via the placenta (where HIV probably does this more commonly than HBV or HCV), most babies become infected with these bloodborne viruses when they inhale HIV-infected blood or other blood-contaminated maternal secretions during delivery. Exposure of the baby's mucous membranes (eyes, nose, and mouth) plus any invasive procedures performed by the obstetric team (e.g. scalp electrodes) where infected maternal blood may enter the baby's bloodstream, are all potential routes for neonatal/perinatal HIV infection. Hepatitis B and C are not usually transmitted transplacentally and nearly all infections are acquired neonatally or perinatally by exposure to infected maternal blood.

Management and prevention

There are several ways to prevent neonatal/perinatal infections with these bloodborne viruses. The initial step is to screen the expectant mother when she attends her first antenatal booking appointment. The timing of this may vary from clinic to clinic, but is generally around 12–16 weeks' gestation. Most clinics in the USA and Europe now screen for rubella (rubella IgG antibodies – the presence of these indicates lifelong immunity), HBV (HBV surface antigen, HBsAg – its presence indicating current HBV infection), and HIV (HIV antibodies – their presence indicating current HIV infection). With rubella (see "Congenital infections: viral" above), if the mother is not immune at this time, there is no recommended intervention (immunizations are contraindicated during pregnancy). She will just have to avoid contact with anyone who seems ill – particularly those with fever and rash illnesses – in the hope that she will not contract rubella infection during her pregnancy.

With HBV, if she is not immune, again, HBV immunization is not recommended during pregnancy (although accidental maternal immunizations with HBV vaccine have so far produced no reported adverse effects on the fetus). Unlike rubella, however, immunization of the baby (not the mother) at birth (then again at 1, 2 and 12 months of age), together with an injection of serum containing high levels of antibodies to HBV (HBV immunoglobulin – HBIG), is known to be effective in preventing HBV infection of the baby. Hence the intervention to prevent HBV infection of the baby can be delayed until the baby is born. Without this intervention, the risks of neonatal HBV infection can be as high as 30% during a normal vaginal delivery. With this intervention, cesarean section is not necessary. Breastfeeding should not be affected as HBV is not normally transmitted in breast milk and the baby will rapidly develop immunity to HBV from the combined HBV immunization and HBV anti-sera given at birth. If babies are infected with HBV at birth (which may occur despite all these preventative measures), >90% of them will remain HBV carriers for life, as the immature neonatal immune system learns to tolerate the virus and therefore does not actively try to eliminate it from the body. Life-long infection with HBV leads to an increase risk of chronic liver diseases, such as cirrhosis and hepatocellular carcinoma later in adulthood (see Chapter 19 and Further reading).

With HIV, there is no vaccine at present or any high-dose neutralizing antibody serum available. However, there are multiple anti-HIV (antiretroviral) drugs available which have been well tested in pregnancy (see Chapter 18). These drugs are given to the mother with newly diagnosed HIV infection, over several weeks to months (depending on whether the mother needs treatment for her HIV infection itself), to reduce the HIV load in her blood to very low levels to reduce the risk of the baby being HIV infected at birth. In addition, babies born to HIV-infected mothers are delivered by cesarean section, to avoid the more difficult vaginal delivery where the baby's eyes, nose, and mouth are exposed to HIV-infected maternal secretions. Also, the mother is advised not to breastfeed her baby, as HIV can be transmitted through breast milk. These three interventions can dramatically reduce the risk of HIV transmission to the newborn from about 30% to less than 5%, depending on how and when they are implemented, and on the nature of the maternal HIV infection. If the neonate is infected with HIV, despite all these precautions, untreated HIV in children has a more progressive, rapid course, though there are now many protocols to treat pediatric HIV/AIDS, however this subject is outside the present scope of this book (some additional detail can be found in the Further reading).

Unlike HBV and HIV, HCV is not routinely tested for at antenatal booking, but can be performed in certain high-risk women, e.g. present or past intravenous drug-users (IVDUs), those with hematological (blood) disorders such as thalassemia who require multiple blood transfusions. This is because HCV was only discovered in 1989 and many such patients have been inadvertently HCV infected from the transfusion of HCV-infected blood products, prior to this date (see Chapter 19). In addition, some hospitals screen for HCV for mothers who have water-births, though the rationale for this is somewhat dubious as HCV is not a waterborne virus infection. There is no vaccine for HCV and no high dose anti-HCV immunoglobulin preparation available. Although there is treatment for HCV infection, the drugs used (interferon and ribavirin) are very toxic to the developing fetus, so this is contraindicated during pregnancy. Fortunately, the efficiency of HCV transmission to the neonate is relatively low (estimated to be 1–5%). Some clinics can offer cesarean section instead of normal vaginal delivery, but this also has an associated risk, and thus some clinics do not offer any special treatment or intervention at all, as there are no universally accepted recommendations at present. Like HBV, HCV is not normally transmitted via breast milk, so breastfeeding is not usually contraindicated in a mother infected with HCV. Should the neonate become HCV-infected, there is currently no universally recommended management protocol and lifelong monitoring of HCV and liver function status may be required. In adults, HCV infection is naturally cleared in 15–20% of individuals, but with the greater immune tolerance of the neonatal immune system, natural HCV clearance may be less likely with HCV infections at birth (see Further reading).

With all of these bloodborne viruses, diagnosis of infection can be made by testing the neonate's blood for the antigen, antibody, or nucleic acid of the virus concerned (HBV, HIV, or HCV), with confirmatory testing performed on a follow-up sample, as required.

Herpes simplex viruses 1 and 2 (HSV-1, HSV-2)

The natural characteristics of human herpes simplex types 1 and 2 (HSV-1, HSV-2) infections have been already described elsewhere in Chapter 7. Virtually all clinically significant HSV infections of the newborn occur perinatally, i.e. during delivery or shortly after. The neonate is most vulnerable in the first month of life to primary HSV infections, where the mother has no pre-existing HSV antibodies to transfer to the newborn. Hence, the most dangerous scenario is if the mother develops a primary HSV infection in the 4–6 weeks prior to delivery, as HSV antibodies normally take this length of time to develop in adult primary HSV infections. Due to the nature of the infection, the most common type of neonatal HSV infection is by HSV-2, as this type most often causes genital herpes around the area of the mother's vagina.

Neonatal herpes manifests in several forms, one predominantly affecting the skin, eyes, and mouth (the cutaneous form), one predominantly affecting the central nervous system (CNS – brain, nerves, spinal cord), and another producing a more disseminated, generalized infection. The last two forms are serious and life-threatening, with a mortality rate of up to 80% without antiviral therapy for the CNS form. In these cases, even if the neonates survive, most of them will have long term neurological sequelae.

Over 90% of women of child-bearing age are already HSV-1 infected, up to 22% of women are HSV-2 infected (either singly or in combination with HSV-1), and of these, 2% may acquire their HSV-2 infection during pregnancy – with primary maternal HSV infection in the third trimester being the highest risk scenario for the neonate. Up to 90% of these women with primary HSV-2 infection may be undiagnosed because they are asymptomatic or any illness is ascribed to other causes.

Management and prevention

Unlike the bloodborne viruses described above, maternal HSV infections are rarely screened for during pregnancy. This is because the lifecycle of HSV infection differs significantly from HBV, HCV, and HIV. Generally with these latter bloodborne viruses, the antenatal screening tests detect markers of current infection, i.e. the mother's blood will contain these viruses if the tests are positive. This is not the case with detection of HSV antibodies, which only indicate previous or recent HSV infection, but not necessarily circulating HSV in the bloodstream. In fact, HSV is often inactive in the human body, even though HSV-1 infects nearly all of us during early childhood before the age of 10 years. Typically, HSV-1 reactivates from either the trigeminal ganglia (where the virus emerges from neurons in the upper spinal cord) and usually causes painful cold sores around and within the mouth. Usually, HSV-2 tends to infect very sexually active individuals (with high numbers of sexual partners) later during their adolescent or young adult years. HSV-2 reactivates from the sacral ganglia (where the virus emerges from neurons in the lower spinal cord) and causes genital herpes. Occasionally, HSV-1 can be found in genital herpes lesions and HSV-2 can be found in cold sores.

Hence, the problem of perinatal/neonatal herpes infections cannot be solved by screening the mother for HSV antibodies, as this does not indicate whether the mother is actively shedding the virus in her genital tract during the perinatal period. Some studies have tried periodic swabbing of the genital area with viral culture/detection during the perinatal period, but it is not practical to swab this region continuously until the time of birth. Although some obstetric teams will actively examine the genital area for signs of genital herpes close to the time of delivery, many cases of neonatal herpes infection occur from mothers who are clinically asymptomatic, i.e. no visible herpes lesions are present around the genital area prior to delivery.

Diagnosis of neonatal herpes infection can be performed by testing swabs (of the eyes, nose, mouth, or skin lesions), or blood (for disseminated infection), or the cerebrospinal fluid for HSV nucleic acid (DNA) using PCR, and/or viral culture for the swabs.

There is no licensed vaccine against HSV-1 or HSV-2 at present, however there is an effective antiviral drug, aciclovir and its related compounds (e.g. valaciclovir). These drugs can be given to the mother if she shows signs of primary HSV infection, particularly in the last trimester, when the risk of adverse effects of the drug on the fetus is minimal, and the benefits in preventing neonatal herpes infection are maximal. The baby can also be delivered by cesarean section and treated with these same drugs from birth to minimize the risk of developing neonatal HSV infection.

In addition, screening of both mother and father for HSV status may be useful. If the father is HSV antibody positive (meaning that he has been HSV infected already), and the mother has not, then there is risk of the father transmitting his HSV infection to the mother (e.g. through kissing or sexual intercourse) during her pregnancy and giving her a primary HSV infection. Maternal abstinence from sexual and oral-genital contact in this situation can prevent HSV infection during pregnancy – though this may be difficult and require a strong will on the part of both parties. If the parents are discordant with regard to the two different types of HSV, i.e. the mother is only HSV-1 infected and the father is only HSV-2 infected, there is some potential cross-protection possible between the antibodies to the two different HSV types, but this may not prevent fetal infection and disease entirely (see also Box 7.3).

Enteroviruses

Conventionally, over 70 different serotypes (each with different antibody specificities) of enteroviruses have been defined. These have been subdivided into different groups: echoviruses (serotypes 1–34), coxsackievirus A (serotypes 1–24), coxsackievirus B (6 serotypes), enterovirus (EV, serotypes 68–72), and poliovirus (3 serotypes). All of them can cause serious primary infection in the newborn, particularly where there is no transferred maternal antibody protection. As the child becomes older, infections with different serotypes of enteroviruses allow some cross-protection against other serotypes, reducing the severity of illness (see also Chapter 7). Enteroviruses can be transmitted to the newborn, during delivery via infected maternal secretions during an acute maternal enterovirus infection. A large variety of neonatal clinical disease can be produced, including hand-foot-and-mouth (HFMD) disease, flaccid paralysis (where the paralyzed limbs become "floppy"), inflammation of the heart ("myocarditis" and "pericarditis"), chest pains ("pleurodynia"), sore mouth and throat ("herpangia," "croup," and "pharyngitis"), inflammation of the brain and/or it's membranes ("encephalitis" and/or "meningitis"), inflammation of the liver ("hepatitis"), red eyes ("conjunctivitis"), and generalized sepsis. In some cases, such neonatal enterovirus infection can be fatal.

Management and prevention

There is no licensed vaccine or antiviral for the prevention or treatment of enterovirus infections at present. Recognition of both maternal and neonatal enterovirus infection can be difficult as the variety of symptoms and signs are so wide. General malaise, a sore throat, a headache, some chest pains, with or without a fever, with or without a rash, in the mother may all be symptoms and signs of an enterovirus infection around the time of delivery; unless enterovirus infection is considered, it may not be tested for and may be missed. Similarly in the infant, nonspecific symptoms can include lethargy, irritability, poor feeding, fever, and/or rash. More serious manifestations include meningitis/encephalitis, hepatitis, pneumonia, and myocarditis, all of which may become life-threatening (see Further reading).

During acute infection, enteroviruses are shed in a variety of body fluids (saliva and other respiratory secretions, stool) and vaginal secretions, so neonatal infection usually comes from the acutely infected mother. For the infected neonate, an experimental, potentially beneficial drug exists (pleconaril, which is still in clinical trials at the time of writing), but where this is unavailable, therapy is supportive – particularly with regard to the respiratory and cardiovascular systems. Immunoglobulin (pooled serum antibodies from multiple blood donors) is also used to treat such neonates, as it may contain some specific or cross-reacting antibodies, but the reported responses have been variable.

Mortality rates of neonatal enterovirus infection range from 0% to over 80%, with damage to the heart and liver accounting for most deaths, though CNS enterovirus infections can lead to a wide range of long term abnormalities including mental retardation, poor motor skills, and seizure disorders. Fortunately, neonates who survive severe enterovirus infections (affecting the liver, heart, and lungs), with the exception of those suffering from neurological disease, generally recover without long term complications.

Emerging infections, pregnancy, neonatal infections

Recently emerging viral infections (some of which are described elsewhere in this book), including West Nile virus, monkeypox, severe acute respiratory syndrome-associated coronavirus (SARS-CoV), agents of bioterrorism, and the viral hemorrhagic fevers, may also have potentially adverse effects on the developing fetus (*in utero*) as well as perinatally (around the time of delivery). In addition, new vaccines developed to combat such emerging infections may also have unknown effects on pregnancy and the neonate. More data and experience is required before any definitive congenital/perinatal syndromes can be determined and protocols developed to deal with these, but some considerations can be found in the Further reading material listed below.

Case study 12.1

A child developed unilateral mucopurulent conjunctivitis 10 days after birth. The child was born by vaginal delivery, and there were no significant intrapartum or postpartum complications. A review of the mother's antenatal history revealed that she had used drugs before pregnancy and had had a recent change in partner.

A conjunctival scraping was inoculated on to McCoy cell lines; iodine staining (40×) of a positive cell culture shows characteristic inclusion bodies:

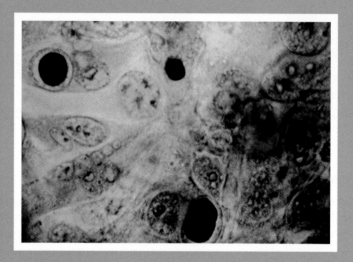

1. What is your probable diagnosis?
2. How did the child acquire this organism?
3. What other eye infection might the child have acquired in a similar manner?

Case study 12.2

A woman presents to the antenatal clinic 4 months pregnant with her first child. She feels very well. Urine microscopy and culture results are as follows:

- Urine microscopy: >50 WBC/mm^3; no RBC; no epithelial cells
- Culture: >10^5 cfu/ml of *E. coli*; typical colonies seen on a MacConkey agar plate are shown below:

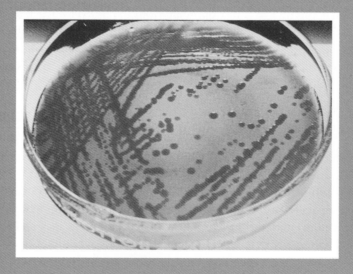

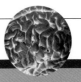

Test yourself

1. Why is the patient asymptomatic?
2. Would you treat in the absence of symptoms?
3. What complications may occur?

Case study 12.3

A pediatrician is called to the postnatal ward to see a baby born 12 hours ago. Labor was long and the delivery difficult, eventually needing the use of forceps. The mother had premature rupture of membranes for 12 hours prior to delivery and a fever of 38.5°C during labor.

On examination the baby is pale and lethargic, has a faint heart murmur, crepitations in both lung fields, and a palpable liver. The following shows the Gram stain of the organism isolated from blood culture:

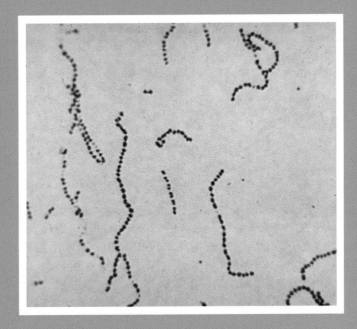

1. What is the baby suffering from?
2. Is this early or late onset disease?
3. Why is this important?
4. What are the predisposing factors in this mother's history?
5. What are the strategies for prevention?

Further reading

Best JM. Rubella. *Semin Fetal Neonatal Med* 2007;12(3):182–192

d'Oulx EA, Chiappini E, de Martino M, Tovo PA. Treatment of pediatric HIV infection. *Curr Infect Dis Rep* 2007;9(5):425–433

Hawkins D, Blott M, Clayden P, et al; BHIVA Guidelines Writing Committee. Guidelines for the management of HIV infection in pregnant women and the prevention of mother-to-child transmission of HIV. *HIV Med* 2005;6(suppl 2):107–148

Kimberlin DW. Management of HSV encephalitis in adults and neonates: diagnosis, prognosis and treatment. *Herpes* 2007;14(1):11–16

Kravetz JD, Federman DG. Toxoplasmosis in pregnancy. *Am J Med* 2005;118(3):212–216

MacLean AB, Regan L, Carrington D (eds). *Infection and Pregnancy*. London: Royal College of Obstetricians and Gynaecologists (RCOG) Press, 2001, 394pp

Mast EE, Margolis HS, Fiore AE, et al; Advisory Committee on Immunization Practices (ACIP). A comprehensive immunization strategy to eliminate transmission of hepatitis B virus infection in the USA: recommendations of the Advisory Committee on Immunization Practices (ACIP) part 1: immunization of infants, children, and adolescents. *MMWR Recomm Rep* 2005;54(RR-16):1–31

Rasmussen SA, Hayes EB, Jamieson DJ, O'Leary DR. Emerging infections and pregnancy: assessing the impact on the embryo or fetus. *Am J Med Genet A* 2007;143(24):2896–2903

Revello MG, Gerna G. Diagnosis and management of human cytomegalovirus infection in the mother, fetus, and newborn infant. *Clin Microbiol Rev* 2002;15(4):680–715

Rittichier KR, Bryan PA, Bassett KE, et al. Diagnosis and outcomes of enterovirus infections in young infants. *Pediatr Infect Dis J* 2005;24(6):546–550

Young NS, Brown KE. Parvovirus B19. *N Engl J Med* 2004;350(6):586–597

Zuckerman AJ, Banatvala JE, Pattison JR, Griffiths P, Schoub B (eds). *Principles and Practice of Clinical Virology*, 5th edition. London: Wiley, 2004, 912pp

Useful websites

Listeriosis and Pregnancy: What is Your Risk? Safe Food Handling for a Healthy Pregnancy. http://www.fsis.usda.gov/Fact_Sheets/Listeriosis_and_Pregnancy_What_is_Your_Risk/index.asp

Prevention of Perinatal Group B Streptococcal Disease Revised Guidelines from CDC. http://www.cdc.gov/mmwr/preview/mmwrhtml/rr5111a1.htm

Specific websites on congenital viral infections

http://www.emedicine.com/med/topic3270.htm

http://virology-online.com/presentations/congenital.htm

Images of various congenital syndromes

Congenital CMV infection. http://www.med.nagoya-u.ac.jp/ped/super/data/IMAGE/CMV.GIF

Congenital varicella syndrome (VZV). http://www.sepeap.es/revisiones/neonatologia/Varicelacongenita.bmp

Fetal hydrops (parvovirus B19). http://www.pathguy.com/lectures/hydrops.jpg

Chapter 13

Infections in the immunocompromised host

D. Mack, N. Shetty

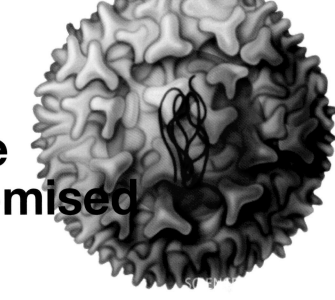

Introduction
   Host defense mechanisms
   The immunocompromised host
   Pathophysiology
Clinical syndromes
   Primary immunodeficiency syndromes
   Hematological malignancies
   Hematopoietic stem cell transplantation
   Solid organ transplantation
   Immunosuppressive medications
   Sepsis induced immunosuppression
   HIV infection
   Mannose binding lectin deficiency

Infecting organisms
   Bacteria
   Fungi
   Viruses
   Parasites
Clinical approach
   History and examination
   Investigations
   Clinical presentations
Prevention and treatment
   Preventative measures

Introduction

Host defense mechanisms

The innate immune system provides largely nonspecific protection against the initiation of infections. Its components include epithelial barriers, phagocytes, complement, and natural killer cells. The adaptive immune system mediates targeted defense against repeated infections. The two arms of this system comprise humoral immunity, directed against extracellular organisms, and cell-mediated immunity, directed against intracellular organisms (see Chapter 3).

The immunocompromised host

The term "immunocompromised host" encompasses a group of patients with diverse and often overlapping conditions which impair various host defense mechanisms, and decrease the patients' ability to respond to infectious diseases. The normal host defenses include the cells of the immune system, immunoglobulins, complement, and various biochemical and physical barriers. Compromise of one or more of these components predisposes the host to a range of infections, depending on the nature of the defect, or defects. Focal defects may result in specific susceptibilities, for example splenic dysfunction predisposes the patient to infections with encapsulated bacteria. In other cases, broad impairment of many components of host defense, such as occurs following bone marrow transplantation, results in susceptibility to infection by a wide range of organisms. The acquired immune deficiency syndrome gives rise to progressive immunocompromise following HIV infection, which predisposes patients to a range of opportunistic infections including cryptococosis and toxoplasmosis.

Pathophysiology

Anatomical barrier defects

Physical barriers to infection include the epithelial of the skin, gastrointestinal tract, and respiratory tract. These epithelia are associated with substances, secretions, and specialized cells with antimicrobial properties. In addition, the barriers are colonized by the commensal microorganisms, in symbiosis with the host.

The physical barriers to infection may be disrupted by trauma, surgery, and the insertion of catheters or other foreign bodies. The integrity of the barriers may be impaired by treatments including chemotherapy, and antibiotic therapy which removes the commensal flora permitting colonization with potentially more virulent organisms. Anatomical barrier defects predispose patients to infections with skin colonizing organisms such as staphylococci, and gastrointestinal tract commensals such as streptococci and *Pseudomonas* species (Table 13.1).

Neutropenia

Neutropenia is defined as an absolute neutrophil count of less than 500 cells/mm^3 or less than 1000 cells/mm^3 but expected to decrease to less than 500 cells/mm^3 within 48 hours. Neutropenia may arise as a consequence of hematological disorders including acute leukemia and aplastic anemia. The use of cytotoxic chemotherapy for the treatment of hematological and solid organ malignancies may give rise to severe and prolonged periods of neutropenia.

As neutophils provide the primary defense against bacterial and some fungal infections, neutropenia predisposes patients to these infections. There is a linear relationship between both the severity and duration of neutropenia and incidence of infections (Figure 13.1).

Most infections are caused by bacteria or fungi from the patient's endogenous flora, the majority arising from the flora of the gastrointestinal tract. Until the early 1980s, most infections in neutropenic chemotherapy patients were caused by Gram negative bacteria, but since this time Gram positive bacterial infections have begun to predominate over Gram negative infections. Reasons for this shift include the increased use of intravascular devices, and the use prophylactic antibiotics with extensive Gram negative cover such as ciprofloxacin. Early in the course of neutropenia, most infections are bacterial in origin, with the emergence of fungal infections usually occurring in the setting of prolonged and profound neutropenia (Figure 13.2).

Innate immune system dysfunction

The innate immune system contributes to the host's rapid, nonspecific defenses against bacterial and fungal organisms. Mechanisms include the complement-mediated activation of neutophils, the opsonization and

Table 13.1 Type of infection related to the immune system and immunosuppressive agents

Immunodeficiency	Causes	Infectious risk
Innate immunity		
Anatomic barrier defects	Trauma Surgery Catheter insertion Prostheses	Bacteria: Gram positive – staphylococci, viridans streptococci, enterococci. Corynebacteria; Gram negative – Enterobacteriaceae, *Pseudomonas* spp., *Acinetobacter* spp. Fungal: *Candida* spp. Viral: Herpes simplex virus
Neutropenia	Acute leukemia Aplastic anemia Cytotoxic chemotherapy	Bacteria: predominantly Gram positive. Enterobacteriaceae, *Pseudomonas* spp. Fungal: *Candida* spp. and *Aspergillus* spp.
Therapy	High dose chemotherapy Corticosteroids Radiotherapy	Bacterial: Gram positive – staphylococci, viridans streptococci, *Nocardia* spp.; Gram-negative – bacilli (*Escherichia coli*, *Klebsiella* spp., *Pseudomonas* spp.) Fungal: *Candida* spp., *Aspergillus* spp.
Adaptive immunity		
Cellular	High dose chemotherapy Radiotherapy Immunosuppressive therapies (corticosteroids, cyclophosphamide, ciclosporin A, tacrolimus, methotrexate, azathioprine, rapamycin, anti-lymphocyte serum, monoclonal antibodies)	Bacterial: *Legionella* spp., *Mycobacterium tuberculosis*, atypical mycobacteria, *Nocardia* species *Listeria monocytogenes*, *Salmonella* spp. Fungal: *Candida* spp., *Aspergillus* spp., *Cryptococcus neoformans*, *Histoplasma capsulatum*, PCP, *Coccidioides immitis* Viral: cytomegalovirus, varicella-zoster virus, herpes simplex virus, Epstein–Barr virus, live viral vaccines (measles, mumps, rubella, poliovirus)
Humoral	High dose corticosteroids, cyclophosphamide, mycophenolate mofetil	Bacterial: Gram positive – streptococci (*S. pneumoniae*, others); Gram negative – *Haemophilus influenzae*, *Neisseria meningitidis*, *Capnocytophaga canimorsus* Viral: enterovirus Parasites: *Giardia lamblia*
Splenic dysfunction	Splenectomy Sickle cell disease	Bacterial: *Streptococcus pneumoniae*, *Haemophilus influenzae*, *Salmonella* infections in sickle cell disease Protozoal: malaria, babesiosis

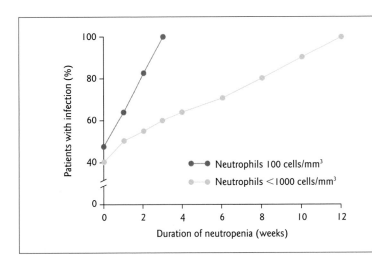

Figure 13.1 Incidence of infection according to duration and severity of neutropenia

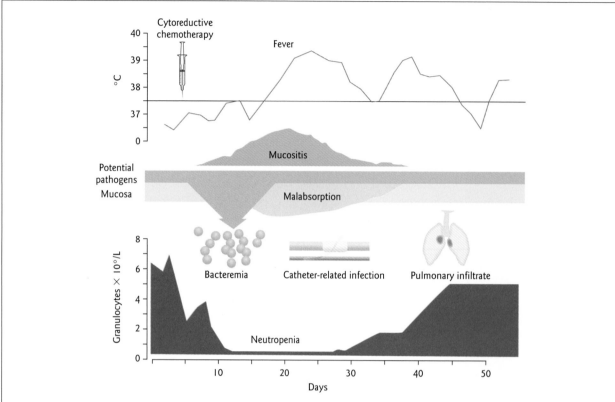

Figure 13.2 The sequence of events during neutropenia. Profound granulocytopenia and mucosal damage usually develop about a week after the start of cytoreductive chemotherapy. Fever develops around a week later, and, if there is bacteremia, it mostly occurs at this time. Signs and symptoms usually manifest themselves during the first few days of fever, that is, during the third week after starting chemotherapy. Infectious complications related to the lung tend to occur a few days later, often being recognized only after 5–6 days of fever.

destruction of bacteria, and the production of soluble inflammatory mediators such as C reactive protein (CRP) and lipopolysaccharide binding protein.

Treatment with chemotherapeutic agents or corticosteroids downregulates the innate immune response, leading to a decrease in phagocytosis and increased host susceptibility to bacterial and fungal infections. Long-term steroid treatment also impairs cell-mediated immunity.

Cellular immune system dysfunction

The cell-mediated immune response includes the recognition of foreign antigen by T cells, and the subsequent proliferation, migration, and activation of T cells in response to infections or inflammation. CD4 T cells are particularly important for the host defense against intracellular pathogens. CD8 T cells play a role in the control of intracytoplasmic viral infections as well as intracellular bacterial infections. Lymphoproliferative disorders, inflammatory disorders, chemotherapeutic agents (e.g. those used to treat organ transplantation recipients), commonly cause impairments of cell-mediated immunity. This results in increased host susceptibility to intracellular pathogens such as *Mycobacterium tuberculosis* and *Salmonella* species, as well as viral and parasitic infections. Infections with viruses including HIV, cytomegalovirus (CMV), and measles may also give rise to impaired cell-mediated immunity.

Humoral immune system dysfunction

The humoral immune response is primarily directed against extracellular bacteria. Components of the humoral immune system including complement and antibody facilitate the internalization and killing of extracellular pathogens by the cells of the innate immune system. Specific antigens give rise to the activation of subsets of B cells. The B cells present these antigens to CD4 T cells, leading to complement-mediated lysis or phagocytosis. B cells are also capable of differentiating into antibody producing plasma cells. Secretory immunoglobulin impairs bacterial motility and adhesion to epithelial surfaces. Immunoglobulin production is decreased in chronic leukemia and multiple myeloma, resulting in increased susceptibility to infection by extracellular bacteria, particularly encapsulated organisms such as *Streptococcus pneumoniae* and *Haemophilus influenzae*.

Splenic dysfunction

An absent or poorly functioning spleen leads to an increased incidence of severe bacterial infections, giving rise to postsplenectomy sepsis (PSS). Functional hyposplenism may occur in a range of autoimmune, hematological (especially sickle cell disease), neoplastic, infiltrative and gastrointestinal disorders, and as a consequence of advanced age, malnutrition, and alcohol excess.

The immunological functions of the spleen include antibody production and the clearance of encapsulated organisms from the bloodstream. PSS is most often caused by encapsulated organisms such as *S. pneumoniae* and *H. influenzae*. PSS typically presents with a short, prodromal febrile illness followed by rapid progression to septic shock with a high mortality rate. The prompt administration of empirical, broad-spectrum antibiotics with activity against encapsulated organisms may be life saving.

Pediatric patients are often given prophylactic oral penicillin V for several years following splenectomy. Such treatment is also used for some adults following splenectomy. Asplenic and hyposplenic patients should be offered immunization with the pneumococcal polysaccharide vaccine, the *H. influenzae* Type B vaccine, the quadrivalent meningococcal vaccine, and yearly trivalent inactivated influenza vaccine immunizations.

Clinical syndromes

The diagnosis of infectious diseases in immunocompromised hosts may be hampered by a lack of typical symptoms and signs of infection, resulting from impairment of the inflammatory response. Microbiological results may not always yield the causative organism, and disease progression can be rapid. Empirical administration of antimicrobial treatment is often required; however, the selection of appropriate agents may be informed by knowledge of the pathogens most commonly associated with various immunocompromised states.

A variety of conditions may give rise to a combination of immune defects which predispose individuals to infections. A variety of primary immune defects have been described. For example, children presenting with severe recurrent septic episodes may have severe combined immunodeficiency (SCID). Patients presenting with abscesses in deep viscera or severe invasive bacterial diseases may have chronic granulomatous disease. Conditions giving rise to secondary immune deficiencies include the extremes of age, pregnancy, diabetes, chronic renal failure, malignancy, chemotherapy, and malnutrition. It is possible to obtain clues regarding the specific immune deficits that may be present based on the clinical syndromes with which patients present (Table 13.2).

Primary immunodeficiency syndromes

The majority of primary immunodeficiencies are diagnosed in infancy; however a proportion remain undiagnosed in to adult life. Approximately 50 000 new cases of primary immunodeficiency are diagnosed in the USA every year. Clues to the diagnosis include:

Table 13.2 Conditions giving rise to immune system deficiencies and associated infections

Conditions	Infections
Primary immunodeficiency syndromes	
Severe combined immunodeficiency (SCID)	Susceptible to overwhelming bacterial sepsis.
Chronic granulomatous disease	Increased susceptibility to bacterial infections, liver abscess, *Burkholderia cepacia* pneumonia, *Nocardia* spp. infections, *Aspergillus* spp. infections
Secondary immunodeficiency syndromes	
Pregnancy, hemodialysis, uremia, intravenous drug use, thalassemia	Meningitis, bacteremia, pneumonia, recurrent infections common
Splenectomy	*Streptococcus pneumoniae, Haemophilus influenzae*
Alcohol abuse	Respiratory infections with *Streptococcus pneumoniae*, TB, *Klebsiella pneumoniae*
Diabetes mellitus	*Staphlococcus aureus* skin infections
Hemochromatosis, iron overload, severe liver disease, myeloma, chronic lymphocytic leukemia, hypogammaglobulinemia	*Streptococcus pneumoniae, Haemophilus influenzae*
Hemotological malignancies, solid organ transplants, e.g. renal	First 6 weeks post-transplant: bacterial infections complicating surgery and urinary tract infections. Gram negative organisms such as *E. coli* and *Pseudomonas*; viridans streptococci, candida species 6 weeks to 6 months "classical" opportunistic infections Later, as the intensity of immunosuppression declines, typical community acquired infections become more common
Hemopoetic stem cell transplantation	Initial neutropenia: bacterial infections After high dose steroids for GVHD: CMV and fungal infections (*Candida, Aspergillus*)
HIV/AIDS	Pneumococcal disease, *Mycobacterium tuberculosis*, (MAI), PCP, *Cryptococcus, Salmonella enteritidis*, toxoplasmosis

CMV, cytomegalovirus; GVHD, graft versus host disease; MAI, *Mycobacterium avium-intracellulare*; PCP, *Pneumocystis pneumania*

- Recurrent infections, for example otitis media, sinusitis, or pneumonia.
- Deep-seated bacterial infections.
- Opportunistic infections, for example PCP (*Pneumocystis* pneumonia; caused by *Pneumocystis jirovecii*), *Giardia, Cryptosporidium*.
- Persistent thrush.
- Lymphandenopathy, hepatosplenomegaly.
- Failure to thrive.
- Family history of immunodeficiency syndromes or early childhood deaths.

Severe combined immunodeficiency

Severe combined immunodeficiency (SCID) results in severe impairment of T and B cell function. Boys are affected more than girls and there is sometimes a family history of the disease. Inheritance is usually

X-linked or autosomal recessive. The genetic defects involved characteristically give rise to abnormalities of T cell cytokine receptors resulting in impaired T cell maturation. In X-linked SCID this results in an absence of peripheral T cells. Peripheral B cells may be normal or increased in number but cannot function normally in the absence of peripheral T cells.

Chronic granulomatous disease

Chronic granulomatous disease (CGD) is caused by defects in the pathway for the production of hydrogen peroxide in the phagosome of phagocytic cells (Figure 13.3). This results in a defective respiratory burst and an impaired response to infections with bacteria, including *Staphylococcus aureus*, and fungi. Patients present with recurrent and often life-threatening infections with such organisms. These infections are often deep-seated, for example hepatic abscesses and suppurative adenitis due to *S. aureus* and infections of the lung involving *Aspergillus* species (Figure 13.4). Granuloma formation is also impaired, which may result in excessive production of granulomatous tissue obstructing viscera, as well as poor scar formation and slow wound healing. Granulocyte transfusions have been used in the treatment of severe infections. Antibacterial and antifungal prophylaxis and interferon gamma have been used to reduce the frequency of infections.

Hematological malignancies

The immune defects arising as consequences of hematological malignancies vary according to the type of disease and the treatments administered. In general, lymphomas give rise to defective cell-mediated immunity, whilst leukemias result in neutropenia and defective neutophil function. Chronic lymphocytic

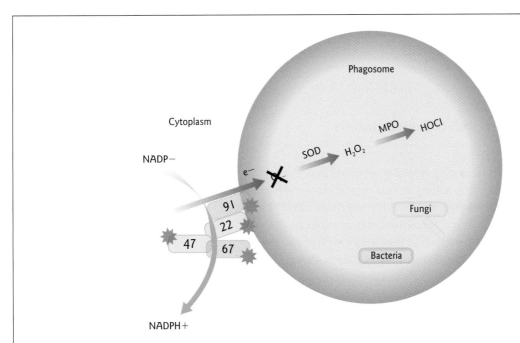

Figure 13.3 The neutrophil oxidative burst is mediated by the structural components of the NADPH oxidase: the membrane-bound components gp91phox and p22phox and the cytosolic factors p47phox and p67phox. In the setting of cellular activation, these factors coalesce on the phagosome membrane and catalyze the transfer of an electron from NADPH to molecular oxygen. This in turn creates superoxide, which is converted to hydrogen peroxide and then to hypochlorous acid (bleach). The genetic absence of any of these structural components causes chronic granulomatous disease (CGD)

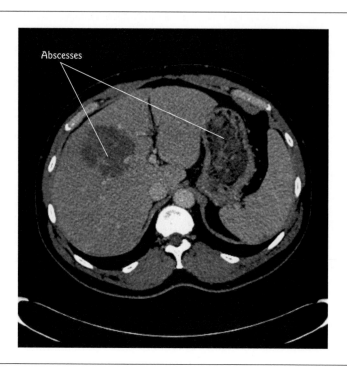

Abscesses

Figure 13.4 Staphylococcal liver abscesses in a patient with chronic granulomatous disease. Note: they are large, diffuse, and multiloculated. Courtesy of University College London Hospitals, UK

leukemia and multiple myloma give rise to defective humoral immunity. In all conditions, treatments with chemotherapy and radiotherapy may result in further immunosuppression. High dose chemotherapy for acute leukemia is intended to eradicate all malignant cells, resulting in severe, prolonged episodes of neutropenia with concomitant mucositis. Such patients frequently have long-term indwelling catheters inserted, further compromising their immune system function. These patients are susceptible to a wide variety of infectious diseases for prolonged periods of time.

Hematopoietic stem cell transplantation

Early infections

During the initial month following hematopoietic stem cell transplantation (HSCT) patients are profoundly neutropenic and often have mucositis. In this period they are particularly susceptible to bacterial infections. Approximately half of the bacteremias in this period are caused by Gram positive organisms arising from the skin or gastrointestinal tract flora. It is sometimes possible to treat indwelling catheter infections due to Gram positive bacteria without line removal. However, infections involving the tunneled sections of the catheter, and line infections caused by fast growing mycobacteria species, usually require line removal for successful treatment. Many Gram negative bacteremias also occur during this period. The incidence of bacteremia due to *Pseudomonas* species has fallen since the introduction of anti-pseudomonal prophylactic antibiotic treatment. Fungal infections may also occur during this period, particularly if engraftment is delayed. Reactivation of herpes simplex virus infections can be prevented by administration of prophylactic aciclovir.

The chemotherapeutic regimens used to facilitate hematopoietic stem cell transplantation give rise to profound and sometimes prolonged immunosuppression. The spectrum of infections seen varies according to the time interval from the commencement of chemotherapy and transplantation, and a range of other factors including:

- Pre-transplant serological tests for infections including viral hepatitis, CMV, and toxoplasmosis.
- The results of cultures of commensal organisms from, for example, respiratory tract samples and stool samples.
- The conditioning chemotherapeutic regimen utilized.

- Complications of transplantation including graft versus host disease (GVHD) and consequent additional chemotherapy.
- Previous infections and antimicrobial prophylaxis.
- The degree and duration of neutropenia.

Infections postengraftment

As the stem cells engraft, the patient's neutophil count recovers, however lymphocyte function remains impaired until approximately day 100 post-transplant. During this second phase patients are at risk of reactivation of CMV, and PCP infections. Both of these infections can be preempted with the routine use of prophylaxis for CMV and PCP. The occurrence of graft versus host disease (GVHD) in this period may require treatment with additional chemotherapy resulting in ongoing immune defects including neutropenia and mucositis, prolonging the risks of serious bacterial and fungal infections, in particular due to *Aspergillus* species.

Late post-transplant infections

Patients without GVHD recover lymphocyte function but do not recover full immune system function for up to 18 months post-transplant. Few further infections occur during this period, however there remains an increased incidence of varicella zoster infections.

Solid organ transplantation

Allowing for variations according to the organ transplanted, most infections following solid organ transplantation occur in the first 4 months post-transplant. In the first month, most of these infections are bacterial, and related to the surgical procedures involved in the transplantation and nosocomial infections. Rarely, infections have been transmitted by the allograft itself, including toxoplasmosis, trypanosomiasis, brucellosis, and recently West Nile Virus. Rates of infections and associated mortalities tend to be higher in heart, lung, and liver transplant recipients than in renal transplant recipients. In the latter group, urinary tract infections are common, and unusual pathogens such as *Mycoplasma hominis* may cause anastamotic breakdown and graft loss.

Following the postoperative period, the immunosuppressive regimens used predispose to reactivations of herpes virus infections; CMV in particular, which may cause severe pneumonitis or colitis. In addition, viral infections including CMV exert immunomodulatory effects, further increasing the degree of immunosuppression and increasing the risk of other infections including opportunistic infections. Opportunistic infections seen in this setting include PCP, *Listeria*, *Nocardia* species, and fungi. Heart transplant recipients who are seronegative for toxoplasmosis prior to transplantation are at risk of disseminated toxoplasmosis should they receive an organ from a seropositive donor. Lung and heart–lung transplant recipients may develop pulmonary viral and *Aspergillus* species infections at a higher rate than other organ recipients. Antiviral and antifungal prophylaxis is widely used in lung transplant recipients to mitigate this risk. Liver transplant recipients have the highest rates of fungal infections amongst solid organ transplant recipients. Life-threatening billiary tract and abdominal infections are also common in this group.

Immunosuppressive treatments are usually tapered after 6 months; however patients continue to be at increased risk of community acquired infections, such as pneumococcal pneumonia, and opportunistic pathogens. Post-transplant lymphoproliferative disease (PTLD) and lymphomas related to Epstein–Barr virus EBV infection may occur more than 1 year after transplant. In cases where significant ongoing immunosuppression is required, the risk of opportunistic infections continues and ongoing prophylaxis may be required.

Immunosuppressive medications

Many immunosuppressive agents have been associated with increased susceptibility to various infectious diseases. These agents are often used in combination. Some of the infectious diseases most commonly associated with a selection of immunosuppressive agents are listed in Table 13.3.

Table 13.3 Immunosupressive agents and associated infections

Agent	Immune component	Infections
Corticosteroids	Decreased phagocytosis and reduced cytokine synthesis	Bacterial infections, fungal infections including *Candida*
	Impairment of T cell function	Herpes viruses, *Strongyloides* hyperinfestation syndrome, opportunistic pathogens with prolonged treatment, e.g. PCP and tuberculosis
Methotrexate	Decreased lymphocyte proliferation	PCP, histoplasmosis, *Listeria*, *Cryptococcus*, MAI
Ciclosporin and tacrolimus	Attenuation of IL-2 and T-lymphocyte expansion	Not associated with increased severe infection when used alone
Mycophenolate mofetil	Decreased lymphocyte clonal expansion	CMV, and EBV associated lymphoproliferative disorder
Anti-TNF agents, etanercept and infliximab	Decreased complement fixation	Bacterial infections, and disseminated infections with *M. tuberculosis*, *Listeria*, *Legionella* sp., *Aspergillus*, CMV
Alemtuzumab	Decreased lymphocyte function	Bacterial infections, reactivation of CMV, respiratory viruses, adenovirus, TB, invasive fungal infections, zoster

CMV, cytomegalovirus; EBV, Epstein–Barr virus; MAI, *Mycobacterium avium-intracellulare*

Corticosteroid administration affects multiple components of the immune system. The risk of infection increases with both the dose and duration of steroid therapy. Bacterial infections reflecting reduced phagocytic function are most commonly seen. With long-term steroid use, impaired cell-mediated immunity gives rise to an increased risk of opportunistic infections including tuberculosis.

Cytoreductive agents such as methotrexate cause neutropenia and mucositis and impaired cell-mediated immunity. Anti-rejection agents such as ciclosporin have little effect on infection risk. Monoclonal antibodies directed against tumor necrosis factor (TNF) are used in the treatment of inflammatory conditions such as rheumatoid arthritis and Crohn's disease. Anti-TNF agents such as infliximab and etanercept have been associated with severe infections due to *Mycobacteria*, *Listeria*, and *Legionella* species. The anti-lymphocyte monoclonal antibody alemtuzumab is used in the treatment of several hematological disorders and may cause lymphopenia lasting several months. Pre-screening for latent infections, and antimicrobial prophylaxis following treatment have been recommended.

Sepsis induced immunosuppression

Following episodes of severe sepsis, an abnormal anti-inflammatory state persists. This may result in a state of relative immunosuppression in some patients, putting them at risk of severe sepsis in response to a "second hit" by a subsequent infection.

Broad-spectrum antibiotic therapy

The use of broad-spectrum antibiotics may be associated with the emergence of specific patterns of resistance. Organisms that are acquired in the hospital setting often have resistance patterns that are the result of sustained selective antimicrobial pressure. Although immunocompromised patients may become colonized by these organisms without becoming ill, the presence of various immune defects increases the risk of clinical infections attributed to such organisms.

Concurrent illness

Several chronic infections may increase the risk of sepsis in immunocompromised patients. CMV causes immunosuppression and predisposes to bacterial infections and opportunistic infections including PCP. Other viral infections may give rise to bone marrow suppression with consequent neutropenia and lymphopenia.

HIV infection

HIV infects a variety of cells involved in the host immune response including CD4 lymphocytes and macrophages. HIV infection impairs the regulation of both the humoral and cellular immune responses to infections. Impaired cell-mediated immunity predisposes patients to infections including PCP, toxoplasmosis, cryptococcosis, infections with herpes viruses, and atypical mycobacterial infections. There is impairment of the response to encapsulated bacteria, giving rise to an increased rate of infections due to *S. pneumoniae*. HIV infection may accelerate the course of viral hepatitis infections, and increases the incidence of Kaposi's sarcoma in concert with human herpes virus 8, and post-transplantation lymphoproliferative disorder in patients co-infected with EBV (see also Chapter 18 on HIV/AIDS).

Mannose binding lectin deficiency

Mannose binding lectin (MBL) is a protein of the innate immune system which is able to bind to mannose-terminated glycoproteins and other carbohydrate structures on the surface of a wide variety of microbial pathogens. Following binding, MBL is able to promote the phagocytosis of microorganisms, and activate the complement system. Several inactivating genetic mutations of the MBL gene are prevalent in the population. Homozygotes for MBL mutations may be predisposed to pneumococcal and meningococcal infections, respiratory tract infections, viral infections including HIV, and serious infections following chemotherapy.

Infecting organisms

Many infections in immunocompromised patients are caused by primary pathogens that commonly cause disease in the immunocompetent host. In addition, immunocompromised patients are susceptible to infections caused by organisms of lower pathogenicity which do not usually cause infections in the immunocompetent and are collectively referred to as opportunistic pathogens. Many opportunistic infections arise from the individual's own flora or local environment.

Bacteria

Neutropenic patients become susceptible to normally nonpathogenic colonizing organisms such as the coagulase negative staphylococci and anaerobes colonizing the skin. Such organisms may colonize indwelling venous catheters leading to bloodstream infections. Viridans group streptococci from the oral cavity may also produce bloodstream infections, particularly in the setting of mucositis. Gram negative bacilli from the gastrointestinal tract may colonize sites such as the airways, and enter the bloodstream during episodes of neutropenia. The organisms implicated include *E. coli* and *Pseudomonas* species which may produce Gram negative sepsis which carries a significant mortality in this setting.

Fungi

The most common opportunistic fungal infections in immunocompromised hosts are caused by commensal *Candida* species. *Candida* colonizing the skin may give rise to intravenous catheter line infections and candidemia which may result in deep-seated fungal infections with spread to organs including the viscera, bone marrow, endocardium, and eye. Inhalation of the spores of molds including *Aspergillus* species may give rise to opportunistic fungal infections, particularly in the period following bone marrow transplantation.

Immunocompromised patients may also be affected by the opportunistic pathogen *Pneumocystis jirovecii*, the fungus responsible for pneumocystis pneumonia (PCP). In endemic areas, dimorphic fungi including *Histoplasma* species and *Coccidioides imitis* may cause respiratory and disseminated infections in the immunocompromised.

Viruses

The herpes viruses may cause infections in the immunocompromised patient as a result of reactivation of latent viral infection. Patients are routinely tested for serological evidence of herpes virus infections prior to transplantation, and given post-transplant antiviral prophylaxis where appropriate. Aciclovir prophylaxis greatly reduces the incidence of HSV oral and genital disease post-transplant. Reactivation of VZV may cause zoster, which should be treated with aciclovir, valaciclovir, or famciclovir in immunocompromised patients. Disseminated primary varicella infection (chicken pox) commonly requires intravenous antiviral treatment in immunocompromised patients.

Parasites

Immunocompromise may lead to the reactivation of chronic parasitic infections, including those caused by *Toxoplasma gondii* and *Strongyloides stercoralis*. Impaired cell-mediated immunity, including the immunocompromise associated with pregnancy, may lead to reactivation of toxoplasmosis and congenital infection. Reactivation of toxoplasmosis may also occur as a result of chemotherapy. Rarely, organ transplant recipients seronegative for toxoplasmosis may acquire the infection from donated organs from seropositive donors carrying the organism. *S. stercoralis* is able to cause autoinfection giving rise to chronic infestations in the immunocompetent. Chemotherapy, for example with corticosteroids, impairs the containment of the autoinfection cycle leading to the hyperinfection syndrome. Complications include meningitis and Gram negative sepsis arising from the larval stages (carrying Gram negative organisms) migrating from gastrointestinal tract (Table 13.4). Leishmaniasis infections may be exacerbated in the setting of immunocompromise, and the reactivation of *Trypanosoma cruzi* infections may occur in such patients.

Clinical approach

History and examination

The presence of immunocompromised states both increases the risk of infection, and decreases the symptoms and signs that usually provide clues to aid the localization and diagnosis of these infections. A detailed history regarding the underlying disease, previous laboratory results, contacts with infectious individuals, travel, and a history of therapies contributing to the immunocompromised state should be obtained. Physical examination should be meticulous as symptoms and signs may be subtle or absent due to the host's impaired inflammatory response. This should include examination of the oral mucosa, perianal area, and venous access sites. Fever is often the only clinical manifestation of infection present, but even this may be absent, for example in patients with infections who have been treated with high doses of corticosteroids. The impaired inflammatory response in neutropenic patients reduces their ability to form pus, for example at the sites of infective skin lesions related to embolic deposits or catheter sites.

Investigations

Cultures of blood, urine, and respiratory secretions may provide clues to the diagnosis. The ease of person to person transmission, both to and from the immunocompromised patient, is increased with increasing levels of immunocompromise, facilitating transmission of organisms such as *Mycobacterium* species. Impaired immune responses to infection result in delays in presentation, by which time the microbiological burden of disease is likely to be high. The range of causative organisms encountered is wider than that for the immunocompetent

Table 13.4 Diagnosis of selected pathogens important in immunocompromised patients

Suspected agent		Methods of diagnosis	Comments
Bacteria	Fastidious or unusual bacteria	2–3 blood cultures with incubation for 7–10 days	
	Legionella species	Urinary antigen Sputum or BAL microscopy DFA and culture PCR	Urinary antigen detects only *Legionella pneumophila* serotype 1
	Nocardia	Respiratory secretions or tissue sample modified acid-fast stain	Blood cultures are frequently negative
	Mycobacterium tuberculosis	Sputum or BAL microscopy and culture Blood culture in selective medium PCR Transbronchial biopsy Bone marrow biopsy	Disseminated tuberculosis may have skin lesions amenable to biopsy
	Nontuberculous mycobacteria	Blood culture in selective medium Biopsy of skin lesions Sputum/BAL in case of lung lesions	Bone marrow stains may allow early diagnosis
Fungi	*Pneumocystis jirovecii*	Direct fluorescence antibody or silver stain from induced sputum or BAL	PCR may be more sensitive, particularly in non-HIV-infected patients
	Candida species	Biopsy of suspicious lesions 2–3 blood cultures plus cultures of catheters or catheter sites Fundoscopy CT scanning for disseminated candidiasis	Blood cultures may be negative in acute disseminated candidiasis, and they are typically negative in chronic disseminated candidiasis
	Cryptococcus neoformans	Detection of cryptococcal antigen in serum or CSF 2–3 blood cultures CSF India ink and culture	
	Histoplasma capsulatum	Stain of tissue samples 2 blood cultures or special fungal bottles Antigen in urine by EIA	Urine antigen positive only in disseminated disease
	Mold infections (*Aspergillus* spp., *Fusarium* spp., *Scedosporium* spp.)	BAL; biopsy of any suspicious lesion Sputum, tracheal aspirate, bronchial brush, galactomannan antigenemia (blood) PCR	Galactomannan antigenemia mainly detects *Aspergillus*, although it may cross react with some other molds such as *Penicillium*; isolation of molds from sputum in intensive care patients is associated with high risk of invasive disease
Viruses	CMV	Quantitative CMV PCR on blood CMV antigen detection Viral culture Cytology may help	Detecting CMV in the blood does not mean it is causing disease; PCR in the BAL is not diagnostic of pneumonia; cytopathic effect seen in cells from BAL may be suggestive
	EBV	EBV PCR on blood Biopsy with immunohistochemistry is required for the diagnosis of EBV-associated lymphoproliferative disease	EBV causes lymphoproliferative disease in some transplant patients, quantitative PCR useful for monitoring viral load

Table 13.4 (cont'd)

Suspected agent		Methods of diagnosis	Comments
	Human herpes virus 6	PCR detection of DNA in CSF Serology	Detection of human herpes virus 6 by PCR in serum does not mean there is active disease. IgG only confirms previous infection
	Adenovirus	Direct immunofluorescence staining and cell culture of secretions PCR in blood BAL Electron microscopy of respiratory secretions	Disseminated adenovirus infection may be diagnosed when adenovirus is found in the blood by PCR or when it is isolated from three different body sites
Parasites	*Toxoplasma gondii*	PCR detection of DNA in blood, BAL, or lung tissue; cysts may occasionally be seen on Giemsa staining of lung or other tissues Serology – IgM often negative, presence of IgG only confirms previous infection	90% of toxoplasmosis disease in intensive care hosts is reactivation; septic shock may occur in AIDS and transplant patients
	Strongyloides hyperinfection	Examination of sputum, BAL, and feces for larvae Detection of adults, larvae, and eggs in histologic sections of intestine by EGD Serology; migration test of larvae by plating stool on blood agar plate	The clinical syndrome of *Strongyloides* hyperinfection includes recurrent or polymicrobial bacteremia with enteric bacteria (Enterobacteriaceae and *Enterococcus* species)

BAL, bronchoalveolar lavage; PCR, polymerase chain reaction; DFA, direct fluorescent assay; GMS, Gomori methenamine silver; CSF, colony-stimulating factor; EIA, enzyme-linked immunoassay; CMV, cytomegalovirus; IgM, immunoglobulin M; EGD, esophagogastroduodenoscopy

population, and alerting the laboratory to the patient's immune status should facilitate more detailed investigations of samples. In addition, cultures from aspirates or biopsy samples of skin lesions may be valuable in identifying the causative organisms, for example where there are emboilic deposits of *Pseudomonas* species (ecthyma gangrenosum) or fungi including *Aspergillus* and *Fusarium* species. The investigation of lymphademopathy may reveal *Mycobacterium* species infections, or lymphoproliferative disorders. However, in many cases of clinically diagnosed sepsis in the immunocompromised, no microbiological diagnosis can be obtained. Additional serological and molecular tests and detailed radiological investigations may provide further evidence to support the diagnosis of infections in immunocompromised patients.

Clinical presentations

Pneumonia

Pneumonia is the commonest infectious cause of death in immunocompromised hosts. The causes of pneumonia vary between patient groups and with the level of immunosuppression encountered. A wide range of causative agents may be implicated (Table 13.5). In most cases it may be possible to narrow down the diagnostic possibilities according to factors in the patient's history and clinical findings, and target investigations and antimicrobial therapy accordingly.

Initial investigations should include chest X-ray, sputum samples, and blood cultures. In cases where the rapid onset of symptoms and signs suggests serious bacterial pneumonia, empirical broad-spectrum antibiotic cover should be commenced after the taking of appropriate cultures. Patients from the community should receive cover for pneumococcal infections, usually with a β-lactam antibiotic, and cover for atypical causes

Table 13.5 Causes of fever and new pulmonary infiltrates in the immunocompromised host

Bacterial infections	
Conventional respiratory pathogens	*S. pneumoniae, H. influenzae, Klebsiella*
Nosocomial pathogens	*E. coli, Pseudomonas* spp.
"Atypical" organisms	*Chlamydia* spp., *Mycoplasma*
Mycobacteria and related organisms	*M. tuberculosis*, atypical mycobacteria, *Nocardia*
Viral infections	
Herpes viruses	Cytomegalovirus, herpes simplex, varicella zoster
Respiratory viruses	Respiratory syncytial virus, parainfluenza, influenza, adenovirus
Fungal infections	
Systemic mycoses	Blastomycosis, histoplasmosis, coccidioidomycosis
Opportunist mycoses	*Candida, Aspergillus, Mucor, Cryptococcus*

of pneumonia, such as mycoplasma, with a macrolide. Hospitalized patients should receive broad-spectrum Gram negative cover including antipseudomonal cover with, for example and antipseudomonal β-lactam antibiotic with or without an aminoglycoside.

When symptom onset occurs more slowly, or when patients fail to respond to first line antibiotic therapy, further useful investigations include CT scanning of the chest. While CT appearances may be nonspecific, bilateral infiltrates may suggest PCP or CMV infection, and mass lesions surrounded by crescents of air may suggest a fungal etiology. Patients may require bronchoscopy with broncho-alevolar lavage (BAL) for viral, mycobacterial and fungal cultures, and cytology for PCP in order to reach a diagnosis. Serological tests may also assist in diagnosis. In some cases, several broad spectrum antimicrobial agents may be instigated to cover bacterial, fungal and viral pathogens if there is no indication as to the causative organism, or if multiple etiologies are suspected.

Neurological infections

Meningitis

Immunocompromised patients are susceptible to a range of primary and opportunistic pathogens which may cause infections of the central nervous system. Acute meningitis may be caused by typical pathogens such as pneumococcus, meningococcus or *H. influenzae*. Patients with defects in cell-mediated immunity have increased susceptibility to intracellular organisms such as *Listeria*, *Legionella*, and *Mycobacterium*, as well as fungal pathogens such as *Cryptococcus neoformans*. Cerebrospinal fluid (CSF) should be examined microscopically and cultures should be made for the likely organisms. In addition, tests for cryptococcal antigen can be performed on blood as well as CSF. Imaging of the chest may reveal concomitant chest disease linked to the central nervous system infection, such as tuberculosis or a lobar pneumonia suggesting pneumococcal infection.

Parenchymal infections

Immunocompromised patients with neurological symptoms or signs should have imaging of the brain performed via CT or MRI scanning. Single or multiple cerebral mass lesions may be caused by bacterial abscesses, tuberculosis, toxoplasmosis, *Nocardia* species, or fungal infections. Multiple lesions with peripheries that enhance with intravenous contrast (ring-enhancing lesions) suggest cerebral toxoplasmosis, but this appearance may also occur with primary or secondary intracerebral malignancies such as lymphomas. Unfortunately serology for toxoplasma is unhelpful in immunocompromised patients. A trial of anti-toxoplasma therapy with pyrimethamine and sulphadiazine may be performed. A good response to such treatment suggests the provisional diagnosis of cerebral toxoplasmosis to have been correct. Rarely, fungal infections may spread from the nose or sinus to the brain parenchyma, causing cerebral mucormycosis. This aggressive infection occurs in neutropenic patients and occasionally diabetic patients. Aggressive surgical debridement of affected tissue is essential to treating the infection, and antifungal treatment usually comprises amphotericin with or without an azole. Despite such measures mortality remains high.

Gastrointestinal infections

Mucositis
Oral mucositis is a common complaint in immunocompromised patients. Cytotoxic chemotherapy may induce mucositis which is followed by secondary bacterial or fungal infections or the reactivation of latent viral infections. *Candida* species and HSV are often implicated, however it is difficult to distinguish the causes of mucositis clinically. *Candida* species and HSV may also cause esophagitis.

Intestinal syndromes
Diarrhea may occur as a consequence of chemotherapy or radiotherapy, or as a manifestation of graft versus host disease in transplant recipients. Bacterial pathogens such as *Salmonella* and *Campylobacter* species may cause prolonged diarrhea in the immunocompromised. *Clostridium difficile* may cause diarrhea and pseudomembranous colitis, particularly following treatment with antibiotics. Cytomegalovirus may cause a severe and prolonged colitis requiring treatment with ganciclovir. Parasitic causes of diarrhea in the immunocompromised include *Giardia*, *Isospora belli*, and *Cryptosporidium* and *Microsporidium* species. *S. stercoralis* hyperinfection syndrome may cause intestinal obstruction as well as septicemia arising from the gastrointestinal tract.

Hepatic syndromes
Disseminated CMV infection and disseminated toxoplasmosis may give rise to hepatitis. Systemic candidiasis may involve the liver and spleen with the formation of multiple abscesses and abnormal liver function tests.

Prevention and treatment

Preventative measures

Physical measures directed towards preventing infections in the immunocompromised host include the use of single rooms and filtered or laminar flow air, as well as barrier protection using gowns and gloves, and practices including hand washing, and aseptic techniques for the placement and access of central venous catheters.

Hematopoietic stem cell transplant (HSCT) recipients seronegative for CMV are given CMV negative and/or leucocyte depleted blood and blood products to reduce the risk of CMV infection post-transplant.

Vaccinations

Vaccination against organisms including *S. pneumoniae* and *H. influenzae* type b should be administered prior to the administration of immunosuppressive medications, where possible, and in the context of increased susceptibility to such infections, for example in hyposplenic patients or those with multiple myeloma.

Prophylactic treatment

Primary prophylactic treatment with low dose trimethoprim-sulfamethoxazole for a variety of immunosuppressed populations significantly reduces urosepsis, PCP, *Listeria* infections, nocardiosis, and toxoplasmosis. Prophylactic treatment with other agents, for example aciclovir, fluconazole, or ciprofloxacin, is sometimes used. Concerns exist regarding the degree to which such prophylactic treatments may encourage the emergence of resistant organisms. Fluconazole prophylaxis is clearly of benefit in reducing the incidence of invasive fungal infections in liver transplant recipients.

Preemptive treatment

Preemptive treatment is targeted at asymptomatic patients who are at high risk of clinical infections, as suggested by laboratory markers or clinical or epidemiological markers. For example, prior testing for asymptomatic carriage of cytomegalovirus in bone marrow and organ transplant recipients permits preemptive treatment with ganciclovir before clinical infection manifests. Patients at very high risk may be given preemptive therapy even in the absence of raised levels of CMV. For HSV-seropositive patients, prophylaxis with oral aciclovir or valaciclovir reduces the incidence of reactivations of HSV infection.

Empirical treatment

For severely neutropenic patients, empirical treatment at the first subtle signs of infection may be beneficial in reducing morbidity and mortality, particularly in the case of Gram negative bacteremia. At the onset of febrile neutropenia, multiple sets of blood cultures should be taken from different sites, prior to the commencement of antimicrobial therapy. Further samples (sputum, urine) should also be taken if indicated by symptoms or clinical findings. In such patients, broad-spectrum antibiotic cover may then be instituted at the first occurrence of an unexplained fever, or other signs of infection. Regimens vary according to local epidemiology and resistance patterns, and agent cost and availability. Initial therapy is aimed at Gram negative organisms, usually including an antipseudomonal penicillin or cepahalosporin, with or without an aminoglycoside, or alternatively an antipseudomonal carbepenem. Should there be a poor response, coverage may be broadened to include Gram positive organisms with the addition of a glycopeptide such as vancomycin. In a therapeutic emergency, Gram positive cover may be initiated at the outset. Regimens may be varied according to a patient's past history of infections and antibiotic treatment, and whether a patient is considered to be at low or high risk of adverse outcomes (see Further reading).

Should there be no response after 2–3 days with the persistence of fever, the possibility of deep-seated fungal infections should be considered, and antifungal therapy may be added to the treatment regimens. In the context of the persistently febrile neutropenic patient there are a variety of causes of persistent fever to be considered (Table 13.6).

Central venous access catheters infected with organisms that are difficult to eradicate such as VRE, MRSA, *Candida* species and *Pseudomonas* species may necessitate catheter removal to effect a cure.

Where causative organisms are identified and patients are improving, treatment regimens may be modified to target the organism and their sensitivities and reduce costs and toxicities. In immunocompromised patients, longer courses of individually tailored antibiotic treatments may be required to affect a cure. In non-neutropenic

Table 13.6 Causes of persistent fever in neutropenic patients

Resistant bacterial infection (e.g. vancomycin-resistant enterococci (VRE))
Bacterial infection associated with tissue necrosis/mucositis (endotoxemia)
Nonculturable or cell wall-deficient bacteria
Other infections (virus, acid-fast bacteria, parasites, e.g. toxoplasmosis)
Malignancy-related fever
Superinfection with fungi
Drug or transfusion fever

immunosuppressed patients, the underlying immune defects may indicate that empirical treatment with appropriate antimicrobials is warranted, after the taking of appropriate samples for culture (Table 13.7).

Immune therapy

Granulocyte colony stimulating factor (G-CSF) has been used to stimulate the production of neutrophils to shorten periods of neutropenia and reduce the incidence of febrile neutropenia. Its use has been recommended in high-risk patients in several guidelines, however this appears to have little impact on mortality.

Table 13.7 Summary of specific immunocompromised states and treatment recommendations

Immunocompromise	Pathogens causing severe sepsis	Recommended empirical regimen for severe sepsis of unknown origin*	Comments
Neutropenia	Enteric Gram negative bacilli, *Pseudomonas aeruginosa*, viridans group streptococci, *Candida* species	Carbapenem or cefepime or piperacillin/tazobactam; quinolone or aminoglycoside + vancomycin	Antifungal coverage should be added if shock develops late in the course of neutropenia or if there is evidence of *Candida* colonization
Splenectomy	*Streptococcus pneumoniae*, *Hemophilus influenzae*, others	Third generation cephalosporin – vancomycin	
Hematopoietic stem cell transplant			
Preengraftment	See "neutropenia" above	See "neutropenia" above	See "neutropenia" above
Before day 100	Without GVHD: catheter-related *S. epidermidis*, *S. aureus*, nonfermentative Gram negative bacilli With acute GVHD: enteric Gram negative bacilli, fungal infection	Very diverse group to make sole recommendation; combination therapy probably appropriate in septic shock	When considering antifungal coverage, septic shock is more commonly caused by *Candida* species, than with mold infection; consider azole-resistant *Candida*
Late	Chronic GVHD: combination of splenectomized and steroid recipients	Third generation cephalosporin – vancomycin	Consider specific immunosuppressive agents being used
Solid organ transplant			
Early	Surgical site source: Gram negative bacilli including *Pseudomonas*, *Staphylococcus aureus* and VRE	Antipseudomonal beta-lactam – linezolid	
Late	Pathogens related to defect in cell-mediated immunity (e.g., *Legionella*, *Listeria*)	Fluoroquinolone – vancomycin or linezolid	
HIV-AIDS	*Pseudomonas aeruginosa*, *S. aureus*, *Streptococcus pneumoniae*, *Salmonella enteritidis*, *Cryptococcus neoformans*; rare but noteworthy: *Toxoplasma gondii*, *Helicobacter*, *Mycobacterium tuberculosis*	Ceftazidime or fluoroquinolone – vancomycin – amphotericin B lipid formulation	Stage of disease and associated risk factors are critical to make the right choice: Neutropenia is a risk factor for *Pseudomonas*, intravenous drug use for *S. aureus*; only advanced AIDS patients are at risk for septic shock caused by *Cryptococcus* and *Toxoplasma*

GVHD, graft-vs.-host disease; VRE, vancomycin-resistant enterococci.

* These recommendations are based on the opinion of experts and are presented as a logical empirical approach. Local patterns of microbial resistance or known colonization with resistant pathogens should influence the choice of empirical regimen.

Test yourself

Infections in the immunocompromised host are among the most challenging both in terms of their study and their management. The case studies described here are designed to help the student get to grips with the most common infections associated with a particular immunocompromised state.

Case study 13.1

A 35-year-old man received a hematopoietic stem cell transplant for lymphoma. He had a persistent high fever and worsening chest symptoms despite broad-spectrum antibiotics. His peripheral neutrophil count was 0.

This high resolution CT scan of his chest showed characteristic lesions; broncho-alveolar lavage grew the organism shown below:

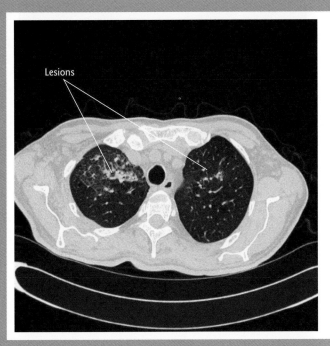

CT scan of a stem cell transplant recipient with chest symptoms. Lesions suggestive of fungal infection. Courtesy of University College London Hospitals, UK

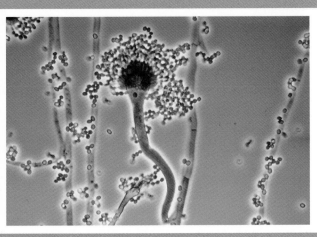

Microscopic image of *Aspergillus fumigatus*, one of the commonest fungi associated with invasive infections in the febrile neutropenic host. Lactophenol cotton blue mount from a culture specimen. Courtesy of University College London Hospitals, UK

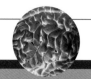

Test yourself

1. Briefly describe the immune suppression that makes a patient vulnerable to such an infection.
2. What measures can be put in place to prevent this happening?

Case study 13.2

A known HIV positive patient presents to the emergency department with severe respiratory tract infection. He has not been taking his anti-retroviral drugs as they make him feel ill. His chest X-ray (below) shows widespread interstitial shadowing. A broncho-alveolar lavage is sent to the laboratory for examination; this organism was found on microscopic examination:

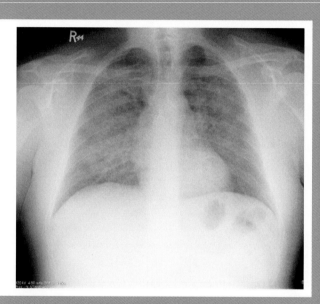

Chest X-ray of an HIV positive patient showing interstitial pneumonia. Courtesy of University College London Hospitals, UK

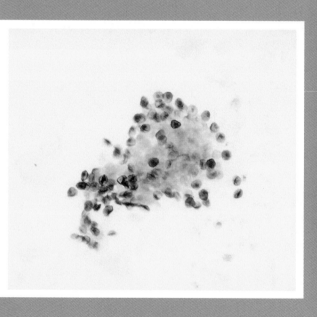

Broncho-alveolar lavage cytology showing *Pneumocystis jirovecii*. Stained by Grocott stain (1000×). Courtesy of Department of Microbiology, University College London Hospitals, UK

Test yourself

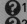 1. Describe the microbiology of the organism. Is infection with this organism an AIDS defining condition?

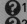 2. What is the disease burden and epidemiology of this organism in the USA (Box 13.1).

Box 13.1 How PCP alerted the world to a new disease entity: AIDS (First Report of AIDS: *MMWR* 1, June 2001)

Twenty years ago, on June 5, 1981, *MMWR* published a report of five cases of *Pneumocystis carinii* pneumonia (PCP) among previously healthy young men in Los Angeles (*1*). All of the men were described as "homosexuals"; two had died. Local clinicians and the Epidemic Intelligence Service (EIS) Officer stationed at the Los Angeles County Department of Public Health, prepared the report and submitted it for *MMWR* publication in early May 1981. Before publication, *MMWR* editorial staff sent the submission to CDC experts in parasitic and sexually transmitted diseases. The editorial note that accompanied the published report stated that the case histories suggested a "cellular-immune dysfunction related to a common exposure" and a "disease acquired through sexual contact." The report prompted additional case reports from New York City, San Francisco, and other cities. At about the same time, CDC's investigation drug unit, the sole distributor of pentamidine, the therapy for PCP, began to receive requests for the drug from physicians also to treat young men. In June 1981, CDC developed an investigative team to identify risk factors and to develop a case definition for national surveillance. Within 18 months, epidemiologists conducted

studies and prepared *MMWR* reports that identified all of the major risk factors for acquired immnodeficiency syndrome (AIDS). In March 1983, CDC issued recommendations for the prevention of sexual, drug-related, and occupational transmission based on these early epidemiologic studies and before the cause of the new, unexplained illness was known.

MMWR has published more than 400 reports about human immunodeficiency virus (HIV) and AIDS and remains a primary source of information about the epidemiology, surveillance, prevention, care, and treatment of HIV and AIDS. This anniversary issue provides new reports on the epidemiologic features and impact of HIV/AIDS on communities in the USA and in other countries. A compilation of notable *MMWR* reports on HIV and AIDS is available at http://www.cdc.gov/mmwr/hiv_aids20.html. A video that includes interviews with participants in these first AIDS investigations and reports and a video summary of each report in this issue is available at http://www.cdc.gov/mmwr.

Reference: CDC. Pneumocystis pneumonia Los Angeles. *MMWR* 1981;30:250–252.

Case study 13.3

A young man recently arrived from Ghana presented with severe headache and visual disturbances. A lumbar puncture was performed and CSF microscopy reported (see below).

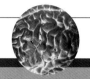

Test yourself

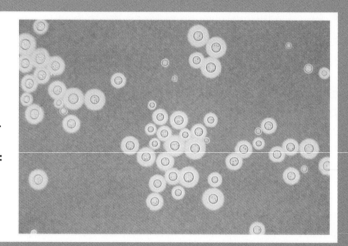

CSF microscopy showing *Cryptococcus neoformans* using India ink negative staining; note thick unstained capsule and budding yeast cells. Provided by Dr Leanor Haley. Courtesy of the Centers for Disease Control and Prevention; from CDC website: http://phil.cdc.gov/phil/details.asp

1. What other test would need to be performed as a matter of urgency?
2. Describe the microbiology of the organism.
3. What is the source of this organism in urban environments?

Case study 13.4

A young Afro-Caribbean boy was seen in the emergency room with overwhelming sepsis. He was wearing a Med Alert bracelet which proclaimed that he was asplenic.

This is his chest X-ray. A Gram stain of his CSF revealed this organism:

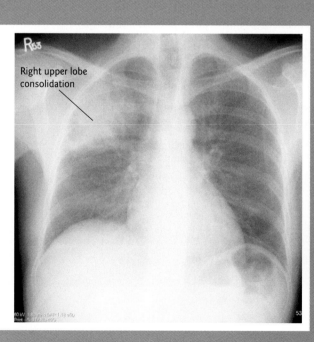

Right upper lobe consolidation

Chest X-ray of a young man with overwhelming sepsis showing right upper lobe consolidation. Courtesy of University College London Hospitals, UK

Test yourself

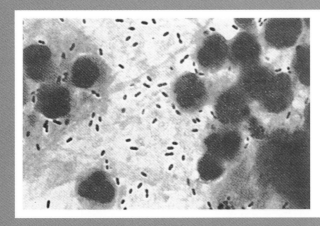

Gram stain of CSF. Courtesy of Department of Microbiology, University College London Hospitals, UK

❓1. List all the organisms that are likely to cause serious infection in such a patient.
❓2. Why are asplenic patients vulnerable to these organisms?
❓3. What is the likely identity of this patient's infecting organism?
❓4. How would you prevent recurrent infections with this organism in such a patient?

Case study 13.5
A renal transplant recipient on long-term immunosuppressive therapy presents with a pain and swelling on his right arm, the overlying skin has broken down with a chronic discharging sinus. Here is an X-ray of the affected arm. Material from the lesion grew the organism on the following page.

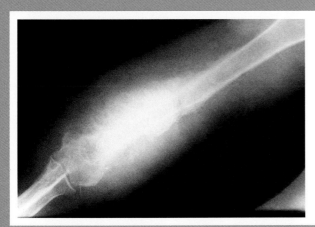

X-ray of an arm showing bony destruction under the cutaneous lesion. Provided by Dr Libero Ajello. Courtesy of the Centers for Disease Control and Prevention; from CDC website: http://phil.cdc.gov/phil/details.asp

Test yourself

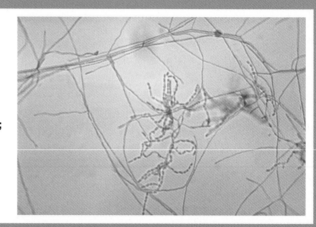

Gram positive aerobic *Nocardia asteroides* as seen growing on slide culture. Provided by Dr Lucille K. Georg. Courtesy of the Centers for Disease Control and Prevention; from CDC website: http://phil.cdc.gov/phil/details.asp

❓1. Describe the immunological dysfunction that predisposes these patients to infections with this organism.
❓2. What is the microbiology and pathogenesis of this organism?

Case study 13.6
An HIV positive man was brought to the emergency room disorientated and confused. His family says that he may have had a convulsion on the way in. This is an MRI of his brain on admission. He has lived alone with his pet cat ever since his partner died of AIDS. A serology report a few days later showed that the Sabin–Feldman dye test was positive; specific IgG titer to the organism was over 2048.

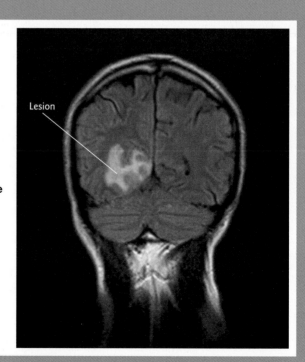

MRI of brain showing lesion adjacent to the left mid-line. Courtesy of University College London Hospitals, UK

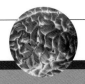

Test yourself

1. What is the organism that may be responsible for this patient's condition?
2. Is it an AIDS defining condition?
3. What could be the role of the pet cat in this case?
4. What other risk factors predispose to infection with this organism?
5. Briefly describe the lifecycle of the organism.

Case study 13.7

A 42-year-old man, born in the USA, was exposed to smear positive TB in 2001 while working as a prison counselor. He had a positive tuberculin skin test (TST) result during the contact investigation and was treated for latent TB infection (LTBI). However, he discontinued treatment because of side-effects. The patient has rheumatoid arthritis and received several infusions of infliximab in December 2006 and February 2007. In October 2007 he sought care for cough, fever, and weight loss. His chest X-ray (see below) revealed upper lobe shadowing with mediastinal lymph nodes, and sputum specimens yielded *M. tuberculosis*. He started standard, four-drug anti-TB therapy and was free of TB disease after the treatment course.

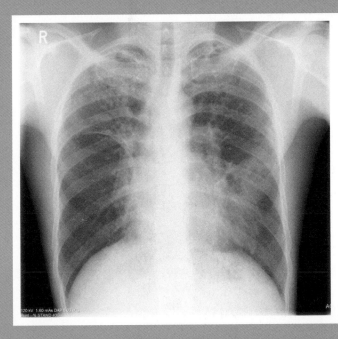

Chest X-ray of a patient on tumor necrosis factor alpha (TNF-α) antagonists – infliximab. Courtesy of University College London Hospitals, UK

1. Explain how you would use screening tests to detect LTBI.
2. What are the CDC recommendations for preventing disease in such individuals?
3. What is the relationship between infliximab and risk of TB?

Read http://www.cdc.gov/MMWR/preview/MMWRhtml/mm5330a4.htm to learn about this interesting group of patients.

Case study 13.8

A severe uncontrolled diabetic patient presented with renal impairment and lesions extending from the maxillary sinuses and orbit of the eye into the brain. A biopsy of the lesion grew a moldy fungus, depicted here in the lacto-phenol cotton blue mount (see following page). Rhinocerebral mucormycoses was diagnosed.

Test yourself

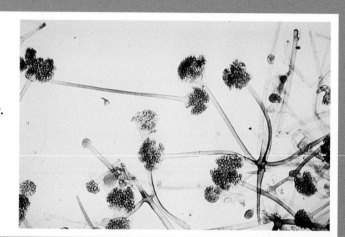

Lactophenol cotton blue mount of mucor.
Courtesy Department of Microbiology,
University College London Hospitals, UK

1. What is the immune dysfunction that severe diabetic patients develop that predisposes them to invasive mold fungal infections?
2. Describe the morphological features of mucor and rhizopus, the common mold fungi that are implicated in this condition.

Case study 13.9
A patient with acute leukemia underwent a bone marrow transplant, as a result of which her neutrophil count went down to zero in the days before the transplant engrafted. During this time she developed systemic signs of sepsis and an ulcerative lesion on her arm (see photograph below). Blood cultures grew *Pseudomonas aeruginosa*.

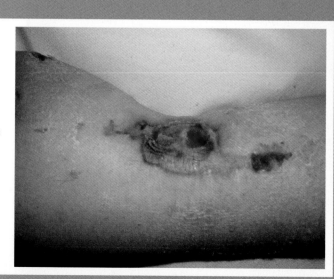

Ecthyma gangrenosum in a neutropenic
patient. Courtesy of University College
London Hospitals, UK

Test yourself

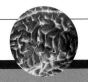

?1. Plot the relationship between the loss of white blood cells and the onset of opportunistic infections.

?2. List the various microorganisms commonly implicated in infections associated with febrile neutropenic patients.

?3. What is the pathogenesis in ecthyma gangrenosum?

Case study 13.10
A patient with chronic granulomatous disease (CGD) presented with a large liver mass, thought to be an abscess. CT-guided aspirate of the lesion showed growth of *S. aureus* from the liver abscess (see CT scan below). The patient required several weeks of antibiotic therapy and granulocyte transfusions to overcome this episode.

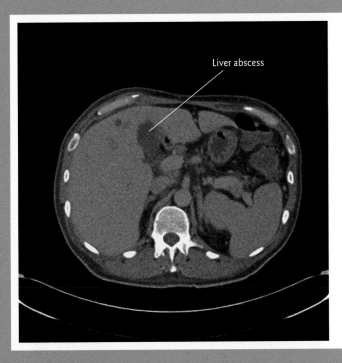

Large liver abscess in a patient with chronic granulomatous disease. Courtesy of University College London Hospitals, UK

?1. What is the immune deficiency in CGD?

?2. What other group of organisms are associated with CGD?

Case study 13.11
A Southeast Asian gentleman recently arrived in USA was admitted with exacerbation of asthma. He was a longstanding asthmatic on steroid therapy. Besides severe asthma he also presented with signs of systemic Gram negative sepsis. Microscopy of expectorated sputum showed these organisms in abundance; most were motile.

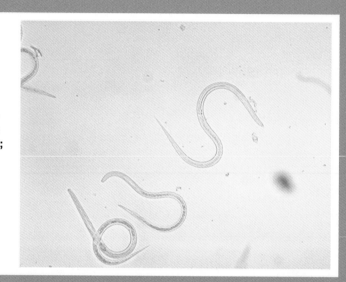

Filariform larva of *Strongyloides stercoralis*. Provided by Dr Mae Melvin. Courtesy of the Centers for Disease Control and Prevention; from CDC website: http://phil.cdc.gov/phil/details.asp

1. Why do we need to bear this organism in mind when treating recent migrants from Southeast Asia?
2. What is the relationship between steroid use and hyperinfection with this organism?
3. What is the mechanism of the associated Gram negative sepsis?

Case study 13.12
A young boy on chemotherapy for acute leukemia developed crops of these lesions just after his last chemotherapy cycle when his neutrophil count was 0.1×10^9/L. Aspirate of the lesion showed this organism on electron microscopy (see following page).

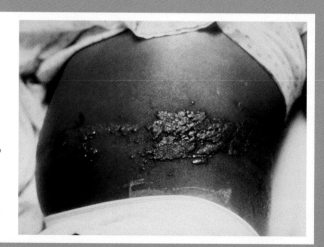

Crops of vesicular lesions across the abdomen. Courtesy of the Centers for Disease Control and Prevention; from CDC website: http://phil.cdc.gov/phil/details.asp

Test yourself

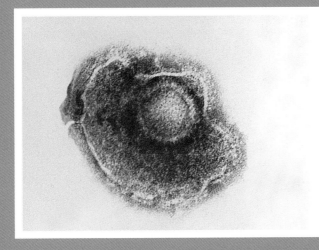

Electron micrograph of a varicella (chickenpox) virus. Provided by: Dr Erskine Palmer/B.G. Partin. Courtesy of the Centers for Disease Control and Prevention; from CDC website: http://phil.cdc.gov/phil/details.asp

1. Why has this happened even though the child has had chickenpox in the past?
2. What is the common name given to this condition?
3. Is the child infectious to other immunocompromised patients?

Further reading

Benson CA, Kaplan JE, Masur HP, Holmes A, King K. Treating opportunistic infections among HIV-infected adults and adolescents. *MMWR* December 17, 2004/53(RR15);1–112. http://www.cdc.gov/mmwr/preview/mmwrhtml/rr5315a1.htm

Gafter-Gvili A, Fraser A, Paul M, van de Wetering M, Kremer L, Leibovici L. Antibiotic prophylaxis for bacterial infections in afebrile neutropenic patients following chemotherapy. *Cochrane Database System Rev* 2005; Issue 4, Art no: CD004386

Gea-Banacloche Sepsis associated with immunosuppressive medications: an evidence-based review. *Crit Care Med* 2004;32(11):S578–S590

General Recommendations on Immunization. *MMWR Recomm Rep* December 1, 2006/55(RR15);1–48

Guidelines for Preventing Opportunistic Infections among Hematopoietic Stem Cell Transplant Recipients. *MMWR* October 20, 2000/49(RR10);1–128

Hughes WT, Armstrong D, Bodey GP, et al. Guidelines for the use of antimicrobial agents in neutropenic patients with cancer. *Clin Infect Dis* 2002;34:730–751

Kaplan JE, Masur H, Holmes KK. Guidelines for preventing opportunistic infections among HIV-infected persons. *MMWR* June 14, 2002/51(RR08);1–46. http://www.cdc.gov/mmwr/preview/mmwrhtml/rr5108a1.htm

Morris A, Lundgren JD, Masur H, et al. Current epidemiology of *Pneumocystis* pneumonia. *Emerg Infect Dis* 2004;10(10):1713–1720

Playford EG, Webster AC, Sorell TC, Craig JC. Antifungal agents for preventing fungal infections in solid organ transplant recipients. *Cochrane Database System Rev* 2004, Issue 3, Art. No: CD004291. DOI: 10.1002/14651858.CD004291.pub2

Recommended Adult Immunization Schedule – United States, October 2006–September 2007. *MMWR* October 13, 2006/55(40);Q1–Q4. http://www.cdc.gov/mmwr/preview/mmwrhtml/mm5540-Immunization1.htm

Sipsas NV, Bodey GP, Kontoyiannis DP. Perspectives for the management of febrile neutropenic patients with cancer in the 21st century. *Cancer* 2005;103(6):1103–1113. http://www3.interscience.wiley.com/cgi-bin/fulltext/109873237/HTMLSTART

Useful websites

CDC. Fact Sheets. Division of Tuberculosis Elimination. Treatment of Latent Tuberculosis Infection (LTBI). http://www.cdc.gov/TB/pubs/tbfactsheets/treatmentLTBI.htm

Doctor Fungus. The Official Website of the Mycoses Study Group. http://www.doctorfungus.org/

Recommendations of the Advisory Committee on Immunization Practices (ACIP). http://www.cdc.gov/mmwr/preview/mmwrhtml/rr5515a1.htm?s_cid=rr5515a1_e

Recommendations of CDC, the Infectious Disease Society of America, and the American Society of Blood and Marrow Transplantation. http://www.cdc.gov/mmwr/preview/mmwrhtml/rr4910a1.htm

Chapter 14
Healthcare associated infections

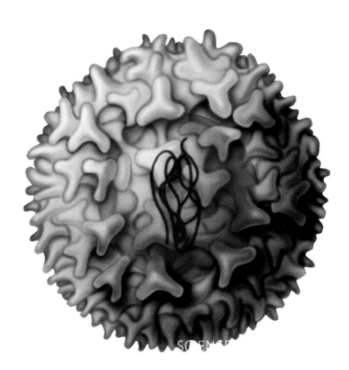

N. Shetty

Definition of a healthcare associated infection
Risk factors for the acquisition of HAI
Source and spread of HAI
Transmission of HAI
Common infections acquired in the healthcare setting

Microbiology of the agents commmonly associated with HAI
Infection control measures
  Handwashing
  Isolation
  Masks, gloves, and aprons
  Injection practices
  Surveillance, education and research

Definition of a healthcare associated infection

Healthcare associated infections (HAIs) are infections that patients acquire during the course of receiving treatment for other conditions or that healthcare workers (HCWs) acquire while performing their duties within a healthcare setting. Specific criteria must be met in order to define an infection as healthcare associated (see Further reading). In general infections are suspected to be hospital acquired if they first appear 48 hours or more after hospital admission in a previously uninfected patient. HAIs are also referred to as nosocomial infections, *nosocomial* comes from the Greek word *nosokomeion* meaning hospital (*nosos* = disease, *komeo* = to take care of).

Within hospitals in the USA, HAIs account for an estimated 2 million infections, 90 000 deaths, and $4.5 billion in excess healthcare costs annually.

Risk factors for the acquisition of HAI

What are the predisposing factors that make one patient more vulnerable to an HAI than another?

Patients come into hospital because they are unwell:

Box 14.1 Premature babies are extremely vulnerable to infection

Baby JJ was born preterm at 26 weeks' gestation (see figure right). She needed immediate surgery for a congenital abnormality of the gut, besides this she needed a long stay central venous catheter for administration of drugs and nutrition as she was unable to feed orally. She was also ventilated intermittently through a tube in her throat. She is typical of the type of patient in hospital who is most susceptible to healthcare associated infections. Let us examine why this is so, what organisms may be implicated, and what we, as healthcare workers, can do to prevent her from suffering further injury through an infection acquired in hospital. Read on to find out more.

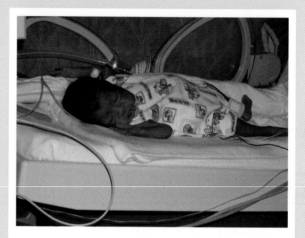

The Departments of Microbiology and Neonatology, UCLH, London are gratefully acknowledged for use of this image

- They may be either very young (like the preterm infant, Baby JJ described in Box 14.1) or very old. Extremes of age carry an inherent risk of poor defence against infection.
- They may have chronic underlying disease that compromises their immune system: diabetes, renal failure, and cancer are just a few examples.
- They may have suffered physical trauma: road accidents, cuts and burns are typical examples when intact skin is breached. We know from earlier chapters that the intact skin is the body's most important defence mechanism against microbial invasion.
- Patients may be on medication that puts them at risk for infection: immunosuppressive and cytotoxic agents are prescribed for a variety of cancers and autoimmune disorders; anti-inflammatory agents such as steroids are known to be immunosuppressive.

Whilst in hospital we may intentionally breach the intact skin or use invasive devices:

- Surgery and subsequent care of the wound is a common entry site for HAIs.
- Indwelling devices: central venous catheters, urinary catheters, endotracheal tubes, and other invasive monitoring devices are routes of entry for infectious agents.

Drugs and other treatments given in hospital may further increase the risk of super-added infection:

- Antimicrobial agents are a perfect example, while they are administered to fight infection, they carry the risk of reducing normal microbial flora and leaving the individual exposed to colonization and infection with resistant "hospital bugs."
- Blood transfusions, parenteral nutrition, and nursing in the recumbent position (ideally the head end should be raised) are all well known risk factors for HAI.

Healthcare staff may be risk factors for HAI:

- All healthcare staff in principle endeavor to follow the paradigm of, "above all else do no harm." However, in reality increasing pressures on healthcare staff combined with ever more complex

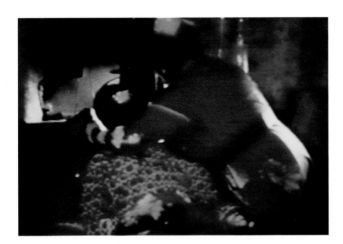

Figure 14.1 The hands of healthcare staff can transmit infection: the greater the need for hands-on care the larger the risk. A colorless fluorescent substance applied on this healthcare worker's hands showed where she placed her hands before she washed her hands. (Note evidence of fluorescence on her tunic pocket, cap, ear, chin and nose and all over the patient and his environment.) It is no wonder that some healthcare staff have eschewed the use of uniforms and caps in favor of scrubs. The Department of Microbiology, UCLH, London is gratefully acknowledged for use of this image

medical/surgical interventions has lead to the recognition that healthcare staff themselves transmit infection from patient to patient. In particular, hands of healthcare staff are well known independent risk factors for the transmission of HAIs (Figure 14.1).

Read the exercise in Box 14.2 for a real life example of a patient at risk of developing an HAI. List all the risk factors that you can identify and come back to this patient after studying the rest of the chapter. Draw up an action plan of care that will minimize his risk.

Box 14.2 Intensive care: a double-edged sword

Mr ATS, a 48-year-old patient, was a victim of a road traffic accident. He suffered a number of pelvic and lower limb fractures, some of them communicating through open wounds to the outside. He needed emergency abdominal surgery to remove an injured spleen and repair lacerations in the liver. He required several blood transfusions in theatre to combat the blood loss from his lacerated liver. He was transferred to the intensive care unit (ICU) for management thereafter (see photograph right). He was mechanically ventilated via an endotracheal tube, he had a central venous catheter for administration of fluids and drugs, a urinary catheter, and an arterial line to monitor arterial pressures. He was a known asthmatic on steroids. In addition, he was prescribed broad-spectrum antibiotics for a "dirty" wound as a result of the road traffic accident.

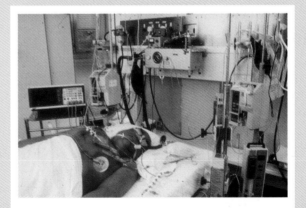

The Department of Microbiology and the ICU, UCLH, London are gratefully acknowledged for use of this image

❓1. List as many risk factors for acquiring an HAI in this patient as you can.

❓2. What can be done to prevent such an infection?

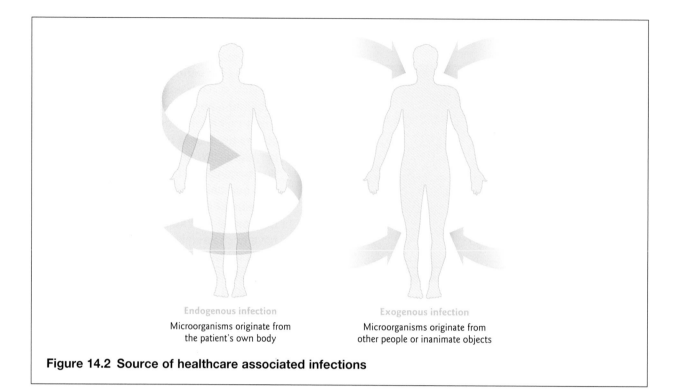

Endogenous infection
Microorganisms originate from
the patient's own body

Exogenous infection
Microorganisms originate from
other people or inanimate objects

Figure 14.2 Source of healthcare associated infections

Source and spread of HAI

All things considered, people are the main source of the organisms causing HAI. Infections can have an endogenous (from within the patients' own flora) or exogenous (from other people or from contaminated surfaces and objects) origin (Figure 14.2).

Transmission of HAI

Microorganisms causing HAI can be transmitted between patients by one or more of four main routes of transmission, in order of importance they are:

Contact

- Direct contact via hands of healthcare staff. Caring of patients necessitates hands-on contact, not only of the patient and their body fluids but also the environment around the patient, i.e. manipulation of intravenous sites, catheters, and administration of drugs. Studies have conclusively shown that hands are heavily colonized with microorganisms, particularly the skin under the often improperly washed, but warm and moist watch strap (Figure 14.3). In the now almost obsolete "Nightingale" ward, where a row of beds lined opposite walls of a long corridor style ward (Figure 14.4), infection spread rapidly often with disastrous consequences.
- Indirect contact involves a contaminated intermediate object: computer key boards and ward telephones are common culprits. Improper use of gloves (Figure 14.5) gives a false sense of security and is commonly incriminated in environmental contamination. Needles that are not disposed off carefully and safely are a particular hazard to healthcare staff (Figure 14.6), as they may transmit blood borne viruses such as HIV and hepatitis C.

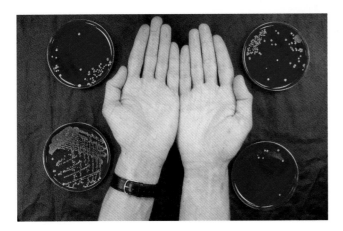

Figure 14.3 Hands are a major source of healthcare associated infections; the area under the watch strap is poorly cleaned and therefore heavily colonized. The bottom left hand culture plate shows a heavy growth of organisms from a skin swab of the area around the watch strap after supervised hand washing. Compare it to the plate on the opposite side. Many hospitals actively discourage the use of wrist watches in clinical areas as part of their infection control policy. Note that hand washing does not eliminate skin bacteria, however it considerably reduces transient flora. The Department of Microbiology, UCLH, London is gratefully acknowledged for use of this image

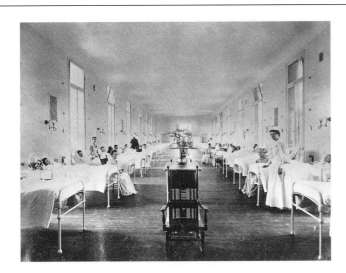

Figure 14.4 A Nightingale Ward with not a hand wash sink in sight, fertile ground for spread of infection. Photograph of women's ward, Royal Victoria Hospital, Montreal, QC, about 1894. © McCord Museum

Droplet

- Large droplets are generated by coughing, sneezing, talking, or during procedures such as suctioning of airways and bronchoscopy. Large droplets are propelled in the air and may land on a patient's nasal or conjunctival mucosa (Figure 14.7). If you are a healthcare worker and have a cold or a runny nose, please do not come to work! Nasal secretions reflexly cause you to take your hands to your nose with or without a tissue. Tens of thousands of viruses abound in these secretions, they contaminate hands and then anything else you may touch, and cause rampant spread in a healthcare setting. In a way this is a type of contact transmission involving droplets.

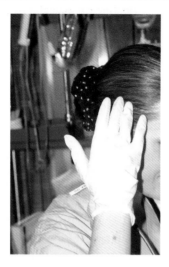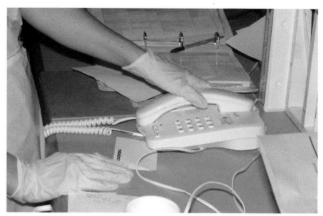

Figure 14.5 The incorrect use of gloves leads to contamination of the environment and spread of infection. A healthcare worker pats her hair into place after touching a patient and then touches the telephone handset with the same pair of gloves. The Department of Microbiology, UCLH, London is gratefully acknowledged for use of these images

Figure 14.6 Improper and unsafe disposal of sharps can cause serious healthcare associated infections in healthcare workers. Note overfull sharps bin and protruding needle attached to a syringe. The Department of Microbiology, UCLH, London is gratefully acknowledged for use of this image

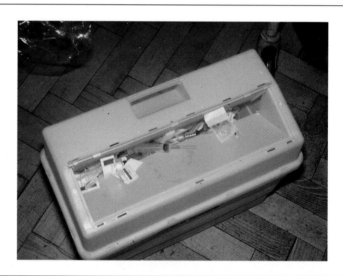

Figure 14.7 Large droplets generated by sneezing. The Department of Microbiology, UCLH, London is gratefully acknowledged for use of this image

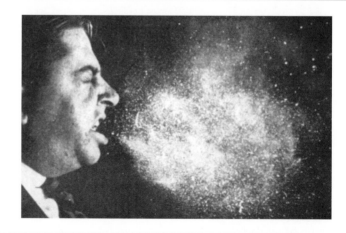

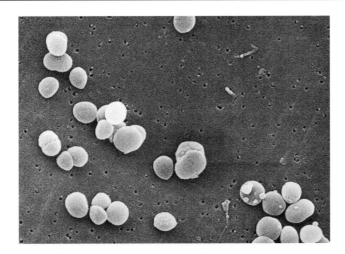

Figure 14.8 Skin scales carrying staphylococci. The Department of Microbiology, UCLH, London is gratefully acknowledged for use of this image

- Small droplets: Transmission by small droplets (<5 μm in diameter) is important in those infections spread via the airborne route. The recent SARS outbreak (see Chapter 22) amply illustrated the rapidity with which airborne organisms can cause widespread disease. Small droplets containing microorganisms remain suspended in the air for long periods of time; special air handling and ventilation units are required to protect susceptible patients from airborne transmission. Respiratory viruses, the chicken pox virus, and *Mycobacterium tuberculosis* are examples of organisms spread by this route.

Skin scales

- Many individuls are heavy skin scale shedders, those suffering from eczema or psoriasis are particularly prone to shedding. Such individuals are also known be heavily colonized with staphylococci. Each skin scale that is shed acts like a miniature magic carpet, carrying organisms into the environment and facilitating transmission (Figure 14.8).

Food and water

- Foodborne transmission of gastrointestinal pathogens is rare in hospitals unless kitchen hygiene has been severely compromised. Waterborne transmission has occurred from time to time and is associated with hydrotherapy pools, birthing pools, air conditoning and humidifying devices, and endoscopy washer disinfectors. Organisms implicated are environmental mycobacteria, environmental Gram negative bacilli, and the *Legionella* species.

Common infections acquired in the healthcare setting

The CDC's National Nosocomial Infections Surveillance (NNIS) system, established in 1970, monitors reported trends in nosocomial infections in acute-care hospitals in the USA. According to published NNIS data, the four most common infections acquired in the healthcare setting are urinary tract infections (UTI), pneumonia (ventilator associated pneumonia in particular), surgical site infection (SSI), and bloodstream infections (BSI), in that order.

The **urinary tract** is the most common site of healthcare associated infection, accounting for more than 40% of the total number reported by acute-care hospitals and affecting an estimated 600 000 patients per year. Most of these infections, 60–80%, follow instrumentation of the urinary tract, mainly urinary catheterization (data from CDC). Although not all catheter associated urinary tract infections can be prevented, a large number could be avoided by the proper management of the indwelling catheter (see Further reading for CDC guidelines for the prevention of catheter associated UTI). Generally UTIs are associated with less morbidity than other infections but can sometimes lead to septicemia and death. Common organisms implicated are the gut associated Gram negative bacilli usually from the patient's own gut flora. They become problematic when the patient becomes colonized and infected with multi-drug resistant organisms.

Pneumonia accounts for approximately 15% of all hospital associated infections and 27% and 24% of all infections acquired in the medical intensive-care unit (ICU) and coronary care unit, respectively. According to NNIS surveillance data it is the second most common hospital associated infection after that of the urinary tract. For hospital associated pneumonia, attributable mortality rates of 20–33% have been reported. The primary risk factor for the development of hospital associated bacterial pneumonia is mechanical ventilation (with its requisite endotracheal intubation). This is also called ventilator associated pneumonia (VAP). The source of the microorganism is often endogenous but may also be exogenous with transfer of an organism via hands of healthcare staff. Gram negative bacteria, including *Pseudomonas*, are the commonest organisms causing infection and many are multi-drug resistant because patients and therefore their flora have been exposed to repeated courses of broad-spectrum antibiotics. The importance of elevating the head of the bed to prevent VAP has been quoted in many studies. For details of CDC guidelines for the prevention of VAP, see Further reading.

Besides ventilator associated pneumonia, respiratory tract infections due to viruses such as varicella, RSV, and influenza/parainfluenza viruses (Table 14.1) pose a problem in pediatric, obstetric and neonatal units and in clinical areas that serve severely immunosuppressed patients (many cancer patients on chemotherapy have no white blood cells as a result of therapy, they are referred to as neutropenic patients).

The neutropenic patient is particularly prone to severe lung infections due to inhaled spores of moldy fungi such as *Aspergillus* species. These spores abound in the dust from building sites. Neutropenic patients nursed adjacent to building and refurbishing sites need to be protected with special air handling and ventilation units (see Further reading for CDC guidelines).

Legionnaires' disease (see also Chapter 9) caused by the waterborne organism *Legionella pneumophila*, has been responsible for HAI over the years. Read an account of legionella and its role in hospitals in Box 14.3.

Surgical site infections cause significant mortality and morbidity in hospitalized patients. CDC surveillance data shows that as of 1999, in the USA alone, an estimated 27 million surgical procedures are performed each year. Based on 1993 NNIS system reports, SSIs are the third most frequently reported nosocomial infection, accounting for 14–16% of all nosocomial infections among hospitalized patients. A surgical infection is indicated by the presence of purulent discharge around the wound or the insertion site of a drain, or by the presence of cellulitis around the wound. Postoperative wounds can become infected at surgery or in the days after. The patient's own skin flora may be the cause of infection, in other cases organisms carried from other patients or from the environment via hands of healthcare staff, are commonly implicated. *S. aureus* including MRSA are by far the commonest organisms cultured from such infections. For details on prevention and control of SSIs see Further reading.

Bloodstream infections represent about 5% of healthcare associated infections. Although they are only a small proportion of nosocomial infections, they have high case-fatality rates, sometimes greater than 50%. The commonest organisms associated with a BSI in hospital form part of the normal flora of the patient's own skin – the coagulase negative staphylococci such as *Staphylococcus epidermidis*. The emergence of *S. epidermidis* as a pathogen has been fueled by the widespread use of catheters, prosthetic joints, valves and other invasive medical devices, and is a growing concern, particularly for immunocompromised cancer patients.

Other infections may occur at the entry site of the intravascular device (Figure 14.9) or along the path of an intravenous catheter (tunnel infection). Although they are only a small proportion of nosocomial infections, they have high case-fatality rates, sometimes greater than 50%. The source of the infectious agents are usually endogenous but can be related to poor hand hygiene of healthcare workers manipulating the catheter. Common infecting organisms include *S. aureus* including MRSA.

Box 14.3 Sustained transmission of nosocomial legionnaires' disease (LD). Arizona and Ohio (report from *MMWR* 1997/46(19);416–421)

In 1996, eight cases of nosocomial LD were diagnosed among cardiac and bone marrow transplant patients at hospital X. Intensified surveillance for nosocomial LD was initiated after the first three case-patients were diagnosed, 25 cases of LD linked to hospitalization during 1987–1996 were identified. All were diagnosed by culture. Most case-patients had received either heart, heart/lung, or bone marrow transplants. Twelve (48%) patients died during their hospitalization; eight of these patients had LD identified on autopsy.

During January–June 1996, nosocomial LD occurred in two patients at hospital Y. Beginning in 1989, as part of surveillance for nosocomial LD, urine samples from all patients with nosocomial pneumonia were tested for *Legionella pneumophila* antigen, a further nine patients with definite nosocomial LD and 29 patients with possible nosocomial LD were identified.

L. pneumophila was isolated from samples obtained from multiple sites in the hot water distribution system during 1994–1996 from both hospitals.

Interventions recommended at the conclusion of this investigation in June 1996 included discontinuing the use of tap water to rinse medical nebulizer equipment, repeating the hyperchlorination procedure as needed in response to positive potable water cultures, increasing the hot water temperature at the point-of-use to at least 120°F (49°C), and identifying "deadlegs" in the potable water plumbing.

Following these interventions, no new cases of nosocomial transmission were identified until February 28, 1997, when a case of possible nosocomial LD occurred in a patient in a critical care unit. *L. pneumophila* isolates from a sample of the patient's lung tissue and from the potable water supply in his room were identical to all previous isolates. Hospital personnel discovered a previously undocumented cross-connection between the hot water tank from an adjacent outpatient-care building and the critical care unit. This tank was cleaned, and the supply system hyperchlorinated. No new cases have been identified at hospital Y since March 1997.

Editorial note: The findings in these and other recent investigations indicate the capacity for legionellae to colonize hospital plumbing systems for long periods and, in the absence of effective preventive measures, to represent an ongoing risk for infection. Colonization rates are higher in large hospitals with older, large hot water tanks in which water is held at lower temperatures.

Nosocomially acquired LD accounts for a substantial proportion of all reported cases of this disease: during 1980–1989, of 3524 cases reported to CDC, 23% were nosocomial, and mortality was 40%, compared with a mortality of 20% in the community.

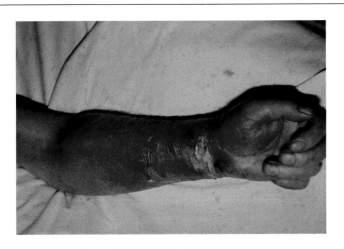

Figure 14.9 Severe soft tissue infection as a result of an infected intravascular catheter entry site. The Department of Microbiology, UCLH, London is gratefully acknowledged for use of this image

Besides the big four infections described above, **gastroenteritis** including antibiotic associated diarrhea (AAD), deserves some mention. Two agents have emerged as problem pathogens causing serious outbreaks of diarrhea in hospitals; they are *Clostridium difficile*, an organism implicated in AAD and the noroviruses.

The primary risk for AAD due to *C. difficile* is obviously exposure to broad-spectrum antibiotics, other risks include gastrointestinal surgery/manipulation, long length of stay in healthcare settings, and advanced age. The spectrum of disease caused by *C. difficile* ranges from asymptomatic colonization, mild, moderate or severe diarrhea, to life-threatening ulceration, inflammation and dilatation of the entire large bowel (otherwise known as pseudomembranous colitis and toxic megacolon). *C. difficile* is shed in feces, it sporulates when outside the body, and spores are widely disseminated in a contaminated environment. Any surface, device, or inanimate object (e.g. commodes, bathing tubs, and electronic rectal thermometers) that becomes contaminated with feces may serve as a reservoir for *C. difficile* spores. *C. difficile* spores are transferred to patients mainly via the hands of healthcare personnel who have touched a contaminated surface or item. Over the past 2 years, several states in the USA have reported increased rates of *C. difficile* associated disease, noting more severe disease and an associated increase in mortality. The increased rates and/or severity of disease may be caused by changes in antibiotic use, changes in infection control practices, or the emergence of a new strain of *C. difficile* associated disease with increased virulence and/or antimicrobial resistance.

Noroviruses are highly contagious, with as few as 100 virus particles sufficient to cause infection. Noroviruses are transmitted primarily through the fecal–oral route; they can also spread via droplets as a result of aerosols generated by, the often explosive, vomiting in affected individuals. In healthcare facilities, transmission can additionally occur through hand transfer of the virus to the oral mucosa via contact with materials, fomites, and environmental surfaces that have been contaminated with either feces or vomitus. The virus spreads rapidly in the healthcare environment often causing entire wards or units to shut down. The attack rate from a single case can be in excess of 80% among patients and staff.

Microbiology of the agents commmonly associated with HAI

Any microorganism that is transmitted from one patient to another can cause an HAI. Table 14.1 lists the most problematical organisms in terms of treatment or control.

Besides the potential to spread and cause serious infections in already sick patients, many of the infectious agents below are resistant to the first line antibiotics commonly used to treat them, *S. aureus* becoming resistant to the β-lactams is a good example. We then rely on second line drugs such as vancomycin, but when even these agents become useless in the face of bacterial resistance, the fear of a completely untreatable staphylococcal infection looms ever closer.

Methicillin resistant *S. aureus* (MRSA)

MRSA is one of the most important nosocomial pathogens worldwide. As its name implies, MRSA is resistant to methicillin and other members of the penicillinase-resistant penicillins including oxacillin, nafcillin, cloxacillin, flucloxacillin, cephalosporins, carbapenems, and other β-lactams. Thus, any *S. aureus* reported as resistant to methicillin should be considered resistant to all classes of β-lactam antibiotics.

MRSA displays resistance to methicillin because it possesses a penicillin-binding protein 2a that has reduced affinity for binding to β-lactam agents. This protein is encoded by the *mec* A gene, which is carried by a large mobile element referred to as staphylococcal chromosome cassette (SCC) *mec*. The SCC *mec* gene has been sequenced, and five types have been identified, designated as I, II, III, IVa, and IVb.

Periodically, "successful" (epidemic) clones emerge which spread locally, nationally, and internationally. Much work on the characterization of such clones has been performed locally and nationally, however there has been little international sharing of data. Unlike plasmid-encoded penicillinase, the methicillin resistance determinant, *mec*, is chromosomally encoded. Horizontal transfer of *mec* is thought to be relatively rare; only a handful of ancestral strains account for all clinical isolates worldwide. Five distinct clones of MRSA have

Table 14.1 Common pathogens that cause HAI

Bacteria	Viruses	Fungi
Gram positive: **Methicillin resistant *S. aureus* (MRSA)** **Vancomycin intermediate *S. aureus* (VISA)** **Coagulase negative staphylococci** **Vancomycin resistant enterococci (VRE)** **Gram negative:** ***Acinetobacter* spp.** ***Pseudomonas* spp.** **ESBL* producing Gram negative organisms** **Anaerobes** ***Clostridium difficile*** **Others** ***Legionella* spp.** ***Mycobacterium* spp.**	**Blood-borne viruses:** Hepatitis B and C HIV **Viruses causing respiratory disease:** Varicella zoster virus (chickenpox, shingles), measles, rubella, parvovirus B19, influenza, adenovirus, parainfluenza, respiratory synctial virus (RSV) **Gastrointestinal viruses:** Noroviruses, rotavirus, enteroviruses, hepatitis A	**Mold:** *Aspergillus* species

* Extended spectrum β-lactamase producing organisms: particularly *E. coli* and *Klebsiella* spp. (see Chapters 3 and 5).

been identified worldwide. In addition to the Iberian clone and the "English" MRSA (EMRSA-15 and 16) clones, the "VISA"(see below) and community clones (Box 14.4) have emerged, changing the epidemiology of MRSA worldwide.

Vancomycin intermediate and resistant *S. aureus* (VISA and VRSA)

Vancomycin intermediate *S. aureus*, or VISA is already showing levels of resistance that, while still manageable, are nonetheless threatening to catapult it into the drug resistant big league (Box 14.5). Risk factors for the acquisition of VISA appear to be prolonged exposure to vancomycin, renal failure requiring dialysis, invasive intravascular devices, and prior infection with MRSA.

The resistance mechanism of VISA has not yet been clarified. Cell wall thickening is a common feature of VISA. Experiments have shown that resistance may be caused by clogging of the thickened cell wall with vancomycin; the cooperative effect of the clogging and cell wall thickening enables VISA to prevent vancomycin from reaching its true target in the cytoplasmic membrane, exhibiting a new class of antibiotic resistance in Gram positive pathogens.

Coagulase negative staphylococci

The coagulase negative staphylococci are Gram positive cocci, they mediate virulence by producing slime or glycocalyx to form a "biofilm" on intravascular catheters and prostheses. A "**biofilm**" consists of layers of bacterial populations adhering to host cells and embedded in a common capsular mass. Bacteria embedded in biofilm can cause serious systemic infections and are difficult to treat as most antibiotics are unable to penetrate or eradicate "biofilms." In addition, multidrug resistant strains are fast becoming major hospital pathogens. Close to 80% of *S. epidermidis* isolates in some US hospitals are methicillin resistant, and recent studies have found resistance to quinolones, cephalosporins, and vancomycin.

Box 14.4   Methicillin-resistant *Staphylococcus aureus* infections among competitive sports participants: Colorado, Indiana, Pennsylvania and Los Angeles County, 2000–2003 (*MMWR*, August 22, 2003/52(33);793–795)

Although outbreaks of methicillin resistant *Staphylococcus aureus* (MRSA) usually have been associated with healthcare institutions, MRSA is emerging as a cause of skin infections in the community.

In February 2003, the Colorado Department of Public Health and Environment was notified about a cluster of MRSA infections among members of a Colorado fencing club. Clusters of MRSA infection among sports team participants were identified in Pennsylvania and Indiana. Affected persons included college and high school-aged football players and wrestlers. They reported large abscesses, requiring admission to hospital, intravenous antibiotics, surgery, and skin grafts. In September 2002, the Los Angeles County Department of Health Services investigated two cases of MRSA skin infection among members of a college football team. Both patients were hospitalized; one received surgical debridement and skin grafts. Isolates from the two players were indistinguishable by molecular testing. Team players reported frequent skin trauma and reported covering wounds approximately half of the time. In addition, health department staff identified the potential for spread through shared items such as balms and lubricants.

Editorial note: This report demonstrates that community acquired MRSA has the potential to spread and cause outbreaks among players of competitive sports, including those sports that involve little skin-to-skin contact among players, such as fencing. Firstly, competitive sports participants might develop abrasions and other skin trauma, which could facilitate entry of pathogens. Even in sports with less direct contact, protective clothing can be hot and might chafe skin, resulting in abrasions and lacerations. Secondly, some sports for which MRSA infections have been reported involve frequent physical contact among players (e.g. football and wrestling). *S. aureus* and other skin flora can be transmitted easily from person to person with direct contact. Thirdly, sports such as fencing have limited skin-to-skin contact but require multiple pieces of protective clothing and equipment, which often might be shared. The use of shared equipment or other personal items that are not cleaned or laundered between users could be a vehicle for *S. aureus* transmission.

Coaches and parents should encourage good hygiene among players, and they should be taught to administer proper first aid, practice appropriate hand hygiene, and implement a system to ensure adequate wound care and to cover skin lesions appropriately before play. Players should be encouraged to practice good hygiene, avoid sharing towels or other personal items, and inform coaches about active skin infections.

Box 14.5   How is a VISA different from a VRSA?

Staphylococcus aureus is classified as VISA or VRSA based on laboratory tests.

S. aureus isolates are routinely tested in microbiology laboratories for their resistance or susceptibility to antimicrobial agents that might be used for treatment of infections. For vancomycin and other antimicrobial agents, tests determine how much of the agent (in µg/ml) is required to inhibit the growth of the organism in culture. The result of the test is usually expressed as a minimum inhibitory concentration (MIC) or the minimum amount of antimicrobial agent that inhibits bacterial growth in culture. Therefore, *S. aureus* is classified as VISA if the MIC for vancomycin is 4–8 µg/ml, and a VRSA if the vancomycin MIC is ≥16 µg/ml.

Infections with VRSA are still a rare occurrence. There have been only six cases of infection caused by VRSA reported in the USA. See http://www.cdc.gov/ncidod/dhqp/ar_visavrsa_FAQ.html#2 for further information on these cases.

Vancomycin resistant enterococci (VRE)

Enteroccocci are Gram positive cocci seen in pairs or short chains, they form part of the normal flora of human intestines and the female genital tract and are often found in the environment. These bacteria can sometimes cause infections particularly in hospitalized and debilitated individuals. Enterococcal species are intrinsically resistant to many antibiotics (cephalosporins, penicillinase-resistant penicillins, clindamycin, and aminoglycosides). For serious enterococcal infections, the combination of a cell-wall active agent (a β-lactam or glycopeptide) and an aminoglycoside is necessary to achieve adequate kill.

Vancomycin or teicoplanin is the glycopeptide that is often used to treat infections caused by enterococci. In some instances, enterococci have become resistant to vancomycin and are thus called vancomycin resistant enterococci (VRE). Most VRE infections occur in hospitals. Read Chapter 5 for the mechanism of resistance to vancomycin. The vancomycin resistance trait in *Enterococcus* species is transferable, through mobile genetic elements carrying the *van* A (high level resistance) or *van* B (low level resistance) genes. Perhaps the greatest threat of VRE is the potential emergence of vancomycin resistance in methicillin resistant *S. aureus* or *S. epidermidis*, through transferable genes – evidence of this is already present in the few cases of VRSA reported from the USA.

Gram negative organisms: *Acinetobacter*, *Pseudomonas*, and ESBL producing organisms

Acinetobacter and *Pseudomonas* spp. are Gram negative rods commonly found in soil and water. *Acinetobacter* can also be found on the skin of healthy people, especially healthcare personnel. *Acinetobacter baumannii* accounts for about 80% of all reported *Acinetobacter* infections. *Acinetobacter* and *Pseudomonas* infections rarely occur outside of healthcare settings.

Outbreaks of *Acinetobacter* infections typically occur in intensive care units and units that care for seriously ill and debilitated individuals. The major issue with *Acinetobacter* and *Pseudomonas* spp. is that they are resistant to many commonly prescribed antibiotics. Decisions on treatment of infections with these organisms should be made on a case-by-case basis after culture and susceptibility results are available.

Infections with multi-drug resistant *extended spectrum β-lactamase (ESBL)* are emerging as important nosocomial pathogens. *Klebsiella* spp., and more recently *Escherichia coli*, are the most commonly implicated organisms harboring a variety of ESBL genotypes. Several outbreaks of ESBL producing organisms in hospital environments have been reported worldwide. Organisms producing ESBLs are able to hydrolyze the third generation cephalosporins; these are among the most widely prescribed β-lactam antibiotics worldwide (see Chapter 5). The mechanism of resistance mediated by ESBL producing organisms is complex. They mediate resistance through the production of different enzymes (called TEM or SHV) coded for by multiple different gene types. At least 130 TEM-type and 50 SHV-type ESBLs have been recognized. More recently, CTX-M-type ESBLs have been detected which preferentially hydrolyze cefotaxime, although mutation can confer ceftazidime activity. These enzymes may sometimes be referred to as cefotaximases. The consequence of an infection with an organism that is an ESBL producer is that the range of available drugs to treat these infections is restricted to the carbapenems.

Clostridium difficile

Clostridium difficle is a Gram positive, rod-shaped, spore forming, opportunistic pathogen. It does not normally cause an infection unless the normal composition of the intestinal flora is altered. These alterations are commonly a result of broad-spectrum antibiotic therapy that decreases the numbers of other colonizing intestinal flora. The most commonly associated antibiotics include: amoxicillin, cephalosporins, and clindamycin, though virtually any antibiotic can be associated with *C. difficile* infection. The severe diarrhea and ulcerative lesions seen in *C. difficile* infection are a result of the action of an enterotoxin. The enterotoxin of *C. difficile* has two components: toxin A causes accumulation of fluid in the bowel lumen, toxin B is cytotoxic and is thought to be primarily responsible for ulceration of the bowel wall. The recent surge of severe *C. difficile* outbreaks in the USA has been linked to a new strain, which appears to be more virulent, probably because they have the ability to produce greater quantities of toxins A and B.

Viruses

Viruses associated with HAI (e.g. HIV, hepatitis B and C, measles, rubella, varicella, parvovirus B19 etc.) are listed in Table 14.1 and are individually discussed in the relevant chapters.

Aspergillus spp.

Invasive aspergillosis has become a devastating opportunistic fungal infection among immunocompromised hosts, with a 357% increase in death rates reported in the USA from 1980 to 1997. The most common cause of invasive aspergillosis is *Aspergillus fumigatus* (Figure 14.10).

The same moldy fungus that grows on food and fruit can infect the lungs and other organs of immunosuppressed patients, especially those who are neutropenic. Building dust is a common source of *Aspergillus* spores; hospital wards close to building sites should ensure the air is passed through special air handling units before admitting vulnerable patients. Invasive aspergillosis commonly manifests as a lung infection (Figure 14.11) and is almost always fatal.

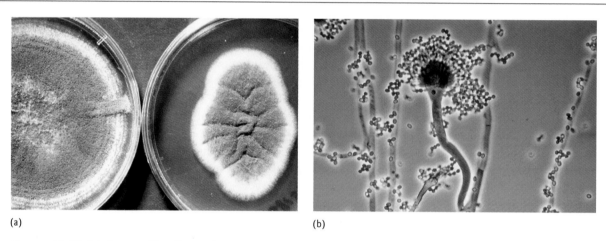

(a)   (b)

Figure 14.10 (a) *Aspergillus flavus* **(left)** *Aspergillus fumigatus* **(right) growing on culture media. (b) Microscopic image of** *A. fumigatus*. **Lactophenol cotton blue stain (40×)**

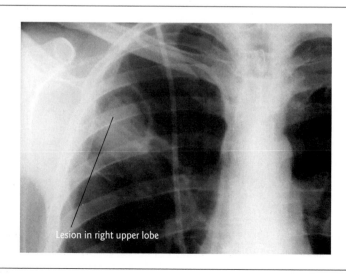

Figure 14.11 Invasive aspergillosis in a neutropenic patient. Note the lesion in the right upper lobe. The Department of Microbiology, UCLH, London is gratefully acknowledged for use of this image

Lesion in right upper lobe

Infection control measures

Handwashing

It may sound like common sense, but it is important to state repeatedly in the healthcare environment that handwashing is one of the most effective methods to prevent the spread of infection. There are two important aspects of hand hygiene that need to be emphasized: hands need to be washed *before* and of course after performing any sort of patient care and proper hand washing technique needs to be practiced in that all surfaces of the hand including the webspaces are thoroughly cleansed. Ideally a clinical handwash basin needs to have elbow operated levers to minimize re-contamination (Figure 14.12).

Many clinical areas have visible and eye catching posters that serve as reminders for healthcare staff to wash their hands (Figure 14.13).

An alternative to handwashing, if washing hands is not feasible because of time constraints or ward design, is to disinfect hands by rubbing with an alcohol solution (Figure 14.14).

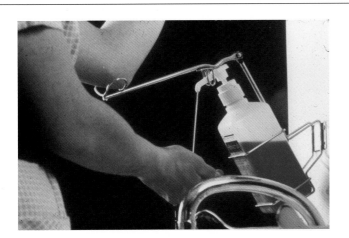

Figure 14.12 Handwashing in a clinical area. Note: elbow operated levers; the taps will have them too. The Department of Microbiology, UCLH, London is gratefully acknowledged for use of this image

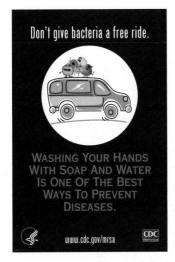

Don't give bacteria a free ride.

WASHING YOUR HANDS WITH SOAP AND WATER IS ONE OF THE BEST WAYS TO PREVENT DISEASES.

www.cdc.gov/mrsa   CDC

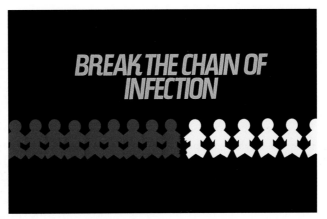

BREAK THE CHAIN OF INFECTION

Figure 14.13 Remember to wash your hands! Courtesy: Educational materials from the CDC, accessed from http://www.cdc.gov/ncidod/dhqp/ar_mrsa_ca_posters.html

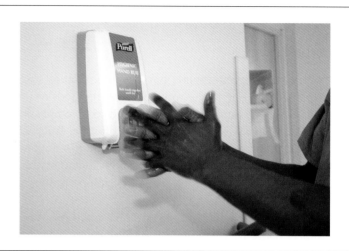

Figure 14.14 Using alcohol hand rub as alternative to handwashing. The Department of Microbiology, UCLH, London is gratefully acknowledged for use of this image

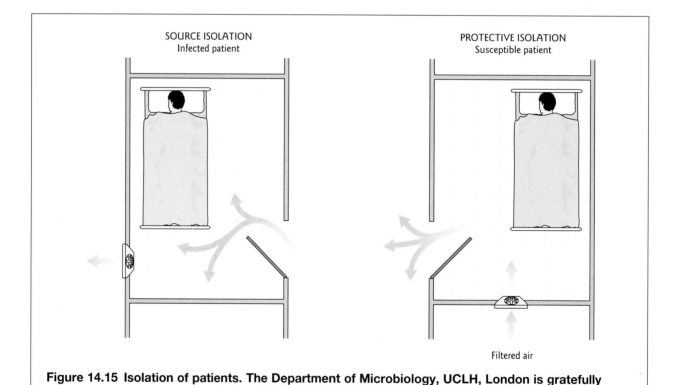

SOURCE ISOLATION
Infected patient

PROTECTIVE ISOLATION
Susceptible patient

Filtered air

Figure 14.15 Isolation of patients. The Department of Microbiology, UCLH, London is gratefully acknowledged for use of this image

Isolation

Appropriate isolation of the patient in a single room plays a critical role in infection control. Isolation facilities may be of two types (Figure 14.15). The isolation of an infected patient is sometimes termed "source isolation." It is important to establish that air flows are directed from the corridor into the room as seen in Figure 14.15. In cases of highly communicable diseases such as chickenpox or tuberculosis, the isolation cubicle is monitored to have negative air pressure in relation to the surrounding areas.

Patients infected by the same microorganism usually can share a room. Such sharing of rooms, also referred to as *cohorting* patients, is useful especially during outbreaks or when there is a shortage of single rooms.

The patient who is not infected, but is especially vulnerable to infection, such as the neutropenic patient, requires "protective isolation." Here the air pressure in the room is under positive pressure as compared to

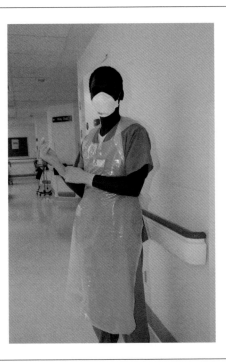

Figure 14.16 Other barriers: the use of masks, gloves, and aprons. The Department of Microbiology, UCLH, London is gratefully acknowledged for use of this image

the corridor and special air handling units ensure that filtered air circulates in the room. For the complete CDC guidance to isolation practices see Further reading.

Masks, gloves, and aprons

Another important group of precautions to prevent the spread of infection is the use of masks, gloves, and aprons (Figure 14.16). Masks that are made of special synthetic material that can filter the air are considered good barriers against microorganisms. Masks made of other material such as wool, gauze, or papers are not considered effective. Masks are used primarily to protect the healthcare worker against airborne agents such as respiratory viruses or *M. tuberculosis*.

Gloves are a necessary barrier when working with patients with a communicable disease. Gloves are used for protection of both the patient and healthcare provider.

Wearing gloves does not replace the need for handwashing. Failure to change gloves between patient contacts is an infection control hazard. Gowns and aprons are worn by personnel during the care of infected patients to reduce the opportunity for transmission of pathogens from patients or items in their environment to other patients or environments; when gowns are worn for this purpose, they should be removed before leaving the patient's environment and hands washed. We often hear the term "universal or standard precautions" (Figure 14.17). Read Box 14.6 for a description of these precautions.

Injection practices

Transmission of blood-borne pathogens is often the result of unsafe injection methods. All staff should be trained in the use of sharps and other needles: to maintain sterility and sterile technique at all times, and to dispose of the used needle and syringe in an appropriate manner, i.e. the use of a sharps container (Figure 14.18).

Surveillance, education, and research

It is mandatory that hospitals in the USA have an infection control committee chaired by the hospital epidemiologist. The committee comprises a multidisciplinary group of individuals (nurses, information

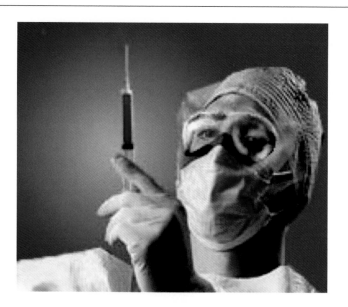

Figure 14.17 Standard precautions. Image from US Department of Labor, Occupational Safety & Health Administration. www.osha.gov/ . . . / hazards/univprec/univ.html

Box 14.6 What are Universal (now called "Standard") precautions

In the summer of 1987, as a result of the AIDS epidemic, the CDC proposed a new concept for isolation precautions called "Universal Precautions," they were designed to minimize the risk of transmission of blood-borne infections especially HIV.

The new term "Standard Precautions" combines the major features of Universal Precautions and Body Substance Isolation (designed to reduce the risk of transmission of pathogens from all moist body substances). These are based on the principle that all blood, body fluids, secretions, excretions except sweat, nonintact skin, and mucous membranes may contain transmissible infectious agents.

Standard Precautions include a group of infection prevention practices that apply to all patients, regardless of suspected or confirmed infection status, in any setting in which healthcare is delivered. These include: hand hygiene; use of gloves, gown, mask, eye protection, or face shield, depending on the anticipated exposure; and safe injection practices. The application of Standard Precautions during patient care is determined by the nature of the healthcare worker–patient interaction and the extent of anticipated blood, body fluid, or pathogen exposure. For some interactions (e.g. performing venipuncture), only gloves may be needed; during other interactions (e.g. intubation), use of gloves, gown, and face shield or mask and goggles is necessary.

Standard Precautions are also intended to protect patients by ensuring that healthcare personnel do not carry infectious agents to patients on their hands or via equipment used during patient care.

In brief:

Hands should be washed promptly and thoroughly as soon as possible after contact with blood or other potentially infectious materials and equipment or articles contaminated by them. Handwashing is necessary because gloves may have inconspicuous holes and because microbial growth may occur due to the moist environment inside gloves.

Standard Precautions employ barrier equipment such as gloves, face shields or masks, eye protection, pocket masks, etc. (Figure 14.18). Barrier equipment is considered appropriate only if it does not permit blood and other potentially infectious materials to pass through to or reach the employee's clothes, skin, eyes, mouth, or other mucous membranes under normal conditions of use.

New elements to Standard Precautions

Three areas of practice that have been added are: respiratory hygiene/cough etiquette, safe injection practices, and use of masks for insertion of catheters or injection of material into spinal or epidural spaces via lumbar puncture procedures (e.g. myelogram, spinal or epidural anesthesia). While most elements of Standard Precautions evolved from Universal Precautions that were developed for protection of healthcare personnel, these new elements of Standard Precautions focus on protection of patients.

Refer to: http://www.cdc.gov/ncidod/dhqp/gl_isolation_standard.html

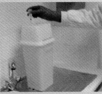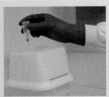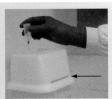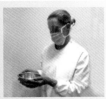

Good Practice

Dispose of sharps immediately after use in a designated sharps disposal bin

Take sharps bin to site of use and dispose of sharps directly into sharps bin after use

Dispose of sharps bin immediately when it is full (indicated by arrow)

Always use universal precautions when at risk of exposure to or when handling, blood, body fluids or tissues

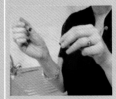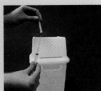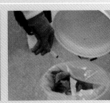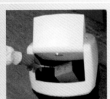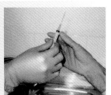

Bad Practice

Regardless of circumstances NEVER recap needles. Do not handle syringes without gloves

NEVER recap needles. You are risking a sharps injury

Do NOT use clinical bins for sharps disposal

Do NOT use general purpose bins for sharps disposal

Used sharps should NEVER be passed by hand between healthcare workers. The user of the sharps has the responsibility for disposal

Figure 14.18 Good practice prevents sharps injuries. Copied from the Health Protection Agency, UK; www.hpa.org.uk

technologists, and statisticians) that oversees the infection prevention and control programs. They advise on hospital cleaning protocols, linen and laundry, and decontamination of invasive devices. They also inspect kitchens, theatres, and the central sterilization unit regularly. This committee is responsible for surveillance, research, and education. It also plays an important role in evaluating infection prevention measures, oversees changes in programs, law, and regulations and reviews new guidelines.

Work with members of your infection control team, they are your greatest allies in the fight against infection.

Test yourself

Case study 14.1

A 60-year-old African man presents with a 4-day history of watery diarrhea, abdominal pain, and distension. No one else in his family is affected, and he has not visited Africa recently. He is known to have chronic obstructive airways disease and 2 weeks ago he was admitted to hospital for worsening cough with a greenish-colored sputum, and breathlessness at rest. Sputum cultures grew *H. influenzae*, sensitive to amoxicillin. He completed the prescribed course of amoxicillin 3 days ago.

On examination he has no fever, although he is breathless and restless. His pulse rate is 100 beats/min and blood pressure 120/80 mm Hg. His abdomen is diffusely tender, with some suggestion of guarding over the lower half. He was referred for a surgical opinion.

Test yourself

1. What is the likely cause of his watery diarrhea?
2. Could this be a healthcare acquired infection?
3. If so discuss the risk factors for a HAI in this patient.
4. What infection control measures would you recommend while he is in hospital so as to decrease transmission of infection?

Case study 14.2

A 68-year-old man had a peripheral intravenous cannula inserted in his left arm at the time of a minor day case surgical procedure. He was 10 kg overweight and cannulation was difficult; he was also diabetic and had previous cardiac problems. As a result of complications the day case procedure had to be converted to an open abdominal surgical operation (a laparotomy). On the fifth postoperative day, he developed fever and complained of pain and redness at the cannula site. The laparotomy wound dehisced due to poor healing and became infected. Blood and wound cultures were sent to the laboratory.

Blood and wound cultures grew MRSA. Looking back through his medical notes, he had a routine preoperative nose screen to establish whether he was an asymptomatic MRSA carrier. These screens were negative at the time of the operation.

1. Could the infection with MRSA be endogenous or exogenous in origin? Justify your answer.
2. What is the major route of transmission of this organism in hospital?
3. How many routes of entry are there in this patient for this organism?
4. Are there any other risk factors that predispose him to infection with MRSA?
5. Do you think the MRSA that we isolated from his cultures were as a result of colonization or infection?
6. What infection control measures would you put in place to protect other patients in his immediate environment?

Case study 14.3

A 72-year-old woman underwent planned coronary artery bypass graft surgery. She gave a history of cigarette smoking for the past 20 years, smoking 10–15 cigarettes a day. She also had chronic osteoarthritis, with limited mobility of the hip joint. She had previously had surgery on her lumbar and cervical spine, with a protracted stay in hospital and several courses of antibiotics for a postoperative chest infection.

The cardiac surgery was uncomplicated, and she was discharged on the eighth postoperative day. A week later, she presented to the hospital with a cough, fever, and pain over the sternal wound. Her respiratory distress became increasingly worse and she was admitted to ICU, where she was intubated and ventilated, she also needed a central venous catheter and a urinary catheter as routine procedures in ICU.

A week into her stay in ICU she became increasingly unwell due to sepsis. Respiratory secretions, urine and blood cultures at this time grew *Acinetobacter baumanii*, susceptible to meropenem and amikacin only. A week later, at a routine review of infections in the cardiac ICU, it was revealed that three other patients in the same bay had contracted *A. baumanii*; one had died. The four isolates of *A. baumanii* were subjected to molecular typing using pulsed field gel electrophoresis. The gel with the dendrogram (a diagram that extrapolates percentage similarity between strains) is shown on the following page. The four isolates from the cardiac ICU are numbered 40, 44, 46, and 47.

Test yourself

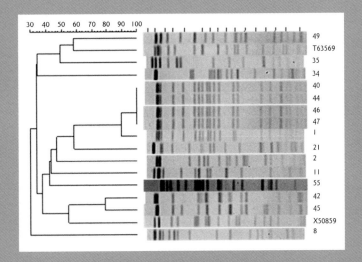

1. List all the risk factors that predispose this patient to a HAI.
2. Could the *A. baumanii* infection be exogenous or endogenous in origin? Justify your answer.
3. After examining the dendrogram do you think there was transmission of *A. baumanii* between the four patients that acquired the infection in the cardiac ICU?
4. What procedures in the care of this patient could have facilitated transmission of the organism within the ICU?
5. How could transmission have been prevented?

Further reading

Garner JS, Jarvis WR, Emori TG, Horan TC, Hughes JM. CDC definitions for nosocomial infections. *Am J Infect Control* 1988;16:128–140

Useful websites

CDC. Guideline for Isolation Precautions in Hospitals. http://www.cdc.gov/ncidod/dhqp/gl_isolation_ptII.html

CDC. Infection Control A–Z Index. Guidelines for the prevention of healthcare associated infections. http://www.cdc.gov/ncidod/dhqp/a_z.html#u

CDC. Infection Control Guidelines: Standard Precautions. http://www.cdc.gov/ncidod/dhqp/gl_isolation_standard.html

Chapter 15
The fever and rash conundrum: rashes of childhood

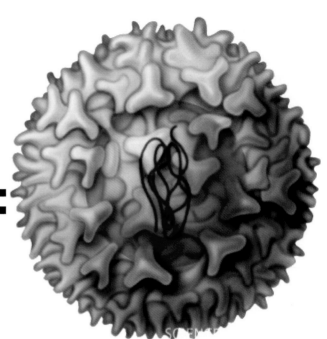

J.W. Tang

Introduction
Characterizing childhood rash illnesses
The naming of childhood rashes
Measles (rubeola, "first disease")
Scarlet fever ("second disease")
Rubella ("German measles," "third disease")

Chickenpox
"Slapped cheek disease" (erythema infectiosum, "fifth disease")
"Sixth disease" (exanthem subitum, roseola infantum)
Other rash illnesses of childhood

Introduction

Febrile rash illnesses in young children are a source of great anxiety to parents, and may be difficult to distinguish clinically, in some cases. Most often, they are self-limiting illnesses in children – the same infections in adults may cause more severe disease – but rarely, they result in some serious complications. As well as the child's health, these childhood rash illnesses have consequences for others around them, as some of them can be very infectious. This is a particularly important consideration when there may be contact with pregnant women – sometimes even the child's mother – as some viral causes of febrile rashes can lead to congenital abnormality, e.g. rubella, chickenpox, and parvovirus B19. These are dealt with in Chapter 12.

Fortunately, nowadays, in most developed countries (including the USA) there are well established childhood immunization programs that protect the majority of children from some of the rash illnesses, e.g. measles, rubella and more recently, chickenpox. The original aim behind these childhood immunization programs was twofold: to protect the children and to protect pregnant women. Nowadays, with an increasing population of immunocompromised individuals (due to HIV/AIDS, cancer patients on chemotherapy, patients on long-term steroids, or patients with organ transplants), there is a third group that benefits from such protection.

Characterizing childhood rash illnesses (see also Chapter 7)

In most cases, childhood febrile rashes present with a prodromal period that may last a few (perhaps 1–3) days, where the child may seem generally unwell with a fever, before the onset of the rash. The skin rash can take several forms: small, red (or **erythematous**), flat spots (a **macular** rash) which are nonitchy, as found in rubella (also commonly known as "German measles"); larger, redder spots that may appear in larger patches that may be raised slightly (a **maculopapular** rash), which may be itchy, as found in measles (also known as **rubeola**); a rash that starts off as red, itchy spots of different sizes and shapes, which become raised and turn into small blisters (or **vesicles**) containing fluid (a **vesicular** rash), as found in chickenpox. In addition, chickenpox has the further distinguishing feature in that not all the vesicles are in the same stage of the development at the same time – some may have just started to form, others may be drying up and falling off. This characteristic used to be one of the main features that allowed doctors to distinguish chickenpox from smallpox before smallpox was finally eradicated in the late 1970s (officially declared eradicated in 1980 (see Chapter 26). The rash may also be blanchable or nonblanchable. This means that if you press on the rash with your fingertip, the redness fades, then when you let go, the redness returns. This distinguishes nonblanchable rashes caused by the bleeding of damaged small vessels under the skin (also known as **petechiae**), caused by more serious illness, such as bacterial septicemia (e.g. meningococcal – see Chapter 7) and viral hemorrhagic fevers (see Chapters 22 and 24), from the more typically blanchable rashes of the more usually benign common childhood infections.

As well as the **character** of the rash, the **distribution** of the rash over the body is an important clinical clue to the possible cause. Most childhood rashes are generalized, i.e. they occur on all the body's skin surfaces – the legs, arms, chest, back, face, and buttocks. Also the type of pattern of the rash can be important, such as the typical "slapped-cheek" appearance of parvovirus B19 (PVB19) infection in childhood. This pattern is less commonly seen in older children and adults when a more "lacy, reticular" pattern (similar to the pattern of the holes in a Swiss cheese – the rash of PVB19 makes up the edges of the holes) may be seen on the arms or legs.

Apart from the character and distribution of the rash, other **associated features or symptoms** may assist in the clinical diagnosis of childhood rashes, e.g. the swelling behind the ears (produced by lymph nodes swelling) in rubella, the red eyes (conjunctivitis) of measles, and the joint pains that may occur in PVB19 infection. The timing of the fever and the subsequent rash and other symptoms may be a more subtle clue to the cause of the rash illness. For example, with PVB19, the fever may settle before the rash and joint pains become manifest. Similarly, in human herpes virus 6 (HHV6) infection (also known as **exanthema subitum** or **roseola infantum**), the fever may be very high, but then settle before the subsequent appearance of the rash. Note that all these aspects of viral rash illnesses can vary in immunocompromised patients, as their lack of a normal immune response allows the virus to replicate unchecked in a way that may produce other disease manifestations not normally seen in immunocompetent individuals.

The naming of childhood rashes

There are several ways to refer to the childhood rashes, and it is useful to mention all of them, as they may be used interchangeably by physicians and other healthcare workers, parents, the media, and textbooks. The most common way is to name them simply by the agent that causes them, e.g. measles (rubeola) and rubella (German measles). Some of the other rashes are referred to by describing their appearance, e.g. chickenpox (caused by varicella zoster virus, VZV), "slapped-cheek disease" (caused by PVB 19), **exanthema subitum**, or **roseola infantum** (caused by HHV6). Finally, an older, less commonly used and more historical way of referring to the childhood rashes just numbers them as "first disease" (caused by measles virus), "second disease" (scarlet fever cause by the Group A beta hemolytic *Streptococcus*), "third disease" (cause by rubella virus), "fourth disease" (considered by some to be caused by the exotoxin of another bacteria *Staphylococcus aureus*), "fifth disease" (caused by PVB19), and "sixth disease" (caused by HHV6).

Table 15.1 lists the different names and features of these common childhood rash illnesses, and summarizes the following sections for the different individual rashes. There is some uncertainty about whether fourth disease is generally accepted as true childhood exanthema, so it has not been included in the following sections.

Table 15.1 Summary of main characteristics of the common childhood rash illness. See corresponding main text sections for more details

Rash illness names Causal agent Transmission route	Typical incubation period*/Rash description	Typical general symptoms	Complications†	Diagnosis	Specific treatment/ Life long immunity/ Licensed vaccine
Measles ("first disease") Measles virus (genus *Morbillivirus*) Via direct contact with infected secretions and small, airborne droplets	10–14 days/Blanchable, erythematous, maculopapular. May be itchy. Starts from the head and descends over the rest of the body. Individual lesions may coalesce and become large blotches. Usually lasts 5–7 days	Viral prodrome: fever (can be high), malaise, flu-like illness, runny nose, coughing, sneezing. With Koplik's spots, and conjunctivitis	Otitis media (7%), pneumonia (6%), encephalitis (0.1%), SSPE (5–10 per million)	Serum measles IgM, paired IgG seroconversion, PCR during acute illness phase	No/Yes/Yes – MMR
Scarlet fever ("second disease") *Streptococcus pyogenes* Via direct contact with infected secretions and short-range, large droplets	A few days/Blanching, erythematous, maculopapular, not usually itchy. Spreads out from the trunk to the rest of the body, including palms of hands and soles of feet. Usually lasts 2–5 days	Typically starts with fever, malaise, coughing, sneezing, "strep sore throat," which may show pus. With "strawberry tongue," redness in joint skin creases	Only in untreated cases: pneumonia, otitis media, bacterial endocarditis, death	*Streptococcus pyogenes* cultured from throat swab	Yes – penicillin-based antibiotics/No – reinfection is possible/ No – not specifically against scarlet fever
Rubella (German Measles, "third disease") Rubella virus (genus *Rubivirus*) Via direct contact with infected secretions and short-range, large droplets	2–3 weeks/Blanchable, erythematous, maculopapular, finer lesions than measles. May be itchy. Usually starts from the head and descends over the rest of the body. Individual lesions do not usually coalesce. Usually lasts about 3 days	May be mild or asymptomatic – with the rash being the first signs of illness. Otherwise, with a typical viral prodrome, with postauricular lymphadenopathy, and arthralgia	Prolonged arthralgia (≤70% adult women), encephalitis (1:6000), hemorrhagic problems (1:3000)	Serum rubella IgM, paired IgG seroconversion, PCR during acute illness phase	No/Yes/Yes – MMR
Chickenpox Varicella zoster virus (genus *Varicellovirus*) Via direct contact with infected secretions and small, airborne droplets	10–21 days/Initially a blanchable, erythematous, maculopapular rash descending from the head to the rest of the body, which soon becomes vesicular. Intensely itchy. Lesions can be found in the mouth and other mucous membranes. Vesicles contain clear fluid. Several generations may appear over 3–5 days. The lesions dry and fall off after 7–10 days	Typical viral prodrome. The vesicular rash is epidermal and fragile (often broken), usually centripetal, with lesions at different stages of development visible at any one time – this distinguishes it from smallpox	Viral and bacterial pneumonia (particularly in smokers, asthmatics), encephalitis (2:10 000), more rarely, involving other organs	Serum VZV IgM, paired IgG seroconversion, PCR during acute phase. Also, direct IFT on vesicle skin scrapings, and viral culture	Yes – aciclovir and other anti-herpesvirus drugs/Yes/Yes – two live-attenuated VZV vaccines are now available

Disease/Virus/Transmission	Incubation/Rash	Clinical features	Complications	Diagnosis	Treatment/Immunity/Vaccine
Slapped-cheek disease (erythema infectiosum, "fifth disease") Parvovirus B19 (genus *Erythrovirus*) Via direct contact with infected secretions and short-range, large droplets	4–20 (usually 14–18 days)/Erythematous, maculopapular, in a "slapped-cheek" pattern in children. Usually nonitchy. Starts from the face and descends over the rest of the body, as a lacy, reticular rash. Variations can be seen, particularly in adults, e.g. a glove-and-stocking distribution, as erythema multiforme "target" lesions, sometimes weeks after the acute infection. Not all lesions may be blanchable as some may be purpuric. The rash usually clears within a few days, but can sometimes recur for several weeks	May be mild or asymptomatic – with the rash being the first signs of illness. Otherwise, with a typical viral prodrome, with a biphasic pattern – first the fever, then the rash and arthralgia	*Aplastic anemia* (red cell destruction), *pancytopenia* (white cell/platelet destruction). Prolonged arthralgia mimicking rheumatoid arthritis	Serum parvovirus B19 IgM, paired IgG seroconversion, PCR during acute illness phase	No/Yes/No
"Sixth disease" (exanthum subitum, roseola infantum) Human herpesvirus 6 (genus *Roseolavirus*) Via direct contact with infected secretions, e.g. saliva	5–15 days/Blanchable, erythematous, maculopapular, "rash of roses". Not usually itchy. Spreads out from the trunk to the rest of the body. Usually lasts a few hours to 1–2 days	Typically starts with an abrupt onset of high fever – sometimes with seizures, with the typical viral prodrome. A biphasic disease, the fever usually subsides before the rash appears. With periorbital edema, a bulging anterior fontanel, swollen glands in the head and neck, and red spots in the mouth	Seizures (6–15%), diarrhea (~70%), meningitis, meningo-encephalitis	Fourfold rise in antibody titers in paired acute and convalescent sera, with PCR during acute illness phase	Yes – aciclovir and other anti-herpesvirus drugs/Not really – HHV6 antibodies do not entirely prevent own HHV6 from reactivating/No

Note: Rubella, chickenpox, and slapped-cheek disease – all may have serious consequences for pregnant women – see Chapter 12. SSPE, subsclerosing panencephalitis; PCR, polymerase chain reaction (not available in all standard diagnostic laboratories); MMR, measles–mumps–rubella vaccine; VZV, varicella zoster virus; IFT, immunofluorescence test.

* Different texts quote different incubation times, which may be an accurate reflection of the natural variation of the infection.

† A higher risk of complications is usually present in adults, and will always exist in immunocompromised patients, who may also manifest some unique complications not seen in otherwise healthy immunocompetent people.

Measles (rubeola, "first disease")

Measles is possibly the oldest of the childhood rash illnesses to be recognized (hence "first disease"), and is also the most infectious. There is still a significant mortality from measles, mainly in developing countries with an estimated 454 000 deaths out of 30 million cases (~1.5% mortality rate) worldwide in 2004, according to the World Health Organization (WHO). In the USA, from 1985 to 1992, the mortality rate from measles was 0.2%, mainly in young children from pneumonia (60% of deaths) and acute encephalitis in adults. Until the start of widespread measles immunization in the 1970s, most children acquired the natural infection. However, since then, the incidence of natural childhood measles infection has decreased dramatically, though there are still sporadic outbreaks in areas where vaccine coverage in that population has dropped below the critical threshold level of around 92–95%. For example, in the USA, before 1963, almost everyone got measles, with about 3–4 million cases being reported each year, with an average of 450 deaths. Measles epidemics occurred every 2–3 years, with more than 50% of the population having had measles by the age of 6 years, and 90% by the age of 15 years. There were almost certainly many more cases occurring than were being reported. However, after the vaccine became available, the number of measles cases dropped by 98% and the epidemic cycles drastically diminished.

Measles is caused by a virus of the *Morbillivirus* genus (Figure 15.1), family Paramyxoviridae. It is extremely infectious, being one of the truly airborne infections and is readily spread by coughing and sneezing, as well as by direct contact with infected body fluids (e.g. saliva, mucus and sputum). The incubation period (the time from infection to the first appearance of symptoms) is about 10–14 days, and infected individuals are probably infectious to others from just before the appearance (during the prodromal period), and throughout the duration of the rash. As with most systemic viral infections, there is usually a prodromal period when the child develops fever (which can be as high as 104–105°F (40–41°C)), headache, coughing, sneezing, red eyes (**conjunctivitis**), a blocked or runny nose. During this early prodromal period, a few days before the onset of the rash, "Koplik's spots" may be seen inside the child's mouth on the inside of the cheek (i.e. on the **buccal mucosa**). These are small bright red spots with blue-white centers, but these are often missed unless the examining physician is thinking specifically of measles.

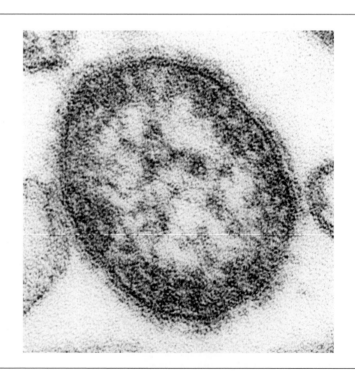

Figure 15.1 Thin-section transmission electron micrograph of a measles virus. It is an enveloped virus containing negative-sense, single-stranded RNA. As with most enveloped viruses, measles virus is rapidly inactivated by heat, light, acidic pH, ether, and trypsin, with a short survival time (<2 hours) in the air, or on objects and surfaces. Provided by Cynthia Goldsmith and William Bellini. Courtesy of the Centers for Disease Control and Prevention; from CDC website: http://phil.cdc.gov/phil/details.asp

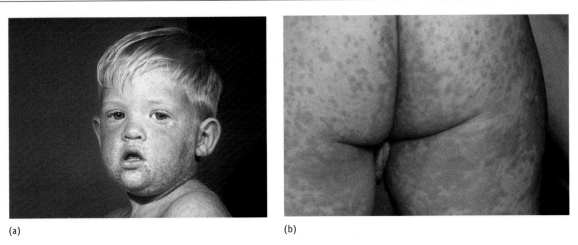

(a)   (b)

Figure 15.2 This child with measles is displaying the characteristic red blotchy pattern on his face (a) and buttocks (b). The rash typically appears first on the face before descending and becoming generalized to involve the rest of the body. It lasts about 5–7 days, before eventually fading from red to brown, and finally flaking off. Courtesy of the Centers for Disease Control and Prevention; from CDC website: http://phil.cdc.gov/phil/details.asp

The blanchable, maculopapular rash that may by itchy, begins 3–5 days after the onset of the prodromal symptoms and lasts for about 5–7 days. It usually starts from the head and moves downwards over the body (Figure 15.2). The individual spots may join together (coalesce) and become confluent, forming larger plaques. The redness of the rash fades to a brown color as the child recovers, and the affected skin flakes off, normally without scarring. Measles is usually a benign illness but in up to 30% of cases, there are complications which include: secondary bacterial or other viral ear infection (**otitis media** – infection of the middle ear in 7% of cases); pneumonia (in up to 6% of cases) either directly from the measles virus, or secondary bacterial infection; and infection of the brain (**acute encephalitis** in up to 0.1% of cases with a case-fatality rate of 15% and long-term damage in up to 25% of survivors). A much rarer form of encephalitis occurs 5–10 years after natural measles infection in 5–10 cases per million measles cases, known as **subsclerosing panencephalitis** (SSPE). This is almost invariably fatal and is characterized by a gradual deterioration in mental function, followed by failure of coordination and movement then death. Complications with measles infections are not uncommon, which may be due to its mildly immunosuppressive effects. Most are self-limiting with appropriate therapy (e.g. antibiotics for secondary bacterial infections). The incidence of acute encephalitis is about 1 in 1000 cases of measles and affected children may suffer long-term brain damage or even death. With SSPE, the incidence is much less (often quoted as 1 in 1 million cases of measles), but the outcome is almost invariably fatal.

Diagnosis is often clinical, as the prodrome and measles rash is quite distinctive. However, laboratory confirmation can be obtained by testing the child's serum for the presence of measles IgM antibody. If paired sera are available (i.e. pre- and post-infection sera), a seroconversion from measles IgG negative to IgG positive, with compatible clinical features, should be sufficient to confirm the diagnosis. This antibody takes several days to appear, and may still be absent on the first days of the rash, in which case a repeat sample should be tested a few days later. Alternatively, in the absence of detectable antibody at this stage, molecular techniques can detect the virus genome directly using the polymerase chain reaction (PCR). However, normally, by the time the patient presents to hospital where such tests can be performed, it is several days after the rash has appeared and antibodies should be present, with little virus left in the bloodstream for the PCR test to detect.

There is no specific antiviral treatment for measles and the mainstay of its control has been with immunization, most recently with the widespread use of the measles-mumps-rubella (MMR) vaccine. Despite long-running controversy, there is no evidence that the MMR vaccine has any causal connection with autism, and the vaccine may prevent measles infection and all its associated complications. Although measles infection in pregnant women does not usually cause a specific congenital abnormality syndrome like other rash illnesses (e.g. congenital rubella syndrome), as with any other cause of a high fever, it may lead to spontaneous abortion. Measles may be more severe in immunocompromised individuals, so any case of measles requires a risk assessment with regard to contact tracing and monitoring the welfare of vulnerable contacts. Postexposure prophylaxis with MMR vaccine within the first 3 days after exposure is recommended by some authorities, though others have found little evidence of its efficacy (see Further reading). After 6 days, postexposure prophylaxis may be attempted with immunoglobulin containing measles IgG. Nowadays, national immunization programs in most countries use the MMR vaccine to protect women of childbearing age against measles. Immunity to measles after wild-type or natural infection is lifelong. There is only one serotype of measles, so this immunity should be protective against exposure from all strains of the measles virus.

Scarlet fever ("second disease")

Scarlet fever is caused by the toxin of Group A beta hemolytic *Streptococcus* species bacteria, which infect the upper airways in children above the age of 4 years, typically beginning with a respiratory infection with a "strep sore throat." It can spread rapidly between children in relatively close (face-to-face) contact (in households and nurseries) via coughing and sneezing, as well as by direct contact with infected body fluids (e.g. saliva, mucus, and sputum). It occurs in about 10% of such streptococcal infections and has become relatively uncommon nowadays, as such "strep sore throats" are often treated early with antibiotics by the family doctor.

Usually the child first presents with a high fever and "flu-like" symptoms, with headache, coughing, sneezing, and a sore throat. Sometimes this is accompanied by nausea, abdominal pain, and vomiting. The rash, which is blanching and maculopapular, usually appears 1–2 days later and spreads out from the trunk to cover the whole body within hours to days, giving the skin a surface texture like sandpaper (Figure 15.3). It is not usually itchy. The area around the mouth is often spared, though the lips, palms of the hand, and soles of the feet may turn bright red. Examination of the throat at this time will reveal redness and sometimes pus (white or yellow fluid containing dead white cells and bacteria that may smell offensive). The tongue may also become swollen and red, giving the appearance of a "strawberry tongue." In addition, red streaks may become prominent in the skin creases over joints, e.g. behind the knees and in the elbow

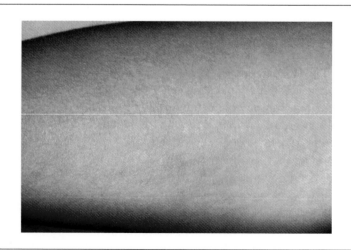

Figure 15.3 Scarlet fever rash on the forearm. This blanching, maculopapular rash first appears on the chest and abdomen then may spread all over the body. Its appearance is similar to that of a sunburn, with a texture like sandpaper. It typically lasts about 2–5 days. Courtesy of the Centers for Disease Control and Prevention; from CDC website: http://phil.cdc.gov/phil/details.asp

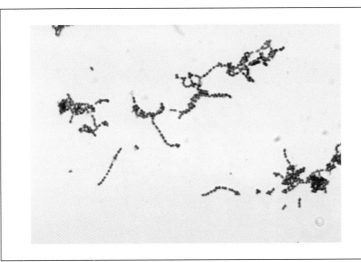

Figure 15.4 Photomicrograph of *Streptococcus* spp. using Gram's stain. The bacteria stain blue as they are Gram positive. Courtesy of the Centers for Disease Control and Prevention; from CDC website: http://phil.cdc.gov/phil/details.asp

creases. Complications are rarely seen nowadays due to prompt antibiotic therapy, but include streptococcal septicemia, bacterial endocarditis (infection and destruction of the heart valves), otitis media, pneumonia, and death.

Diagnosis is important for the appropriate treatment to be given. It is easily obtained using a cotton swab to rub the back of the child's throat, which is then cultured on the appropriate bacterial culture medium and examined microscopically after 24 hours using specific stains (e.g. Gram's stain), for the presence of the causative streptococcal species: *S. pyogenes* (a Group A beta hemolytic *Streptococcus* species, Figure 15.4). Treatment lasts 10–14 days and is usually penicillin-based. Children with penicillin allergy may be given an alternative drug, such as erythromycin. "Strep sore throat" can recur and recurrent infections may raise the possibility of an underlying immunodeficiency, the cause of which requires further specialist investigations.

Rubella ("German measles," "third disease")

Clinically, rubella is a mild illness, with up to 50% being asymptomatic or subclinical, and if it were not for the devastating effects on the fetus, it would probably have remained a relatively minor viral exanthem. However, instead, it has become the major impetus for national childhood immunization programs around the world. In the USA during a rubella epidemic in 1964–1965, there were about 12.5 million cases of rubella resulting in about 20 000 cases (0.2%) of congenital rubella syndrome (see Chapter 12). The epidemic alone at the time was estimated to cost about US$ 840 million, which did not include the cost of caring for these handicapped children, which is estimated to be >US$ 200 000 by today's standards.

In the USA, there was previously no predominant age group at which rubella infection occurred, e.g. from 1982 to 1992, about 30% of cases occurred in each of these three age groups: <5 years, 5–14 years, and 15–39 years of age. Adults older than 40 years of age usually accounted for less than 10% of cases. However, since 1993, people of 15–39 years of age have made up more than 50% of all reported cases, and in 2003, this increased to 71%. Since the mid-1990s, many reported rubella cases in younger adults in the USA have occurred in young Hispanic adults, who have presumably imigrated from areas where childhood rubella vaccine is not routinely given. It may also be a consequence of much more comprehensive rubella vaccine coverage in the younger child and adult age groups.

Rubella is caused by a virus in the genus *Rubivirus* (Figure 15.5), family *Togaviridae*. Like measles, it is also transmitted by droplets, as well as by direct contact with infected body fluids (e.g. saliva, mucus, and sputum), but is less transmissible and is not considered a truly airborne infection. As with measles, rubella is probably transmissible from just before the onset of the rash (during the prodromal period) and during the rash illness phase, though this will decrease substantially with the appearance of serum antibodies.

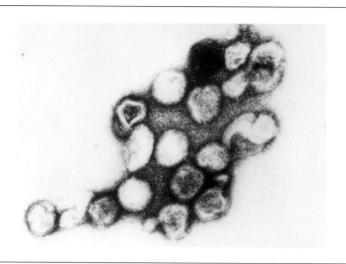

Figure 15.5 Transmission electron micrograph of several rubella viruses. This is an enveloped virus containing negative-sense, single-stranded RNA. Provided by Dr Erskine Palmer. Courtesy of the Centers for Disease Control and Prevention; from CDC website: http://phil.cdc.gov/phil/details.asp

After an incubation period of around 2–3 weeks, there may be a mild illness in the child, consisting of low-grade fever, some upper respiratory tract symptoms, such as cough, runny nose, general malaise, and lymphadenopathy ("swollen glands") – characteristically, those behind the ears (postauricular, Figure 15.6). This prodromal period may last up to a week before the onset of the rash. Often the first sign of illness may be the rash, which appears within 1–3 days after the prodromal period, and lasts for about 3 days. Like the rash of measles, it is usually blanchable, maculopapular and occasionally itchy, but the spots are finer and

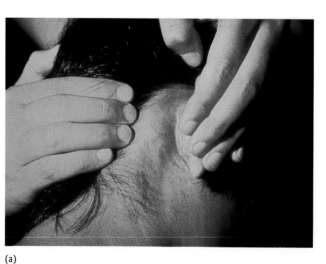

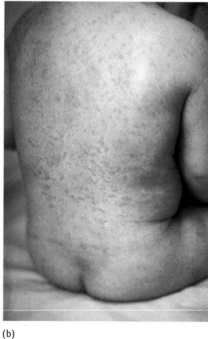

(a)   (b)

Figure 15.6 Rubella prodrome – the neck of a male patient with rubella. Postauricular (behind the ears) lymph nodes are chracteristically swollen in rubella (a). Rash of rubella on skin of child's back. Note that the distribution is similar to that of measles but the lesions are less intensely red, and there is little or no coalescing of individual spots (b). Courtesy of the Centers for Disease Control and Prevention; from CDC website: http://phil.cdc.gov/phil/details.asp

there is little or no coalescing to make the large blotchy appearance of the rash, typical of measles (compare Figures 15.2 and 15.6). In addition, the associated symptoms are quite different between rubella and measles. Rubella does not usually produce the intensely red conjunctivitis (red eyes) typically seen in measles, but does typically cause joints pains – particularly in adults with rubella – a feature not typical of measles.

Complications with rubella infection are relatively rare, compared to measles, and mostly occur in adults. These may take the form of prolonged joint pains (**arthralgia**) in up to 70% of adult women (but rarely in children or adult males), encephalitis (about 1 in 6000 cases, mainly in adults, with a mortality of 0–50%), as well as bleeding (**hemorrhagic**) problems (up to 1 in 3000 cases, more often in children than adults). The latter complication is due to the action of the rubella virus on some components (e.g. platelets causing **thrombocytopenia**) of the clotting system. However, the main complications of rubella infection are its effects on the fetus. This is discussed elsewhere in Chapter 12. Suffice it to say here that any confirmed case of rubella requires urgent contact tracing to see if any susceptible pregnant women has been exposed and possibly infected. Rubella infection in the immunocompromised may take longer to clear and prolong the duration of any related complications.

Diagnosis is usually made by the detection of rubella IgM in the serum, or if paired sera are available (i.e. pre- and post-infection sera), a seroconversion from rubella IgG negative to IgG positive, with compatible clinical features, should be sufficient to confirm the diagnosis. If a case of rubella is suspected early on during the prodromal period, and serum rubella IgM and IgG is absent at this stage, a molecular PCR test for rubella virus genome can be performed if available. The presence of rubella virus RNA in the patient's serum is good evidence for current infection with rubella.

There is no specific antiviral treatment for rubella, with the main method of control being immunization – now mainly with the MMR vaccine. Unlike measles, the MMR vaccine is not useful as postexposure prophylaxis for rubella, probably because the anti-rubella antibodies do not appear rapidly enough in response to the vaccine. Immunoglobulin is not generally used for rubella post-exposure prophylaxis. As with measles, immunity to rubella after wild-type or natural infection is lifelong and there is only one serotype of rubella, so this immunity should be protective against exposure from all strains of rubella virus.

Chickenpox

Chickenpox is caused by **varicella zoster virus** (VZV, Figure 15.7), in the genus *Varicellovirus*, family *Herpesviridae*. It is one of the major childhood rash illnesses that, historically, has not been given a numerical name. Its importance came from its similarity to smallpox, particularly in the early and mid 20th century, as there was a move towards the development of a smallpox vaccine with an aim to eradicating this ancient disease. From this section, it will be seen there are several important clinical features that distinguish chickenpox from smallpox (see also Chapter 26).

In the USA, in the pre-vaccine era, chickenpox was endemic, with virtually everyone having experienced chickenpox by adulthood. Hence, the number of annual chickenpox cases could be estimated by the annual birth rate – approximately 4 million cases per year. Chickenpox was removed as a nationally notifiable disease in the USA in 1981, but some states continued reporting cases to the Centers for Disease Control and Prevention (CDC). Data collected from 1990 to 1994, showed that the majority of cases (about 85%) occurred in children <15 years old, with the highest age-specific incidence of chickenpox occurring in children 1–4 years old, making up 39% of all reported cases. This age distribution was probably due to their early exposure to VZV in pre-school and child care groups. Slightly older children of 5–9 years accounted for 38% of cases, with adults older than 20 years accounting for only 7% of cases.

Perhaps contrary to popular belief, chickenpox has a significant associated morbidity and mortality. For example, in the USA prior to the availability of the VZV vaccine, about 11 000 hospital admissions annually occurred for chickenpox, with 2–3 per 1000 cases being healthy children and 8 per 1000 cases being adults. The mortality rate was about 1 in 60 000, with 103 deaths reported annually during 1990–1996. Most of these deaths occurred in children and adults with normal immune systems (i.e. they were **immunocompetent**). Since the introduction of the VZV vaccine in the USA in 1996, the number

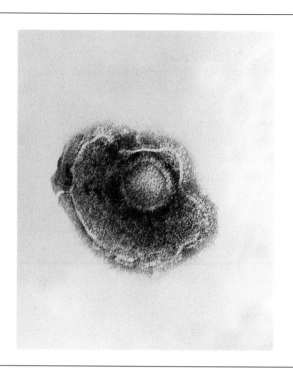

Figure 15.7 Electron micrograph of varicella zoster virus (VZV) that causes chickenpox. This is an enveloped virus containing double-stranded DNA. Provided by Dr Erskine Palmer and B.G. Partin. Courtesy of the Centers for Disease Control and Prevention; from CDC website: http://phil.cdc.gov/phil/details.asp

of admissions and deaths from chickenpox has decreased by more than 90%. In addition, the risk of complications from chickenpox increases with age, being rare in healthy children, but increasing in teenagers, the mortality rate rising from 1 per 100 000 in 1–14 year olds, to 2.7 per 100 000 in 15–19 year olds, to 25.2 per 100 000 in adults aged 30–49. Adults make up only 5% of reported chickenpox cases, but around 35% of the deaths. Very young children, less than 1 year old, have a higher mortality, particularly neonates (in the first 28 days of life) who have no protective maternally acquired VZV IgG antibodies, when neonatal VZV infections may have an overwhelming VZV infection with a mortality rate of 30%. The other vulnerable group is the immunocompromised patient, when uncontrolled VZV replication may have multi-organ involvement from disseminated VZV, resulting in rapid death if not treated appropriately, early and aggressively. In addition, and in contrast to the previous childhood rashes illness described so far, chickenpox has a lifelong implication for those infected. Unlike measles and rubella, VZV has not disappeared from the body when recovery from chickenpox is complete – it remains in the body and may cause disease many years later (Box 15.1).

In children, after an incubation period ranging from 10 to 21 days, primary VZV infection usually begins with a short 1–2 day prodromal period before the onset of the rash. Like other viral prodromes, clinical symptoms include fever (up to 102°F, 39°C), headache, malaise, flu-like symptoms, before the rash appears. Again, in children, this may be the first sign of the disease. Like measles and more so than rubella, chickenpox is considered to be transmitted by the airborne route, as well as by direct contact with infected body fluids (e.g. saliva, mucus, and sputum). It is, therefore, extremely infectious. Even recurrent infection – facial shingles or disseminated zoster in immunocompromised patients – are considered as infectious via the airborne route. The rash usually starts from the head and descends rapidly to cover the rest of the body, being concentrated mainly on the trunk in a centripetal distribution. This is the opposite of smallpox and is one of the clinically important distinctions between the two diseases. Chickenpox lesions begin as erythematous, raised (i.e. maculopapular) and itchy before becoming vesicular, and several generations of lesions usually appear on the body over several days with as many as 200–500 spots appearing with each generation (Figure 15.8). Lesions can be found on mucus membranes, such as inside the mouth, and may affect the eyes in severe cases. The vesicles contain clear fluid and these will eventually dry up, crust and fall

Box 15.1 A lifetime of varicella zoster virus infections

Although this chapter is primarily on childhood infections, it is important to note that the main economic and health burden from VZV infection is not from its primary infection that causes chickenpox in young children and (some adults), but from its recurrent infection that causes **herpes zoster** of shingles. After primary infection causing chickenpox, like other members of the human herpes virus family, VZV remains latent in the human body – for VZV this is specifically in the sensory, dorsal root ganglia (DRG) of the spinal cord. It may activate as painful herpes zoster ("shingles") at times of reduced immunity, particularly in the immunocompromised and the elderly. This reactivation or **recurrent** infection is caused by the migration of VZV down the sensory nerves from the DRG to the particular patch on the skin (or **dermatome**) that they supply. Since there are left-sided and right-sided DRGs and VZV from only one of these reactivates at any one time in normal immunocompetent individuals,

shingles usually occurs only on one side of the body. The exception to this is VZV reactivation in immunocompromised patients, when VZV may reactivate from multiple dermatomes at the same time and produce a form of shingles indistinguishable from chickenpox, often referred to as **varicelliform** or "disseminated" zoster, which can be lethal in such patients, if untreated. The problem with shingles is not the vesicular rash that may occur on that dermatome, but the pain that precedes it, and which may persist for long after the shingles rash has disappeared. This **postherpetic** pain or **neuralgia** can be severely debilitating, leading the sufferers (usually the elderly) to depression that may lead to more severe forms of treatment, such as surgically severing the sensory nerve roots supplying that affected area of skin. Pain complaints and attempts at its control for such patients may require frequent hospital admissions and long-term medication.

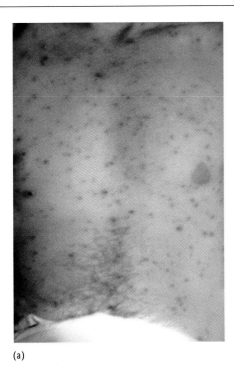
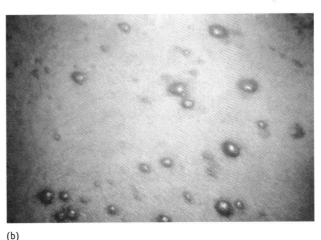

(a)   (b)

Figure 15.8 This patient with chickenpox developed lesions on the skin of his chest and torso (a). It usually starts on the face first then descends over the rest of the body, being most concentrated on the trunk. Several generations of lesions occur over 1–5 days, each generation producing 200–500 itchy blisters, which are fragile and easily broken (close-up, b). Such broken lesions may become secondarily infected with bacteria as a consequence of repeated scratching. Provided by Dr K.L. Hermann; Courtesy of the Centers for Disease Control and Prevention; from CDC website: http://phil.cdc.gov/phil/details.asp

off, after several days. This continuous cycle of rash appearance and crusting may continue for up to 5 days, with the last lesions being shed after 7–10 days. Hence, a second distinguishing feature from smallpox is that the rash of chickenpox exhibits lesions in various stages of this cycle at the same time, whereas smallpox lesions develop and scab over more or less simultaneously, in synchrony with each other. Also, whereas the vesicles of chickenpox are epidermal, fragile and burst readily, those of smallpox are dermal, much tougher and less easily broken.

In normal children, chickenpox is usually self-limiting, requiring no treatment in most cases. However, in infants in the first year of life (in the absence of maternal VZV antibody), adults, the immunocompromised and the elderly, chickenpox can be more severe with various complications. These can range from secondary bacterial skin infections (especially at broken vesicle sites), to viral or secondary bacterial pneumonia, to encephalitis (in about 2 cases per 10 000 VZV cases). Pneumonia is the most common complication, especially in smokers and others with some pre-existing lung condition, e.g. asthma, cystic fibrosis. Other rarer complications include those involving the brain, heart, liver, kidneys, eyes, joints, and the clotting system.

The diagnosis of chickenpox is usually made clinically, but laboratory confirmation can be performed using serology by the detection of VZV IgM, though this may be negative during the first few days of the rash. Seroconversion from VZV IgG negative to positive status is also definitive of primary VZV infection if pre- and post-infection sera are available for testing. A scraping of the skin from the base of a vesicle collected on a swab and cultured in human embryonic lung (HEL) cells) after 10–14 days' incubation, with confirmatory VZV identification using a VZV-specific immunofluorescence test (IFT), will also confirm the diagnosis of chickenpox. Alternatively, the skin scraping collected directly onto a glass slide, can be tested directly using the VZV-IFT. If there is sufficient VZV in the sample, this can give a more rapid diagnosis, rather than waiting for the VZV to grow for 10–14 days – and often VZV does not grow in culture. Electron microscopy (Figure 15.7) alone can only make a diagnosis of a herpesvirus but not the specific VZV species, whereas VZV-specific PCR testing of the vesicle skin scraping can give a direct diagnosis also – usually within 24 hours.

Box 15.2 Vaccination against chickenpox – a blessing or a time-bomb?

The increasingly widespread use of the live-attenuated VZV vaccines (one produced by GlaxoSmithKline – Varilrix – and one produced by Merck – Varivax), worldwide, mainly in the developed countries at present, will gradually reduce the incidence of wild-type, natural chickenpox infection. This has some interesting implications for the natural history of chickenpox and shingles, as well as other recurrent VZV-related disease. Natural chickenpox infection in children boosts the natural immunity of nearby adults, such as parents and relatives, to their own naturally acquired VZV. This has the effect of increasing their immune system control of their own latent VZV in their dorsal root ganglia (DRG). This boosting effect may delay the onset of any shingles for several more years or longer. If all the children receive the VZV vaccine, then this boosting effect will be lost and adults infected with the wild-type VZV may develop shingles earlier – perhaps during their working lives. This will place an increasing burden on society, if these working parents need to take time off work to treat their shingles and the postherpetic neuralgia that may be severe in some cases. One solution to this is to give the VZV vaccines to the adult also, to boost their own immunity to compensate for the loss of immune boosting from exposure to natural VZV. At the same time, it is unknown how long the VZV vaccine-induced immunity will last. If it does not last more than 20 years, then children who have received the VZV vaccine may become more susceptible to wild-type VZV (e.g. acquired from abroad, from countries where the VZV vaccine is not widely used or available), and they may develop severe adult chickenpox with significant risk of serious complications or even death.

Specific antiviral therapy using aciclovir-based drugs (e.g. valaciclovir, famciclovir, penciclovir) is available for treating chickenpox and other related VZV diseases, including those related to recurrent VZV infections, such as shingles and encephalitis. The dosage and duration of treatment can be adjusted according to the severity of the disease and in some cases, where available, quantitative PCR results. Although the VZV IgG antibody acquired after primary VZV infection (chickenpox) provides lifelong immunity against other VZV infections, it does not always prevent a person's own VZV from reactivating from the dorsal root ganglias to cause disease. This is partly due to the cellular arm of the immune system (T-cell-mediated) also playing a role in the control of latent VZV, as well as the antibody or humoral (B-cell-mediated) arm. However, usually the immune control of latent VZV in immunocompetent individuals should last from their first, primary VZV infection (chickenpox), into their middle- and old- age. With the recent introduction and increasingly widespread use of the live-attenuated VZV vaccines, the natural history of VZV infection and reactivation is changing, but as yet, we are not sure of all the consequences because they have only been in widespread use for about 10 years now (Box 15.2).

"Slapped cheek disease" (erythema infectiosum, "fifth disease")

"Slapped cheek disease" is caused by parvovirus B19 (PVB19). This virus was accidentally discovered during investigations for hepatitis B virus, and is a small, nonenveloped virus containing a single strand of positive-sense DNA belonging to the genus *Erythrovirus*, family *Parvoviridae* (Figure 15.9).

This virus is slightly different from the other childhood infections discussed so far, in that measles, rubella and VZV (now all vaccine-preventable diseases) in the pre-vaccine era, had a very high seropositivity (i.e. IgG antibody positive) rate in the adult population – as much as 80–90%. This is not the case for PVB19. In the USA, the seroprevalence of PVB19 infection is only 5–10% by 2–5 years, 50% by 15 years, 60% by 30 years, and 90% by 60 years of age. Worldwide, the seroprevalence rates are similar. Like rubella, the transmission of PVB19 is by small droplets of short distances, as well as by direct contact with infected body fluids (e.g. saliva, mucus, and sputum). Like the other viruses, its transmission is facilitated by coughing and sneezing during its prodromal stage of infection. As a consequence of this epidemiology, the importance of PVB19 infection is not only in the childhood population, but adults with various underlying medical conditions are also quite commonly infected with various potentially severe consequences (Box 15.3).

After an incubation of 4–20 (usually 14–18) days, an infected child experiences a typical viral, febrile, flu-like prodrome that may last 5–7 days. However, up to 20% of those infected may not experience any

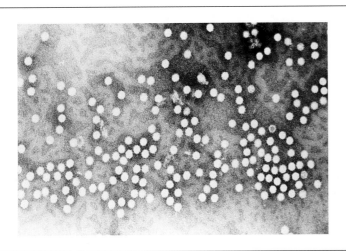

Figure 15.9 An electron micrograph (EM) showing numerous small (22–24 nm in diameter) parvoviruses from the *Parvoviridae* family. The appearance of parvovirus B19 is very similar under EM. They are nonenveloped viruses containing a positive-sense, single-stranded DNA genome. Courtesy of the Centers for Disease Control and Prevention; from CDC website: http://phil.cdc.gov/phil/details.asp

Box 15.3 The complications of parvovirus B19 infections are not mainly confined to children

Parvovirus B19 (PVB19) infects cells expressing an antigen called the "P" blood antigen. This antigen is found on various cells of the hematological (blood-forming) system, including red cells (**erythrocytes**) and some white cells (**leukocytes**), but particularly the early dividing precursor (**blast**) cells of these lineages that are mainly found in the bone marrow. Infection of these cells by the virus leads to destruction of the cell, with the release of millions and millions of PVB 19 viruses – as many as 10^{12} viruses/ml blood can be found in acute PVB19 infections. Those groups of individuals particularly affected by PVB19 infections are:

Pre-existing hematological conditions

People with pre-existing hematological conditions that shorten the natural lifespan or reduce the oxygen-carrying capacity of the red cells, e.g. sickle-cell anemia, or thalassemia or autoimmune hemolytic anemias. In these people, acute PVB19 infection can destroy many of their remaining red cells, but particularly those precursor red cells (**reticulocytes**) that would normally replace these mature red cells, which have been destroyed by the virus, or have a shortened lifespan due to their underlying hematological disease. This rapid destruction and failure of replacement of these red cells causes an "aplastic crisis," i.e. so many red cells are destroyed and not being replaced quickly enough, that the hemoglobin (Hb) levels drop to dangerously low levels, such that there is insufficient to transport oxygen around the body. Such aplastic crises may lead to painful and incapacitating ischemia in limbs and vital organs, resulting in emergency blood transfusions, amputation, and even death.

Prolonged PVB19 infection

Those with immunodeficiency may have a prolonged PVB19 infection, some lasting many years, as their immune system cannot clear the virus from the circulation. Such patients require regular red cell transfusions as their bodies cannot make new red cells due to the persistent PVB19 infection destroying red cell precursors in the bone marrow. Without regular transfusions (which also has associated risks), the Hb of these patients will continue to drop until they die of multiple organ ischemia, probably slipping into a coma first (the brain requires the most oxygen of any body organ) before the other organs fail. In some cases intravenous immunoglobulin (IVIG), produced by pooling the purified sera from many blood donations, may help as this IVIG contains some PVB19-specific IgG antibodies that will neutralize some of the PVB19 virus for a while. However, without the endogenous production of the patient's own PVB19 antibodies, the virus continues replicating and its numbers will eventually rise to its previous levels and continue to cause the same problems.

Persistent, postinfectious, symmetrical arthritis

An added complication of PVB19 infection is persistent, postinfectious, symmetrical arthritis. This is most common in adults, particularly women, and less common in children or male adults and may start with the acute PVB19 infection and continue after the acute infection has resolved. The small joints of the hands and feet are usually affected and may mimic other arthritic diseases such as rheumatoid arthritis (RA), though unlike RA actual bone and joint damage is not observed. There is some evidence of PVB19 antigen in joints and the arthritis of PVB19 infection, like the rash, is thought to be immune-mediated, i.e. the body has an inappropriate response to the PVB19 infection, and in some cases, ends up attacking itself.

symptoms. Like rubella where the infection may also be subclinical or asymptomatic, this is of concern in pregnant women who will not know then that they have acquired an infection which could potentially damage their fetus. Interestingly, although males and females are usually infected in equal ratios, females seem to be infected more frequently in outbreak situations, and females also tend to have prolonged, postinfectious, arthritic symptoms.

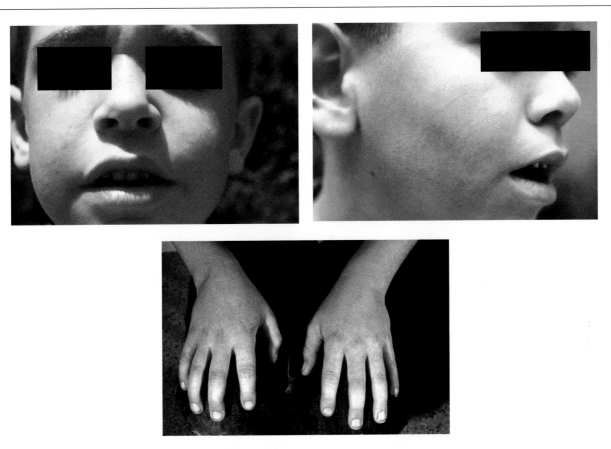

Figure 15.10 The face of a boy showing symptoms of acute parvovirus B19 infection, also known as erythema infectiosum and "fifth disease." Note the red "slapped cheek" appearance, which is another common name for this disease. Although the "slapped-cheek" appearance on the face is the most distinctive feature, the PVB19 rash may also manifest on other parts of the body in various forms – in this case, as a red, blotchy rash on the hands. Courtesy of the Centers for Disease Control and Prevention; from CDC website: http://phil.cdc.gov/phil/details.asp

After the prodromal illness, during which time the child may feel quite well, the characteristic bright, red, erythematous, maculopapular, "slapped-cheek" rash appears on the face, followed by a more lacy, reticular, usually nonitchy rash over the rest of the body, spreading out towards the limbs (Figure 15.10). The rash usually appears and disappears within a few days but occasionally it can recur for several weeks. In adults, it is during this second phase of this "biphasic" infection that joint pains may appear. Together with the rash, the joint pains are thought to be immune mediated, as the body develops an IgM antibody response to the virus. As with rubella, which is also a mild or asymptomatic infection in some cases, the rash may be the first symptom of the disease. The rash of PVB19 is perhaps the most variable of the childhood rashes. Besides the typical "slapped-cheek" appearance, other patterns have been described, including a more purpuric (nonblanchable, bruise-like) rash that may be itchy, or a rash consisting of "target-like" lesions mimicking another rash often seen with other infections or drug reactions, called **erythema multiforme**. Rarely, in some individuals, a later rash may appear, some time after the acute PVB19 infection, taking the form of a "glove-and-stocking" distribution. This has been described as an erythematous, papular rash on the hands and feet, with a distinct border at the ankles and wrists, respectively. It is accompanied by pain and swelling (**edema**).

Some complications of PVB19 infection have been described in Box 15.3. As the rash and joint pains are mainly due to the immune response, particularly the appearance of PVB19 IgM antibodies, immunocompromised children and adults with PVB19 may not experience these symptoms and the first indication of PVB19 infection is a drop in their Hb levels. Other organs may be the target of PVB19 infections, and this can also be seen in severe infections caused by the other viruses described here. Due to its P-antigen receptor on cells of the hematological system, PVB19 infection may cause damage to the clotting system and the small blood vessels in many vital organs, causing diseases like thrombocytopenia (platelets), vasculitis (the blood vessel lining), glomerulonephritis (the kidneys), encephalitis (the brain), myocarditis (the heart) as well hemophagocytic syndrome (cells within the bone marrow).

Diagnosis of acute PVB19 infection is usually made by the detection of PVB19 IgM in the serum, or if paired sera are available (i.e. pre- and post-infection sera), a seroconversion from PVB 19 IgG negative to IgG positive, with compatible clinical features, should be sufficient to confirm the diagnosis. Unlike the other viral exanthems that may be IgM negative in the first few days of the rash, PVB19 IgM should be present once the rash appears, as the rash is immune mediated. A fall in Hb levels is often the first sign of acute PVB19 infection in immunocompromised patients who may not develop typical rash or arthralgia symptoms, as they may not develop a detectable PVB19-specific antibody response. However, in such patients, the PVB19 DNA levels should be very high and easily detectable by PCR. Although not routinely used diagnostically, an electron microscopic (EM) examination of the sera from such patients will probably demonstrate many parvoviruses (as shown in Figure 15.9). Like measles and rubella, PVB19 is not routinely cultured in most diagnostic laboratories, as the cell culture systems for these viruses are not routinely maintained, except in specialist virology reference laboratories.

There is no specific antiviral drug to treat PVB19 infection, but PVB-specific IgG (convalescent) antibodies from pooled blood donors in IVIG can be used as a temporary supply of neutralizing antibodies. There is only one serotype of PVB19, and like rubella, measles and chickenpox, after recovery from the acute infection, these antibodies should protect the individual against all strains of PVB19 for life. Presently, there is no licensed vaccine against PVB19, but this is urgently needed, since, like rubella and chickenpox (and to a lesser extent, measles), there is potential for damage to the fetus (causing **hydrops fetalis** – see Chapter 12) when susceptible pregnant women are infected with PVB19. There is no universally accepted postexposure prophylaxis for PVB19 infection, and contact tracing is problematic. By the time the rash appears, the patient is no longer infectious as this is an immune (antibody)-mediated rash. The period before the appearance of the rash (and antibodies), during the 5−7 day prodromal period in which the virus is infectious, is the time within which contact tracing is required. However, few people can remember in detail what they have been doing and where they have been during these previous 5−7 days. Often, this period is further back in the past, as these infected patients may present to healthcare workers only after the rash has been there for a few days – they may have felt relatively well throughout this time. Unlike measles and chickenpox, and more like rubella, the mortality from acute parvovirus B10 infection and its complication rate, in children, is minimal.

"Sixth disease" (exanthem subitum, roseola infantum)

The viral cause of "sixth disease" has only been found relatively recently, in the late 1980s, though the clinical disease has been described for over 100 years. The cause has been assigned to another member of the human herpesviruses (HHV), a virus in the genus *Roseolavirus*, family *Herpesviridae*, simply named HHV type 6 (HHV6). As with VZV, the other human herpesvirus already discussed here, HHV6 is an enveloped virus containing double-stranded DNA, with a similar electron microscopic (EM) appearance (Figure 15.7). It is not possible to reliably distinguish between the individual members of the herpesvirus family using EM alone. HHV6 has two subtypes or strains, HHV6A and HHV6B. The rash illness is usually caused by HHV6B in children under the age of 2 years. Another beta herpesvirus, HHV7, has been suspected to cause a similar rash illness in slightly older children (≥2 years old). The rashes due to HHV6B and HHV7 are usually clinically indistinguishable. Transmission is thought to be via direct contact with body fluids, most commonly saliva, particularly between parents and children. Like VZV, HHV6 (and HHV7) remain latent in the human body after primary infection – in this case, mainly in some of the white cell species – monocytes and lymphocytes.

In the USA, about 86% of children have been infected with HHV6 by 1 year of age, and almost 100% have been infected by 4 years old. Maternal antibody may offer some protection for the first few months after birth, but the majority of HHV6 infections occur between 6 and 18 months of age, which is a pattern that is similar worldwide. However, most HHV6 infections are asymptomatic. In the USA, only about 12–30% of all HHV6-infected children are thought to exhibit the typical **exanthem subitum** rash.

The illness in children is distinctive because of the rapid, biphasic presentation. After an incubation period of around 5–15 days, symptoms appear abruptly, with a sudden onset of high fever (up to 104°F, 40°C), with associated prodromal symptoms (malaise, irritability, and cough), which may last 3–6 days. As the fever subsides, the characteristic, blanchable, nonitchy, maculopapular "rash of roses" (**roseola infantum**) appears, normally appearing first on the trunk then sometimes extending to the head and limbs (Figure 15.11). The lesions are similar to those of rubella in that they usually remain separate and do not coalesce. The rash is short-lived, and may disappear within a few hours to 2 days. Other associated symptoms include swelling around the eyes (**periorbital edema**, 30% of cases), and a palpable bulge on the front of the skull (**bulging anterior fontanel**, 26%), as well as erythematous spots in the mouth (Nagayama spots, 65%) and swollen glands on the head and neck (cervical, postoccipital and postauricular lymphadenopathy, 31%). Usually the infection is without complications, but the high fever, rash and other associated symptoms may alarm parents into bringing their child into hospital, where observation and reassurance is usually all that is required.

Nevertheless, complications can occur and include seizures (6–15%) and diarrhea (~70%), which are generally self-limiting in normal immunocompetent children, but can lead to more serious meningitis or meningo-encephalitis in immunocompromised children and adults. Complications may occur with primary HHV6 infection in children and reactivated HHV6 infection in immunocompromised older children and adults.

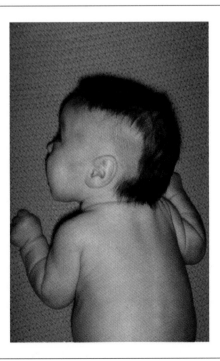

Figure 15.11 Typical erythematous, maculopapular rash of "sixth disease" (also known as exanthem subitum or roseola infantum) caused by human herpesvirus 6B (HHV6B). From the slide collection at Department of Microbiology, University College London Hospitals, London

Diagnosis of primary HHV6 infection is not routinely available in most standard (usually hospital-based) diagnostic laboratories. In a child younger than 2 years old with compatible symptoms at presentation, a clinical diagnosis can be made. Serum taken at this time can be tested for both HHV6 antibodies and DNA (using PCR). Ideally, a sample taken very early in the illness (e.g. just after the onset of the high fever), then another sample taken 10–14 days later after recovery (a convalescent sample), should show a fourfold antibody titer rise in HHV6-specific antibody, with HHV6 DNA PCR being positive in the first acute sample. To add to the difficulty of laboratory diagnosis, in infants less than 1 year old the maternal HHV6 antibodies may be still detectable, and there is some cross-reactivity possible with HHV7 antibodies in the HHV6 antibody detection assay. HHV6 DNA can also be detected in saliva during primary or reactivated infection, so both the site and timing of the samples are important for making an accurate diagnosis of primary HHV6 infection.

Therefore, above the age of 2–3 years, it is likely that HHV6 DNA detectable in the blood or saliva may well be due to reactivation, which is usually asymptomatic, unless the patient is immunocompromised, when it may be a significant pathogen. In such patients, HHV6 may reactivate to cause encephalitis and can be treated by specific anti-herpes antiviral agents, such as aciclovir, foscarnet, ganciclovir, and cidofovir. Some of these drugs have severe side-effects and should only be used under expert guidance usually in close collaboration with the diagnostic laboratory that can assay the response to treatment. There is no vaccine against HHV6 as yet, and this may be difficult to utilize even if it is developed, as the age of infection is so young (6–18 months old), and maternal antibodies may interfere with the action of any vaccine at this age of life.

Other rash illnesses of childhood

This chapter has only covered the most common, childhood febrile rash illnesses. Other infections may cause rashes in some children, such as infectious mononucleosis (glandular fever) caused by Epstein–Barr virus (EBV), and very occasionally, cytomegalovirus (CMV) which can cause a similar syndrome. Often the rash of EBV is precipitated by an antibiotic (usually ampicillin and occasionally, other penicillin-based drugs), so it is not a true viral exanthema. One important, common childhood rash illness that has not yet been described is hand-foot-and-mouth disease.

Hand-foot-and-mouth disease (HFMD) is caused by a few members of the enteroviruses (a large family of nonenveloped, positive-sense, single-stranded RNA viruses), usually by coxsackie A16 but also by enterovirus 71. It is relatively common in children (<10 years old), but also in adults in whom it may cause other associated systemic symptoms. It should not be confused with the "foot-and-mouth disease" of livestock (cattle, sheep, and pigs), which is a different disease of animals caused by a different virus that rarely infects humans. Viruses that cause HFMD are transmitted by direct contact with infected body fluids, and also over short distances by coughing and sneezing, during the viral prodromal illness when the infected person is contagious. Spread between all susceptible family members within one household is not unusual. These symptoms occur after a short incubation period of about 3–7 days. One to two days later, small, red, painful blisters may appear in the mouth, on the palms of the hands or the soles of the feet. They are not usually itchy, but are tender to touch and may ulcerate. Normally, recovery is complete after 1–2 weeks, without further complications, but as there are so many species of enteroviruses, recurrent disease with other members of this virus family may occur later. The diagnosis is usually made clinically, with laboratory tests being rarely requested, but a swab may be taken from one of the lesions for viral culture with or without enterovirus PCR testing. The lesions of HFMD may be easily confused with those caused by human herpes simplex virus 1 or 2 (HSV 1 or HSV 2) that can also cause painful, oral lesions or ulcers. Laboratory testing can easily distinguish between these two types of virus. Primary infection with HSV 1 or 2 can occur in this same age group of children, so confusion may not be so uncommon. Specific, licensed antiviral treatment for HFMD is not available, but occasionally, enteroviruses can cause severe systemic infection and organ damage (e.g. myocarditis, meningitis, encephalitis, hepatitis), requiring intensive care – and in some rare cases organ transplantation. An unlicensed drug called pleconaril may be made available for such severely ill children, but may not be easily obtained in all healthcare centers. There is no licensed vaccine available for HFMD, at present.

Enteroviruses do not cause specific congenital syndromes in pregnant women who are infected by them. However, newborn babies may acquire the infection from the mother and some of them may suffer overwhelming, life-threatening illnesses. This is rare and usually affects neonates younger than 2 weeks (see Chapter 12 on neonatal viral infections).

Test yourself

One of the main problems with childhood rash illnesses is trying to distinguish between them and it can be notoriously difficult to do this, clinically – though some diseases are more easily identified than others, e.g. chickenpox and measles. This is important when it comes to infection control as the modes of transmission differ between these viruses and this has consequences for the subsequent management of any exposed, susceptible individuals – particularly in a busy hospital with both pregnant women and many different groups of immunocompromised patients. The following is based on a real case and illustrates this problem in a typical hospital pediatric clinical setting.

Case study 15.1
A 6-month-old boy is brought to the pediatric emergency room with a four- to five-day history of fever and rash that presented more or less at the same time. The child is in mild distress but otherwise quite alert, without conjunctivitis (i.e. no red eyes) or other significant clinical symptoms or signs.

The child's rash is a generalized, erythematous, macular, papular rash that appeared on the head and neck first then spread downwards to the legs, with relative sparing of the palms of the hands and soles of the feet. The boy is admitted for observation directly into an isolation room, accompanied by the mother. All healthcare workers attending to the child are known to be immune to rubella, measles, and chickenpox. Some blood tests are performed.

The child remains well overnight and the mother requests for him to be discharged home the next morning.

1. What is your differential diagnosis of this child with an acute fever and rash? What else would you like to know?
2. If you were the child's pediatrician, what specific tests would you request?
3. Usually the tests may take several days to complete. Therefore, how would you respond to the mother's request for discharge?

Further reading

Banatvala JE, Brown DW. Rubella. *Lancet* 2004;363(9415):1127–1137

Brisson M, Edmunds WJ, Gay NJ. Varicella vaccination: impact of vaccine efficacy on the epidemiology of VZV. *J Med Virol* 2003;70(suppl 1):S31–S37

Broliden K, Tolfvenstam T, Norbeck O. Clinical aspects of parvovirus B19 infection. *J Intern Med* 2006;260(4):285–304

Campadelli-Fiume G, Mirandola P, Menotti L. Human herpesvirus 6: an emerging pathogen. *Emerg Infect Dis* 1999;5(3):353–366

Hall CB, Caserta MT, Schnabel KC, et al. Characteristics and acquisition of human herpesvirus (HHV) 7 infections in relation to infection with HHV-6. *J Infect Dis* 2006;193(8):1063–1069

Kerdiles YM, Sellin CI, Druelle J, Horvat B. Immunosuppression caused by measles virus: role of viral proteins. Rev Med Virol 2006;16(1):49–63

Mandell GL, Bennett JE, Dolin R (eds). *Principles and Practice of Infectious Diseases*, 6th edition. Philadelphia: Churchill Livingstone, 2005

Morens DM, Katz AR, Melish ME. The fourth disease, 1900–1881, RIP. *Lancet* 2001;357(9273):2059

Morens DM, Katz AR. The "fourth disease" of childhood: reevaluation of a nonexistent disease. *Am J Epidemiol* 1991;134(6):628–640

Rentier B, Gershon AA; European Working Group on Varicella. Consensus: varicella vaccination of healthy children – a challenge for Europe. *Pediatr Infect Dis J* 2004;23(5):379–389

Weisse ME. The fourth disease, 1900–2000. *Lancet* 2001;357(9252):299–301

Welsby PD. Chickenpox, chickenpox vaccination, and shingles. *Postgrad Med J* 2006;82(967):351–352

Zuckerman AJ, Banatvala JE, Pattison JR, Griffiths P (eds). *Principles and Practice of Clinical Virology*, 5th edition. London: Wiley, 2004

Useful websites

There are many useful websites for childhood rashes. These are just a selection of them.

CDC. Epidemiology and Prevention of Vaccine-Preventable Diseases, 10th edition. Atkinson W, Hamborsky J, McIntyre L, Wolfe S (eds). Washington DC: Public Health Foundation, 2007. http://www.cdc.gov/nip/publications/pink/

CDC. National Center for Immunization and Respiratory Diseases. Division of Viral Diseases. http://www.cdc.gov/ncird/dvd.htm

DermIS. An online dermatology atlas with photographs of most rash appearances, though you need to know the name of the rash illness you are looking for (or suspecting). http://dermis.multimedica.de/dermisroot/en/list/all/search.htm

EMedicine from WebMD. Emergency Medical Articles. http://www.emedicine.com/emerg/PEDIATRIC.htm

Hardin MD. Childhood Skin Rashes. Another useful site combining text and images with multiple links to other relevant websites, but you still have to know the name of the rash you are looking for (or suspecting). http://www.lib.uiowa.edu/hardin/md/skinrashes.html

Patient UK. Common Childhood Rashes. A useful website for both patients and doctors to differentiate and recognize different childhood rashes (but no photographs). http://www.patient.co.uk/showdoc/40000396/

Part 4

Infections of global impact

Chapter 16
Tuberculosis

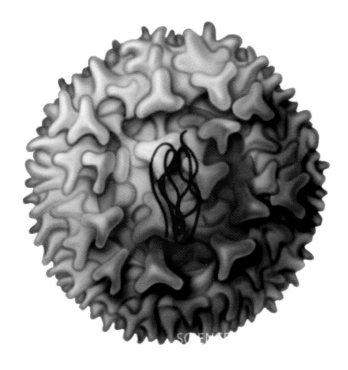

S. Srivastava, N. Shetty

Public health perspectives of tuberculosis: global and regional
Epidemiology of tuberculosis in the USA
Pathogenesis and clinical presentation: The Great Destroyer
Clinical features of tuberculosis
Primary TB
Post-primary pulmonary TB
Extrapulmonary TB

Pathogenesis and virulence
The innate immune system in tuberculosis
Acquired immunity against *M. tuberculosis* infection
Pathogenesis in TB–HIV co-infection
Genetic variability in *M. tuberculosis*
Diagnosis of tuberculosis
Management of a case of tuberculosis

When John Bunyan, the Christian writer, preacher and author of the *The Pilgrim's Progress* used his now famous epithet ". . . captain of all these men of death . . ." little did the world realize that tuberculosis would continue to be a major killer over four centuries later. The history of tuberculosis (TB) can be traced to the earliest history of mankind. Egyptian mummies from 5000 BC showing deformities consistent with tuberculosis have been discovered. Other historical references include Chinese literature (4000 BC), Indian literature (2000 BC), Hippocrates (400 BC), and Aristotle (350 BC). The "Great White Plague" of 1600 BC which started in Europe and continued for more than 200 years referred to tuberculosis.

The English physician Benjamin Marten published *A New Theory of Consumption* in 1720 in which he referred to the etiological agent of TB as wonderfully minute living creatures. Robert Koch identified the causative agent of TB on 24 March 1882 and called it the tubercle bacillus due to the presence of small rounded bodies or tubercles found in diseased tissue.

In the USA the peak mortality figures due to TB were recorded at 1600 per 100 000 population in New England in 1880. The introduction of sanatorium cure was one of the first steps towards control of TB. Hermann Brehmer, a Silesian botanist, who recovered from TB, is credited with having designed the first sanatorium. The sanatorium movement was pioneered in the USA by Edward Livingston Trodeau, a physician who had also recovered from TB, in Saranac Lake, New York, in 1886. Dr. Herman Biggs of New York started the mandatory reporting of TB cases in 1892. His recommendations laid the groundwork for a campaign called "*War on Consumption*." In 1904 a voluntary health agency was organized under the National Association for the Study and Prevention of Tuberculosis, later renamed the National Tuberculosis Association (NTA) and now known as the American Lung Association.

Streptomycin was administered for the first time for the treatment of TB in 1944. Since then many other agents have been trialled successfully against TB. These were important because monotherapy resistant mutants began to appear within a few months. However, no new anti-TB drugs have been discovered in the last 30 years and researchers are looking for new drug targets against the causative agent.

Public health perspectives of tuberculosis: global and regional

Tuberculosis (TB) is the leading cause of death associated with infectious diseases globally. Based on surveillance and survey data, WHO estimates that there were 8.9 million new cases of TB in 2004 (140 per 100 000 population), including 3.9 million (62 per 100 000 population) new smear-positive cases. Country-wide estimates of the incidence rate of TB in 2005 are shown in Figure 16.1. The incidence of TB will continue to increase substantially worldwide because of the interaction between the TB and

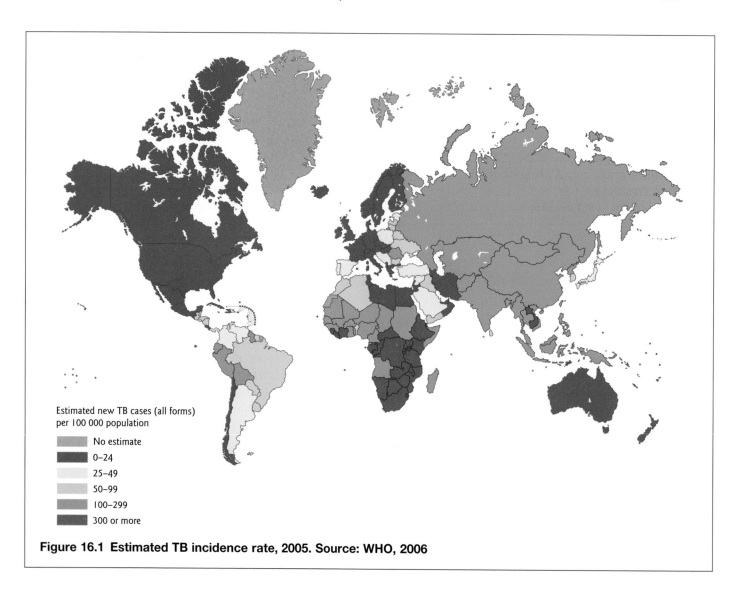

Estimated new TB cases (all forms) per 100 000 population

- No estimate
- 0–24
- 25–49
- 50–99
- 100–299
- 300 or more

Figure 16.1 Estimated TB incidence rate, 2005. Source: WHO, 2006

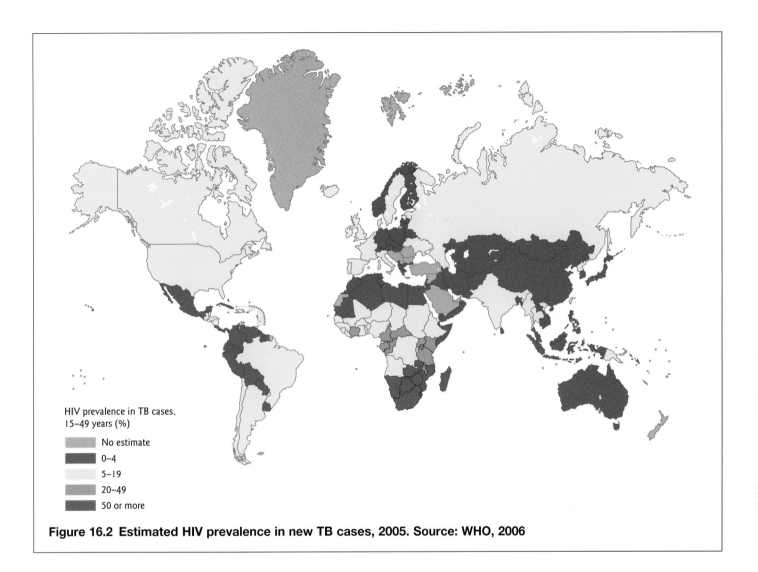

Figure 16.2 Estimated HIV prevalence in new TB cases, 2005. Source: WHO, 2006

HIV prevalence in TB cases, 15–49 years (%)

- No estimate
- 0–4
- 5–19
- 20–49
- 50 or more

HIV epidemics (Figure 16.2). An estimated 1.7 million people (27/100 000 population) died from TB in 2004, including those co-infected with HIV (248 000). The African Region alone accounts for 81% of the estimated 741 000 cases of TB among HIV positive people in the world, but for only 4% of those reported to have begun antiretroviral therapy (ART) in 2003. The region of the Americas (mainly Brazil), on the other hand, accounts for 3% of the estimated cases but for 96% of the 9388 people reported to have started on ART in 2003.

In many developing countries, TB is mainly a disease of young adults affecting carers and wage-earners in a household, thus placing a huge economic burden on society as a whole. Chemotherapy, if properly used, can reduce the burden of TB in the community, but because of the fragile structure of treatment programs in many countries TB cases are not completely cured and patients remain infectious for a much longer time. Another important consequence of poor treatment compliance is development of drug resistance in many developing countries.

Resistance to TB drugs is probably present everywhere in the world. If an isolate of *Mycobacterium tuberculosis* is resistant to rifampin and isoniazid it is classed as multi-drug resistant. The total number of multi-drug resistant TB (MDR-TB) cases estimated to have occurred worldwide in 2004 is 424 203 or 4.3% of all new and previously treated TB cases. In the same year, 181 408 MDR-TB cases were estimated to have occurred among previously treated TB cases alone. Three countries – China, India, and the Russian

Box 16.1 Tuberculosis trends and the extensively drug resistant tuberculosis in the United States, 1993–2006 (report from *MMWR* March 23, 2007/56(11);250–253)

The current definition of MDR-TB is the resistance to at least rifampin and isoniazid.

The definition of XDR-TB in the USA requires resistance to at least isoniazid and rifampin among first-line anti-TB drugs, resistance to any fluoroquinolone, and resistance to at least one second-line injectable drug (amikacin, capreomycin, or kanamycin). Between 1993 and 2006; a total of 49 cases (3% of evaluable multi-drug resistant (MDR) TB cases) met the revised case definition for XDR-TB. Of these, 17 (35%) were reported during 2000–2006.

Editorial note: After approximately 30 years of declining trends, a TB epidemic occurred in the USA during 1985–1992. From 22 201 cases in 1985 (9.3 per 100 000 population), reported TB increased to 26 673 cases in 1992 (10.4 per 100 000 population). Although the incidence of MDR-TB in the USA was largely unknown before 1993, the number of cases began increasing in New York City in the early 1980s, and numerous outbreaks of MDR-TB were described in the late 1980s and early 1990s. TB-control activities included improving laboratory services for rapid, accurate culture and drug susceptibility testing and improving infection control.

Characteristics of XDR-TB cases changed during 2000–2006 in parallel with the changing epidemiology of TB in general and MDR-TB in particular. These changes included an overall decrease in the number of cases, a decrease in the proportion of cases in HIV-infected persons, an increase in the proportion of cases among foreign-born persons, and an increase in the proportion of Asians among persons with XDR-TB, compared with 1993–1999.

Federation – accounted for 261 362 MDR-TB cases, or 62% of the estimated global burden. Eastern Europe reported the highest prevalence of MDR-TB among new cases, and figures from former Kazakhstan and Israel both had an MDR prevalence rate of 14.2%. Other high prevalence areas include Uzbekistan (13.2%), Estonia (12.2%), and China's Liaoning Province (10.4%).

Worldwide attention was focused on South Africa when in October 2006 a research project publicized a deadly outbreak of XDR-TB in the small town of Tugela Ferry in KwaZulu-Natal. XDR-TB is the abbreviation for extensively drug resistant TB. This strain of *M. tuberculosis* is resistant to first- and second-line drugs, and treatment options are seriously limited. Of 536 TB patients at the Church of Scotland Hospital, which serves a rural area with high HIV rates, some 221 were found to have multi-drug resistance and of these, 53 were diagnosed with XDR-TB. Fifty-two of these patients died, most within 25 days of diagnosis. Of the 53 patients, 44 had been tested for HIV and all 44 were found to be HIV positive. The patients were receiving anti-retrovirals and responding well to HIV-related treatment, but they died of XDR-TB. Since the study, 10 more patients have been diagnosed with XDR-TB in KwaZulu-Natal. Only three of them are still alive. Read Box 16.1 for the information on resistance in the USA. See Further reading for air travel and the risk of TB including XDR-TB after an air passenger from the USA traveled to Europe after being diagnosed with XDR-TB.

Directly observed treatment (where a designated person is given the responsibility by mutual consent to observe a patient swallowing his medication) is the most effective strategy available for controlling the TB epidemic today. Directly observed treatment, short course (DOTS) uses sound technology and packages it with good management practices for widespread use through the existing primary healthcare network (Box 16.2). It has proven to be a successful, innovative approach to TB control in countries such as China, Bangladesh, Vietnam, Peru, and countries of West Africa. However, new challenges to the implementation of DOTS include health sector reforms, the worsening HIV epidemic, and the emergence of drug-resistant

> # Box 16.2 "TB anywhere is TB everywhere." Theme for World TB Day: 24 March 2007 (report from MMWR: Public Health Dispatch: tuberculosis outbreak in a homeless population – Portland, Maine, 2002–2003. 3 December 2005/52(48);1184–1185)
>
> During June 2002–July 2003, seven men with active pulmonary TB disease in Portland, Maine, were reported to the Maine Bureau of Health (MBH). Six were linked through residence at homeless shelters; four had matching *Mycobacterium tuberculosis* genotypes. The median age of patients was 51 years (range: 39–66 years); Culture specimens from all seven patients were positive for *M. tuberculosis* and all isolates were susceptible to first-line drugs. Three (43%) patients had cavitary pulmonary disease, three (43%) were infected with hepatitis C virus, and one patient was infected with human immunodeficiency virus and hepatitis C. Six (86%) patients had a history of alcoholism.
>
> Prompt investigation and identification of approximately 1100 likely contacts prevented further spread of TB. DOTS is probably the single most effective method to ensure compliance and restrict spread in vulnerable patient groups such as the homeless.

strains of TB. The technical, logistical, operational and political aspects of DOTS work together to ensure its success and applicability in a wide variety of contexts. Worldwide, 183 countries were implementing the DOTS strategy by the end of 2004, and 83% of the world's population was living in regions where DOTS was in place.

For a summary of the worldwide status of TB and targets for the future see Box 16.3.

> # Box 16.3 A summary of the problem and targets for the future
>
> ### TB facts, 2006
>
> - TB is curable but kills 5000 people every day
> - TB is a disease of poverty and affects the poorest and the most malnourished
> - Worldwide 2 billion people are affected with TB bacilli
> - 1 in 10 people with the TB bacilli will become sick with active TB in their lifetime; the risk is even higher for patients with HIV/AIDS
> - TB is contagious and spreads through the air. Each untreated person will infect 10–15 people every year
> - TB is a worldwide epidemic; the highest rates per capita (29%) are seen in Africa; about half of all new cases of TB appear in six Asian countries (India, Pakistan, Bangladesh, China, Phillipines, Indonesia)
> - MDR-TB is defined as resistance to rifampicin and isoniazid. MDR-TB is present in 109 countries
>
> - 450 000 new cases of MDR-TB occur every year. The highest rates of MDR-TB are in countries of former Soviet Union and China
> - XDR-TB is the extensively drug resistant tuberculosis that is resistant to isoniazid, rifampicin, any fluoroquinolone and at least one of the three injectable second-line agents (capreomycin, kanamycin, and amikacin)
>
> ### TB targets
>
> - 2005: the World Health assembly targets to detect 70% of sputum smear positive cases and successfully treat 85% of detected cases
> - 2015: Millenium Development Goals target is to halt and reverse incidence trend of TB
>
> The Stop TB Partnership hopes to halve the prevalence of and deaths due to TB by 2015 in comparison to 1990.

Epidemiology of tuberculosis in the USA

In 2006, a total of 13 767 TB cases (4.6 per 100 000 population) were reported in the USA, representing a 3.2% decline from the 2005 rate. The TB rate in 2006 was the lowest recorded since national reporting began in 1953, but the rate of decline has slowed since 2000. Foreign-born persons and racial/ethnic minority populations continue to be affected disproportionately by TB in the USA. In 2006, the TB rate among foreign-born persons in the USA was 9.5 times that of US-born persons. The TB rates among blacks, Asians, and Hispanics were 8.4, 21.2, and 7.6 times higher than rates among whites, respectively. TB is a nationally notifiable disease in the USA.

Among US-born persons, the number and rate of TB cases continued to decline in 2006. The US-born TB rate was 2.3 per 100 000 population (5924 or 43.3% of all cases with known origin of birth), representing a 7.0% decline in rate since 2005 and a 68.6% decline since 1993. Among foreign-born persons, the number of TB cases increased in 2006, but the rate decreased. The foreign-born TB rate in 2006 was 21.9 per 100 000 population, representing a 0.5% decline in rate since 2006 and a 35.8% decline since 1993. In 2006, approximately half (55.6%) of TB cases among foreign-born persons were reported in persons from five countries: Mexico (1912), the Philippines (856), Vietnam (630), India (540), and China (376).

Human immunodeficiency virus (HIV) contributes to the TB pandemic because immune suppression increases the likelihood of rapid progression from TB infection to TB disease.

A total of 124 cases of multidrug-resistant TB (MDR-TB) were reported in 2005, the most recent year for which complete drug-susceptibility data are available. The proportion of MDR-TB cases remained constant at 1.2% from 2004 (129 of 10 846 TB cases) to 2005 (124 of 10 662). In 2005, MDR-TB continued to disproportionately affect foreign-born persons, who accounted for 101 (81.5%) of 124 MDR-TB cases.

Pathogenesis and clinical presentation: The Great Destroyer

As a general rule the term "tuberculosis infection" refers to a positive TB skin test (see below) with no evidence of active disease. "Tuberculosis disease" refers to cases that have positive microscopy or culture for *Mycobacterium tuberculosis* or a radiographic and clinical presentation of TB.

M. tuberculosis (MTB) and the other members of the *M. tuberculosis* complex – *M. bovis*, *M. africanum*, and *M. microti* – primarily affect the lungs. During infection droplet nuclei containing the organism are inhaled and deposited on the bronchial mucosa, the organisms are ingested by macrophages and transported into the pulmonary lymphatic system. In the majority of people exposed to infected droplet nuclei, the pulmonary macrophages do not destroy the organism; organisms are able to inhibit macrophage phagocytosis and continue to replicate within the macrophages whilst being transported to regional lymph nodes or the pleura. This replication occurs before the development of effective cell-mediated immune responses, which normally take between 6 and 12 weeks and is demonstrated by tuberculin skin test conversion (see below). This stage is called **primary TB infection**.

In highly susceptible persons, as in children and the immunosuppressed, extensive lymphatic and blood-borne spread can occur in this period, resulting in widespread disease. Seeding of MTB is sometimes referred to as miliary TB because on imaging the individual seeded lesions resemble millet seeds (Figure 16.3). This seeding can occur in virtually every organ in the body (hence the reference to "The Great Destroyer"): the lungs, brain, lymph nodes, and other organs such as the bones and kidneys. Miliary TB, tuberculous meningitis, and TB septicemia are life-threatening consequences and still represent major causes of death from TB around the world.

In most exposed people, however, the pulmonary macrophages remain contained at the site of infection and in the local regional lymph nodes because of the development of a cell-mediated immune response. As a result, a primary granulomatous lesion (Gohn focus) develops comprising a local area of lung inflammation,

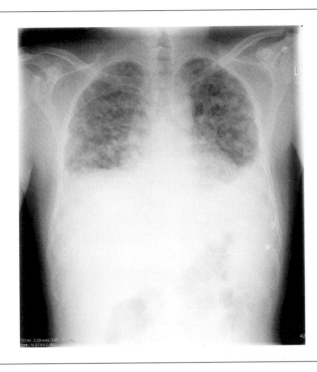

Figure 16.3 Miliary TB; note the characteristic "millet seed" nodular infiltrates. Courtesy University College London Hospitals, UK

adjacent to the terminal bronchus, with swelling of regional lymph nodes. In time, healing by resolution, scarring, and the eventual deposit of calcium within the scar tissues ensues.

Although the human immune response is highly effective in controlling primary infection resulting from exposure to *M. tuberculosis* among the majority of immunocompetent persons, all viable organisms might not be eliminated. Residual infected macrophages can be identified containing bacilli that have gone into a state of "dormancy". *M. tuberculosis* is thus able to establish latency (referred to as **latent TB infection or LTBI**), a period during which the infected person is asymptomatic but harbors *M. tuberculosis* organisms that might cause disease later.

This state of latency can last for many decades, often until the death of the host (unless some event impairs the cell-mediated defence mechanisms). This ability of *M. tuberculosis* to change its metabolic state to dormancy over many decades accounts for the persistence of the organism within the macrophage environment, and for the potential for reactivation at any time, resulting in possible transmission to other individuals. The mechanisms involved in latency and persistence are not completely understood.

When cell-mediated defence mechanisms are impaired, the bacilli may become metabolically active again, replicate, and move outside the macrophage into the surrounding tissues. This is known as **reactivation or post-primary TB**, which is the usual pattern of disease development in most cases of active TB in our community. Once a person has contracted LTBI, the risk for progression to TB disease varies. The greatest risk for progression to disease occurs within the first 2 years after infection, when approximately half of the 5–10% lifetime risk occurs. Multiple clinical conditions are associated with increased risk for progression from LTBI to TB disease. HIV infection is the strongest known risk factor. Other key risk factors in the US population are diabetes mellitus and acquisition of LTBI in infancy or early childhood. A recent addition to the known risk factors for progression from LTBI to TB disease is the use of therapeutic agents that antagonize the effect of cytokine tumor necrosis factor alpha (TNF-α). These agents have been proven to be highly effective in treating autoimmune-related conditions such as Crohn's disease and rheumatoid arthritis. Cases of TB have been reported among patients receiving all three licensed TNF-α antagonists (i.e. infliximab, etanercept, and adalimimab).

Clinical features of tuberculosis

Primary tuberculosis

It is rare for primary TB to cause symptoms. When they do occur, they are usually related to underlying immuno-suppression or in very young children. Symptoms are often localized to the site(s) of disease, accompanied by systemic symptoms including malaise, fever, anorexia, weight loss, and night sweats.

Post-primary pulmonary tuberculosis

This is the most common form of TB and is often referred to as reactivation TB. The patient may be symptom free initially, the onset is often insidious and typically the patient will have been ill for weeks to months before seeking help.

Symptoms include cough, sputum, breathlessness, and (much less frequently) hemoptysis. Often this is accompanied by weight loss and night sweats. A characteristic of post-primary pulmonary TB is that there are few symptoms or signs despite extensive lung disease. Abnormal chest signs are usually the result of lung fibrosis, cavities, or pleural disease (Figure 16.4). Tuberculosis can also affect the pleura (the sac or lining that covers the lung).

Extrapulmonary TB

Virtually any organ system in the body can be affected in TB. Common extrapulmonary sites are.

Lymph node

The commonest form of extrapulmonary TB is that of the lymph nodes. Any lymph node in the body may be involved. TB of the cervical and supraclavicular lymph nodes is common. Patients seek medical help

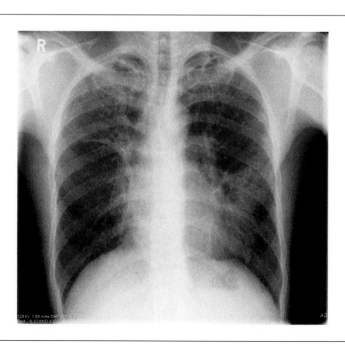

Figure 16.4 Characteristic changes on chest X-ray in a patient with post-primary pulmonary TB, showing apical fibrosis and cavitation. Courtesy University College London Hospitals, UK

Table 16.1 Classification of nontuberculous mycobacteria (report from *MMWR* March 23, 2007/56(11);250–253)

Species	Runyon group	Pigment formation	Collective designation of complex
M. kansasii	I		
M. marinum	I	Photochromogens	–
M. simiae	I		
M. scrofulaceum	II		
M. szulgai	II	Scotochromogens	–
M. gordonae	II		
M. avium	III		
M. intracellulare	III	Nonchromogens	MAC (*M. avium* complex)
M. ulcerans	III		
M. fortuitum	IV		
M. chelonae	IV	Rapid growers	*M. fortuitum–chelonae* complex

because of a mass in the neck; nodes in the neck may break down and drain spontaneously. In adults, granulomatous lymphadenitis is almost invariably caused by *M. tuberculosis*; in children, especially those younger than 5 years of age, nontuberculous mycobacteria are more common (Table 16.1 and Box 16.4). Diagnosis is established by performing acid-fast stains and appropriate culture on material obtained by needle aspiration or surgical biopsy, or from draining fluid.

Box 16.4 Clinical importance of nontuberculous mycobacteria

- Clinically, pulmonary disease caused by nontuberculous mycobacteria is very similar to TB. *M. kansasii* is most commonly associated with TB-like lung disease
- Disseminated infection is usually limited to immunocompromised patients, particularly HIV-infected individuals, in whom the *M. avium–intracellulare* complex is responsible for more than 90% of cases

- Cervical lymphadenitis due to infection with *M. scrofulaceum* is seen especially in children younger than 5 years
- Granulomatous skin lesions and soft tissue infections are usually associated with *M. marinum* (swimming pool granuloma) or *M. ulcerans*
- Generally, nontuberculous mycobacteria are resistant to first line anti-TB drugs (see Further reading)

Bone and joint

TB can affect bones and joints causing arthritis and osteomyelitis. Fever and localized pain are common. The lower spine and weight-bearing joints are most often affected; there may be multiple osteolytic lesions (break down of bone structure). About half of these patients do not have evidence of pulmonary involvement. Skeletal disease is commonly seen in the elderly.

Meninges

TB meningitis is a serious and potentially fatal condition that is associated with long-term sequelae in those who survive. The disease has an insidious onset and patients present with abnormal behavior, headaches, or convulsions. The organism gains access to the central nervous system through the bloodstream.

Meningitis is frequent in infants and small children as an early complication of primary infection, but it may be seen in any age group. Usually, the cerebrospinal fluid has a low glucose content (compared with simultaneous blood glucose), increased protein, increased cells (commonly lymphocytes), and no growth of common bacterial pathogens (see Table 10.2). There may not always be a positive reaction to a tuberculin skin test.

Genitourinary

Genitourinary TB needs to be considered when patients present with recurrent urinary tract infections with no growth of common bacterial pathogens; pyuria without bacteriuria; unexplained hematuria; recurrent fever without explanation; or evidence of abnormalities in the kidney, ureters, or bladder, especially when multiple areas are involved. Men may also present with a beaded vas deferens on palpation, a draining scrotal sinuses, epididymis (particularly with calcification), or induration of the prostate or seminal vesicles. Women may present with irregular menses, amenorrhea, pelvic inflammatory disease (salpingo-oophoritis or endometritis), or infertility. A diagnosis is generally obtained with repeated cultures of first-voided early morning urine specimens or is made on the basis of culture and histologic examination of biopsy material. Some patients with pulmonary TB (5–10%) have urine cultures positive for *M. tuberculosis* even though there are no abnormal findings in the genitourinary tract.

Peritoneum and intestines

Tuberculous peritonitis is characterized by ascites (free fluid in the abdomen) and fever; a "doughy" abdomen or abdominal mass is occasionally noted. Concomitant pleural effusion is common. The majority of patients have no lung parenchymal abnormality visible on chest radiograph. The ascitic fluid usually has a high protein content in the region of 3 g/L.

Diagnosis is established by histologic staining methods with the identification of a caseating granuloma (see "Granuloma formation" below) in tissue that is usually obtained surgical means. Tissue obtained for biopsy should also be stained and cultured for mycobacteria. The diagnosis may also be established by culture of peritoneal fluid; yields are results from swallowing sputum containing *M. tuberculosis* or by drinking unpasteurized milk from cows infected with *M. bovis*. The mucosal epithelium of the small intestine is studded with granulomatous lesions and intestinal obstruction is a common complication. This type of TB is common in endemic areas, particularly the Indian subcontinent and Africa.

Pericardium

Tuberculous pericarditis is an uncommon condition and is associated with high mortality. The majority of patients with tuberculous pericarditis have extensive pulmonary involvement with concomitant pleural involvement. Diagnosis is difficult and requires an invasive procedure where a needle is inserted into the pericardial sac to aspirate fluid and to perform a pericardial biopsy.

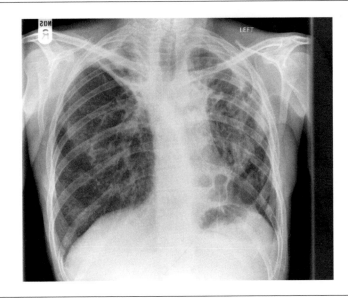

Figure 16.5 Chest X-ray of an HIV positive patient with TB. Note bilateral lung infiltrates. Courtesy University College London Hospitals, UK

Larynx

Occasionally, patients with TB first seek medical attention for hoarseness, a sore throat, or both. Laryngeal involvement with TB is usually associated with extensive pulmonary involvement; patients expectorate a large number of organisms in the sputum.

Other organs

TB may involve nearly any organ or structure in the body and produce signs and symptoms related to the specific site as well as systemic illness. For example, adrenal involvement may result in adrenal insufficiency. Chronic granulomatous skin infections with deep tissue penetration may result from mycobacterial infection.

Tuberculosis in the AIDS patient

The diagnosis of TB usually precedes or coincides with the diagnosis of AIDS but may also follow it. The clinical presentation of TB in an HIV-infected person may differ from that in persons with relatively normal cellular immunity who develop reactivation TB. Apical pulmonary disease with cavitation, a classic finding in immunologically normal persons, is less common. Patients may present with infiltrates in any lung zone, often associated with mediastinal and/or hilar lymphadenopathy (Figure 16.5).

Extrapulmonary disease occurs in 40–75% of patients, often in the presence of pulmonary disease. Lymphatic and hematogenous TB are especially common among persons with HIV infection. Central nervous system (CNS) involvement, including brain abscesses, has been reported and may be especially difficult to diagnose when it occurs in conjunction with other opportunistic CNS infections such as toxoplasmosis.

Pathogenesis and virulence

Microbiology and classification

By definition, species belonging to the genus *Mycobacterium* are acid-alcohol fast and have abundant mycolic acids in their cell walls (see Figures 2.6 and 2.7). *Mycobacterium tuberculosis* is the prototype species within the

Mycobacterium tuberculosis complex, comprising *M. tuberculosis*, *M. africanum*, *M. bovis*, and *M. microti*. A "complex" refers to closely related species and is defined as two or more species whose distinction is of little or no medical importance. Hence, TB caused by *M. africanum* is treated in the same manner as that caused by *M. tuberculosis*.

The species within the genus *Mycobacterium* fall into two main groups based on growth rate. The slowly growing species require more than 7 days forming visible colonies on solid media, whereas the rapid growing species require fewer than 7 days. *M. tuberculosis* complex belongs to the slow growing group.

M. tuberculosis is the most common species to cause TB in humans. It is an obligate pathogen and cannot multiply outside host cells. Human to human transmission is most common. *M. bovis* is transmitted from infected cows to humans via the consumption of unpasteurized milk. Although the transmission is still reported in developing countries, with the advent of pasteurization and bovine TB eradication programs in most industrialized countries, transmission of *M. bovis* has now become rare. The other mycobacteria belonging to the *M. tuberculosis* complex rarely cause human disease.

Virulence

Virulence mechanisms of *M. tuberculosis* are poorly understood; most appear to relate to cell wall structure and to the secretion of **soluble factors** that enable the organism to survive in a hostile intra-cellular environment. Examples are superoxide dismutase (**SodA**) and catalase peroxidase (**KatG**), which degrade reactive oxygen intermediates and are important for intracellular survival of *M. tuberculosis*.

Immunodominant proteins such as the heat shock protein X, Esat6 and CF-10, the 19-kD protein and glutamine synthase are thought to play a role in latency or persistence of *M. tuberculosis* and contribute to virulence as seen in animal models.

Cell surface components: Mycobacteria possess a unique set of proteins, lipids, and carbohydrates on their cell surface. Some of these are potent virulence factors unique to pathogenic mycobacteria.

Enzymes involved in general cellular metabolism: Pathogenic mycobacteria require essential nutrients and co-factors such as sources of carbon, amino acids, purines, pyrimidines, and divalent metals such as Mg^{2+} and Fe^{2+} during infection. Hence, enzymes required for the uptake and metabolism of these factors and for lipid and fatty acid metabolism are important for the survival and virulence of pathogenic mycobacteria.

Immune response mechanisms and pathogenesis

M. tuberculosis is an obligatory aerobic intracellular pathogen, which has a predilection for lung tissue rich in oxygen supply. The tubercle bacilli enter the body via the respiratory route. The infection begins when the organisms reach the pulmonary alveoli (air sacs) and infect alveolar macrophages, where the mycobacteria replicate exponentially. From the alveolar macrophages the bacteria are taken up by dendritic cells and then carried over to the regional lymph nodes and then through the bloodstream to distant tissues where TB could potentially develop giving rise to the pulmonary and extrapulmonary forms of TB. Extrapulmonary TB occurs in about 15% of TB patients. Only 10% of TB infection progresses to TB disease, but if untreated, the death rate is 51%.

The innate immune system in tuberculosis

Efficient intracellular killing of *M. tuberculosis* depends on successful interaction between infected macrophages and antigen specific T cells. T cell subsets contribute to host defences by secreting macrophage activating cytokines such as tumor necrosis factor (TNF) and interferon gamma (IFN-γ); they also lyse the infected host cell. Released mycobacteria can then be taken up by newly recruited macrophages. Activation of Toll-like receptor-2 leads to intracellular killing of *M. tuberculosis*.

Macrophage–*Mycobacterium* interaction

Binding of *M. tuberculosis* to monocyte/macrophages involves complement receptors (CR1, CR2, CR3, and CR4) and mannose receptors (MR) on the macrophages and lipoarabinomannan (LAM) on the mycobacterial surface. Cytokines can upregulate and downregulate the expression of receptors and ligands.

Phagocytosis of tubercle bacilli by alveolar macrophages is the first step in the host–pathogen relationship that decides the outcome of infection. Within 2–6 weeks there is development of cell-mediated immunity heralded by the influx of lymphocytes and activated macrophages in the lesion, resulting in granuloma formation. Since the pathogen is intracellular, humoral immunity is inadequate in dealing with the infection and the significance of relevant antibodies remains lacking. It has been shown that patients with impaired T cell function (e.g. HIV/AIDS, corticosteroids, old age) are at increased risk of developing clinically manifest TB, whereas patients with defective humoral immunity (e.g. sickle cell disease, multiple myeloma) show no increased predisposition to TB. Macrophages engulf the bacteria and the exponential growth of bacteria is checked. However, mycobacteria are able to survive and multiply within macrophages.

Intracellular survival of tubercle bacilli

Macrophage parasitism is the predominant feature of infection with *M. tuberculosis*. Intracellular survival of the microorganism rests upon the ability of tubercle bacilli to interfere with phagolysosome biogenesis (see Chapter 3 for a description of normal phagocytosis). The most prominent characteristics of the *M. tuberculosis* phagosome are its incomplete luminal acidification and absence of mature lysosomal hydrolases.

Inefficient antigen processing capacity is another important aspect of the mycobacterial phagosome. Mycobacterial protein and lipid products have been identified to prevent phagosome maturation.

The role of other cell types

The role for neutrophils has been suggested by their increased accumulation in the TB granuloma and increased chemotaxis. Neutrophils provide agents such as defensins which are absent in macrophage-based killing.

Natural killer (NK) cells are capable of activating phagocytic cells at the site of infection. Different types of TB are associated with different degrees of depression of NK cell activity. Multi-drug resistant TB is associated with a significant reduction in NK cell activity.

Acquired immunity against *M. tuberculosis* infection

Humoral immune response

It appears from various studies that the humoral immune response may not be relevant in protecting against TB.

Cellular immune response

As an intracellular pathogen, the immunological response to *M. tuberculosis* is predominantly intracellular. The tuberculous granulomas contain both CD4⁺ and CD8⁺ T cells that interact with antigen presenting cells (APCs). This interaction helps to contain the infection within the granuloma and prevent reactivation.

Readers may recall from Chapter 3 that since tubercle bacilli are phagocytosed by macrophages and reside within phagosomes they require MHC class II molecules for antigen processing and presentation. Following antigen presentation to CD4⁺ T cells, the activated CD4⁺ cells produce Th 1 cytokines such as IL-2 and IFN-γ sufficient to activate macrophages. The recruitment of CD8⁺ T cells requires antigen processing and presentation by MHC class I molecules. For this the antigen must be present in the cytosol of infected cells. Reports provide evidence for a mycobacteria-induced pore or break in the vesicular membrane of the phagosome that might allow mycobacterial antigen to enter the cytoplasm of the infected cell and hence induce MHC class I mediated pathway.

Spontaneous T cell apoptosis or apoptosis induced by mycobacteria can cause T cell hyporesponsiveness. In TB, CD95-mediated Th 1 depletion occurs resulting in attenuation of protective immunity against *M. tuberculosis*, thereby enhancing disease susceptibility. Necrotic centers in tuberculous granulomas have shown the presence of apoptotic T cells.

Th1 and Th2 dichotomy in tuberculosis

Th1 cytokines include IL-2 and IFN-γ, and Th2 cytokines include IL-4, IL-5, IL-10, and IL-13. Th1 cytokines activate macrophages, NK cells, cell-mediated immunity, and certain immunoglobulin isotypes. Th2 cytokines activate humoral immunity and depress macrophages and cell-mediated immunity. Patients with TB have a Th2-type response in peripheral blood compared to tuberculin positive patients who have a Th1-type response in peripheral blood. At the site of disease only Th1-type response is seen without enhancement of Th2 responses. The strength of Th1-type immune response is directly related to the clinical manifestations of the disease. Low levels of circulating IFN-γ in peripheral blood are associated with severe clinical TB. Patients with limited TB have an alveolar lymphocytosis in infected regions of the lung and these lymphocytes produce high levels of IFN-γ. In patients with far advanced or cavitary disease Th1-type lymphocytosis is not present.

Granuloma formation

A successful host inflammatory response to mycobacteria at the infected focus requires chemokines and adhesins for cell migration, localization, priming, and differentiation of T cell responses. The inflammatory cells form a granuloma, wherein CD4+ T cells are prominent, followed by CD8+ T cells, dendritic cells, and epithelioid cells. Proliferation of mycobacateria occurs in the lymphocyte and macrophage derived cells in the granuloma. Differentiated epithelioid cells produce extracellular matrix proteins (osteopontin, fibronectin) that provide a cellular anchor in the granuloma. The dead macrophages form a caseum (gray-white amorphous material) and bacilli are contained in the caseous centers of the granuloma. Bacilli may remain dormant in the granuloma (latent TB) or may get re-activated when the host becomes susceptible leading to clinically manifest reactivation TB. When bacilli are discharged into the airways because a granulomatous focus in the lung has burst into a main bronchus (airway), it results in the highly transmissible form of TB known as "open" or "smear positive" TB. The lymph nodes in draining the region may be hyperplastic, reactive, hyporeactive, or nonreactive.

The tuberculin skin test

We have seen that the immune defence response against TB largely entails cell-mediated immunity (CMI). Delayed-type hypersensitivity (DTH), a closely related but not identical phenomenon to CMI, is manifested clinically as a type IV immune response mediated by lymphocytes. If a patient has been exposed to TB antigens primed lymphocytes produce a characteristic indurated response to the intradermal injection of protein from the cell wall of the tubercle bacillus. The most commonly used test employs the Mantoux technique wherein a small amount of tuberculoprotein (purified protein derivative, or PPD) is introduced into the intradermal tissues with a small-gauge needle. The amount of induration is measured between 2 and 5 days later. See the section "Diagnosis of tuberculosis" below for the diagnostic interpretation of a tuberculin skin test.

Pathogenesis in HIV-TB co-infection

In the present era of HIV/AIDS, HIV-TB co-infection merits further study since it has implications for the prognosis of both infections. About 60–70% of HIV positive patients will develop TB in their lifetime with a higher proportion of extrapulmonary disseminated disease, a higher frequency of false negative tuberculin skin tests, atypical features on chest radiographs, fewer cavitating lung lesions, a higher rate of adverse drug reactions, presence of other AIDS-associated manifestations, and a higher death rate.

The features of TB infection in HIV/AIDS patients are nonspecific due to immunodeficiency. TB is the most common life-threatening opportunistic infection among patients with HIV/AIDS. About 25–65% of patients with HIV/AIDS have TB of any organ. About 50% of HIV-TB co-infection cases are negative by acid-fast staining. Chest radiographs do not manifest with characteristic fibrosis and cavitation and can be normal in up to 10–20% of patients with HIV/AIDS.

In patients with relatively intact immune function (CD4$^+$ count >200/mm^3), characteristic pulmonary TB (Figure 16.4) is more frequently seen than extrapulmonary TB. Sputum smears are often positive. As immunosuppression progresses, extrapulmonary TB becomes increasingly common with involvement of two or more noncontiguous organs concomitantly.

HIV causes a decline in the numbers and function of CD4$^+$ T cells, which reflects the integrity of granuloma. Both HIV and TB infections are intracellular. HIV gp120 binds to T cell receptors on CD4$^+$ T cells. This prevents the uptake of mycobacteria by the receptors and causes hyporesponsiveness to soluble tubercle antigens. HIV infection also downregulates the Th1 response which enhances the susceptibility to many intracellular infections including TB. The Th2 responses are unaffected or not increased. Recurrence of TB is more frequent in HIV/AIDS patients due to both endogenous reactivation and exogenous re-infection.

TB in turn accelerates the progression of HIV/AIDS infection. Infected macrophages within a granuloma produce TNF-α in response to tubercle bacilli. TNF-α is a potent activator of HIV replication. The sites of active TB infection act as foci of HIV replication and evolution independent of systemic HIV disease activity.

Genetic variability in *M. tuberculosis*

Although much is known about factors that contribute to the risk for transmission of *M. tuberculosis* from person to person, the role of the organism itself is only beginning to be understood. Genetic variability is believed to affect the capability of *M. tuberculosis* strains to be transmitted or to cause disease once transmitted, or both.

A family of *M. tuberculosis* isolates that were genetically similar was first identified in patients from China, and named the Beijing family. The Beijing family has been identified in most countries, and appears to be spreading globally. The *M. tuberculosis* W-strain family, a member of the Beijing family, is a group of clonally related multi-drug resistant organisms of *M. tuberculosis* that caused nosocomial outbreaks involving HIV-infected persons in New York City during 1991–1994. W-family organisms, which have also been associated with TB outbreaks worldwide, are believed to have evolved from a single strain of *M. tuberculosis* that developed resistance-conferring mutations in multiple genes. The growth of W-family organisms in human macrophages is four- to eightfold higher than that of strains that cause few or no secondary cases of TB; this enhanced ability to replicate in human macrophages might contribute to the organism's potential for enhanced transmission.

Diagnosis of tuberculosis

Since 1995, CDC has provided approximately $8 million/year to state and local public health laboratories to improve TB laboratory services in the USA, and has placed increased emphasis on reliable and prompt results. The latter included efforts to reduce the delays associated with laboratory testing for *M. tuberculosis*, to improve communication between laboratories and healthcare providers, and to maintain a trained workforce. Recommendations developed during the mid-1990s for TB laboratory services remain valid and include:

- Prompt delivery of specimens to the laboratory
- Use of rapid, state-of-the-art methods (e.g. fluorescence microscopy, liquid media, and rapid identification methods)
- Reporting of smear results to healthcare providers within 1 day
- Reporting of culture identification of *M. tuberculosis* complex within 21 days
- Reporting of drug-susceptibility test results within 30 days, and
- Reporting of all positive test results to the specimen submitter within 1 working day from the date of report.

Acid-fast smear

The Ziehl–Neelsen carbolfuchsin or Kinyoun carbolfuchsin stains have been essential in TB diagnosis for nearly 100 years. Although less sensitive than culture, the acid-fast smear is a rapid and inexpensive test that can be performed with a minimum of equipment and is very specific for mycobacteria. Depending on the bacterial load, a single sputum smear has sensitivity between 22% and 80%, but the yield is improved when multiple sputum specimens are examined and concentration methods used. See Figures 2.6 and 2.7 for a description of the acid-fast cell wall and staining characteristics.

Fluorochrome stains

Most laboratories in the USA use fluorochrome stains, such as auramine-rhodamine stain. With these techniques, mycobacteria fluoresce with a bright orange color and can be easily seen on low-power microscopy, increasing the sensitivity of the smear detection.

Nucleic acid amplification

Direct tests of nucleic acid amplification are rapid, widely available, and can be performed in a day.

Gene probes

The Amplified *Mycobacterium tuberculosis* Direct Test (Gen-Probe) targets mycobacterial ribosomal RNA. The test uses DNA probes that are highly specific for *M. tuberculosis* species. It is best used (and only approved for use) in patients in whom acid-fast bacilli smears are positive and cultures are in process. Since specificity is less than 100%, even in patients with positive smears, occasional false positive results do occur, usually in patients with nontuberculous mycobacterial infections.

Gene probes for rifampin resistance

Different insertion, deletion and missense mutations within a hypervariable region of *rpoB*, the gene encoding the β-subunit of the DNA-dependent RNA polymerase of *M. tuberculosis*, contribute to the development of resistance to rifamycins. This feature is exploited in molecular tests that can rapidly detect the potential for resistance to rifampin in the organism. High frequency mutations in codons 531, 526 and 516 may serve as predictors of resistance to rifampin. This in itself is a useful surrogate marker for MDR-TB as surveillance studies have shown that >90% of rifampin resistant isolates of *M. tuberculosis* are also resistant to isoniazid.

PCR testing

This technique amplifies even very small portions of a predetermined target region of *M. tuberculosis*-complex DNA. The test uses an automated system that can rapidly detect as few as one organism from sputum, bronchoalveolar lavage, blood, cerebrospinal fluid, pleural fluid, or other fluid and tissue samples and has shown sensitivity and specificity of nearly 90% in pulmonary disease. However, the interpretation of a PCR result must always be used in conjunction with a smear result and clinical suspicion of disease (Table 16.2).

Table 16.2 Interpretation of PCR results in the diagnosis of tuberculosis (reproduced from CDC)

Smear	PCR	Clinical suspicion	Comment
Positive	Positive	High/low	Diagnosis: active TB
Negative	Negative	High/low	Cannot exclude active TB
Negative	Positive	High	Suspect *M. tuberculosis*; start treatment and review therapy when culture results are final
Negative	Positive	Low	Active TB, old TB, or contaminant; consult specialist
Positive	Negative	High	*M. tuberculosis* or nontuberculous mycobacteria; start therapy and review when culture results are final
Positive	Negative	Low	Most likely nontuberculous mycobacteria but cannot exclude *M. tuberculosis*; consider initiating TB therapy until culture results are final

Culture techniques

The ability to culture mycobacteria is the "gold standard" in the diagnosis of TB and is a more sensitive method than smear diagnosis. Löwenstein–Jensen culture medium is the most commonly used solid medium, but mycobacterial growth may take up to 6 weeks. Therefore many laboratories simultaneously culture specimens in a broth-based medium that takes only 2–3 weeks for mycobacterial growth. Mycobacteria grown in liquid media are usually speciated and subcultured in the presence of different antimycobacterial agents to assess drug sensitivity. One of the newest and fastest techniques for growing *M. tuberculosis* is the Mycobacterial Growth Indicator Tube. The advantage of this system is the rapidity with which it detects growth.

The CDC and the World Health Organization recommend initial susceptibility testing for all *M. tuberculosis* isolates because of the emergence of drug resistance worldwide.

Tuberculin skin tests

The Mantoux test is the preferred and standard skin test for detecting TB. It involves injection of 1–5 tuberculin units (TU) of purified protein derivative (PPD, tuberculin), usually 0.1 ml, intradermally. Induration is then assessed at 48–72 hours. The extent of induration (not erythema) should be measured across two diameters at right angles and the two measurements then averaged.

About 20% of patients with active TB may have negative skin tests, and some populations have an even higher incidence of false negative results. For example, false negative rates up to 50% have been reported in patients with advanced HIV infection. Alternately, false positive results may occur in patients infected by other nontuberculous mycobacteria (e.g. *Mycobacterium avium* complex). Therefore, a negative skin test never rules out TB, and a positive skin test alone does not establish the diagnosis.

BCG vaccine and skin testing

The skin test reactivity associated with BCG (Bacille Calmette–Guérin, a highly modified strain of *M. bovis*) vaccination in childhood usually diminishes in 5 years. A positive skin test in a person vaccinated with BCG more than 5 years before skin testing should be considered as caused by *M. tuberculosis* infection and not attributed to BCG vaccination. Many of these patients are from countries in which TB is prevalent, and the likelihood of infection is high.

Table 16.3 Recommendations for the interpretation of the tuberculin skin test (reproduced from CDC)

Skin test interpretation depends on:
- the measurement in millimeters (mm) of the induration and
- the person's risk of being infected with TB and/or progression to disease if infected.

The following three cut points should be used to determine whether the skin test reaction is *positive*. A measurement of 0 mm or anything below the defined cut point for each category is considered *negative*

Induration of ≥5 mm is considered positive in:	Induration of ≥10 mm is considered positive in:	Induration of ≥15 mm is considered positive in:
• HIV positive persons • Recent contacts of TB case patients • Persons with chest X-ray evidence of prior TB • Patients with organ transplants and other immunosuppressed patients	• Recent immigrants from high-prevalence countries • Injection drug users • Residents and employees of high risk congregate settings, i.e. prisons, nursing homes/elderly care homes, all healthcare facilities, residential facilities for AIDS patients, homeless shelters • Mycobacteriology laboratory personnel • Persons with silicosis, diabetes mellitus, chronic renal failure, cancer patients, weight loss of 10% of ideal body weight, gastrectomy, and jejunoileal bypass • Children <4 years of age, or infants, children and adolescents exposed to adults at high risk	• Persons with no known risk factors for TB

Booster effect

Although repeated exposure to tuberculin itself will not sensitize an uninfected person, it may sensitize patients who were infected previously and have experienced waning immunity. This is termed the booster effect and can occur with a second skin test even a year after the first test. This makes it difficult to assess whether the reaction represents new conversion or boosting of an old infection. Recommendations for skin test interpretation are outlined in Table 16.3. Converters and reactors are not contagious to others unless active TB develops.

Interferon gamma release assays

In 2005, a new *in vitro* test, QuantiFERON-TB Gold (QFT-G, manufactured by Cellestis Limited, Carnegie, Victoria, Australia) received final approval from the US Food and Drug Administration (FDA) as a diagnostic test for *M. tuberculosis* infection, both latent tuberculosis infection (LTBI) and active tuberculosis (TB) disease. This enzyme-linked immunosorbent assay (ELISA) test detects the release of interferon gamma (IFN-γ) in fresh heparinized whole blood from persons who have been exposed to *M. tuberculosis*. When their blood is incubated with mixtures of synthetic peptides simulating two proteins present in *M. tuberculosis*: early secretory antigenic target-6 (ESAT-6) and culture filtrate protein-10 (CFP-10) sensitized T cells release IFN-γ. The presence of IFN-γ therefore indicates that the patient has been exposed to *M. tuberculosis* at some time. ESAT-6 and CFP-10 are secreted by all *M. tuberculosis* and pathogenic *M. bovis* strains. Because these proteins are absent from all BCG vaccine strains and from commonly encountered nontuberculous mycobacteria (NTM) except *M. kansasii*, *M. szulgai*, and *M. marinum*, QFT-G is expected to be more specific for *M. tuberculosis* than tests that use tuberculin purified protein derivative (PPD) as the antigen.

QFT-G represents one type of IFN-γ release assay (IGRA). Tests such as QFT-G measure the IFN-γ released by sensitized white blood cells after whole blood is incubated with antigen. Tests such as ELISpot enumerate cells releasing IFN-γ after mononuclear cells recovered from whole blood are incubated with similar antigens.

Before QFT was approved in 2001, the tuberculin skin test (TST) was the only test available for detecting latent TB infection. QFT-G results can be available <24 hours after testing without the need for a second visit, whereas a TST requires a second encounter to read the result 48–72 hours after administration of the test. As a laboratory-based assay, QFT-G is not subject to biases and errors of TST placement and reading. However, errors in collecting or transporting blood specimens or in running and interpreting the assay can decrease the accuracy of QFT-G.

Injection of PPD for the TST can boost subsequent TST responses, primarily in persons who have been infected with NTM or vaccinated with BCG. Compared with the TST, QFT-G might be less affected by boosting from a previous TST.

QFT-G is a new test; more information is needed regarding:

- Interpretation in young children, especially those aged <5 years
- Performance in persons with impaired immune systems, including persons with HIV/AIDS, those who will be treated with TNF-α antagonists, and others
- Determination of the subsequent incidence of TB disease after LTBI has been either diagnosed or excluded with QFT-G
- Length of time between exposure, establishment of infection, and emergence of a positive QFT-G test result
- Economic evaluation and decision analysis comparing QFT-G with TST
- Changes in QFT-G results during therapy for both LTBI and TB disease
- Ability of QFT-G to detect reinfection after treatment for both LTBI and TB disease, and
- Performance of QFT-G in targeted testing programs (e.g. for recent immigrants from high-incidence countries) and contact investigations.

Until these questions are answered, QFT-G needs to be used in conjunction with clinical, radiological, microbiological and epidemiological factors associated with each case. See Further reading for detailed guidance issued by the CDC on the use of these new tests.

Management of a case of tuberculosis

Excellent guidelines are available from the World Health Organization, the American Thoracic Society, the Infectious Diseases Society of America, and CDC for the management of cases and contacts of TB. See Further reading to access this information.

Test yourself

Case study 16.1

A 12-year-old schoolgirl was reported by her teacher when she was unable to play games at school and was falling behind in her studies. She was of Haitian origin, born in the USA of first generation Haitian parents. She lived in an extended family with her grandmother and her uncle and his family of three children aged between 6 months and 4 years.

At the local healthcare facility a more detailed history revealed that she had had a cough for several weeks with a low grade temperature, night sweats, and loss of weight.

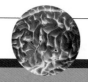

Test yourself

The chest X-ray and a CT scan of the lung are shown below:

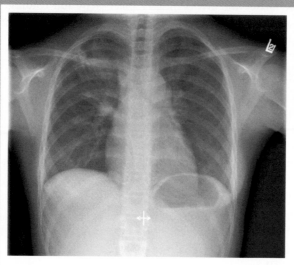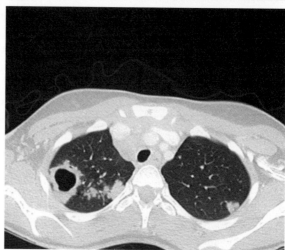

Both figures courtesy University College London Hospitals, UK

A sputum examination revealed moderate acid-fast bacilli on auramine staining. Several weeks later the sputum grew *M. tuberculosis* sensitive to first line anti TB drugs.

Her parents are very concerned and have several questions. Read the literature in the Further reading section and try and answer their queries.

1. Is she an infection risk to her family and classmates at school?
2. Does she need to stay away from school and if so for how long?
3. Does she need to be admitted to hospital and for how long?
4. She has been very close to her young cousins, playing with them after school and kissing and holding them, what do we need to do to make sure that they have not been infected? Currently they are completely well.
5. Parents of the other children in her class have been phoning the school voicing their concerns. Put in a plan of action to make sure that the children are managed appropriately.
6. What is the role of TST and the new IGRA tests in the management of close contacts (family and classmates).

Further reading

Horsburgh CR, Feldman S, Ridzon R. Practice guidelines for the treatment of tuberculosis. *Clin Infect Dis* 2000;31:633–639

Useful websites

CDC. Division of Tuberculosis Elimination. Fact Sheets. Treatment of Latent Tuberculosis Infection (LTBI). http://www.cdc.gov/TB/pubs/tbfactsheets/treatmentLTBI.htm

CDC. Guidelines for Using the QuantiFERON®-TB Gold Test for Detecting *Mycobacterium tuberculosis* Infection, USA. MMWR December 16, 2005/54(RR15);49–55. http://www.cdc.gov/mmwr/preview/mmwrhtml/rr5415a4.htm

CDC. Treatment of Tuberculosis. American Thoracic Society, CDC, and Infectious Diseases Society of America. MMWR June 20, 2003/52(RR11);1–77. http://www.cdc.gov/MMWR/preview/mmwrhtml/rr5211a1.htm

WHO. A World Free of TB. http://www.who.int/tb/en/

WHO. Investigations into USA Air Passenger with XDR TB. http://www.who.int/tb/features_archive/tb_and_airtravel/en/index.html

Chapter 17
Malaria

D. Mack

The epidemiology and burden of malaria
The parasite and its lifecycle
  Exoerythrocytic phase
  Erythrocytic phase
  Vector phase
Clinical features and pathogenesis

Diagnosis
Treatment
Prevention
Vector control
Immunization
Global malaria control

The epidemiology and burden of malaria

Malaria is an infectious disease of global importance caused by several species of *Plasmodium* parasites which belong to the apicomplexa group of single celled, eukaryotic protozoa. There are four main species of *Plasmodium* capable of causing human infections: *P. falciparum*, *P. vivax*, *P. ovale*, and *P. malariae*. Malaria can be transmitted by approximately 70 species of female *Anopheles* mosquitoes during feeding. Rare routes of transmission include exposure to infected blood or blood products, organ transplantation, and vertical transmission giving rise to congenital infection.

Malaria is transmitted in:

- Large areas of Central and South America
- The islands of Hispaniola (including Haiti and the Dominican Republic)
- Africa
- Asia (including the Indian subcontinent, Southeast Asia, and the Middle East)
- Eastern Europe
- The South Pacific.

See Figure 17.1a and b.

In Africa, Papua New Guinea, and Haiti, *P. falciparum* is the predominant malaria species. *P. vivax* causes most infections in Southeast Asia, the Indian subcontinent, Central and South America, North Africa, and the Middle East. *P. ovale* is found in West Africa and Asia, while *P. malariae* is found in most endemic areas.

Malaria infections cause up to 500 million episodes of febrile illness annually. Almost all deaths result from *P. falciparum* infections which cause an estimated 700 000 to 2.6 million fatal infections annually. Most fatalities occur in sub-Saharan Africa in children under the age of five and in pregnant women. Repeated *P. falciparum* infection may also give rise to severe anemia in children and pregnant women. Children who survive episodes of severe malaria may have developmental abnormalities. *P. vivax*, *P. ovale*, and *P. malariae* cause nonfatal infections but collectively have a wider geographical distribution than *P. falciparum*. Up to 40% of the world's population lives in malaria-endemic areas and approximately 5% of the world's population is infected at any given time.

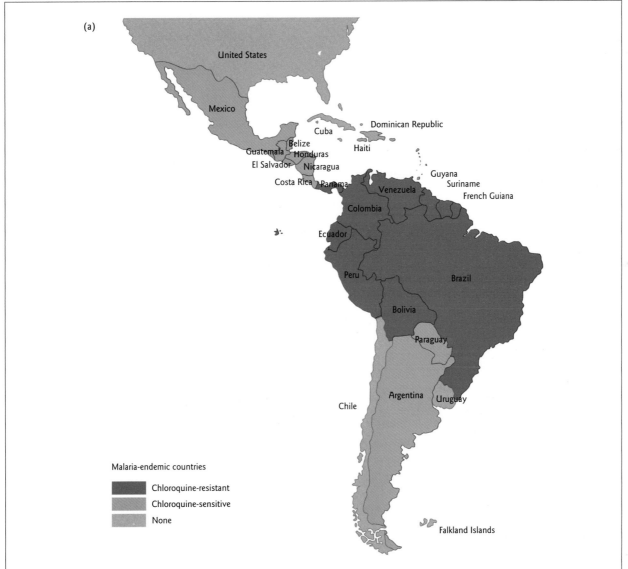

Figure 17.1 Worldwide prevalence of malaria. (a) Malaria-endemic countries in the Western Hemisphere.

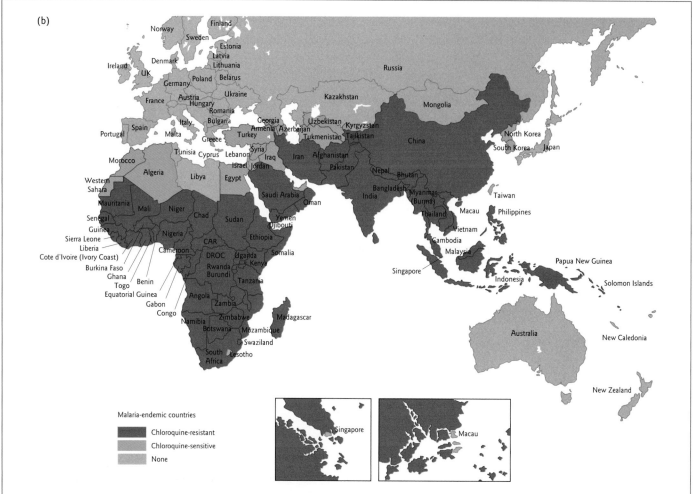

(b)

Malaria-endemic countries

- Chloroquine-resistant
- Chloroquine-sensitive
- None

Figure 17.1 (*cont'd*) (b) Malaria-endemic countries in the Eastern Hemisphere. Courtesy Centers for Disease Control; from: http://wwwn.cdc.gov/travel/yellowBookCh4-Malaria.aspx

The infection and mortality rates are both rising, in association with drug resistance in the parasites, and insecticide resistance in the mosquito vector. The economic burden of malaria upon African countries has been estimated at US$12 billion per year. The burden inflicted by malaria on a particular population is the product of a complex interplay between parasite, host, and vector. This burden is borne disproportionately by vulnerable segments of society including children, pregnant women, and the poor.

Every year up to 50 million people travel from nonendemic countries to malaria endemic areas and are at risk of contracting malaria. Endemic malaria was eradicated from the USA in the 1950s. Almost all recent cases in the USA have been imported by persons travelling from endemic areas. Rarely, cases arise from local mosquito-borne transmission. Each year approximately 1200 cases of malaria in US civilians are reported to the Centers for Disease Control (CDC). Most of these infections are acquired in Africa, followed by Asia and the Caribbean and Central and South America. Most infections acquired by travelers to Africa are due to *P. falciparum* while those acquired in other endemic regions are predominantly caused by *P. vivax*.

The parasite and its lifecycle

. . . With tears and toiling breath,
I find thy cunning seeds,
O million-murdering Death.

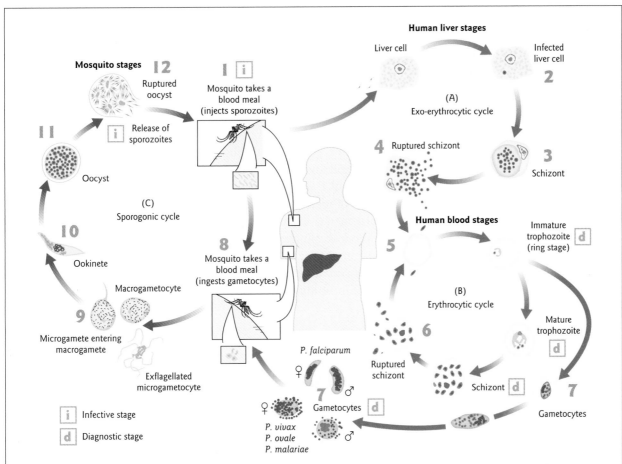

Figure 17.2 The malaria parasite lifecycle. The malaria parasite lifecycle involves two hosts. During a blood meal, a malaria-infected female *Anopheles* mosquito inoculates sporozoites into the human host (1). Sporozoites infect liver cells (2) and mature into schizonts (3), which rupture and release merozoites (4). (Of note, in *P. vivax* and *P. ovale* a dormant stage (hypnozoites) can persist in the liver and cause relapses by invading the bloodstream weeks, or even years later.) After this initial replication in the liver (exo-erythrocytic schizogony (A)), the parasites undergo asexual multiplication in the erythrocytes (erythrocytic schizogony (B)). Merozoites infect red blood cells (5). The ring stage trophozoites mature into schizonts, which rupture releasing merozoites (6). Some parasites differentiate into sexual erythrocytic stages (gametocytes) (7). Blood stage parasites are responsible for the clinical manifestations of the disease. The gametocytes, male (microgametocytes) and female (macrogametocytes), are ingested by an *Anopheles* mosquito during a blood meal (8). The parasites' multiplication in the mosquito is known as the sporogonic cycle (C). While in the mosquito's stomach, the microgametes penetrate the macrogametes generating zygotes (9). The zygotes in turn become motile and elongated (ookinetes) (10) which invade the mid-gut wall of the mosquito where they develop into oocysts (11). The oocysts grow, rupture, and release sporozoites (12), which make their way to the mosquito's salivary glands. Inoculation of the sporozoites into a new human host perpetuates the malaria life cycle (1). Provided by Alexander J. da Silva, PhD/Melanie Moser. Courtesy of the Centers for Disease Control and Prevention; from CDC website: http://phil.cdc.gov/phil/details.asp

The piece above is a fragment of a poem by Ronald Ross, written in August 1897, following his discovery of malaria parasites in *Anopheles* mosquitoes fed on malaria-infected patients.

The lifecycle of malaria has several phases (Figure 17.2). The exoerythrocytic and erythrocytic phases take place in the human host, and sexual reproduction takes place in the mosquito vector. The presence of malaria parasites in the blood of affected individuals was first noted by Charles Louis Alphonse Laveran, a French army surgeon, in 1880. Dr Ronald Ross, a British medical officer working in India, proved that malaria was transmitted by mosquitoes in 1898. The latent hepatic hypnozoites of *P. vivax* and *P. ovale* were not observed until the 1980s.

Exoerythrocytic phase

Infective sporozoites are injected from the salivary glands of the mosquito into the human host as the mosquito prepares to take a blood meal. Sporozoites are carried through the circulation to the liver. They enter hepatocytes where they multiply asexually and asymptomatically to produce thousands of merozoites within each infected hepatocyte. In *P. falciparum* and *P. malariae* infections, all infected hepatocytes rupture after 6–16 days, each releasing tens of thousands of merozoites into the bloodstream. Most *P. vivax* and *P. malariae* merozoites are released after a similar incubation period, but a proportion remain latent in the liver for months to years before emerging to produce clinical episodes of malaria. The merozoites enter erythrocytes via a process involving the apical complex of the protozoa, and invagination of the red blood cell membrane. The binding of merozoites of *P. vivax* to erythrocyte membranes requires the presence of the Duffy blood group antigens. In West Africa, most individuals lack these antigens and are protected from *P. vivax* infection.

Erythrocytic phase

Once inside the red blood cell, the trophozoites initially assume a characteristic "ring form" morphology before enlarging to become mature trophozoites. Maturing trophozoites are highly metabolically active, consuming glucose from the host's plasma, and erythrocyte contents including hemoglobin. Toxic degradation products from the proteolysis of hemoglobin are stored within the parasite food vacuole as the malaria pigment hemazoin. The parasites undergo multiple rounds of asexual nuclear division as they develop into schizonts. Approximately 48 hours after erythrocyte invasion in *P. falciparum*, *P. vivax*, and *P. ovale* infections, or 72 hours in *P. malariae* infections, the infected red blood cells are lysed (schizogony), releasing 16–32 merozoites into the bloodstream. Simultaneously, the contents of the parasitized erythrocyte are released into the circulation, triggering the production of cytokines which contribute to the clinical symptoms of malaria.

In *P. falciparum* infections, each merozoite is capable of infecting new erythrocytes of any age, resulting in an exponential increase in parasite biomass. The first half of the *P. falciparum* asexual erythrocytic cycle takes part in circulating red blood cells. Parasite derived *P. falciparum* erythrocyte membrane protein 1 (*Pf*EMP1) then appears on the surface of the infected red blood cells and facilitates attachment to vascular endothelium (cytoadherence). Most *P. falciparum* infected erythrocytes then become sequestered in the microvasculature throughout the body, including the brain, viscera, and placenta, where they are able to avoid destruction by the spleen and reach high densities.

P. vivax and *P. ovale* merozoites can only infect reticulocytes, limiting the levels of parasitemia attained in these infections. In these infections, erythrocytes exhibit granules which stain red (Schüffner's dots). Red blood cells infected with *P. vivax* enlarge, while those infected with *P. ovale* take on an oval appearance. Some *P. ovale* trophozoites take on a rectangular, or "band" appearance. The merozoites of *P. malariae* predominantly infect old red blood cells and only low levels of parasitized red blood cells are reached. Untreated, malaria infections may persist for several years, or even decades in the case of *P. malariae*. Sequestration does not occur in non-*P. falciparum* infections.

During erythrocytic development, some merozoites differentiate into sexual forms known as male and female gametocytes. Gametocytes do not undergo further multiplication and do not cause clinical symptoms. Some gametocytes may survive in the peripheral blood for up to several weeks, providing an extended opportunity for onward transmission of malaria by the mosquito vector. Key clinical and microscopic features of *Plasmodium* species infections in humans are summarized in Table 17.1.

Table 17.1 Clinical and microscopic features of *Plasmodium* species infections in humans

	P. falciparum	*P. vivax*	*P. ovale*	*P. malariae*
Clinical features				
Erythrocytic cycle (days)	2	2	2	3
Hypnozoites	No	Yes	Yes	No
Erythrocytes invaded	All ages	Reticulocytes	Reticulocytes	Old erythrocytes
Duration of untreated infection (years)	2	4	4	40
Mean incubation period (days)	13	13	14	35
Microscopic features (see Figure 17.4)				
Infected RBC size and shape	Normal	Enlarged	Enlarged, oval	Normal
Schüffner's dots	None	Present	Present	None
Multiple parasites per RBC	Common	Rare	Rare	Rare
Schizonts in peripheral blood	Rare, 8–24 merozoites	12–24 merozoites	8–12 merozoites	6–12 merozoites
Gametocytes	"Crescent" shaped	Round or oval	Round or oval	Large and oval

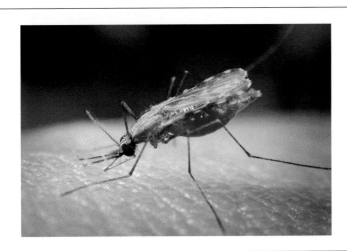

Figure 17.3 A female *Anopheles* mosquito feeding on a human host. Courtesy of the Centers for Disease Control and Prevention; from CDC website: http://phil.cdc.gov/phil/details.asp

Vector phase

Female *Anopheles* mosquitoes capable of transmitting malaria ingest gametocytes while taking a blood meal (Figure 17.3). In the mosquito mid-gut the male and female gametocytes are released from the erythrocytes and cross-fertilize to form zygotes. The zygotes develop through a mobile ookinete phase into oocysts containing numerous sporozoites. The oocysts rupture, releasing the sporozoites, which migrate via the mosquito lymph system to the salivary glands. There the sporozoites can be injected into a new human host as the mosquito takes another blood meal. The sexual reproductive cycle takes 1–2 weeks to complete in the vector host and can only occur where temperatures are maintained between 16°C and 33°C, and at altitudes below 2000 m above sea level. The distributions and behaviors of different female *Anopheles* mosquito species vary, and even among single species, feeding and resting behaviors may differ in closely related geographical locations and environments. Environmental changes including deforestation, migration, new agricultural practices, and climate change may influence vector behavior and malaria transmission.

Clinical features and pathogenesis

The regular, intermittent paroxysms of fever caused by malaria infections were first clearly described by Hippocrates. The use of deliberate infection with malaria as means of inducing fever to treat neurosyphilis in the early 20th century provided information about the natural history of untreated malaria. Malaria infections typically have incubation periods ranging from 13 to 28 days (Table 17.1) but this may extend to several months, particularly in the case of *P. malariae* infections.

The symptoms of malaria are temporally related to the release of parasites and erythrocyte contents into the circulation during shizogony, and the release of host inflammatory mediators in response to this event. The principal inflammatory mediator released is tumor necrosis factor (TNF), the levels of which are related to disease severity in *P. falciparum* infections. The mild prodromal symptoms include malaise, headache, back pain, nausea, vomiting, and diarrhea. These are followed by the onset of paroxysmal chills and rigors, followed by high fevers, followed by profuse sweats. Paroxysms of fever may occur with regular periodicity coinciding with the rupture of schizonts and the release of TNF in response. This process gives rise to 48-hour (*P. falciparum*, *P. vivax* or *P. ovale*) or 72-hour (*P. malariae*) cycles or symptoms. The differential diagnosis of malaria includes typhoid fever, dengue fever, influenza, leptospirosis, meningococcal disease, and pneumococcal disease.

Anemia

The destruction of both infected and uninfected erythrocytes gives rise to a progressive normochromic, normocytic anemia and jaundice. Infected erythrocytes are removed by the spleen, or destroyed by the process of schizont rupture. The spleen is capable of "pitting" the parasites out, and returning previously infected erythrocytes to the circulation. Unfortunately uninfected erythrocytes also undergo changes and become less deformable. The uninfected cells may be removed by the spleen in large numbers, or undergo intravascular hemolysis. Uncommonly, massive intravascular hemolysis may lead to "blackwater fever" with the passage of dark urine. Bone marrow suppression may further contribute to anemia, and may take weeks to recover following infection. In young children, recurrent infections lead to severe, prolonged anemia and iron deficiency. Thrombocytopenia resulting from increased splenic clearance is common, and a coagulopathy may develop in cases of severe *P. falciparum* disease.

Severe *P. falciparum* malaria

In untreated *P. falciparum* infections in nonimmune subjects, the multiplication and sequestration of parasites results in multi-organ failure and death within weeks of initial infection. The underlying mechanism of severe *P. falciparum* disease is thought to be microvascular obstruction by the parasitized red blood cells. Severe manifestations of *P. falciparum* infections include cerebral malaria, respiratory and renal failure, and severe malaria of pregnancy (Table 17.2). Renal impairment arises from acute tubular necrosis, while pulmonary edema results from increased vascular permeability. Metabolic acidosis, tissue hypoperfusion, hypoglycemia, and secondary bacterial infections (particularly *Salmonella* septicemias) contribute to mortality. Hypoglycemia arises from the increased demand for glucose due to the metabolic demands of the illness and glucose consumption by the parasites. Hepatic glycogen stores are rapidly depleted, especially in children, and gluconeogenesis fails. Quinidine treatment stimulates insulin secretion by the pancreatic beta-cells, compounding hypoglycemia.

P. falciparum in pregnancy

In pregnancy, the immune response to malaria is suppressed, and a large number of infected erythrocytes become sequestered within the placenta. These processes combined with maternal anemia result in placental insufficiency and intrauterine growth retardation. In highly endemic areas, recurrent infections

Table 17.2 Indicators of severe *P. falciparum* malaria (based on the World Health Organization criteria for severe malaria, published in 2000)

Manifestation	Features
Cerebral malaria	Glasgow Coma Scale score ≤9 Coma for ≥30 minutes following a seizure
Severe anemia	Hematocrit <15% or hemoglobin <50 g/L in presence of parasite count >10 000/µl
Renal failure	Low urine output, raised creatinine
Pulmonary edema or acute respiratory distress syndrome	Hypoxemia, positive end-expiratory pressure
Hypoglycemia	Blood glucose <2.2 mmol/L (<40 g/dl)
Circulatory shock ("Algid malaria")	Low blood pressure, cold clammy skin
Coagulopathy	Spontaneous bleeding, disseminated intravascular coagulation
Repeated convulsions	3 or more in a 24-hour period
Acidemia/acidosis	Arterial pH < 7.25 or acidosis (plasma bicarbonate <15 mmol/L)
Marcoscopic hemoglobinuria ("Blackwater fever")	Not secondary to G6PD
Hyperparasitemia	>5% parasitized erythrocytes or >250 000 parasites/µl in nonimmune patients
Hyperpyrexia	Core body temperature >40°C
Hyperbilirubinemia	Total bilirubin >43 µmol/L (>2.5 mg/dl)
Impaired consciousness	Rouseable mental condition
Prostration or weakness	

lead to reductions in birth weight. In areas of intermediate and low *P. falciparum* transmission, severe maternal malaria is more common. Severe malaria in pregnancy is often complicated by hypoglycemia and pulmonary edema; maternal mortality is high and fetal loss common.

Cerebral malaria

The sequestration of infected erythrocytes occurs to the greatest extent in the brain. Autopsy studies reveal small vessels packed with erythrocytes containing the mature asexual parasites not often seen in the peripheral circulation. Infected and uninfected erythrocytes exhibit decreased deformability, and uninfected cells adhere to infected erythrocytes – "rosetting." The resulting microcirculatory obstruction reduces oxygen and substrate supply to the brain resulting in anaerobic glycolysis, lactic acidosis, and cellular dysfunction. Cerebral malaria is characterized by seizures, confusion, and the development of coma. The onset may be insidious, or abrupt. Alternative diagnoses including hypoglycemia, status epilepticus, and bacterial meningitis should be considered. In patients with cerebral malaria there are usually no focal neurological signs and the neck stiffness characteristic of meningeal irritation is absent. Decerebrate or decorticate posturing may occur and there may be a divergent gaze with equal, reactive pupils. Flame shaped hemorrhages may be observed on fundoscopy. At lumbar puncture, the opening pressure is often raised in children but is usually normal in adults. Examination of the cerebrospinal fluid reveals a normal protein and white blood cell count. Untreated, cerebral malaria is uniformly fatal. Those successfully treated may be left with neurological deficits including hemiparesis and cortical blindness.

Immunity to *P. falciparum*

The genome of *P. falciparum* contains many genes encoding antigens expressed on the surface of infected red blood cells. These genes include the *var* gene family which encode the *Pf*EMP1 proteins which, in addition to being instrumental in cytoadherence, are a major antigenic determinant of the parasite. Alterations in *var* gene expression are common and alter parasite antigenicity as the organism "changes its spots." In the chronically infected patient who has developed a degree of immunity to one set of antigens, a switch in *var* gene expression alters the *Pf*EMP1 antigens causing a recurrence of malaria symptoms. This and other mechanisms, including a degree of impairment of cell-mediated immunity, delay the development of complete immunity by the human host. Over time, the levels of cytokines released during infections decreases, reducing the symptoms experienced during infections. Following repeated infections with a variety of local strains exhibiting differing antigens, immunity to these local strains becomes established (premunition).

The intensity of malaria transmission in a particular setting determines the age at which premunition commonly develops, and hence the clinical features seen across different age groups. In areas of high transmission, babies are usually protected from severe malaria by maternal antibodies. Repeated infections in early childhood lead to the development of premunition. In such circumstances, the main manifestation of infection is severe malaria anemia arising from the destruction of parasitized red blood cells and bone marrow suppression in repeatedly infected young children. In older children and adults who have developed premonition, most infections are short lived and asymptomatic (Table 17.3).

In the setting of variable or intermittent *P. falciparum* transmission, immunity does not become well established and older children develop severe malaria including cerebral malaria, which carries a 20% mortality. In locations where malaria transmission is seasonal or rare, and in travelers to endemic areas, premonition does not occur. In these circumstances, all age groups are susceptible to clinical malaria and cerebral malaria is a common manifestation of severe malaria at all ages.

Genetic traits including sickle cell trait, thalassemia, and glucose-6-phosphate dehydrogenase deficiency (G6PD) provide variable degrees of protection against infection with malaria. Conversely, several tumor necrosis factor (TNF) promoter polymorphisms have been associated with severe *P. falciparum* disease.

P. vivax and *P. ovale*

P. vivax and *P. ovale* cause similar illnesses with fevers every second day (tertian malaria). Fever periodicity may facilitate transmission by the night-biting mosquitoes. Chloroquine does not treat the latent hypnozoites which may reactivate after months or years to cause recurrent clinical episodes of malaria. Treatment with primaquine is required to eradicate the hypnozoites and prevent relapses.

P. malariae

In *P. malariae* infections, fevers occur every third day (quartan malaria). The incubation period may stretch to 30 days or more before the onset of symptoms. Symptoms may be mild and persistent untreated infections

Table 17.3 Malaria transmission and clinical features for different age groups. The pattern of disease in travelers to any endemic area corresponds to that seen in areas of low endemicity

Endemicity	Transmission	Clinical features			
		Infants	Children	Adults	Pregnancy
High	Stable	Anemia	Mild symptoms	Asymptomatic	Anemia, low birth weight, prematurity
Intermediate	Intermediate	Anemia	Cerebral malaria	Usually asymptomatic	Cerebral malaria
Low (and travelers)	Unstable	Cerebral malaria and anemia	Cerebral malaria	Cerebral malaria, renal failure	Cerebral malaria, low birth weight, anemia

may lead to recurring symptoms over years to decades. Chronic infections may lead to the production of circulating immune complexes which may cause nephritic syndrome.

Relapses and recrudescences

Inadequate treatment of *P. falciparum* infection may lead to a recrudescence of symptoms after several weeks. Infections due to *P. malariae* may persist for years or even decades as the erythrocytic cycle can continue at low levels almost indefinitely before producing symptoms. *P. vivax* and *P. ovale* can cause relapses of infection following treatment, due to the reactivation of hypnozoites in the liver.

Diagnosis

Any person presenting with a febrile illness who has spent time in an area where malaria transmission occurs in the months prior to presentation should be assumed to have malaria until proven otherwise. In travelers, inadequate malaria prophylaxis may prolong the incubation time of infection, as may premunition in semi-immune individuals. In the presence of symptoms, malarial prophylaxis should be discontinued while urgent diagnostic tests for malaria are conducted. Malaria is a notifiable disease and should be reported to state health departments, which in turn report cases to the CDC.

Microscopy

The microscopic examination of appropriately stained thick and thin blood films for malaria parasites remains the accepted standard for malaria diagnosis. Common stains include Giemsa's and Field's stains. Thick film examination is more sensitive than thin film examination for the detection of parasites. Should the initial film be negative, several further films should be examined at 12-hour intervals in order to detect low level parasitemias. Thin films allow differentiation of *Plasmodium* species and calculation of the parasite density, usually expressed as the percentage of red blood cells containing parasites. The ring form, trophozoite, schizont and gametocyte stages are all distinguishable by microscopy (Figure 17.4). Whilst microscopy provides good sensitivity and specificity, it is labor intensive and requires technical skill. The limit of detection of malaria infection by blood film examination is a parasitemia of approximately 0.001%, equivalent to 50 parasites per microliter of blood. In the USA, assistance and "telediagnosis" of digital microscopic images is available through the CDC.

P. falciparum

In *P. falciparum*, while thin ring forms are commonly seen, trophozoites and schizonts are rarely identified in peripheral blood films due to the sequestration of the late stage asexual parasites in the microcirculation. One consequence of this sequestration is that estimation of total parasite burden from examination of a peripheral blood film is unreliable. Two similar peripheral blood parasite counts may correspond to sequestered parasite biomasses differing by as much as 100-fold. This disparity is reflected in the poor correlation between admission parasitemia and disease outcome in *P. falciparum* infections.

Other species

In *P. vivax*, *P. ovale*, and *P. malariae* infections, sequestration does not occur, and consequently all morphological stages circulate in the peripheral blood. In *P. vivax* and *P. ovale* infections, thick rings forms, amoeboid trophozoites, schizonts, and round gametocytes are seen in the peripheral blood smears (Figure 17.4). As the trophozoites of *P. vivax* and *P. ovale* develop, the parasitized erythrocytes enlarge and develop red-staining Schüffner's dots. Some *P. malariae* trophozoites take on a rectangular or "band" form within the erythrocytes. Mixed infections (commonly *P. falciparum* with one of the other species) may occur, and the successful treatment of one species may be followed by symptoms occurring because of the second.

Problems with microscopy

The interpretation of blood film microscopy is complicated by the fact that in endemic areas, individuals with premunition sustain parasitemias asymptomatically. In the absence of microscopy, overdiagnosis and subsequent overtreatment for malaria may result in morbidity and mortality due to other missed alternative diagnoses, and the overuse of antimalarial drugs in immune individuals whose parasitemia is not the cause of their presenting symptoms. In nonendemic counties, failure to consider diagnostic tests for malaria may have rapidly fatal consequences in cases of imported *P. falciparum* infection.

Rapid diagnostic tests (RDTs)

The measurement of circulating specific products of parasite metabolism offers an alternative means of estimating total parasite biomass, including that of sequestered parasites. In the early 1990s, a variety of malaria rapid diagnostic tests (RDTs) were developed. These devices are intended to provide simple, swift and accurate diagnosis of malaria in circumstances where microscopic diagnosis is unavailable or unreliable. The tests have been designed to detect various products of malaria metabolism. Most tests are presented as immunochromatographic assays in the form of card or cassette tests, or dipstick tests. Where the coverage of accurate microscopic services is poor, RDTs offer an alternative and potentially cost saving means of malaria diagnosis. RDTs have also been marketed in kit form for use by travelers to endemic areas for self diagnosis. The metabolic products targeted include *P. falciparum* histidine-rich protein 2 (HRP-2), aldolase, and *Plasmodium* lactate dehydrogenase (PLDH).

HRP-2 tests

Plasmodium falciparum HRP-2 is thought to play a role in hemozoin formation by the parasite. HRP-2 is produced by *P. falciparum* only and is released from erythrocytes at schizont rupture. The antigenic activity of HRP-2 in the bloodstream may persist for up to 4 weeks after the resolution of a malaria infection following successful treatment. This makes HRP-2 detection impractical for the monitoring of response to treatment, or the diagnosis of treatment failure or re-infection.

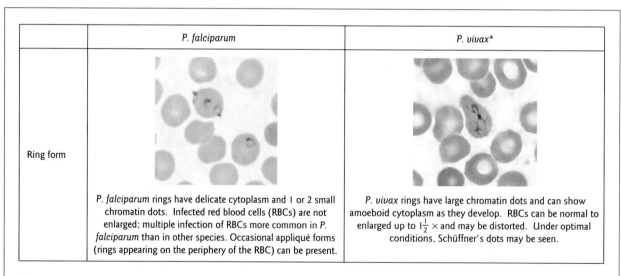

	P. falciparum	*P. vivax**
Ring form	*P. falciparum* rings have delicate cytoplasm and 1 or 2 small chromatin dots. Infected red blood cells (RBCs) are not enlarged; multiple infection of RBCs more common in *P. falciparum* than in other species. Occasional appliqué forms (rings appearing on the periphery of the RBC) can be present.	*P. vivax* rings have large chromatin dots and can show amoeboid cytoplasm as they develop. RBCs can be normal to enlarged up to $1\frac{1}{2} \times$ and may be distorted. Under optimal conditions, Schüffner's dots may be seen.

Figure 17.4 Appearances of *P. falciparum* and *P. vivax* malaria parasites in thin film, stained preparations of peripheral blood. *Comparisons with *P. ovale* and *P. malariae* are described where appropriate. Courtesy Centers for Disease Control; from: http://www.dpd.cdc.gov/dpdx/HTML/ImageLibrary/Malaria_il.htm

	P. falciparum	*P. vivax**
Trophozoites	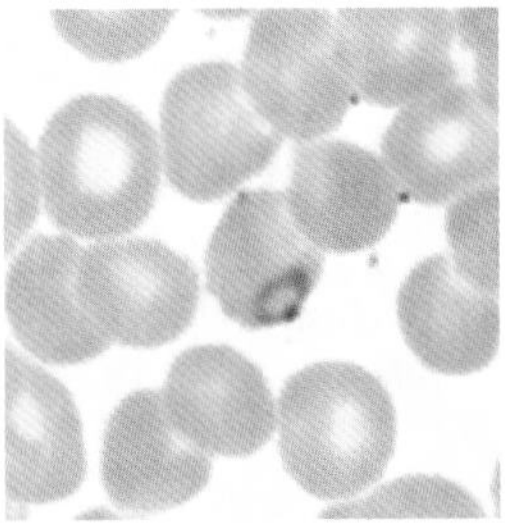 Rarely seen in peripheral blood, older, ring stage parasites are referred to as trophozoites. The cytoplasm of mature trophozoites tends to be thicker and more dense than in younger rings. Growing trophozoites in *P. falciparum* can appear slightly amoeboid in shape	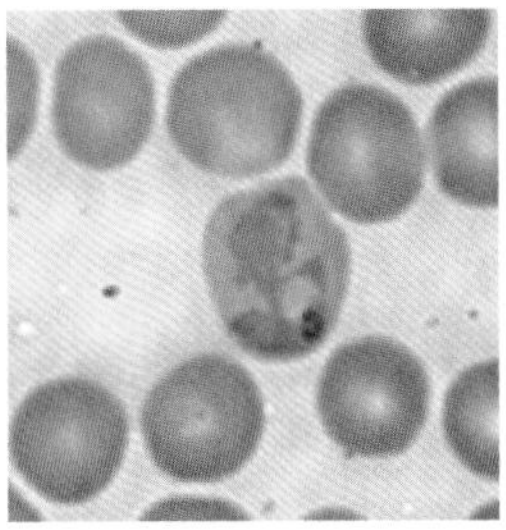 Trophozoites show amoeboid cytoplasm, large chromatin dots, and have fine, yellowish-brown pigment. RBCs are enlarged $1\frac{1}{2}$ to $2\times$ and may be distorted. Under optimal conditions, Schüffner's dots may appear more fine than those seen in *P. ovale* 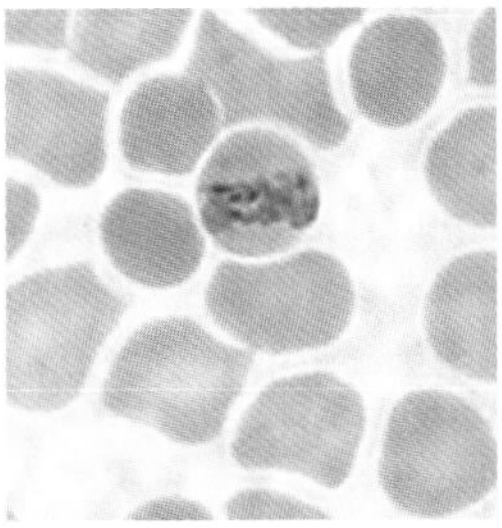 Note band forms in *P. malariae*
Schizonts	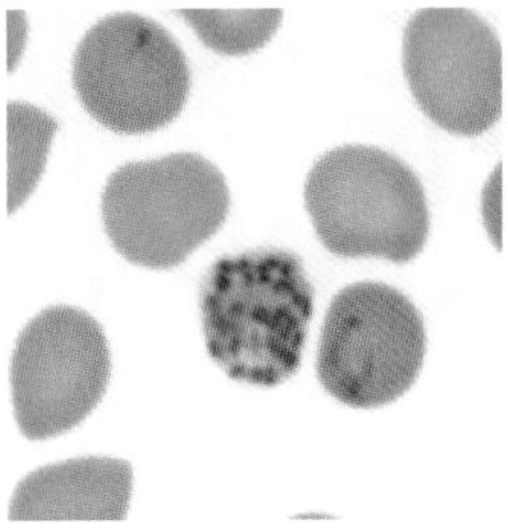 Schizonts are seldom seen in peripheral blood. Mature schizonts have 8 to 24 small merozoites; dark pigment, clumped in one mass	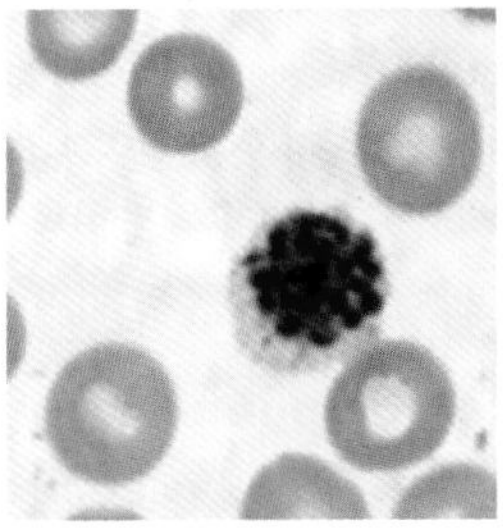 Schizonts are large, have 12 to 24 merozoites, yellowish-brown, coalesced pigment, and may fill the red blood cell (RBC). RBCs are enlarged $1\frac{1}{2}$ to $2\times$ and may be distorted. Under optimal conditions, Schüffner's dots may be seen
Gametocytes	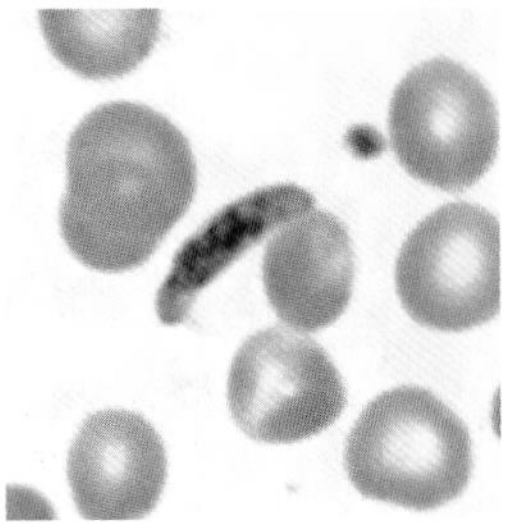 Note crescent shaped gametocytes and distortion of RBC	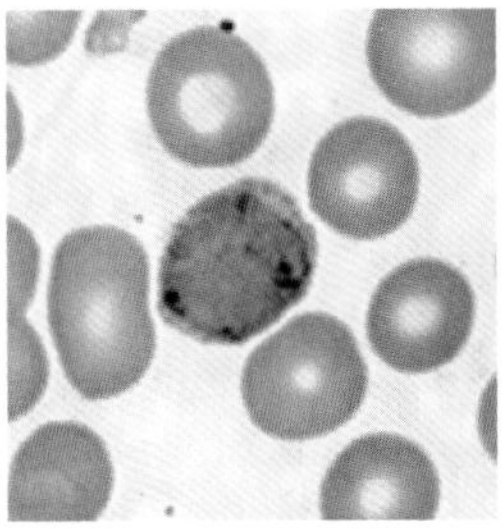 Gametocytes are round to oval with scattered brown pigment and may almost fill the RBC. RBCs are enlarged $1\frac{1}{2}$ to $2\times$ and may be distorted. Under optimal conditions, Schüffner's dots may appear more fine than those seen in *P. ovale*

Figure 17.4 (*cont'd*)

PLDH tests

During the asexual erythrocytic cycle, malaria parasites utilize large amounts of glucose via glycolysis. This process involves the conversion of pyruvate to lactate which is catalyzed by *Plasmodium* lactate dehydrogenase (PLDH). The four species of *Plasmodium* produce distinct isomers of PLDH. All isomers differ from human LDH and can be collectively or specifically detected by rapid diagnostic tests utilizing monoclonal antibodies against PLDH isomers. *Plasmodium falciparum* LDH (*Pf*LDH) is produced at high levels during the asexual erythrocytic cycle, particularly by the trophozoite stage parasites. *Pf*LDH levels correlate well with microscopic parasitemia, making this metabolite useful for monitoring response to treatment.

Aldolase tests

Plasmodium aldolase is an enzyme active in the glycolytic pathway of all four *Plasmodium* species. Detection of the pan-malarial aldolase antigen may be combined with detection of the *P. falciparum* specific HRP-2 antigen on a single test device to enable the differentiation of *P. falciparum*, non-*P. falciparum* (usually *P. vivax*), and mixed *P. falciparum*, non-*P. falciparum* infections. One such device, the BinaxNOW malaria RDT, was approved for use laboratories in the USA by the Food and Drug Administration in June 2007.

Nucleic acid-based tests

A variety of nucleic acid-based tests for the detection of malaria parasites have been developed. These tests may be significantly more sensitive than microscopy for the diagnosis of malaria infection and may be used for accurate identification of *Plasmodium* species. Because such tests are expensive and require technical expertise, they are not widely available.

Treatment

The choice of antimalarial agents for the treatment of malaria infections will be informed by the species present, the drug resistance pattern where the infection was acquired, the patient's ability to absorb oral medication, and the severity of disease and level of parasitemia in the case of *P. falciparum* infections.

Quinoline-like compounds

Powdered preparations of cinchona bark were used to treat febrile illnesses in the 16th century. Quinine was first isolated from cinchona bark in 1820. The quinoline-like compounds accumulate in the parasite food vacuole where they are thought to interfere with heme degradation. The development of related synthetic antimalarials began in the 1920s and led to the production of primaquine, and the related compounds amodiaquine, mefloquine, halofantrine, lumefantrine, hydroxychloroquine, and chloroquine.

Chloroquine

Chloroquine became the mainstay of malaria treatment in the 1950s, however by the 1960s resistance to this agent in *P. falciparum* started to spread across the tropics. Chloroquine resistance in *P. vivax* has emerged in Papua New Guinea and Indonesia. Chloroquine resistance arises through point mutations in the chloroquine resistance transporter gene which result in a reduction in chloroquine levels within the parasite food vacuole.

Mefloquine

In Southeast Asia chloroquine resistance led to the introduction of mefloquine for the treatment of *P. falciparum*. Subsequently resistance to mefloquine in *P. falciparum* emerged in the late 1980s in areas around the border between Thailand and Cambodia. The use of mefloquine for malaria prophylaxis has been limited by reports of psychiatric side-effects.

Primaquine

Primaquine is still used routinely for the eradication of the hypnozoite stages of *P. vivax* and *P. ovale* to prevent relapse.

Quinine and quinidine

Quinine is used orally and intravenously to treat *P. falciparum* infections. Quinidine is an isomer of quinine that is more active, but more cardiotoxic. It is used in the USA for the intravenous treatment of severe *P. falciparum* malaria. Quinine and quinidine are also active against the other species of human malaria but do not eradicate hypnozoites. Resistance to both agents remains rare.

Anti-folate agents

The biguanides, including proguanil, were discovered in the 1940s. Active metabolites of these compounds inhibit parasite dihydrofolate reductase, as does the purine analog pyrimethamine. Pyrimethamine is commonly used in a synergistic combination with sulfadoxine, an agent that inhibits a second enzyme in the malaria folate synthesis pathway. This combination is referred to as SP and has been marketed as Fansidar. The anti-folate agents preferentially inhibit parasite folate synthesis. Unfortunately resistance to anti-folate agents has emerged through successive point mutations in the genes encoding the target enzymes. Resistance to SP is now widespread in Africa, making this combination unreliable for the empirical treatment of *P. falciparum* infections in affected areas.

Other agents

The novel antimalarial drug atovaquone is an analog of co-enzyme Q and acts on the parasite electron transport chain, interfering with parasite respiration and pyrimidine synthesis. When used alone, point mutations rapidly give rise to resistance. Atovaquone has been used in combination with proguanil as a safe and highly effective treatment for malaria, and for malaria prophylaxis. This combination is marketed as Malarone. Resistance to this combination of agents is rare; however Malarone is relatively expensive, limiting its use in resource-poor settings. Several antibacterial drugs also have significant antimalarial activity, including doxycycline and clindamycin. They are used in combination with agents such as quinidine for the treatment of malaria in the USA. Doxycycline may also be used for malaria prophylaxis.

Artemisinins

The plant *Artemesia annua* is known as qinghao in China, and sweet wormwood in the USA. Extracts from the leaves of this plant (qinghaosu, or artemisinin) have been used for the treatment of fever in China for many centuries. Artemisinin and its derivatives, artemether and artesunate, are rapidly effective in the treatment of malaria and significant resistance is yet to emerge. The mechanism of action of these agents involves the production of free radicals which are toxic to the malaria parasites. The artemesinins are being used widely in the tropics both orally, in combination with other agents (artemisinin combination therapy, or ACT), and parenterally or *per rectum* for the treatment of *P. falciparum* disease. Treatments using combinations of drugs with differing modes of action are being promoted to maximize treatment effectiveness and reduce the emergence of further drug resistance. For example, combination treatment with artesunate and mefloquine has proved highly effective for the treatment of *P. falciparum* in Southeast Asia. Other ACT regimens include artemether in combination with lumefantrine, and artesunate in combination with amodiaquine. Barriers to effective ACT programs include the relatively high cost of the drugs, and the marketing of counterfeit tablets. Because many deaths from malaria occur in the home setting, these treatments need to become widely available at a community level in order to facilitate the home-based management of malaria infections.

Treatment of severe *P. falciparum* infections

Infection with *P. falciparum* is a medical emergency as severe complications may develop within hours. Urgent laboratory confirmation of malaria infection should be followed by the immediate commencement of appropriate treatment. In the USA, returned travelers with malaria should usually be admitted until a satisfactory response to therapy has been observed. Blood films should be repeated every 12 hours until negative. Intravenous therapy is indicated for patients with signs of severe disease including prostration, coma or impaired consciousness, respiratory distress, or in those in whom vomiting makes the absorption of oral medication unreliable (Table 17.2).

Hypoglycemia should be anticipated and promptly corrected with intravenous dextrose. For adults with severe malaria, fluid resuscitation should be carefully titrated to reduce the risk of pulmonary edema. Deterioration in respiratory function may also be caused by bacterial pneumonia, or aspiration pneumonia. Seizures should be treated with anticonvulsants. Regular acetaminophen should be prescribed to control pyrexia. Adults may develop acute tubular necrosis requiring renal replacement therapy. In patients with cerebral malaria, radiological imaging and lumbar puncture should be performed to detect concomitant bacterial meningitis or intracerebral hemorrhage. Exchange blood transfusion should be considered where parasitemia is estimated to be greater than 10% or other markers of severity are present.

For CDC guidelines to treat severe *P. falciparum* malaria see Further reading.

Treatment of nonsevere malaria infections

Uncomplicated *P. falciparum* infections and infections due to other species can usually be treated with oral medication, unless the patient is vomiting.

Following the initial treatment of *P. vivax* and *P. ovale* infections, a 2-week course of primaquine should be given to eradicate the hepatic stage hypnozoites in order to prevent relapses. Patients should be screened for glucose-6-phosphate dehydrogenase deficiency prior to treatment with primaquine so that the risk of intravascular hemolysis in patients with this deficiency may be avoided. These patients should be counseled about the risk of relapse, and prophylaxis with chloroquine may be considered when primaquine is contraindicated. Treatment regimens for uncomplicated malaria recommended by the CDC are outlined on their website: http://www.cdc.gov/malaria/diagnosis_treatment/index.htm

Treatment of malaria in pregnancy

Chloroquine, pyrimethamine, proguanil, and quinine are safe in pregnancy, and artemisinins are thought to be safe after the first trimester. Hypoglycemia is very common during the treatment of *P. falciparum* infections. The tetracyclines and primaquine are contraindicated in pregnancy. Pregnant women with *P. vivax* or *P. ovale* infections may be treated with chloroquine prophylaxis during pregnancy and breastfeeding to prevent relapse. Primaquine treatment should be delayed until after the completion of breast feeding.

Prevention

Residents of and travelers to malaria endemic areas are advised to avoid mosquito bites if possible. Preventive measures include:

- Wearing full length clothing at peak biting times (between dusk and dawn)
- Sleeping in air-conditioned or mosquito-screened rooms
- Using bed nets impregnated with an insecticide such as permethrin
- The use of mosquito repellents such as DEET (*N, N*-diethylmetatoluamide) applied topically to exposed skin
- Permethrin and DEET may be applied to clothing, shoes, and camping gear.

Recommendations regarding chemoprophylaxis for travelers are provided by the CDC in the "Health Information for International Travel" book ("The Yellow Book," see Further reading). Prophylaxis should be started before travel, and continued throughout the period of exposure and for a variable period after leaving malaria-endemic areas. Travelers should be made aware that adherence to a prophylactic regimen does not guarantee protection from malaria infection. If travelers develop symptoms consistent with malaria they should seek prompt diagnosis and treatment. In most cases, civilians diagnosed with malaria in the USA have not complied with an appropriate prophylactic regimen. Targeted chemoprophylaxis delivered as intermittent preventive treatment (IPT) for residents of high and medium transmission areas may also carry benefits, particularly for pregnant women and young children.

Vector control

Indoor residual spraying of insecticides

Insecticides such as dichloro-diphenyl-trichloroethane (DDT) have been used since the 1940s in programs aimed at the eradication of malaria through control of the mosquito vector. DDT is very effective when used for indoor residual house spraying. DDT kills the female *Anopheles* mosquitoes as they rest indoors after taking a blood meal. Although concerns exist about the side-effects of DDT on pregnancy and lactation, and resistance has appeared, it continues to be used in certain areas to improve malaria control.

Insecticide-treated nets (ITNs)

Trials of the use of bed nets impregnated with insecticides such as pyrethroids have shown reductions in overall child mortality and episodes of clinical malaria. Most bed nets require repeated re-treatment to remain effective. Despite their benefits, the widespread adoption of ITNs has been hampered by cost and distribution barriers. Resistance to pyrethroids has developed, and alternative agents are in development, some of which can be incorporated into the bed net fibers during manufacture, avoiding the need for re-treatment.

Other measures

The future uses of insecticides may be limited by emerging resistance in insect populations. In specific environments, other measures which have been used to control the *Anopheles* mosquito population include the drainage of breeding sites and the use of larvivorous fish to control mosquito larvae. Socioeconomic development such as improvements in housing may aid malaria control. The potential uses of genetically modified mosquitoes which are unable to be infected with *Plasmodium* species are being investigated.

Immunization

Several immunizations designed to provide protection against *P. falciparum* and *P. vivax* infections are in development. Most vaccines have been targeted at the malaria sporozoite and merozoite antigens with the intention of preventing hepatocyte invasion or to trigger the destruction of infected hepatocytes. The SPf66 subunit vaccine containing *P. falciparum* merozoite surface proteins has proved partially effective in South America but subsequent trials elsewhere yielded conflicting results. The RTS,S/ASO2A vaccine, which contains *P. falciparum* sporozoite protein analogs, has been shown to provide significant, though short-term protection against *P. falciparum* clinical infection, and severe disease. Trials of this vaccine have demonstrated 40% protection in nonimmune subjects. In semi-immune individuals the vaccine reduced clinical episodes of malaria and severe disease.

Further subunit vaccine development will focus on antigen selection, the use of adjuvants, and the public health benefits of a partially protective vaccine. Other possible subunit targets include the *P. falciparum* erythrocyte membrane proteins (*Pf*EMPs). Immunization with γ-irradiated sporozoites provides protective immunity by limiting the development of the liver stage parasites but there are significant practical barriers to the widespread use of a live, attenuated strain of *P. falciparum* in an immunization program. A novel approach is the generation of an antibody response against gametocyte and ookinete surface proteins to block the sexual reproductive cycle within the *Anopheles* vector in the form of a transmission-blocking immunization.

Global malaria control

Improvements in the global control of malaria will require the effective implementation of measures already known to be effective as well as research into new treatments and control strategies. International organizations contributing to global malaria control include the World Health Organization's Global Malaria Program, the Bill & Melinda Gates Foundation, the Global Fund to Fight AIDS, Tuberculosis and Malaria, and the US President's Malaria Initiative. Large scale, collaborative efforts are being directed at multipronged approaches to sustainably reduce the terrible morbidity and mortality inflicted by human malaria infections. Priorities include the provision of diagnostic tools and effective treatments such as ACTs, and the reduction of malaria transmission through vector control measures including insecticide treated bed nets and insecticide spraying programs. Research into new drug treatments and immunization candidates continues. Sustained investments in medical personnel and healthcare infrastructure are required to ensure the tools to control malaria are made available to the vulnerable populations most affected by this disease.

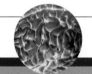

Test yourself

Case study 17.1
A 43-year-old man presents to his local hospital with a 5-day history of high fevers and headaches following a flu-like illness which began 3 weeks after he returned to the USA after visiting friends and relatives in his home country of Nigeria. He has been taking some tablets labeled as "Coartem" (artemether and lumefantrine) which he bought from a street vendor in Nigeria.

1. On examination he appears drowsy and disorientated. He vomits in the emergency department. What steps would you take next?

Case study 17.2
A 28-year-old woman has been back in the USA for 3 months after spending 2 months working as a freelance photojournalist in Afghanistan. She did not take any malaria prophylaxis. After 1 month in Afghanistan she developed a fevers and chills. She took some tablets of Malarone (atovaquone and proguanil) which were given to her by a colleague, without having any blood tests performed, and her symptoms resolved.

1. You are her family doctor and she presents to you complaining of fevers, sweats, headache, and backache. How will you manage this patient?

Case study 17.3
You are working for a medical relief organization and are responsible for the provision of medical services to a refugee camp in sub-Saharan Africa. Adults and children in the camp have been diagnosed with severe *P. falciparum* malaria. In the host country, extensive resistance of *P. falciparum* to chloroquine has been reported, and occasional failures of Fansidar observed.

1. What empirical treatments for malaria would you consider instituting in the refugee camp?

Further reading

Centers for Disease Control and Prevention. *Health Information for International Travel 2008*. Atlanta: US Department of Health and Human Services, Public Health Service, 2007

Chen LH, Wilson ME, Schlagenhauf P. Controversies and misconceptions in malaria chemoprophylaxis for travelers. *JAMA* 2007;297:2251–2263

Griffith KS, Lewis LS, Mali S, Parise ME. Treatment of malaria in the United States: a systematic review. *JAMA* 2007;297:2264–2277

Matuschewski K, Mueller A-K. Vaccines against malaria – an update. *FEBS J* 2007;274(18):4680–4687

Thwing J, Skarbinski J, Newman RD, et al; Centers for Disease Control and Prevention. Malaria surveillance – United States, 2005. *MMWR Surveill Summ* 2007; Jun 8;56(6):23–40

White NJ. Malaria. In: Cook GC, Zumla AI (eds) *Manson's Tropical Diseases*, 21st edition. London: Saunders, 2002, chap 71

World Health Organization. Severe falciparum malaria. *Trans R Soc Trop Med Hyg* 2000;94(suppl 1):S1–S90

World Health Organization. *WHO Guidelines for the Treatment of Malaria*. Geneva, Switzerland: WHO Press, 2008

Useful websites

CDC. Malaria Topic Home. http://www.cdc.gov/malaria/index.htm

CDC. Traveler's Health Yellow Book. Health Information for International Travel. http://wwwn.cdc.gov/travel/contentYellowBook.aspx

Malaria programs

http://www.fightingmalaria.gov/index.html

http://www.gatesfoundation.org/GlobalHealth/Pri_Diseases/Malaria/

http://www.malariavaccine.org/

http://www.mmv.org/rubrique.php3?id_rubrique=15

http://www.rollbackmalaria.org/

http://www.who.int/malaria/

Chapter 18

Human immunodeficiency virus (HIV) and acquired immunodeficiency syndrome (AIDS)

J.W. Tang

Epidemiology
Classification
Virology
Natural history of HIV infection
Clinical features

Laboratory diagnosis
Treatment
Vaccines
Confidentiality and public health
Summary

Epidemiology

The human immunodeficiency viruses 1 and 2 (HIV-1, HIV-2) originated from the simian immunodeficiency viruses (SIVs) of primates and probably spread initially to the local indigenous populations of Central and Western Africa during their hunting, killing, and butchering of such primates for meat. Research has shown that HIV-1 arose from the SIV of chimpanzees (SIV_{cpz}) and that HIV-2 arose from the SIV of the sooty mangabey monkey (SIV_{sm}). HIV-1 was first isolated in 1983, followed by HIV-2 in 1986, and they represent two distinct epidemics. Studies using phylogenetic analyses of HIV sequences estimate that HIV-1 appeared in the human population in 1931 and HIV-2 in 1940. After this initial species barrier-crossing event, individuals infected with these primate SIVs then transmitted the human form of these viruses (HIV-1, HIV-2) to others in their communities who then disseminated these viruses worldwide (see Further reading).

In the 1980s, the HIV/AIDS epidemic in western countries initially spread rapidly amongst the sexually promiscuous, high risk groups. These included intravenous injecting drug users (IDUs) who shared needles and men-who-have-sex-with-men (MSM) who routinely practiced anal intercourse that was more traumatic and bloody than vaginal intercourse. Unfortunate victims of this early HIV epidemic were those patients requiring regular infusions of blood products, e.g. patients with hemophilia and hematological malignancies, who were inadvertently transfused with HIV-contaminated blood products. Elsewhere during the later stages of the HIV/AIDS epidemic, especially in Africa, heterosexual intercourse was the main route of HIV transmission, with the epidemic affecting men, women, and ultimately their children. Although the risk from blood products was rapidly reduced after the introduction of commercial HIV antibody screening assays in 1985, not all countries have implemented stringent screening of their blood supply probably due to a lack of resources and appropriately skilled manpower. In addition, the blood product screening programs in some countries that rely only on HIV antibody to detect HIV-infected donations may miss those donations from patients who are HIV infected but have not yet developed their HIV antibodies ("HIV seroconversion patients"). Nowadays, antigen and molecular tests are being implemented in blood product screening programs to detect HIV antigen and nucleic acid (RNA) to avoid HIV-contaminated donations entering the blood supply. Safe sex messages and related programs have helped to reduce the sexual transmission of HIV, but it will be impossible to entirely eliminate promiscuity and the availability of commercial sex, with some clients inevitably refusing to use condoms. The introduction of antiretroviral therapy (ART) for HIV-infected pregnant women has also reduced the rate of vertical, perinatally acquired mother-to-child HIV infection.

The Joint United Nations Program on HIV/AIDS (UNAIDS) estimated that by the end of 2005, there were about 40 million people living with HIV worldwide: 38 million were adults including 17.5 million women and 2.3 million children (under 15 years old). During 2005 there were 4.9 million new cases of HIV infection (4.2 million adults and 0.7 million children), and 3.1 million AIDS-related deaths (2.6 million adults and 0.57 million children). Compared to 2003 when approximately 42 million were living with HIV, and 2002 when approximately 5.5 million new HIV infections and 3.2 million AIDS-related deaths were reported, it seems that we have not made much progress in reducing the size of the HIV pandemic (see Further reading and online Table at www.wiley.com/go/shettyinfectiousdisease).

Classification

Both HIV-1 and HIV-2 belong to the family of retroviruses, in the genus *Lentivirus*. Retroviruses have been discovered in a variety of vertebrate species (animals and man), associated with various disease manifestations, including malignancies, autoimmune diseases, immunodeficiency syndromes, aplastic and hemolytic anemias, bone, joint and central nervous system diseases.

The many different strains of HIV-1 have been categorized into major (M), new (N), and outlier (O) groups. These may represent three separate zoonotic transmission events from chimpanzees in these areas. Groups N and O are found mainly in West and Central African countries (Gabon and Cameroon), but infected individuals have been found worldwide due to the widespread availability and convenience of international travel. Group M HIV strains are mainly responsible for the HIV/AIDS pandemic. They are so diverse that they have been subdivided into subtypes (or clades) A–K, including some circulating recombinant forms (CRF 01 AE/B and CRF 02 A/G). Such a large viral diversity has made the development of diagnostic tests that can detect all HIV-1 subtypes more difficult. The diversity of HIV-2 is not as great as HIV-1, although subtypes A–H have been used (see Further reading).

Virology

It is important to understand the processes involved in HIV replication in some detail, as these have been targeted for various therapeutic interventions.

The human immunodeficiency viruses are lipid enveloped with a diameter of approximately 100 nm. Transmembrane glycoproteins are embedded in this membrane, including gp41, which is attached to a surface glycoprotein (gp120). These two viral proteins are responsible for attachment to the host cell and are encoded by the HIV *env* gene. Beneath the envelope are viral coded proteins: p17 (the matrix protein), p24 and p6 (the core proteins) and p7 (the nucleocapsid protein bound to the viral RNA). These proteins are all encoded by the HIV *gag* gene. Two copies of the ~10 kilobase (kb), positive-sense, HIV RNA genome (i.e. it is a diploid RNA retrovirus), together with the protease, integrase and reverse transcriptase (RT) enzymes (all coded for by the HIV *pol* gene), are contained in the central core region (Figure 18.1).

Other HIV-1- and HIV-2-coded proteins with various regulatory or immunomodulatory functions, include *vif* (viral infectivity protein), *vpr* (viral protein R), *tat* (transactivator of transcription), *rev* (regulator of viral protein expression), and *nef* (negative regulatory factor). Some other protein-coding differences between HIV-1 and HIV-2 are: *vpu* (viral protein U) present in HIV-1 but not in HIV-2, and *vpx* (viral protein x) present in HIV-2 and not in HIV-1 (see Further reading).

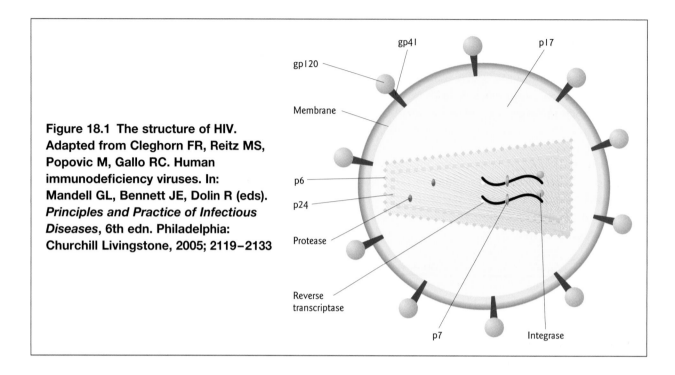

Figure 18.1 The structure of HIV. Adapted from Cleghorn FR, Reitz MS, Popovic M, Gallo RC. Human immunodeficiency viruses. In: Mandell GL, Bennett JE, Dolin R (eds). *Principles and Practice of Infectious Diseases*, **6th edn. Philadelphia: Churchill Livingstone, 2005; 2119–2133**

Human immunodeficiency virus initially attaches with its gp120 membrane protein to the CD4 molecule present on CD4+ T (helper) lymphocytes, macrophages, and microglial cells. This triggers a conformational change in the host-cell envelope allowing the binding of another HIV co-receptor in the host-cell membrane, either CCR5 or CXCR4, which is required for successful virus and host-cell fusion. Once inside the host-cell, the HIV-encoded RT transcribes its viral RNA into double-stranded DNA (dsDNA), which is subsequently integrated into the host-cell genome under the action of the viral integrase (Figure 18.2).

This integrated viral DNA ("provirus") then acts as a template for the transcription of HIV genomic and messenger RNA by the replicating machinery of the host cell. Recombination between the two HIV RNA strands and the high error rate involved in the RT step during viral replication, account for the extremely high genetic diversity of HIV.

It is the integration of the linear HIV provirus dsDNA into the host-cell genome which establishes a lifelong infection in man. New HIV progeny are produced during host-cell replication, which is enhanced

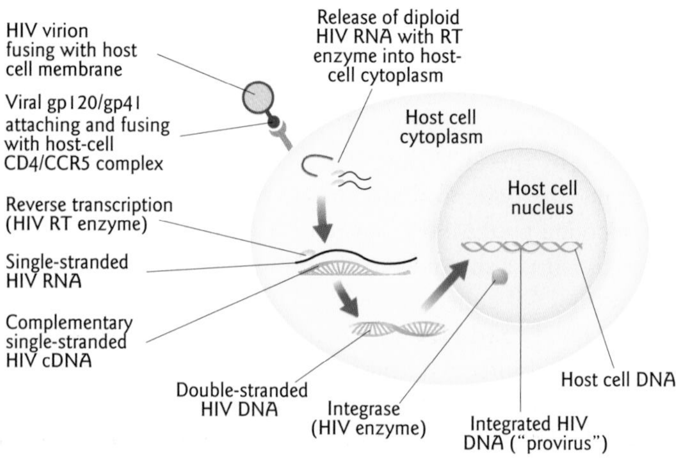

Figure 18.2 The formation of HIV provirus in a host cell. Adapted from Cleghorn FR, Reitz MS, Popovic M, Gallo RC. Human immunodeficiency viruses. In: Mandell GL, Bennett JE, Dolin R (eds). *Principles and Practice of Infectious Diseases*, **6th edn. Philadelphia: Churchill Livingstone, 2005; 2119–2133**

by several factors, e.g. coinfection with other organisms, inflammatory cytokines, and cellular activation. When the host-cell replicates, the HIV provirus is also transcribed by the host-cell RNA polymerase II enzyme, to produce the HIV viral messenger RNA (vmRNA) and HIV genomic RNA, which are carried along with the host-cell mRNAs to be translated into proteins by the host-cell ribosmes. This HIV vmRNA codes for a long *gag-pol* precursor polypeptide that is cleaved by the HIV-encoded protease enzyme to produce the HIV *gag* and *pol* proteins. This vmRNA is also spliced to produce other vmRNAs that code for the HIV proteins *tat, rev, vif, vpr, vpu* (for HIV-1 or *vpx* for HIV-2). The structural *env* precursor polypeptide is also translated into a precursor polypeptide that is cleaved by cellular (not viral) proteases, to produce the envelope glycoproteins gp41 and gp120. The final complete HIV virion is produced when these viral proteins and the replicated diploid HIV genomic RNA are assembled in the host-cell cytoplasm and given an envelope by budding through the host-cell membrane, producing complete HIV virions (Figure 18.3).

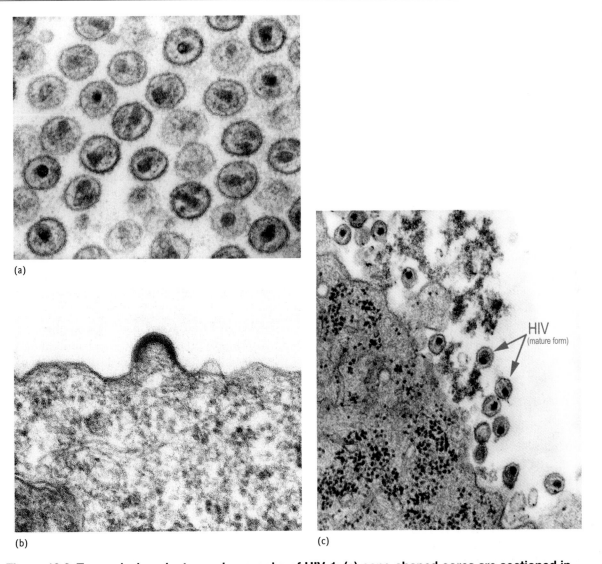

(a)

(b)

(c)

Figure 18.3 Transmission electron micrographs of HIV-1: (a) cone-shaped cores are sectioned in various orientations showing the electron-dense wide end of the core containing viral genomic RNA; (b) HIV-1 budding from a cultured lymphocyte; (c) mature forms of HIV in a tissue sample. Courtesy of the Centers for Disease Control and Prevention. From CDC website: http://phil.cdc.gov/phil/details.asp

Natural history of HIV infection

The progression of HIV infection can be essentially characterized by declining peripheral blood CD4 lymphocyte counts, opportunistic infections, generalized wasting with systemic and specific system diseases.

Only about 50% of individuals with primary HIV infection are symptomatic, e.g. presenting with fever, rash, and lymphadenopathy. After seroconversion and the resolution of these initial "seroconversion illness" symptoms, there may follow a variable length asymptomatic period of anything between 2 and 15 years, during which HIV replication continues. Despite the presence of HIV antibodies, this viral replication occurs at a high rate (up to 10^{10} infectious virions/day) resulting in approximately 10^8–10^9 lymphocytes/day being infected. These infected lymphocytes are quickly replaced, providing more cells susceptible to HIV infection. It is this rapid turnover of the huge number of HIV virions that generates a wide viral diversity, making it extremely difficult to achieve long-lasting antiviral and vaccine effectiveness.

Several mechanisms serve to deplete the number of HIV-infected lymphocytes: (i) direct cytopathic effects of HIV; (ii) immune destruction of HIV-infected cells by cytotoxic CD8 T lymphocytes; and (iii) apoptosis in the presence of specific cytokines, which may occur in nearby, but non-HIV-infected, lymphocytes (see Further reading). The monitoring of HIV load and CD4 counts are essential to determine the progression of a patient's HIV disease and in the absence of ART, the natural course of HIV infection has been well characterized.

During primary HIV infection (PHI), which is included in the Centers for Disease Control (CDC) classification Stage 1, the virus replicates at high levels in the absence of antibodies to HIV. The HIV RNA load and p24 antigen (Ag) levels rise to a maximum during PHI, then fall to a "set-point" level during the early asymptomatic phase. The actual level of this set-point depends on the aggressiveness of the individual's immune response. After this, there is a gradual rise in the HIV RNA load and HIV p24 antigen (Ag) which accelerates during the symptomatic phase, generally about 2 years after the PHI. It has been found that the CD4 count and HIV RNA levels attained at the "set-point," during the early asymptomatic phase of HIV infection, are highly predictive of disease progression. In an almost reciprocal relationship, the CD4 lymphocyte counts drop rapidly for a short period, then recover to almost normal levels. The asymptomatic phase of HIV infection may last 2–15 years (CDC stages 2/3) during which there is a steady drop in CD4 counts. As a consequence of this, the patient becomes more immunocompromised and susceptible to opportunistic infections. Eventually, CD4 counts decrease even more rapidly as the patient develops full-blown AIDS and approaches end-stage disease (Figure 18.4).

It can be seen that HIV antibodies (Ab) rise to maximum levels within the first 3–6 months after PHI and normally remain detectable throughout the lifetime of the patient. However, these antibodies may wane with time, becoming more difficult to detect in patients who maintain their HIV RNA loads at undetectable levels (<50 genome copies/ml) for many years using highly active antiretroviral therapy (HAART). "Rapid-progressors" are patients who experience an accelerated form of these stages of HIV disease, such that HIV RNA and p24 Ag levels remain high throughout their infection and their CD4 counts rapidly drop, leading to end-stage AIDS within five years. By contrast, "long-term nonprogressors" are patients who remain clinically well, maintaining a normal CD4 count and low or undetectable HIV RNA loads, despite not being on HAART. These patients essentially remain in the asymptomatic phase of HIV infection for a much longer period of time than expected. Both these extremes may simply represent a population's normal distribution of immune responses to HIV infection (see Further reading).

Clinical features

The clinical manifestations of HIV infection may not be apparent for some time, maybe even years. Perhaps only 30–40% of HIV-infected individuals experience a seroconversion illness as HIV antibodies start to appear (fever, lymphadenopathy, and rash) and others may not become ill until they acquire or develop an AIDS-defining illness. After seroconversion, there is a slow decline in their specialized T-helper (CD4$^+$)

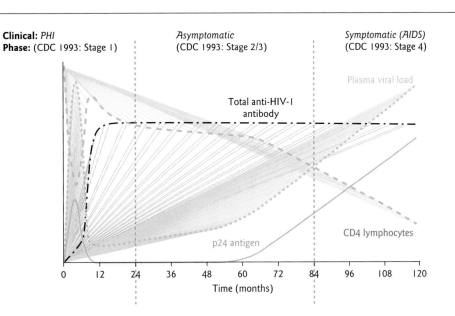

Figure 18.4 The natural progression of untreated HIV infection. Adapted from Weiss RA, Dalgleish AG, Loveday C, Pillay D. Human immunodeficiency viruses. In: Zuckerman AJ, Banatvala JE, Pattison JR, Griffiths PD, Schoub BD (eds). *Principles and Practice of Clinical Virology***, 5th edn. Chichester: John Wiley, 2004; 721–757**

lymphocyte count as their HIV RNA and p24 Ag levels gradually rise. During this time, the individual may remain and feel relatively well, and continue his/her normal lifestyle including sexual activity. This is one reason why HIV is so difficult to control – infected individuals are infectious but may not feel sick and can therefore transmit the virus to others who do likewise, and so on. This time interval between being **infected** and being **infectious** to others often determines how easy it is to control an outbreak of this disease (see Further reading).

When the HIV RNA levels have risen high enough, and their CD4 counts have fallen low enough, if untreated, the individual develops acquired immunodeficiency syndrome (AIDS). What this means is that the bacteria, viruses, and parasites that we are exposed to from the environment and other people in our everyday lives, and which are normally controlled by the body's immune system, are able to cause clinical disease and even death. These "opportunistic" infections (i.e. those that do not normally cause disease in healthy people) can now infect and cause illness in a patient with HIV infection who has now developed AIDS, as their immune system is too crippled to defend them. It has been said that HIV infection attacks the "conductor" of the immune system "orchestra" when it attacks the T-helper (CD4⁺) lymphocyte. Such opportunistic infections include viruses such as cytomegalovirus (CMV) that can damage the eye (CMV retinitis) and oral hairy leukoplakia (Figure 18.5a) caused by Epstein–Barr virus (EBV, which also causes glandular fever); fungal infections, such as disseminated candidiasis (caused by *Candida albicans*) (Figure 18.5b); and various cancers, including Kaposi's sarcoma (Figure 18.5c) caused by human herpes virus 8 (HHV8, also called Kaposi's sarcoma herpes virus, KSHV), which is a cancer of the cells lining the blood vessels (the endothelial cells).

Other common opportunistic infections in patients with AIDS are *Pneumocystis* pneumonia (PCP), toxoplasmosis, tuberculosis and other *Mycobacterium* species infections, cryptococcosis, JC virus progressive multifocal leukoencepahlopathy (JCV-PML), reactivated herpes simplex (extremely painful oral ulcers and genital herpes) and varicella zoster virus (disseminated shingles) infections, and various lymphomas and cancers. Any of these opportunistic infections or cancers can cause death if not promptly treated. A description of each of these opportunistic infections is discussed in Chapter 13.

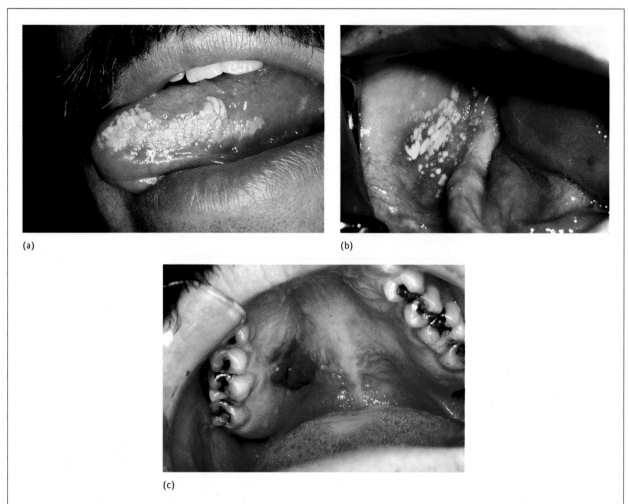

(a)

(b)

(c)

Figure 18.5 Some common presentations of opportunistic infections in AIDS in HIV-infected patients: (a) advanced oral hairy leukoplakia (OHL) on the lateral border of his tongue, which is due to EBV replication under immunosuppressed conditions; (b) oral pseudomembranous candidiasis (*Candida albicans*) infection; (c) intraoral Kaposi's sarcoma of the hard palate, caused by HHV8 (KSHV), which occurs in about 7.5–10% of AIDS patients, and can range in appearance from small asymptomatic, flat purple-red to larger nodular growths. Provided by JS Greenspan, University of California, San Francisco; Sol Silverman, Jr. Courtesy of the Centers for Disease Control and Prevention; from CDC website: http://phil.cdc.gov/phil/details.asp

Laboratory diagnosis

The laboratory diagnosis of HIV involves detecting the presence of HIV RNA and/or HIV p24 Ag and/or HIV Ab. This can be performed using various commercial or in-house assays and should include a highly sensitive screening assay (designed to detect all truly HIV-positive samples, though there may be some false positive results as a consequence of the test's high sensitivity), followed by a highly specific confirmation assay (designed to detect all truly HIV-negative samples, though there may be some false negative results as a consequence of the test's high specificity). The most common approach, recently, is to use screening assays that can detect HIV Ab and/or HIV p24 Ag with confirmation tests that detect HIVAb and/or HIV p24 Ag and/or HIV RNA. In addition, there are specific assays used to measure HIV RNA loads in patients known to be HIV infected who are on HAART. These viral assays are not designed to be used to diagnose new infections and can give false positive results, so should not be used for the initial screening of new samples from suspected cases of HIV infection (see Further reading).

Assays for detecting HIV Ab or HIV p24 Ag are usually based on enzyme immunoassay (EIA) technology where patient samples are added to a microtiter plate or other solid phase receptacle. Any HIV Ab or HIV p24 Ag in the patient sample will bind to capture antigens or antibodies, respectively, bound to the solid phase. After a wash-step to remove excess, unbound sample, an indicator antibody or antigen is added to the solid phase. If the patient is HIV infected, the indicator regent will form an immune complex (Ab–Ag) "sandwich" that will remain after further washing and produce a signal (e.g. a color change or fluorescence) when the final indicator substrate is added. Nowadays, more rapid, yet still relatively accurate tests are available to encourage more frequent HIV testing in the general population (Figure 18.6).

Molecular tests use the principal of target amplification (e.g. the polymerase chain reaction, PCR), or signal amplification (e.g. hybridization) to detect the presence of HIV RNA. These are the most sensitive forms of detection assay, but need to be performed in more specialized, better equipped laboratories with highly skilled personnel to avoid contamination, false positive or negative, or inaccurate quantitative results. Such sensitive, accurate molecular techniques are required for the quantification of HIV RNA for monitoring patients on HAART. In order to put patients on the appropriate HAART regimen, tests are also available to identify any drug-resistance-associated mutations in the HIV genome. Such HIV resistance tests allow clinicians to put the patient on the most optimum drug regimen at the very start of their

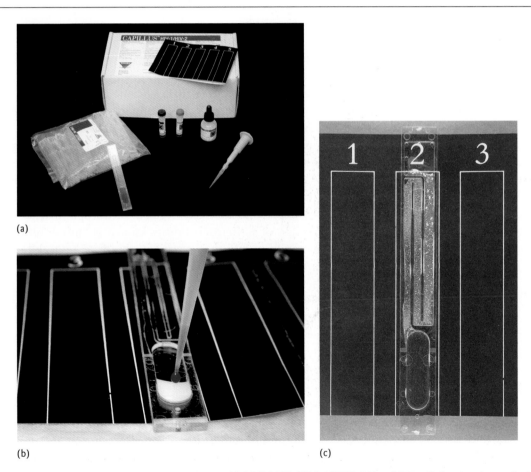

(a)

(b)

(c)

Figure 18.6 An example of a rapid HIV test (CAPILLUS HIV-1/HIV-2 Rapid Test) for testing whole blood, serum, or plasma (a). The blood sample is added to the capillary slide well and mixed with the reagent (b). If HIV-1/HIV-2 specific antibodies are present, the HIV-1 and HIV-2 protein-coated polystyrene latex beads will aggregate, forming white clumps on the slide (c). Provided by Cheryl Tryon; Stacy Howard. Courtesy of the Centers for Disease Control and Prevention; from CDC website: http://phil.cdc.gov/phil/details.asp

treatment (similar to the use of antibiotic sensitivity results). The majority of these HIV resistance tests involve "genotyping" the HIV genome and require the sequencing of certain parts of the HIV genome (mainly on the *pol* gene) to detect the presence of any mutations that will make certain drugs or drug classes ineffective. Alternatively, and much more expensive and difficult to perform, are phenotyping resistance assays. These involve attempting to grow HIV in *in vitro* cultures, in the presence of various concentrations of the drug of interest. The results are then expressed as a "-fold drug resistance" as compared to a laboratory, fully sensitive, HIV strain, grown in the presence of the same concentrations of the same drug. Unfortunately (again, similar to the use of antibiotics against bacteria), the increasing availability of HAART for treating HIV has given rise to an increased prevalence of drug-resistant HIV strains, including an increasing incidence of the transmission of such resistant HIV strains to susceptible individuals. This has made HIV resistance testing of newly diagnosed HIV patients more common in some countries where most of their HIV patients are taking HAART. The lack of strict adherence to HAART regimens has generated such drug-resistant HIV strains, making HIV diagnosis, therapy, and monitoring more expensive and problematic (see Further reading).

Generally, HIV is not cultured for the routine diagnosis of HIV infection, but is reserved for drug-resistance assays and research purposes, such as vaccine development and molecular epidemiology studies. Similarly, electron microscopy (EM) is also not used in routine HIV diagnostic testing, though it has been used to investigate HIV pathogenesis (Figure 18.3).

Treatment

There is now a formidable arsenal of drugs to treat HIV infection and a detailed discussion of these drugs and their use in combination regimens is outside the scope of this text. Most of them are based on the "false substrate" principle whereby the drug molecule acts as the normal substrate for the HIV RT enzyme, leading to chain termination and incomplete formation of the HIV DNA provirus. This prevents integration into the host-cell genome, transcription and translation of HIV proteins, ultimately inhibiting the formation of new HIV virions. Such drugs fall into one of the following classes: nucleoside RT inhibitors, e.g. AZT (azidothymidine), 3TC (lamivudine), d4T (stavudine); non-nucleoside RT inhibitors, e.g. efavirenz, nevirapine and, most recently, etravirine; nucleotide RT inhibitors, e.g. tenofovir; protease inhibitors, e.g. ritonavir, indinavir, saquinavir. Most recently, the fusion process between the HIV gp120/gp41 surface glycoproteins and the host-cell CD4/co-receptor molecules has been targeted for disruption with a drug called T-20/enfuvirtide, which is the first in the class of antiretroviral drugs known as "fusion inhibitors." Unlike the RT inhibitors which can all be taken orally as pills, gels or syrups, this drug has to be injected, and is considerably more expensive (at the moment) than the RT inhibitors. It is usually used with other the other drugs as a form of "salvage therapy," rather than as part of a first line treatment regimen for HIV patients who require therapy for the first time. Other fusion inhibitors are also being developed and target different components of the HIV–host-cell receptor fusion complex. In 2007, two new classes of anti-HIV drugs have been licensed, an integrase inhibitor (raltegravir by Merck Inc.) and a CCR5 receptor inhibitor (maraviroc by Pfizer Inc.), adding to the rapidly expanding arsenal of new anti-HIV drugs that are available.

Often, treating the HIV infection itself to reduce the HIV RNA levels and increase the CD4 lymphocyte count will help to control the opportunistic infections, but this may take some time. Unfortunately, this "immune reconstitution" process and the body's subsequent immune response to some opportunistic infections, such as tuberculosis, may make the patient worse and can cause death. This is why, in some cases, it is important to treat and control the specific opportunistic infection first, before starting antiretroviral drugs to treat HIV. Specific treatments are therefore also required for each individual opportunistic infection. Again, the details of such therapy are outside the scope of this book, but see Further reading.

Vaccines

The development of an effective HIV vaccine has been problematic, to say the least (see Further reading). One of the major problems is that HIV infection does not produce an antibody that enables the human body to clear the viral infection, i.e. the antibody produced is not neutralizing. Hence any vaccine must do better than just producing a similar antibody response, which is clearly ineffective. In fact, it is uncertain exactly what combination of immune responses (humoral and/or cellular) is required to clear HIV from the body, since there have been no documented cases of an individual clearing the virus and "recovering from HIV." Live vaccines have been used to elicit both the specific (humoral and cellular) arms of the immune response, but with the case of HIV and its inherent rate of mutability, any live attenutated virus vaccine may revert to virulence and cause AIDS. Even the traditional first step of an inactivated whole virus vaccine approach for HIV may be too risky, as it is difficult to ensure that every single virion has been inactivated. Subunit or subvirion vaccines using just one or more HIV proteins without containing the whole virus are possible but any such vaccine would have to somehow overcome the high genetic mutation rate and therefore antigenic protein variability of HIV. The error rate inherent in replicating the HIV genome is estimated to be about 1 base error for every 10 kb copied, i.e. almost 1 base error for every full HIV genome replicated (HIV has a genome of about 9 kb in length). This means that an extremely conserved HIV protein must be used for a vaccine to produce a long-lasting immunity. However, HIV exists as a quasispecies (i.e. the replication process is so inaccurate, that each HIV virion may be genetically unique) even within the same individual, so that it is unlikely that a vaccine directed against any particular protein will protect everyone from every HIV virion to which he/she is exposed. Finally, any protective HIV vaccine has to be 100% effective because if a single virion manages to infect a lymphocyte and integrate its provirus into the cell genome, it will always have the potential to produce more HIV virus, even though all other circulating HIV virions have been cleared by the vaccine-primed immune system. This then goes back to the problem of how to protect all CD4 lymphocytes in the body against infection from every HIV virion in the quasispecies of HIV contained in the infecting inoculum (e.g. from an HIV-contaminated needle shared amongst intravenous drug users, or from HIV-infected semen during traumatic, bloody anal intercourse).

Confidentiality and public health

Case study 18.1 in the "Test yourself" section below deals with some of the issues of confidentiality and public health that a clinical team may have to confront when treating a patient who has been diagnosed with HIV infection. It is based on a true case.

Read Boxes 18.1 and 18.2 for other legal/ethical aspects of HIV.

Box 18.1 Deliberate transmission of HIV as a criminal offence

At least one man in the USA and one man in England has been convicted under criminal law of deliberately transmitting HIV to a partner. The US case involved a man (a doctor) who deliberately injected his girlfriend (a nurse) with blood from a patient under his care who was known to be HIV infected (see Further reading). In the UK, an HIV-infected man was convicted of grievous bodily harm when two women accused him of knowingly transmitting HIV to them (see Further reading). In such cases, sequencing of the HIV RNA and phylogenetic analysis (i.e. comparing the nucleic acid sequences) from each of the HIV-infected people involved, may reveal a connection between the accused and accusing parties. However, without a definite time of exposure and a known previous HIV-negative status, it is difficult to show who transmitted the virus to whom. In the US case, the girlfriend was a regular blood donor, and was known to be HIV negative up to 4 months before she was injected by her doctor boyfriend. However, in the English case, neither of the women had such careful documentation of their previously HIV-negative status. Hence, to convict in such cases, other evidence is required to ascertain the sequence of events leading up to HIV infection in the alleged victims of such attacks. Another, earlier case from Scotland with some discussion of the relevant legal issues, is also listed in Further reading.

Box 18.2 Accidental transmission of HIV through needlestick injury and postexposure prophylaxis

Healthcare workers (HCWs) caring for HIV-infected patients are always at some risk of injury from HIV-contaminated body fluids, tissues and healthcare equipment. The most common form of injury leading to possible HIV infection in HCWs is a needlestick injury (NSI). Taking blood from an HIV-infected patient must be performed with great care, but occasional injuries are not uncommon, due to sudden patient movements, attempted re-sheathing of needles, simple carelessness, fatigue, distraction, etc. Needlestick injuries from needles used to give drugs pose less risk as blood is not purposely drawn into the needle that causes the injury, though there will be more risk from needles used for intravenous as opposed to intramuscular or subcutaneous injections. The first stage in dealing with an NSI is to wash the wound (soap and water should be fine) and encourage bleeding from the injury site. This will hopefully minimize the number of HIV virions that enter the bloodstream. A baseline blood sample should also be taken and stored, which may be tested later to show that the HCW was not already HIV-infected at the time of injury (from some other, non-work-related, source).

The risk of transmission depends on several factors: the volume of blood transmitted in the injury, the HIV level in that blood, the time taken to wash and clean the area, and the delay in taking HIV postexposure prophylaxis (PEP) drugs. The general risk of transmission of HIV through NSIs has been generally estimated as about 1:300. This is less than the risk of acquiring two other common bloodborne viral infections: hepatitis B (HBV) and hepatitis C (HCV). The chance of acquiring HBV from a high-infectivity HBV carrier is about 1:3, and that of acquiring HCV from an HCV-viremic patient, about 1:30. These risks will vary with the actual viral loads of the patients at the time of the injury, as well as the nature of the injury and the amount of blood transmitted. For blood splashes to mucous membranes, such as the eyes, nose, mouth, the risk of HIV, HBV and HCV transmission has been estimated to be about **10 times less** than via a NSI (blood-to-blood) exposure. The risk of HIV acquisition probably depends on the number of susceptible cells (e.g. macrophages, lymphocytes) that can be infected by HIV, which are at highest concentration in the bloodstream itself.

Drugs used for HIV PEP usually include a triple combination of zidovudine (AZT), lamivudine (3TC), and nelfinavir, though these may vary depending on the local prevalence of HIV drug resistance. The first two drugs are reverse transcriptase (RT) enzyme inhibitors to prevent the formation of the HIV provirus. The last drug is a protease inhibitor that prevents formation of the proteins required for final HIV virion assembly. It has been shown that in monkeys, HIV can integrate and disseminate throughout the body in a few hours, so HIV PEP should be given as soon as possible after NSI from a known or strongly suspected HIV-infected patient or other source. Normally, HIV PEP will continue for up to 28 days, under the careful monitoring of an HIV physician, until repeated laboratory testing demonstrates that no HIV infection has occurred. Nonoccupational exposure to HIV occurs in the general public through sexual intercourse, sharing of needles between intravenous drug users, etc., but in these situations, there may be more delays in attending hospitals, and this may lessen the effectiveness of taking HIV PEP. In addition, whereas in occupational exposure situations it is possible to test the source of the blood for HIV, in nonoccupational exposure events, this may be more problematic. The drugs given for HIV PEP are not given lightly, so whenever possible, it is important to establish the HIV status of the source blood before making the decision whether or not to give HIV PEP, as the side-effects can be serious, sometimes even fatal (see Further reading).

Summary

For those living in developed countries that can afford the cost of HAART, it is likely that HIV infection will become a chronic disease, like insulin-dependent diabetes mellitus (IDDM), requiring a drug therapy regimen throughout life that must be strictly followed and monitored, to avoid complications and death. Unlike IDDM, however, HIV infected patients may need to change drugs at fairly regular intervals to avoid resistance and treatment failure. This requires that new drugs be always available meaning that there will be continuing arms race between the virus and the ingenuity of pharmaceutical companies, as well as governments and non-governmental organizations that need to find the money to pay for these lifelong treatment regiments. Already, the HIV/AIDS pandemic is hitting the poorer, developing nations the hardest. Continued negotiations between pharmaceutical companies and these countries, together with mediators, such as the World Health Organization, the UN and the richer nations, are required to ensure that these antiretroviral drugs are made available to them at an affordable price. It has been argued that the development of a safe, cheap, effective, protective HIV vaccine would allow people to practice unsafe sex methods again (see Further reading), more freely, but this should not be an obstacle to this goal.

Test yourself

Case study 18.1

A 55-year-old man is brought to the emergency room (ER) after collapsing at home. He began having continuous seizures in the ambulance on the way to the hospital. He was given anticonvulsants to control his seizures and an attempt to stabilize him was made in the ER. However, he went into respiratory failure and had to be admitted to the intensive care unit (ICU) for sedation, intubation, and mechanical ventilation. Intravenous anticonvulsants were continued on the ICU because an electroencephalogram (EEG) showed continuous seizure activity in his brain.

1. What is the most likely diagnosis in this type of presentation?

His wife gave a 6-month history of her husband gradually losing weight and becoming generally unwell. Most recently, he had developed a cough and shortness of breath in the 2 weeks prior to this admission. He had not collapsed or had seizures before. They had been married for over 20 years and had two children. They had not traveled abroad in the last 12 months and had not had any mosquito bites recently. There had been no reports of West Nile fever cases in their area in the past several months.

2. Does this new information narrow down the possible likely (differential) diagnoses? How?

The ICU (intensive care unit) team found a low lymphocyte count on his routine blood tests and his chest X-ray (CXR) showed a picture suspicious of *Pneumocystis* pneumonia (PCP).

3. Now, what is a likely diagnosis? Is there any test you would now like to do?

The team decided to perform an HIV test to assist their medical management, despite the patient being sedated and unconscious and unable to give consent. The result came back as HIV positive. A bronchoscopy obtained a broncho-alveolar lavage (BAL) specimen that confirmed a diagnosis of PCP, as suggested on the CXR.

4. Given this new HIV diagnosis, are there any other issues you would like to clarify here? What are they and why?

Test yourself

The ICU team now had a dilemma. Should they tell his wife of his HIV diagnosis? Bear in mind they performed the HIV test without the patient's consent in the first place. Or should they wait until the patient recovers enough to discuss this with him first?

5. Given the ICU team's actions to test for HIV (under the guise of "best medical care" for the patient), now, what are the pros and cons of these options and why?

Each country, state, or institution may have their own guidelines for such situations. Therefore, local legal (and perhaps ethical) counsel should be sought in such cases from the local hospital management to avoid any lawsuit. However, in most situations, still, HIV testing requires explicit (written) consent from a patient (although the CDC is trying to make HIV testing more routine and less stigmatizing now).

In some cases unconscious patients may be tested if the clinical team believes that this will significantly alter (and improve) the patient's medical management and possible outcome. However, the results of the HIV test should not be revealed to others (even to members of his/her own family) by the clinical team without the patient's explicit consent, and before the patient is given a chance to do so.

This is the dilemma of the patient's right to confidentiality versus public health, i.e. the welfare of those in the community. The patient should be encouraged to reveal his/her HIV status to allow his/her partner to be tested (and treated if necessary) as early as possible. In the event that the patient refuses to inform his/her partner about his/her new HIV status then clinical teams may breach this confidentiality as the patient is then putting his/her rights above that of his/her partner, which is now recognized to be unacceptable (see Further reading).

In this scenario, the clinical team could not foresee the patient recovering within a reasonable time from his HIV-related neurological illness, and therefore, whether he would be mentally competent to discuss his new HIV status with his partner, or even to give consent for the clinical team to do this for him. His wife was finally informed, but fortunately, eventually tested HIV negative. The patient died on the ICU without ever recovering from his HIV disease, so in retrospect the ICU team's decision was appropriate.

Further reading

Clinical and basic research into HIV/AIDS is a rapidly developing field and it is likely that many of these references will be slightly outdated by the time this text goes to press. Readers are encouraged to search the literature for more up-to-date information (and updated editions of the textbooks) on areas of particular interest.

Textbooks

Cleghorn FR, Reitz MS, Popovic M, Gallo RC. Human immunodeficiency viruses. In: Mandell GL, Bennett JE, Dolin R (eds). *Principles and Practice of Infectious Diseases*, 6th edition. Philadelphia: Churchill Livingstone, 2005, pp 2119–2133

Dolin R, Masur H, Saag MS (eds). *AIDS Therapy*, 2nd edition. Philadelphia: Churchill Livingstone, 2002

Jeffery K, Pillay D. Diagnostic approaches. In: Zuckerman AJ, Banatvala JE, Pattison JR, Griffiths PD, Schoub BD (eds). *Principles and Practice of Clinical Virology*, 5th edition. Chichester: John Wiley, 2004, pp 1–21

Weiss RA, Dalgleish AG, Loveday C, Pillay D. Human immunodeficiency viruses. In: Zuckerman AJ, Banatvala JE, Pattison JR, Griffiths PD, Schoub BD (eds). *Principles and Practice of Clinical Virology*, 5th edition. Chichester: John Wiley, 2004, pp 721–757

Papers

Deeks SG. Challenges of developing R5 inhibitors in antiretroviral naïve HIV-infected patients. *Lancet* 2006;367:711–713

Escoto-Delgadillo M, Vazquez-Valls E, Ramirez-Rodriguez M, et al. Drug-resistance mutations in antiretroviral-naive patients with established HIV-1 infection in Mexico. *HIV Med* 2005;6(6):403–409

Fraser C, Riley S, Anderson RM, Ferguson NM. Factors that make an infectious disease outbreak controllable. *Proc Natl Acad Sci USA* 2004;101(16):6146–6151

Gallo RC. The end or the beginning of the drive to an HIV-preventive vaccine: a view from over 20 years. *Lancet* 2005;366(9500):1894–1898

Hammer SM. Clinical practice. Management of newly diagnosed HIV infection. *N Engl J Med* 2005;353(16):1702–1710

Korber B, Muldoon M, Theiler J, et al. Timing the ancestor of the HIV-1 pandemic strains. *Science* 2000;288(5472):1789–1796

Lemey P, Pybus OG, Wang B, et al. Tracing the origin and history of the HIV-2 epidemic. *Proc Natl Acad Sci USA* 2003;100(11):6588–6592

Pillay D, Bhaskaran K, Jurriaans S, et al. The impact of transmitted drug resistance on the natural history of HIV infection and response to first-line therapy. *AIDS* 2006;20(1):21–28

Sax PE, Islam R, Walensky RP, et al. Should resistance testing be performed for treatment-naive HIV-infected patients? A cost-effectiveness analysis. *Clin Infect Dis* 2005;41(9):1316–1323

Smith RJ, Blower SM. Could disease-modifying HIV vaccines cause population-level perversity? *Lancet Infect Dis* 2004;4(10):636–639

Tang JW, Pillay D. Transmission of HIV-1 drug resistance. *J Clin Virol* 2004;30(1):1–10

Wensing AM, van de Vijver DA, Angarano G, et al. Prevalence of drug-resistant HIV-1 variants in untreated individuals in Europe: implications for clinical management. *J Infect Dis* 2005;192(6):958–966

Forensic investigations involving HIV transmission chains

Several cases of HIV transmission between individuals have been reported in the academic literature, some of which describe how the genetic analyses of the virus have led to criminal prosecutions. However, such sequence (or "phylogenetic") evidence is not sufficient alone to convict a person of deliberately transmitting HIV to another with intent to harm. This is another expanding area of applied HIV research that will be useful, if carefully applied.

Bird SM, Brown AJ. Criminalisation of HIV transmission: implications for public health in Scotland. *BMJ* 2001;323(7322):1174–1177

Chalmers J. The criminalization of HIV transmission. *Sex Transm Infect* 2002;78(6):448–451

Dyer O. Man convicted of grievous bodily harm for infecting two women with HIV. *BMJ* 2003;327:950

Metzker ML, Mindell DP, Liu XM, Ptak RG, Gibbs RA, Hillis DM. Molecular evidence of HIV-1 transmission in a criminal case. *Proc Natl Acad Sci USA* 2002;99(22):14292–14297

Pillay D, Rambaut A, Geretti AM, Brown AJ. HIV phylogenetics. *BMJ* 2007;335(7618):460–461

HIV patient confidentiality, disclosure, and public health

This is obviously a sensitive issue and there have been many guidelines written to assist physicians on how to handle such difficult cases. These papers/websites give some idea of the scale of the dilemmas sometimes encountered by physicians.

Ateka GK. HIV status disclosure and partner discordance: a public health dilemma. *Public Health* 2006;120(6):493–496. Also available online at: http://www.pubmedcentral.nih.gov/articlerender.fcgi?&pubmedid=16690093

A study on HIV confidentiality/disclosure in the context of pregnancy

CDC. Attachment H: Technical Guidance for HIV/AIDS Surveillance Programs.
http://www.cdc.gov/hiv/topics/surveillance/resources/guidelines/guidance/attachment_h.htm

Useful CDC website on aspects of HIV data/confidentiality on PCs, laptops, data transmission

Confidentiality of human immunodeficiency virus status on autopsy reports. Council on Ethical and Judicial Affairs,
American Medical Association. *Arch Pathol Lab Med* 1992;116(11):1120–1123. Also available online at:
http://www.ama-assn.org/ama1/pub/upload/mm/369/ceja_ca92.pdf

An interesting early US debate and recommendations on the maintenance of HIV confidentiality after death – on post-mortem reports

Department of Health. Comprehensive UK guidelines for HIV status confidentiality/disclosure.
http://www.ahpn.org/downloads/policies/DHConfidentiality&DisclosureConsultation.pdf

Does HIV status influence the outcome of patients admitted to a surgical intensive care unit? A prospective double
blind study. *BMJ* 1997;314(7087):1077–1081; discussion 1081–1084. Also available online at: http://www.bmj.com/
cgi/content/full/314/7087/1082

An early debate about the ethics of HIV/AIDS consent/confidentiality for research studies

Vernillo AT, Wolpe PR, Halpern SD. Re-examining ethical obligations in the intensive care unit: HIV disclosure to
surrogates. *Crit Care* 2007;11(2):125. Also available online at: http://www.bioethics.upenn.edu/pdf/
wolpe_hivdisclosure.pdf

*A useful summary of the US situation, directly relevant to the case scenario presented above. A useful debate on the above paper from
the US viewpoint can be found at*: http://ccforum.com/content/11/3/416

Useful websites

Again, these are continuously updated, so there may be some new data/guidelines by the time this text goes to press.

WHO

The WHO has many links from its websites on HIV/AIDS, which are updated regularly. http://www.who.int/hiv/en/;
http://www.who.int/hiv/topics/en/

CDC

Similarly, the CDC has a comprehensive, continuously updated website on HIV/AIDS. http://www.cdc.gov/hiv/
resources/factsheets/

Including, **for healthcare workers:**

Updated US Public Health Service Guidelines for the Management of Occupational Exposures to HBV, HCV,
and HIV and Recommendations for Postexposure Prophylaxis. *MMWR* June 29, 2001/50(RR11);1–42.
http://www.cdc.gov/mmwr/preview/mmwrhtml/rr5011a1.htm

For the general public:

Antiretroviral Postexposure Prophylaxis After Sexual, Injection, Drug Use, or Other Nonoccupational Exposure to
HIV in the United States. *MMWR* January 21, 2005/54(RR02);1–20. http://www.cdc.gov/mmwr/preview/
mmwrhtml/rr5402a1.htm

United Nations

The United Nations (UN) website is a massive website touching on all aspects of the HIV/AIDS pandemic, including
the politics, social and economic aspects, with supporting data. http://www.unaids.org/en/; http://www.unaids.org/
en/KnowledgeCentre/HIVData/default.asp

Chapter 19
Viral hepatitis

J.W. Tang

Clinical features
Hepatitis A (HAV)
Hepatitis B (HBV)
Hepatitis C (HCV)

Hepatitis D (HDV)
Hepatitis E (HEV)
Other hepatitis viruses

There are five recognized, established viruses (A, B, C, D, and E) that cause acute and sometimes chronic hepatitis (i.e. acute and chronic liver inflammation). These viruses are perhaps unique compared to the other pathogens in this book, in that the damage they cause is not directly due to the virus themselves. Rather, the body's immune response to viral-infected liver cells (hepatocytes) results in destruction of these cells, and release of the virus to infect other surrounding hepatocytes. Hence, the outcome of viral hepatitis infections depends mainly on the strength of the host immune response. Too strong, and the host immune response may kill the host by rapidly destroying all viral-infected hepatocytes (known as fulminant hepatitis). Too weak, and the host may not be able to remove the virus from the body, resulting in chronic viral infection of the liver, and a long-term cycle of inflammation/damage/repair or fibrosis/inflammation, etc. that may result in severe scarring of the liver (cirrhosis) and even cancer (hepatocellular carcinoma), when the repair mechanisms fail and some cells become transformed and immortalized.

Clinical features

It is useful to describe the clinical features of viral hepatitis here as they are similar amongst and difficult to distinguish between the different hepatitis viruses. The different hepatitis viruses have different incubation periods, but once symptoms begin, they usually take the form of malaise, lethargy, sometimes weight loss, low-grade fever, and loss of appetite. Later, the urine becomes dark (like tea without milk), and the stools become pale and may become unusually foul-smelling and difficult to flush away. During this time, the whites of the eye and the skin may become yellow in color (Figure 19.1), and sometimes various types of rashes can be seen (Figure 19.2).

Figure 19.1 Clinical signs of acute viral hepatitis include a yellowing of the whites (sclera) of the eye and skin called icterus or jaundice. These signs are more often seen in adults and teenagers than children, due to the more mature and vigorous host immune response to the virus in the older age groups, which is the actual cause of the liver damage. Provided by: Dr Thomas F. Sellers. Courtesy of the Centers for Disease Control and Prevention; from CDC website: http://phil.cdc.gov/phil/details.asp

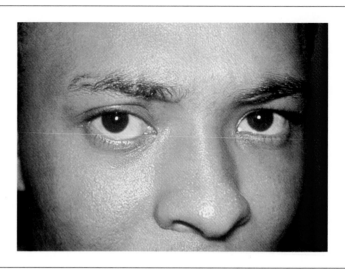

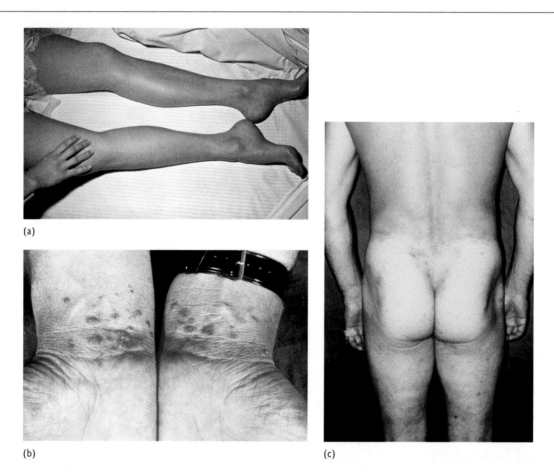

(a)

(b)

(c)

Figure 19.2 This patient with viral hepatitis presented with this fine macular rash over her legs (a). Patients with hepatitis C may also develop a more specific form of rash called lichen planus. This can be intensely itchy and appears as raised, red, scaly, flattened bumps, often on the wrists (b) and ankles and torso (c). Other causes of this unusual skin disorder include stress-related factors and autoimmune diseases. Provided by Susan Lindsley. Courtesy of the Centers for Disease Control and Prevention; from CDC website: http://phil.cdc.gov/phil/details.asp

The outcomes of human infections by the various hepatitis viruses differ, and can be divided into the acute-only hepatitis viruses (types A and E) that are also mainly fecal–orally transmitted and waterborne, and the acute-with-chronic hepatitis viruses (B, C, and D) that are also mainly transmitted via infected blood and are thus referred to as bloodborne. Each of these will now be described in more detail.

Hepatitis A (HAV)

Discovered in the early 1970s, this is a hardy, small (27 nm), nonenveloped virus, with a single strand of positive (mRNA)-sense RNA. It is a member of the Picornavirus family (Figure 19.3). It is widespread throughout the world, being more common in developing countries (where ~90% of the population may have been exposed) than developed countries (30–40% may have been exposed). In the USA, HAV used to account for about 150 000 new cases of viral hepatitis per year during the 1980s, but this has now declined to below 50 000 since 2004.

It has an average incubation period of 30 days (range 15–50), and is transmitted via the fecal–oral route, i.e. poor hand hygiene after using the toilet where HAV is shed in the stool, leaves HAV on hands, which is then transferred to food when cooking or preparing drinks, and consumed by others. Other routes of transmission include via sex and indirectly via fomites (contaminated inanimate objects). Food may not be contaminated in the kitchen, but at source, such as HAV-contaminated water or ice, or shellfish caught in HAV-contaminated seawater – particularly around coastlines where untreated sewage is dumped directly into the sea.

Hepatitis A is more symptomatic in older patients due to the maturity of their immune response (<10% symptomatic in <6 year olds; 40–50% in 6–14 year olds; 70–80% in >14 years). It can occur sporadically in individuals, or in outbreaks usually due to food or water contamination. Most infections are self-limiting with no long-term sequelae or carrier state, though there is occasionally a serious case of fulminant hepatitis (about 100 cases/year in the USA) that may cause death (very rare ~0.1–0.3% of HAV cases, though this can be as high as 1.8% in >50 year olds). Other complications include a prolonged or relapsing course of illness lasting as long as 6–9 months in about 10% of cases, though in most cases, clinical recovery is complete within 2 months.

Diagnosis is usually by testing for anti-HAV IgM and should be positive by the time the patient presents with symptoms. Viral culture, electron microscopy (EM), and molecular detection for viral RNA (polymerase chain reaction, PCR, testing) are not usually required nor performed in normal diagnostic laboratories. Other tests for HAV include testing for an enzyme (alanine amino transferase, ALT) released

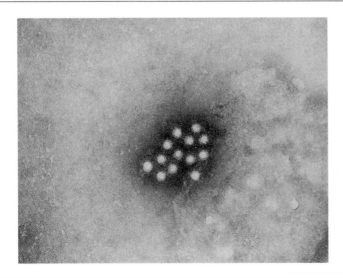

Figure 19.3 An electron micrograph of the hardy hepatitis A virus (HAV), which can survive up to a month at room temperature. This virus enters an organism by ingestion of water and food contaminated by human feces, and reaches the liver through the bloodstream. HAV infection is endemic in third world countries, and is prevalent in the Far East. Provided by Betty Partin. Courtesy of the Centers for Disease Control and Prevention; from CDC website: http://phil.cdc.gov/phil/details.asp

by dying hepatocytes. The ALT levels sharply increase to several thousand international units per milliliter (IU/ml), at the same time as symptom onset and the rise in anti-HAV IgM. At this time, HAV is shed in the stool and can be transmitted to others if careful fecal–oral hygiene is not observed. With clinical recovery, the ALT normalizes and the virus disappears from the stool, though the anti-HAV IgM may remain detectable for 3 months or more. By this time the level of protective anti-HAV IgG is already rising and should remain detectable and confer lifelong protection.

There is no specific antiviral therapy for HAV. For those who have not yet been exposed, there is an effective protective vaccine, consisting of inactivated cell cultured virus, given by intramuscular injection in two doses at least 6 months apart. If exposed to HAV, immunoglobulin (pooled immune sera from multiple donors) can be given within 7–28 days of exposure. In some cases, the HAV vaccine may also be given in the first week after contact, depending on local guidelines.

Hepatitis A is not usually a risk for mother-to-child-transmission (MTCT) during delivery, or in blood donors, as the viremic period is so short and occurs during the symptomatic period, when donation is usually refused.

Hepatitis B (HBV)

Although the clinical presentations of acute HAV and HBV may be similar, the similarities really end there. Discovered in the late 1970s, hepatitis B is the only member of the Hepadnavirus family, and is a small (42 nm), lipid-enveloped, partially double-stranded DNA virus (Figure 19.4). It is widespread, with an estimated 300 million infected worldwide. In the USA, it used to account for 200 000–300 000 new hepatitis cases per year in the 1980s, but this has now declined to about 60 000 per year since 2004. Unlike HAV, HBV has a long-term carrier state, and there are about 1.25 million HBV carriers in the USA (about 0.4% of the population). Its ability to produce a carrier state means that it stays infectious in those individuals for much longer than with HAV, however the mode of transmission for HBV is more restricted.

Hepatitis B has a significantly longer incubation period than HAV, being anything between 1 and 6 months, though the average is around 2–3 months. It is transmitted mainly through blood, though other body fluids, such as semen, are also efficient carriers of the virus. Hence, HBV can be transmitted through sharing needles amongst intravenous drug users (IVDUs), through accidental needlestick injuries (usually to

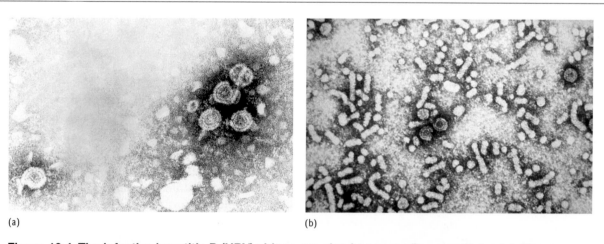

(a)   (b)

Figure 19.4 The infective hepatitis B (HBV) virions are also known as Dane particles (a). These particles measure 42 nm in their overall diameter, and contain a DNA-based core that is 27 nm in diameter (the smaller circles, seen on the right). HBV produces many extra surface and core proteins that may act as immunomodulators that appear as the other linear forms (b). Provided by Dr Erskine Palmer. Courtesy of the Centers for Disease Control and Prevention; from CDC website: http://phil.cdc.gov/phil/details.asp

healthcare workers, HCWs), blood transfusions (from poorly screened blood donations), sexual intercourse and tattoos, piercing and acupuncture with HBV-contaminated needles.

Again, as with HAV, HBV has an age-dependent distribution for symptomatic infection, being symptomatic in only 10% of <5 year-olds, but in 30−50% of >5 year olds. Many HBV-infected individuals remain asymptomatic, unlike HAV where the majority (80−90%) of adult cases are symptomatic. Although the mortality rate from acute HBV infection is similar to that of HAV at 0.5−1%, the main morbidity and mortality from HBV arises from the long-term complications in the HBV carriers.

Being asymptomatic means that there is a higher chance that the HBV will not be cleared from the body, as the symptoms generally arise from the strength of the host immune response in destroying viral-infected cells. Therefore, chronic infection (leading to the long-term HBV carrier state) tends to occur in the <5 year olds that are asymptomatically infected with HBV (30−90%), but rarely (only in 2−10%) in the >5 year olds who generally develop symptoms with HBV infection. The HBV carriers then are at further risk (15−25%) of morbidity and mortality from liver cirrhosis with liver failure, and liver cancer (hepatocellular carcinoma) that has a very poor prognosis. Hence, ironically, with acute HBV infection, the more sick you become (as long as you do not die from fulminant hepatitis), the more likely that you will clear the virus and not develop the long-term carrier state with all its related complications.

Diagnosis of HBV infection, like HAV, relies on serology and HBV antigen detection – but it is much more complicated, as HBV produces many different immunogenic viral proteins. Viral culture and EM are not routinely used in diagnosis, and HBV DNA detection is usually used to monitor the response to therapy, rather than to diagnose new cases of HBV, though there are exceptions (Box 19.1).

There are several HBV antigens that stimulate a specific host antibody response. The acute markers of HBV infection are the appearance of HBV surface antigen (HBsAg), the IgM antibody to the HBV core antigen (anti-HBc IgM). In patients who develop a very strong immune response, the HBsAg may be rapidly cleared within a few days after the onset of symptoms, such that by the time the patient presents with clinical acute hepatitis, the HBsAg test may be negative. However, the anti-HBc IgM will be positive for several months and serves as a marker of recent acute HBV infection.

The definition of an HBV carrier requires that the HBsAg remains positive for more than 6 months. There can be two types of HBV carrier. In a highly infectious HBV carrier (i.e. higher HBV replication rate and serum level), another part of the HBV core antigen, the HBe antigen (HBeAg), remains detectable. This is also normally present for a short while during acute HBV infection, but is soon cleared by the appearance of anti-HBe antibodies during recovery. This may also happen in an HBV carrier, denoting a drop in the level of HBV replication and perhaps a sign of final HBsAg clearance and serological immunity to HBV infection. This is signaled by the appearance of anti-HBs antibodies, which neutralize the HBsAg.

Normally, the appearance of anti-HBs in levels >10 mIU/ml (milli-international units per ml) signifies lifelong immunity to HBV, as there is only one serotype of HBV (like HAV). Therefore, in the recovered and immune patient, there will be detectable anti-HBs, anti-HBe, and anti-HBc (antibody to HBV core protein). However, there are exceptions to this rule that can make it difficult to truly know a person's HBV status. This can be particularly important if the person concerned is a healthcare worker, such as a surgeon or dentist, who may transmit his/her own HBV to their patients (Box 19.1). Finally, after long-past infection, and in the absence of any further exposure to HBV, sometimes, naturally immune patients may only retain the anti-HBc antibodies as their marker of previous HBV infection. This can also be a nonspecific reaction in some individuals, i.e. a false positive result.

There is specific antiviral treatment, as well as preventative vaccination and immunoglobulin postexposure prophylaxis (PEP) for HBV. Specific antiviral drugs include lamivudine (3TC), interferon (Box 19.2 and Further reading), and adefovir, which are well established drugs for treating HBV. Newer drugs, some of which may already be licensed by the time this text goes to press, are: tenofovir, emtricitabine, telbuvidine, and clevudine. Some of these drugs (lamivudine, tenofovir, and emtricitabine) are also active against HIV and may be used in HIV-HBV coinfected patients.

The HBV vaccine is a recombinant (i.e. a protein expressed by insertion of the specific viral gene into individual fungal or bacterial cells that are labeled with drug-resistant or other markers, to allow selection

Box 19.1 Transmission of hepatitis B between patients and doctors

There are numerous published reports of the transmission of bloodborne viruses (BBVs): HIV, hepatitis B (HBV) and C (HCV) between patients and their doctors. During surgery, if a doctor accidentally cuts his/her hand with a clean scalpel blade, it is possible for his/her blood to drip into the patient – even if gloves are worn. If the cut is made with a scalpel that has already been used on the patient, there is the risk that any BBVs may be transmitted to the doctor from the patient, but, the doctor may still bleed into the patient, if he/she does not scrub out immediately and wash the bleeding, cut area.

Activities with sharp instruments, or any environment within which sharp edges may be encountered, which cannot be seen by the operator in a direct line-of-sight, have been termed "exposure-prone procedures" (EPPs). Such EPPs have the highest risk for transmitting BBVs between healthcare workers and patients. This includes not only surgeons and dentists, but also midwives who frequently must insert their hands into the womb to assist in the baby's delivery. During such procedures, the midwives' hands may not be visible, and any injury may go unnoticed until the hands are withdrawn and the gloves inspected – or during final hand-washing, after the procedure is over.

To prevent healthcare worker-to-patient transmission, all healthcare workers should be immune to HBV (there is no vaccine for HIV or HCV, as yet), which is the most transmissible of the BBVs via sharps (mainly needles and scalpels) injuries. The HBV vaccine consists of recombinant (fungal- or bacterial-expressed) HBsAg protein that induces a specific host immune response to that particular protein. This immunity is reliable and long-lasting (see the main text).

However, some individuals may become naturally infected with so-called mutant HBVs that express an HBsAg during their replication that is not neutralized by the vaccine-induced anti-HBs antibodies, so the mutant HBV can continue to replicate in the presence of the vaccine-induced anti-HBs – at least until the body can produce its own antibodies to this mutant virus.

Another type of mutant HBV has been found. Previously, in some countries, such as the UK, HBV carriers who had no HBeAg (i.e. HBsAg positive, HBeAg negative), were deemed to have a sufficiently low serum HBV copy number (viral load) to allow them to continue working with EPPs (e.g. surgery or midwifery). However, it became clear after a series of doctor-to-patient transmission events that some of these HBeAg positive HBV carriers had very high HBV levels. Further investigation revealed that there are some "pre-core" mutant HBVs that do not produce HBeAg, even when replicating to very high levels. Therefore, now in the UK, an HBV DNA testing check is required annually and must be under 10^3 copies/ml, for such healthcare HBV carrier healthcare workers who continue performing EPPs. A further allowance in the UK guidelines is that if such healthcare workers are on HBV treatment, and if their initial pre-treatment HBV levels were between 10^3 and 10^5 copies/ml, such healthcare workers require 3-monthly HBV level checks, all of which must be below 10^3 copies/ml, to allow them to continue performing EPPs.

Unfortunately, to prevent patient-to-HCW transmission of BBVs, the only foolproof method is to avoid accidental injury with contaminated sharps, as well as splashes of potentially BBV-contaminated body fluids to healthcare workers' mucous membranes (eyes, nose, mouth) and other potential portals of entry through the skin (e.g. patches of eczema, psoriasis, unhealed/poorly healed wounds). As well as avoidance of sharps injuries, this can also be partially achieved by wearing the appropriate personal protective equipment (PPE), such as gloves, gowns, masks, face and eye shields.

Box 19.2 Interferon therapy for viral hepatitis

Interferons (IFNs) are naturally produced proteins and form part of the innate (nonspecific) human immune response. They were discovered in the 1950s and were found to be produced in response to the presence of foreign nucleic acid in cells. The IFN protein is then secreted by the infected cell to stimulate the surrounding (uninfected) cells to resist further infection by the virus. One of the main abilities of interferons is to inhibit cell division, which acts to prevent viral replication, as well as cancer growth. Interferons are also cytokines (cellular messengers) that stimulate the body, preparing it to fight the infection and cancer – hence the name "interferon" describing its "interfering" action.

There are at least two recognized classes of IFNs, depending on the receptors they bind. Type I IFNs all bind to the IFN-α receptor. There are several type I IFNs, but of these, IFN-α and IFN-β are currently used for treating medical conditions. Various forms of IFN-α are used to treat chronic hepatitis B and C, mainly IFN-α 2a and 2b. A more recent form of these two interferons has had a side chain added (polyethylene glycol, PEG), to greatly increase the half-life of these IFNs (i.e. pegylated-IFNs) in the body, so that they can be given by weekly (by self-administered intramuscular or subcutaneous injection), instead of daily. This has increased the tolerance and effectiveness of these IFNs for treating chronic hepatitis. Similarly, various forms of IFN-β (IFN-β 1a and 1b) are used to treat some forms of multiple sclerosis. In the body both IFN-α and IFN-β are naturally secreted by many cell types including **lymphocytes** (natural killer – **NK cells**, **B cells**, and **T cells**), as well as macrophages, fibroblasts (that make connective tissue), endothelial cells (that line blood vessels), and osteoblasts (that produce bone). They stimulate both **macrophages** and NK cells to elicit an antiviral response, and are also active against **tumors**.

Type II IFNs contain just one member – IFN-γ – that binds to the IFN-γ receptor. **IFN-γ regulates** the immune and inflammatory responses, and there is only one type in humans. It is produced in a more restricted range of cells (only in activated T cells and NK cells), and it has some weak antiviral and anti-tumor effects. However, this is not its main role. The main role of IFN-γ is that of a **cytokine**, i.e. to enhance the effects of the type I IFNs, including IFN-α and IFN-β. IFN-γ recruits **leukocytes** to a site of infection, resulting in increased inflammation. It also stimulates **macrophages** to kill bacteria that have been phagocytosed. Since IFN-γ is so vital for the regulation of the host immune response, it may also, inadvertently, lead to **autoimmune disorders**.

and purification of the specific viral protein) HBsAg protein vaccine and is very safe and efficacious. It is given in three doses, at 0-, 1-, 6-month intervals, and can be given as part of a childhood immunization program (Figure 19.5, the first dose being given at birth) in HBV endemic areas, or in adults who are traveling to or working in high-risk HBV countries or environments. Healthcare workers are routinely required to have HBV immunization if they are not immune to HBV before starting work in healthcare facilities in developed countries such as the USA and Europe. The vaccine may also be given in an accelerated dose form at 0, 1, 2 and 12 months, such as for the prevention of MTCT when the mother is an HBV carrier, or in healthcare workers who are either non-HBV vaccine responders or who have not had the HBV vaccine yet. In both regimens, the final dose is considered to be a booster.

Vaccine response is tested by testing serum for anti-HBs antibodies between 1 and 2 months post-HBV immunization. This interval is important, as the guidelines for effective levels of anti-HBs post-vaccine apply to samples taken within this time-frame. The anti-HBs antibodies will wane with time, so it is no good taking a post-vaccine serum to check for anti-HBs antibodies 6–12 months later, when they may have become undetectable in some individuals. Within this time-frame, any response with an anti-HBs level of >10 mIU/ml is considered to be an indication of life-long vaccine-induced immunity to HBV infection. This is because the long-term memory T cell (cell mediated) immunity has been demonstrated to have been stimulated in these individuals, so that even if there is very little detectable anti-HBs in the future, an initial

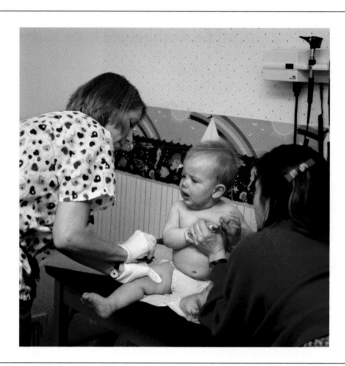

Figure 19.5 A physician's assistant administering a hepatitis B vaccination to a 9-month-old infant. Courtesy of the Centers for Disease Control and Prevention; from CDC website: http://phil.cdc.gov/phil/details.asp

anti-HBs response of >10 mIU/ml has been found to signify the capacity for a sufficiently rapid cell-mediated response to generate adequate levels of neutralizing anti-HBs antibodies to prevent HBV infection.

For HBV PEP, in a healthcare worker who is unresponsive to the vaccine, or has just not had time to be immunized against HBV yet, HBV immunoglobulin (HBIG) can be given to neutralize part or all of the HBV to which he/she has been exposed. This is almost always given in conjunction with the accelerated HBV vaccine regimen. Examples of such situations include: needlestick injury from an HBeAg positive HBV carrier to a nonimmune (anti-HBs negative) healthcare worker, to prevent MTCT in an HBeAg positive HBV carrier mother, where the HBV vaccine and HBIG PEP is given to the baby at birth. As with all immunoglobulins produced from pooled human sera from blood donations, there is always the risk of unidentified viruses or other infections (e.g. prions) being transmitted with the immunoglobulin, so some people refuse the HBIG and just take the accelerated HBV vaccine in such situations.

Hepatitis C (HCV)

Discovered in 1989 by complex molecular methods, hepatitis C is caused by a small (~50 nm diameter), lipid-enveloped, single-stranded, positive sense RNA member of the flavirus family. It is a major health problem in the world today, with between 150 million and 200 million people infected worldwide. In the USA HCV used to account for 240 000 new cases of viral hepatitis per year in the 1980s, but this has now declined to about 26 000 per year since 2004. Currently, it is estimated that about 3.2 million people (1.6% of the US population) are still chronically infected with HCV, with a total of 4.1 million having been infected.

Like HBV, HCV is primarily a bloodborne virus and is transmitted mainly by direct blood-to-blood contact. However, it differs significantly from HBV in that it is relatively inefficiently transmitted via sexual intercourse and through MTCT. The most common and efficient means of transmitting HCV is via the sharing of needles amongst IVDUs, but also in some cases, iatrogenically (i.e. by the action of doctors), in healthcare services (Box 19.3). One unfortunate consequence of its relatively recent discovery, coupled with the fact that it can produce a life-long infectious, relatively asymptomatic carrier state, meant that thousands of people were infected through blood and blood product transfusions, particularly during the 1970s and 1980s. This has led to some sufferers receiving compensation for this "accident," though by no means all.

For some authorities, it was difficult to award compensation for an infectious agent that was unknown to science at the time such transfusions were given – often for life-threatening conditions (Box 19.3).

Hepatitis C has an average incubation period of 6–7 weeks – somewhere between that of HAV and HBV, though the range is similar to HBV, between 2 and 26 weeks. However, unlike HAV and HBV, HCV infection is much more insidious and less often symptomatic. Therefore, HCV-infected individuals may feel quite well, but are infectious, and may inadvertently spread the virus to others whenever others are exposed to the individual's HCV-infected blood. This may be during an activity as innocuous as sharing toothbrushes, which may cause transient bleeding during vigorous (or even more gentle) brushing,

---

Box 19.3 Iatrogenic (doctor-induced) transmission of hepatitis C: compensation and irony?

HCV transmitted by donated blood

When hepatitis C (HCV) was discovered in 1989 and found to be a bloodborne virus (BBV) similar to HIV and HBV, the USA began screening their blood donations for HCV the following year in 1990. The UK delayed this screening process for another year to 1991 in order to improve the HCV screening assays that were initially by anti-HCV antibody only. This difference in screening policy partially contributed to the UK government making *ex-gratia* (voluntary without admitting any legal liability or obligation) payments to people infected with HCV who were still alive on August 29, 2003, where their HCV infection could be attributable to UK National Health Service (NHS) treatment with blood or blood products (e.g. clotting factors such as VIII or IX) before September 1991. Each patient received an initial lump sum payment of £20 000 (GBP), with those developing more serious stages of disease, such as liver cirrhosis or liver cancer, receiving a further £25 000. This also applied to those who contracted HCV through someone else infected with HCV during this period.

HCV transmitted inadvertently through protection against a parasite

Blood transfusions are one form of iatrogenic ("caused by doctor") infection related to HCV. Another, now rather infamous, example occurred in Egypt. During 1950–1980, a nationwide campaign was carried out to eliminate schistosomiasis (an endemic parasitic infection by flatworms, also known as bilharzias, that causes chronic infection in the bladder that may lead to bleeding and cancer). This was performed by healthcare teams traveling between villages to treat infected

individuals with an intravenous injection of tartar emetic (potassium antimony tartrate). Unfortunately, due to the large numbers of people requiring treatment, the needles were often reused without adequate sterilization, and in some cases HCV-infected blood was transmitted between individuals by such needles. The injection treatment required 12–16 doses, each given once a week, so that those infected with HCV from the first injection would have become HCV viremic by the second to fourth weeks and then able to act as sources for further HCV transmission. This was further compounded due to the mostly asymptomatic nature of HCV acute infection, where about 80% of those infected do not feel unwell. With a population of about 67 million, eventually about 15–20% became HCV infected. With the gradual availability and use of oral treatments for schistosomiasis, the need for injection disappeared by the early 1980s. However, now, Egypt remains the country with the world's highest prevalence of HCV. The irony is that the original cause of the schistosomiasis outbreaks in Egypt was likely to be the construction of the Aswan Dam that opened in 1970. This was a technical achievement of huge benefit to the country, but it also enhanced the number of breeding sites for schistosomiasis throughout the year.

In these two examples, both blood transfusion and schistosomiasis treatment were well-meaning and undoubtedly life-saving, however, sadly, the stories of the inadvertent and iatrogenic transmission of HCV seems to have eclipsed the underlying necessary reasons for these treatments in the first place.

depending on the state of the gums. Only about 20% of individuals may develop jaundice, but most (~60–85%) will develop chronic HCV infection, of which 10–70% will develop some form of chronic liver disease, including cirrhosis in ~5–20% of these, with ~1–5% eventually dying of complications from this. The progression to liver failure from HCV, like HAV and HBV, is age-related, with the >40 year olds progressing quickly, which is exacerbated with the drinking of alcohol, male gender, and HIV and/or HBV coinfection.

In addition to the typical clinical features of acute viral hepatitis described above, HCV infection has also been associated with more unusual features, such as unusual skin rashes (see Figure 19.2), unusual behavior of the blood ("cryoglobulinemia" – when abnormal proteins in the blood cause it to solidify and become gel-like in cold temperatures), generalized inflammation of the blood vessels ("systemic vasculitis") that can mimic other autoimmune disorders, and even an association with some types of cancer (non-Hodgkin B-cell lymphoma) in some studies (see Further reading).

The diagnosis of HCV is problematic. In HAV, the IgM test is a reliable indicator of acute infection and should be positive when the patient presents with symptoms. The same can be said for HBsAg and anti-HBc IgM for HBV. However, there is no commercially available anti-HCV IgM test, the antibody test for HCV detects all antibodies (IgG and IgM) but this may not become positive for several months after infection. Also, during this period, most HCV-infected individuals may feel quite well and not seek medical help and will therefore not be tested for HCV. There are some HCV core antigen test kits commercially available, but the preferred test for the diagnosis of acute HCV infection is the HCV RNA polymerase chain reaction (PCR) test that detects the HCV RNA genome. This is usually positive within 2–4 weeks of HCV infection, and sometimes earlier, depending on the sensitivity of the assay used and the host immune control of the HCV replication. Like HAV and HBV, viral culture and EM are not routinely used in HCV diagnosis. Nowadays, in developed countries, HCV RNA testing is used to screen blood donations to avoid missing any HCV-infected and infectious, but still anti-HCV negative donors. To reduce the cost of such screening, individual donations are not screened separately, but in pools of varying size (e.g. samples from 10 to 100 donors may be mixed and tested for HCV RNA, depending on the sensitivity of the PCR test used).

There is currently no vaccine or immunoglobulin available for preventing or for use as PEP for HCV infection. Part of the reason for this is that the anti-HCV antibody, unlike in HAV and HBV, is not able to neutralize and remove the virus, often coexisting with replicating HCV in the blood chronic HCV carriers. Treatment of HCV infection is complex, with many associated drug side-effects. A successful outcome is not guaranteed, and is dependent on many factors, including the "genotype" of the virus, as well as age, alcohol use, and coinfection with the other bloodborne viruses, HIV and HBV.

Hepatitis C has been classified into six major genotypes (1–6). Of these, genotypes 2 and 3 respond best to combination therapy lasting between 24 and 48 weeks, with interferon (of which there are now several formulations, see Box 19.2 and Further reading) and ribavirin (an antiviral drug most effective against RNA viruses), with a possible cure rate of 70–80%, depending on their baseline liver state. Genotype 1 is the most difficult to treat with a response rate of around 50–60%, and genotypes 4, 5 and 6 have an approximate intermediate response rate between 60% and 80%. There are many side-effects with therapy, and the outcome (i.e. successful HCV clearance) is not guaranteed.

Unlike HAV, HBV, and HIV, there is no recommended PEP for HCV exposure. A few studies have shown that treatment of HCV in the acute phase (within about 6 months of exposure and subsequent infection) can be very successful. However, the potentially severe side-effects from the treatment (interferon can muscle pains, headaches, fatigue, depression, weight loss, sleep disturbance, irritability, and a decrease white cell count; ribavirin can cause reversible anemia by destruction of the red cells that may be severe) make it difficult to recommend for every exposure to HCV.

Hepatitis D (HDV)

Hepatitis D is caused by an incomplete or defective member of the Circovirus family, a negative sense, single-stranded, closed, circular DNA virus. It is defective in the sense that it cannot replicate without the presence of HBsAg, which forms the lipid envelope of HDV. It is necessarily distributed in regions where HBV is present, but surprisingly is uncommon in the HBV-endemic countries in Southeast Asia, such as China and the Pacific islands. Relatively high prevalences of HDV are seen in the Middle East and some neighboring countries of the former Soviet Union, as well as in some countries in central Africa and the northwestern parts of South America along the Amazon river basin.

Since HDV is dependent on HBV for its replication, it is transmitted in the same way as HBV, as it cannot cause disease without it. Interestingly though, perinatal HDV infection is unusual. The importance of HDV comes from HBV-HDV coinfection (i.e. acquiring both viruses together), or HBV-HDV superinfection (i.e. being an HBV carrier, first, then becoming infected with HDV later). These two modes of infection have different clinical consequences.

With HBV-HDV coinfection, the symptoms and signs of acute infection are similar to acute HBV infection alone, but can be much more severe, with 2–20% developing fulminant hepatitis with risk of death. However, they are more likely to clear their HBV-HDV coinfection than in HBV-HDV superinfection, where the risk of chronic infection with liver cirrhosis is much higher (70–80%) than with HBV chronic infection alone (15–30%). Often, HDV is suspected when a previously asymptomatic HBV carrier develops acute hepatitis, which may be due to a sudden flare-up of his HBV (i.e. a sudden increase in HBV replication causing increasing levels of ALT, general malaise, and jaundice, occasionally with abdominal pain), or perhaps, superinfection with HDV.

The diagnosis of HDV infection in the presence of HBV is made by testing for anti-HDV total and anti-HDV IgM antibodies. Hepatitis D surface antigen (HDsAg) can also be detected during acute HDV infection. Viral culture, EM and PCR testing are not normally used, except in research settings. In HBV-HDV coinfection anti-HDV IgM and anti-HDV total antibodies are usually detectable throughout infection, and disappear after recovery, eventually leaving no marker of past HDV infection.

In HBV-HDV superinfection, as most cases become chronically infected, anti-HDV IgM and anti-HDV total antibodies generally remain detectable as long as HBV infection persists. In addition, HDsAg and HDV RNA can be detected in these patients. The HBsAg levels fall as HDsAg appears, probably due to utilization by HDV during its replication.

There is no specific treatment for HDV. The treatment for HBV will also treat the HDV. In the same way, immunization against HBV will also protect against HBV-HDV coinfection. However, there is no way to prevent HDV superinfection of an existing HBV carrier, except by education to avoid the risk of HDV through high-risk behaviours, such as injecting drug use and promiscuous sex.

Hepatitis E (HEV)

Hepatitis E is caused by a small (32–34 nm) diameter, nonenveloped single-stranded, positive sense RNA virus (Figure 19.6). It was formerly considered to be a member of the Calicivirus family (same as noroviruses), but it has now been reclassified in its own family *Hepeviridae* (genus Hepevirus). It is endemic in many developing countries worldwide, particularly South (India, Pakistan, Bangladesh) and Southeast Asia (China) and parts of North Africa and the Middle East. There is also a hotspot in Central America. There are four recognized genotypes of the virus of which genotypes (showing slight differences in their genetic sequences) 1 and 2 are found exclusively in humans, and genotypes 3 and 4 can be found in animals, such as pigs. These animal HEV genotypes have also been shown to act as zoonoses, with the potential to transmit to humans (see Further reading).

It is very similar to HAV in terms of its transmission route (fecal–oral and waterborne, e.g. via the ingestion of contaminated poorly cooked food and drink), and presents with a clinical picture similar to all the hepatitis viruses. Its mean incubation period is about 40 days (range 15–60), and it has been found in the stool approximately 4 weeks after infection, remaining detectable (and therefore transmissible) for about 2 weeks thereafter. Like HAV, there is no documented long-term sequelae or chronic infection or carrier status as there is with HBV and HCV. Unlike HAV, there is relatively little person-to-person transmission with HEV, and serious outbreaks often occur during widespread flooding in HEV-endemic areas when

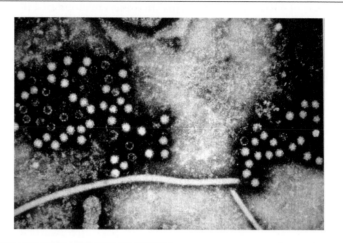

Figure 19.6 This electron micrograph depicts hepatitis E viruses (HEV), provisionally classified as members of the Caliciviridae family. Hepatitis E virus (HEV), the major etiologic agent of enterically transmitted non-A hepatitis worldwide, is a spherical, nonenveloped, single-stranded RNA virus that is approximately 32–34 nm in diameter. Courtesy of the Centers for Disease Control and Prevention; from CDC website: http://phil.cdc.gov/phil/details.asp

HEV-infected sewage and floodwater act to carry the virus over wide areas, exposing large numbers of people to infection. Most cases of HEV in the USA are imported, i.e. occurring in travelers returning from HEV-endemic areas, such as India.

Interestingly, infection with HEV results in a higher mortality in pregnant women, up to 15–25%, which is much higher than the 1–3% for other infected individuals. It is not entirely clear why this is. With HEV, like other hepatitis viruses, mortality increases with age of infection.

Diagnosis is made by detection of anti-HEV IgM with or without total anti-HEV antibodies. As in most cases, IgM antibodies remain detectable for around 2–3 months after acute infection (though in some cases longer than this), and the IgG may last sometime and offer some protection to reinfection while it lasts. As with the other hepatitis viruses, culture and EM are not routinely used in diagnostic testing, though PCR can detect HEV RNA in serum and stool during acute illness and for at least 2 weeks after illness onset. As with the other hepatitis viruses, the rise in ALT more or less coincides with the rise of IgM antibodies, but normalizes well before the IgM disappears (Figure 19.7).

There is an initial viremia after infection, which does not cause any symptoms during the incubation period, which varies between the different viruses (from several weeks to several months). Then there is a sharp rise in the ALT levels, together with the appearance of IgM and IgG (which often appear very closely together, but the rise in IgM is much faster), which trigger the onset of symptoms. During this acute illness phase, the virus is often present and the patient is infectious, i.e. is able to transmit the virus to others. After

Figure 19.7 An overview of the serological and antigenic events surrounding acute viral hepatitis infection

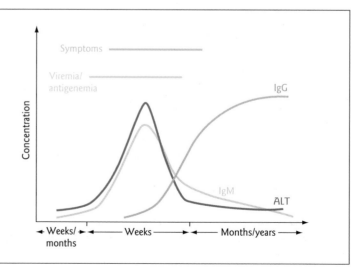

this acute illness period which may last days to weeks, clinical recovery begins with a gradual normalization of the ALT, a waning of the IgM, persistence of the IgG, and disappearance of the viral antigen and nucleic acid (RNA or DNA) from the patient. If there is a carrier state (e.g. in chronic HBV, HCV or HDV infection), there is persistence of the viral antigen and nucleic acid, even in the presence of antibodies, which may last for more than 6 months to many years. Some patients remain carriers for life, if untreated.

There is no specific antiviral therapy for acute HEV infection, though there is a promising vaccine in development. Although most cases of HEV are self-limiting and the mortality is relatively low, a large outbreak in an HEV-endemic country, most of which are classified as low-income, will be a severe public health and economic burden. The availability of a cheap, effective vaccine will be of great benefit to these countries.

Other hepatitis viruses

There are other viruses that were thought to be linked to hepatitis, sometimes referred to as hepatitis viruses F and G. Hepatitis F is now actually nonexistent. It was thought to be a new virus by some Japanese researchers in the early 1990s, but was subsequently not confirmed by others. Hepatitis G (HGV) is also known as GBV, and is often referred to as HGV/GBV. It was discovered in the mid-1990s, and it is still uncertain whether this virus has any role in human disease. It is a member of the Flavivirus family (like hepatitis C). Interestingly, it seems to replicate in lymphocytes and not hepatocytes, so it is unlikely to be a cause of viral hepatitis. More intriguing is that in some studies it has been found to reduce HIV replication in coinfected patients, though this has not been confirmed in all studies. Finally, another virus called transfusion-transmitted virus (TTV) was discovered in the late 1990s. It is a member of the Circovirus family, a nonenveloped, single-stranded DNA virus. It was thought to be a new non-A to E hepatitis virus, as it was discovered in a patient with hepatitis, but now its association with human disease is unclear (see Further reading).

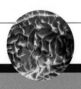

Test yourself

Case study 19.1

A 27-year-old woman, thought to be about 35 weeks pregnant, is brought to the emergency room (ER) after being found collapsed in the street. She is unkempt and dirty and has obviously been living on the street. She seems semiconscious and is incoherent, with a strong smell of alcohol about her. Her skin has a yellow tinge as do the whites of her eyes, and needle tracks can be found on both arms as well as in her groins, where there are several infected abscesses. The admitting doctor makes a quick differential diagnosis of alcohol-induced liver failure with encephalopathy, and admits her for rehydration, a urine drug screen, vitamin B$_1$ (thiamine, essential in alcoholics to reduce the chance of permanent brain damage), and an obstetric review of her pregnancy. The obstetrician is concerned that she may not have had any antenatal checks, orders an urgent rubella, HIV and HBV screen, as well as a fetal ultrasound, as she cannot feel any fetal movement or detect any fetal heart beat. Since she has evidence of intravenous drug use, an HCV screen is also ordered.

The ultrasound shows very small-for-dates fetus, with an erratic heart beat and poor respiratory movements. The drug screen shows evidence of recent heroine use, and the blood alcohol is grossly elevated. There is some suspicion that she was attempting suicide by drug and alcohol overdose. Her blood results come back as positive for HBV (HBsAg and HBeAg positive), HCV (anti-HCV, later confirmed to be HCV RNA positive), and HIV (anti-HIV and p24 Ag positive). Her CD4 count is only 50 cells/μl. Vaginal examination shows evidence of chronic trauma and scarring, probably due to long-term street prostitution, and the decision is made to deliver the baby by cesarean section, both to avoid HIV perinatal transmission as well as concern that the maternal heroine levels may be dangerously suppressing the fetal respiration.

Test yourself

Unfortunately, during the cesarean section, one of the obstetricians sustains a deep scalpel wound, and quickly removes herself from the operative field, squeezes the wound and washes it thoroughly with soap and water, then attends the ER for HIV PEP. Both the mother and baby received triple antiretroviral therapy (ART) for their HIV infection/exposure, with the baby receiving accelerated HBV vaccination and HBIG to prevent HBV transmission also. They are referred to a multidisciplinary HIV/HBV/HCV bloodborne virus specialist clinic, for further long-term followup and testing – particularly for the baby to monitor whether there is any HIV/HBV/HCV infection diagnosed, postnatally. The mother is given specific instructions not to breastfeed the baby and to stop drinking alcohol and to consider entering an alcohol and drug rehabilitation program.

The doctor who sustained the needlestick injury took 28 days of HIV PEP (stavudine, lamivudine, and nelfinavir) with relatively few side-effects, and remained anti-HIV/p24 Ag negative 3 months later. She was already immune to HBV through immunization. Her main concern, besides the HIV, was contracting HCV, as the mother's HCV load came back as 10 million copies/ml. Although the mother's HIV load on admission was about 100 000 copies/ml, it appears that her use of double gloves and immediate washing and taking of the HIV PEP, prevented HIV infection. Unfortunately, she seroconverted for anti-HCV 3 months later and underwent an intensive, high dose interferon treatment regimen to try to cure her HCV infection. Although the virus was HCV genotype 1, she managed to clear her HCV after 24 weeks of interferon therapy alone. However, she could not work during this time, as she felt so unwell, though the hospital allowed her to retain her post until she recovered and finally returned to work, with no long-lasting sequelae.

1. What do you think of the ER doctor's initial diagnosis?
2. What are the concerns for the baby?
3. Do you think the doctor who sustained the needlestick injury was lucky not to have contracted HIV?

Further reading

Any clinical virology textbook should have good summaries of these hepatitis viruses.

Arie J, Zuckerman, et al. (eds). *Principles and Practice of Clinical Virology*, 5th edition. Chichester: Wiley, 2004

Gerald L, Mandell JE, Bennett RD (eds). *Principles and Practice of Infectious Diseases*, 6th edition. Edinburgh: Churchill Livingstone, 2004

Some interesting papers on specific aspects of viral hepatitis

Shepard CW, Finelli L, Alter MJ. Global epidemiology of hepatitis C virus infection. *Lancet Infect Dis* 2005;5(9):558–567

Shepard CW, Finelli L, Fiore AE, Bell BP. Epidemiology of hepatitis B and hepatitis B virus infection in United States children. *Pediatr Infect Dis J* 2005;24(9):755–760

Shepard CW, Simard EP, Finelli L, Fiore AE, Bell BP. Hepatitis B virus infection: epidemiology and vaccination. *Epidemiol Rev* 2006;28:112–125

Stapleton JT. GB virus type C/hepatitis G virus. *Semin Liver Dis* 2003;23(2):137–148

US Public Health Service. Updated US Public Health Service Guidelines for the Management of Occupational Exposures to HBV, HCV, and HIV and Recommendations for Postexposure Prophylaxis. *MMWR Recomm Rep* 2001 Jun 29;50(RR-11):1–52

Useful websites

CDC. Viral Hepatitis. http://www.cdc.gov/ncidod/diseases/hepatitis/slideset/index.htm

Health Protection Agency, UK. Topics A–Z. All aspects of viral hepatitis. http://www.hpa.org.uk/topics/index_i.htm

WHO. Immunization Safety. Viral Hepatitis Prevention Board. Prevention of viral hepatitis. http://www.who.int/immunization_safety/safety_quality/vhpb/en/

Chapter 20
Influenza

J.W. Tang, P.K.S. Chan

Introduction
Epidemiology
Classification and nomenclature
  The virus
  Antigenic variation

Transmission
Clinical features
Laboratory diagnosis
Antivirals
Vaccines
Avian influenza A(H5N1)

Introduction

Influenza epidemics have been reported as early as during the times of ancient Greece and Rome, making influenza one of the oldest infections known to man. It is one of the most common human viral infections and one of the most infectious human respiratory viruses. The changing nature of the virus gives rise to seasonal epidemics causing significant health and economic impact to humans. For this reason, it requires continuous surveillance worldwide by the World Health Organization (WHO). Antivirals are available for prophylactic and therapeutic uses. However, the therapeutic window is narrow and vaccination remains the mainstay of control for influenza. The efficacy of the vaccine depends on the matching between vaccine components and the circulating strains. When a new strain has successfully adapted to human-to-human transmission, a pandemic may occur, with subsequent substantial health and economic impact. This chapter introduces various aspects of this important pathogen and presents a hypothetical (but not unrealistic) pandemic influenza case scenario (see "Test yourself" section).

Epidemiology

Influenza viruses are endemic in wild birds, particularly waterfowl, in which it replicates, often asymptomatically, and is shed in the droppings, from where it can infect other birds. Therefore, in the bird population, multiple strains of the virus can mix and infect multiple avian hosts. The transmission of this virus to man is commonly believed to involve the infection of an intermediate, nonavian, domesticated animal, such as the pig, before it crosses over into man, possibly undergoing further host-adaptive mutations on the way. Sometimes the virus will transmit to man without any noticeable human-specific adaptive mutations, such as can be seen in the current cases of avian H5N1 influenza that have been occurring since the end of 2003. This natural history defines influenza as a zoonosis (i.e. a microbe which infects man from an animal reservoir). All three of these hosts (wild birds, domesticated animals, and humans) may well live close together, such as in the traditional farms that can still be found in China. This is why China has often been considered the origin or epicenter of new influenza strains.

In the USA, on average, each year, 5–20% of the population is infected with seasonal influenza, with more than 200 000 people being hospitalized for influenza-related complications, and about 36 000 deaths. The more vulnerable members of the population, such as the elderly, the very young, and those with chronic medical problems, are at highest risk for serious illness or dying from influenza-related illness. Unfortunately, because of its wide distribution in both animal and human hosts, unlike smallpox, polio and measles where man is the only host, it is unlikely that influenza will ever be eradicated.

Classification and nomenclature

Influenza viruses are classified into three genera – **influenza A, B, and C** – based on the antigenic differences of nucleoprotein and matrix protein. Influenza C only causes trivial infections and is not regarded as clinically important. Both influenza A and B are clinically important and associated with substantial health and economic burden. Influenza A viruses are further divided into subtypes based on the antigenic differences found in its surface or envelope glycoproteins hemagglutinin (H) and neuraminidase (N). So far, 16 H and 9 N subtypes have been identified.

Influenza A viruses have much wider host specificities. In addition to the humans, birds, and pigs that can be infected, it can also infect dogs, cats, whales, and seals. Influenza B infection is mainly restricted to humans, though the virus has been isolated from seals.

The nomenclature system for influenza viruses takes into consideration the host of origin, location, and year of first isolation, e.g. A/goose/Guangdong/1/96(H5N1) refers to the influenza "A" virus isolated from a "goose" in "Guangdong" and belonging to subtype "H5N1" which was the first isolate collected in 1996. When the animal species is not specified, e.g. A/New Caledonia/20/99(H1N1), it implies the virus was isolated from human.

The virus

Influenza viruses are classified under the family Orthomyxoviridae. The virion is an 80–120 nm spherical pleomorphic (i.e. of multiple shapes and sizes), enveloped particle (Figure 20.1).

Influenza virus contains single-stranded, negative-sense (i.e. anti-mRNA sense), RNA in eight separate segments, with each segment closely associated with multiple nucleoproteins forming ribonucleoprotein complexes. The ribonucleoprotein complexes are surrounded by a layer of matrix protein which forms the core of the virion. The external layer or envelope is inserted with approximately 500 spike-like projections formed by the glycoproteins hemagglutinin (H) and neuraminidase (N) (Figures 20.2 and 20.3).

Antigenic variation

There are two ways that influenza viruses can change their antigenic properties, and therefore escape their recognition by the human immune system. The first one is known as "antigenic drift" that may result in more serious seasonal epidemics occurring around the world, perhaps every few years. This is because any previous existing immunity may only partially protect the people against this new strain. The second one is "antigenic shift" that results in severe outbreaks, worldwide (i.e. a pandemic) due to the complete absence of any partial pre-existing immunity in the human population to this completely new influenza strain. So far

Figure 20.1 Electron micrograph of influenza viruses. Influenza viruses are pleomorphic particles of sizes ranging from 80 to 120 nm in diameter. The appearance of different genera, i.e. influenza A, B, and C, or different subtypes, e.g. H3N2, H1N1, and H5N1, are indistinguishable from each other. The outer covering layer appearing as a fringe is the envelope of the virus, comprising two important surface glycoproteins, the hemagglutinin (H) and the neuraminidase (N). These proteins are critical in determining the characteristics of the virus, and are used for classifying the different subtypes. Image courtesy of the Department of Microbiology, The Chinese University of Hong Kong

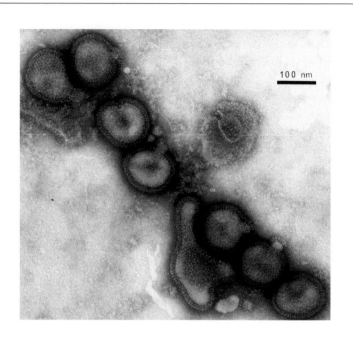

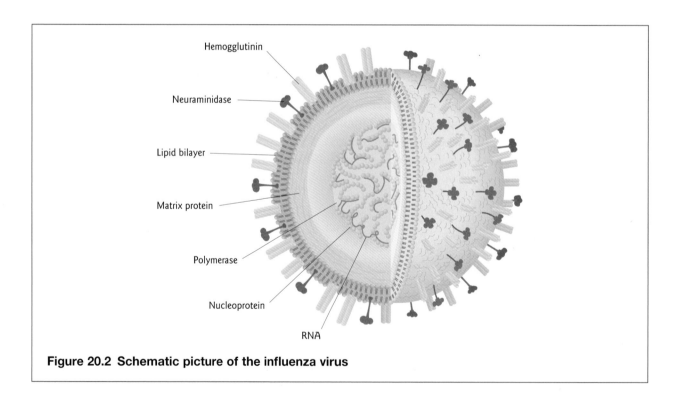

Figure 20.2 Schematic picture of the influenza virus

this has occurred three times in the last 100 years: 1918, 1957, and 1968. Some scientists believe that a new influenza pandemic is long overdue already.

The underlying basis for antigenic drift originates from minor changes to the amino acid sequences of the H and N glycoproteins as a result of mutations in viral genome generated during normal viral replication. When mutations involving critical positions occur, it may render the human immunity accumulated from exposure to previous strains less protective. When significant antigenic drift has accumulated, the number of persons

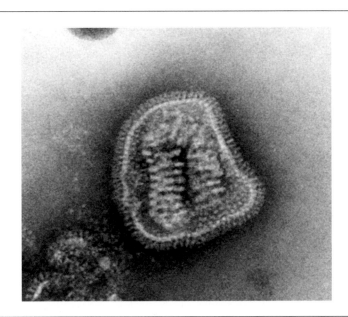

Figure 20.3 Ultrastructure of an influenza virion. This magnified electron micrograph of a single influenza virion shows several aspects of its ultrastructure very clearly, including its surface glycoproteins (hemagglutinin and neuraminidase), lipid bilayer, matrix protein, and segmented ribonucleoprotein. Provided by Dr Erskine L. Palmer and Dr M. L. Martin. Courtesy of the Centers for Disease Control and Prevention; from CDC website: http://phil.cdc.gov/phil/details.asp

infected and their severity of illness tends to increase. Significant antigenic drifts may occur every few years, and are reflected as a more serious (more people becoming sick or dying) and longer-lasting seasonal epidemic. This may result in a change in the following season's WHO seasonal influenza vaccine's composition.

The more significant antigenic shift results from an introduction of a new influenza subtype to humans. Of the 16 H and nine N subtypes that exist in nature, so far, only, a few e.g. A(H3N2) and A(H1N1), are currently adapted to infecting and circulating among humans. Since all subtypes of influenza A are found in aquatic birds, they serve as a reservoir for the influenza gene pool and a source of recombination of influenza viral RNA segments derived from different influenza subtypes (Figure 20.4). If a new reassortment results in a completely new influenza strain that can adapt to efficient human-to-human transmission, and for which there is no pre-existing immunity, a pandemic may occur. Since there will be no protection from existing human immune systems, this new virus will spread rapidly and globally, and often with high morbidity (the number of people who become sick) and mortality (the number of people who die). Such influenza pandemics have occurred in 1918 – the "Spanish flu" caused by influenza A(H1N1); 1957 – the "Asian flu" caused by influenza A(H2N2); and 1968 – the "Hong Kong flu" caused by influenza A(H3N2).

In addition, recent research has shown that pure avian influenza strains have been infecting humans for some years now, including influenzas A(H9N2), A(H7N7), and A(H5N1). Also, research has shown that the original 1918 influenza A(H1N1) was also probably a purely avian influenza virus that transmitted to humans with no specific adaptations, i.e. the virus isolated from infected humans and birds was virtually identical (see Further reading).

Transmission

Influenza is mainly transmitted by the aerosol route via droplets. These infectious droplets are generated by coughing and sneezing, and therefore the infectivity of an infected person is related to the intensity of upper respiratory tract symptoms. Since droplets have a certain weight, they cannot go too far. In practice, the potential infectious zone is taken as 1 m, though there are reports in the literature of occasional more long-distance transmission. The virus can survive in hands and fomites (inanimate objects, such as toys, utensils, table tops, etc.) for a considerable period of time (several hours, even days when contained in biological material, such as sputum and saliva). These contaminated objects can be an important source of indirect transmission. The infectious period following the onset of illness varies with age. Young children with primary infection shed a higher titer of viruses, and for a longer period of around 10 days. There is some evidence that influenza

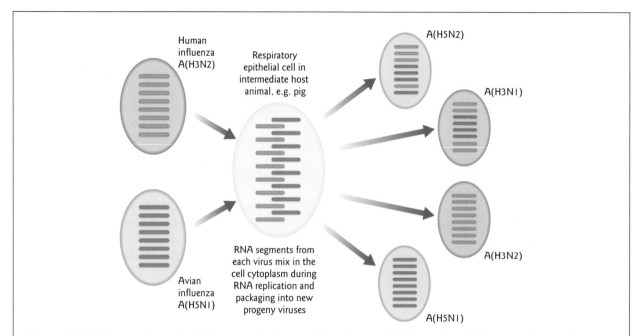

Figure 20.4 Reassortment of influenza A viruses. The characteristics of an influenza virus are determined by the amino acids coded by the nucleic acid sequences in the eight genetic segments. If two different influenza viruses infect an individual host at the same time, their RNA segments may mix and reassort in a new combination in any new progeny viruses. A wide variety of possible new reassorted progeny viruses can therefore be generated. If one of these reassorted viruses can be transmitted efficiently between humans then an influenza pandemic may occur

may be infectious for up to 1 day before the onset of symptoms in some people, which makes the identification of infectious individuals, and therefore infection control, more problematic (see Further reading).

Clinical features

Influenza has an incubation period of around 2–4 days. The clinical course ranges from a mild upper respiratory tract illness to a severe, even fatal pneumonia. The classical presentations are often in adults, though this is less common and symptoms may be more atypical in young children and the elderly. These symptoms include an abrupt onset of high fever, chills, headache, dry cough, myalgia, and anorexia (loss of appetite), with upper respiratory symptoms such as rhinorrhoea, nasal congestion, and sore throat. The illness may last for 1–2 weeks in healthy adults.

Pneumonia, either primary viral or secondary due to bacterial infections (particularly *Staphylococcus aureus*, *Streptococcus pneumoniae*, and *Haemophilus influenzae*), is the most common complication seen in the high risk group, including elderly, patients with chronic illnesses (e.g. patients on renal dialysis, patients with diabetes, asthma, chronic obstructive pulmonary – COPD, and ischemic heart disease), immune suppression, and pregnant women. In particular, the exacerbation of pre-existing pulmonary conditions (e.g. asthma, COPD, and cystic fibrosis) is an important cause of hospitalization for influenza. Otitis media is a common complication seen in young children.

Less common complications include: myositis (muscle tissue inflammation), rhabdomyolysis (muscle tissue breakdown), myocarditis and pericarditis (inflammation of the heart muscle and its covering membrane – see Chapter 9), and encephalopathy (see Chapter 10). Reye's syndrome is seen mainly in children and is characterized by encephalopathy and fatty liver degeneration. It is a rare condition preceded by a number of viral infections including influenza. It has been quite strongly associated with the use of aspirin in children with influenza, and for this reason, the use of aspirin is contraindicated in children under the age of 16 years.

Laboratory diagnosis

A number of other respiratory infections can mimic the presentations of influenza. Diagnosis solely based on signs and symptoms is unreliable, the sudden onset and muscle aches is quite distinctive for influenza infection. Although the use of the term "influenza-like illness" is acceptable for surveillance purposes, a specific diagnosis for influenza requires laboratory testing and confirmation.

There are three commonly used approaches to detect influenza viruses. The first of these is virus isolation, in which the clinical sample is inoculated into a cell culture system consisting of a monkey kidney-derived cell monolayer grown on the side of a glass tube (Figure 20.5). This cell culture tube is then examined regularly (daily or every other day) under a light microscope for a characteristic influenza viral cytopathic effect (CPE – a distinctive pattern of cell death) in the cell monolayer. Virus isolation is sensitive but may take 5–10 days before any characteristic CPE is seen.

The second option is by using direct detection methods, which use influenza virus-specific antibodies to stain virus-infected cells collected in the clinical specimen (e.g. a nasopharyngeal aspirate – NPA, a saline wash of the nose that contains infected cells). Infected cells can be seen under an ultraviolet (UV) light microscope as they light up with a (usually) green fluorescence under UV light (Figure 20.6). The main advantage of direct detection is that it is quick, with results being available within a few hours – or even less than 15 minutes for some rapid test kits. Since there is no prior amplification in this direct detection approach, the sensitivity relies heavily on the quality of the clinical specimen (i.e. how many infected cells can be collected in the NPA).

The third approach is by using molecular amplification and detection, which applies molecular techniques such as the polymerase chain reaction (PCR) to amplify the viral RNA (Figures 20.7 and 20.8). This is a highly sensitive and highly skilled technique that requires well trained and experienced laboratory workers in order to minimize the possibility of cross-contamination among different specimens.

Antivirals

Two classes of antiviral agents are available for treating influenza. The M2 ion channel blockers amantadine (Symmetrel, Lysovir, Symadine) and rimantadine (Flumadine) are the first generation anti-influenza agents. These compounds interfere with the pH-dependent uncoating of viral genome, and induce a premature

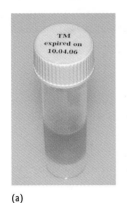
(a)
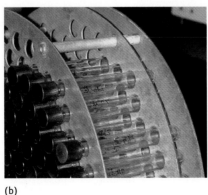
(b)
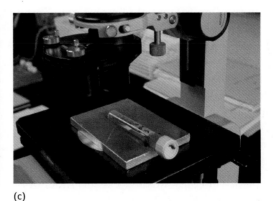
(c)

Figure 20.5 Viral isolation involves the collection of a clinical sample in special virus transport medium (pink liquid, a), inoculation into and incubation with a permissive cell monolayer, e.g. Madin-Darby canine kidney (MDCK) cells for growing influenza virus (b), then examining them regularly under a light microscope (c) for a characteristic influenza viral cytopathic effect (CPE). Images courtesy of the Department of Microbiology, The Chinese University of Hong Kong

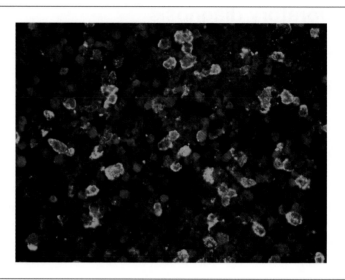

Figure 20.6 Immunofluorescence of influenza virus antigen (green color) using an influenza-specific monoclonal antibody-based direct detection test. Image courtesy of the Department of Microbiology, The Chinese University of Hong Kong

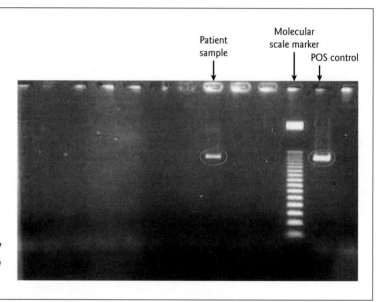

Figure 20.7 Influenza virus detection using the polymerase chain reaction (PCR) to amplify the viral RNA (to its complementary DNA). The older form of this assay uses gel electrophoresis to reveal the presence of any PCR products. The red circles show that the PCR product bands of the positive control and the patient sample have traveled the same distance from the top of the gel, meaning that they are the same size (molecular weight) and therefore represent the same influenza virus genome fragment. Images courtesy of the Department of Microbiology, The Chinese University of Hong Kong

conformational change of the H protein. These two steps are essential in the virus replication cycle. Amantadine and rimantadine are effective against influenza A but not against influenza B since the M2 protein is not present in the latter.

Central nervous system disturbances and gastrointestinal upset are the two most commonly observed adverse effects of M2 channel blockers. Patients may experience anxiety, insomnia, dizziness, headache, and difficulty in concentrating. Patients should be warned against driving or operating dangerous machines while taking these drugs. Dosage adjustment is required for the elderly or those with poor renal function. More severe central nervous system adverse events may occur in overdose.

Zanamivir (Relenza) and oseltamivir (Tamiflu) are newer anti-influenza agents. These compounds are neuraminidase inhibitors (NAIs). By inhibiting the normal function of the viral neuraminidase (N), they interfere with the normal release of progeny viruses from infected cells. The released virions form aggregates, further decreasing their efficiency in spreading to other parts of the respiratory tract. Neuraminidase inhibitors are effective against both influenzas A and B.

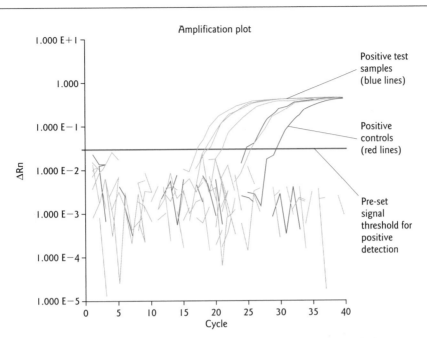

Figure 20.8 More modern PCR techniques can now show the presence of the PCR product as the PCR reaction proceeds in "real-time." Such real-time PCR assays attach a specific fluorescent signal molecule to the strands of any target RNA present in the sample, so that, as the number of amplified target RNA (as complementary DNA) molecules increase, so does strength of this fluorescent signal. The more target molecules that are present in the sample to start with, the earlier the fluorescent signal reaches a pre-defined threshold fluorescent level signifying a positive detection result. Hence, with the appropriate calibration controls, it is also relatively easy to quantify the mount of viral genome in the original clinical sample using real-time PCR. Since the real-time PCR shows the presence or absence of the PCR product during the PCR reaction, there is no need for a second "gel electrophoresis" detection step afterwards, so real-time PCR is also faster than the older "conventional" PCR methods. Images courtesy of the Department of Microbiology, The Chinese University of Hong Kong

Neuraminidase inhibitors have a better safety profile than M2 channel blockers. Oseltamivir is available, orally, either as a capsule or liquid suspension. Both forms are well tolerated. Mild nausea and vomiting are the most frequent adverse effects seen in a small proportion of patients, which can be minimized somewhat by taking the drug with food. Dosage adjustments are required if there are kidney problems.

Zanamivir is available as orally inhaled powder. The most notable adverse effect is the induction of bronchospasm (i.e. a sudden onset of shortness of breath due to constriction of the upper airways) in patients with underlying airway disease, such as asthma and COPD. Hence, zanamivir is not recommended for these patients, though if the drug has to be used, a fast acting bronchodilator (to rapidly dilate or open up the airways) should be at hand.

In general, like most antivirals, anti-influenza agents should be started within 48 hours of illness onset to achieve maximum treatment efficacy. Prophylactic use of anti-influenza agents (e.g. oseltamivir) may be considered when the risk of exposure is high (e.g. frontline healthcare workers). Due to recent data on the widespread prevalence of amantadine resistance in circulating influenza viruses in the USA and elsewhere, amantadine and rimantadine were not recommended by the Centers for Disease Control and Prevention (CDC: http://www.cdc.gov/flu/han011406.htm) for influenza prophylaxis and/or treatment during the 2005/2006 US influenza season (see Further reading).

Vaccines

The first generation of influenza vaccine was prepared by inactivating whole viruses harvested from embryonated chicken eggs. Due to excessive local reactions at injection sites and more systemic side-effects associated with these "whole-virus" vaccines in 1960s, they were later replaced by so-called "split-virus" vaccines. These vaccines are composed of specific viral proteins selected and purified from disrupted whole virus particles. Since the 1980s, influenza vaccines have been further purified to contain mainly just the surface glycoproteins H and N with a small, nonspecified amount of the viral core proteins. These "subunit" vaccines have a much better safety profile, though they are less immunogenic than the whole virus vaccines. Hence such split-virus and subunit vaccines require "adjuvants," various inert chemicals, to be added to enhance the immunogenicity of these vaccines. Most recently, in the 2000s, a live, attenuated (weakened) influenza vaccine has been developed and licensed in the USA and elsewhere though most of the currently used influenza vaccines are subunit vaccines (Box 20.1).

The usual annual, seasonal influenza vaccines are trivalent and are composed of two influenza A subtypes (currently H1N1 and H3N2) and one influenza B subtype. To achieve the maximum protective effect, the strains selected as these vaccine components should match with the current circulating strains. This matching of strains is presently coordinated by the WHO, which has established an international surveillance network to continuously monitor and collect circulating influenza strains from different parts of the world. In February and September each year, for both northern and southern hemispheres, respectively, the WHO

Box 20.1 A summary of the types of influenza vaccine available

Inactivated vaccines

Inactivated vaccines consist of either: whole virus (containing intact, inactivated virus), subvirion or split-product vaccine (containing purified virus disrupted with detergents) and subunit or surface antigen vaccines (containing purified hemaglutinin and neuraminidase glycoproteins, only). The seasonal influenza vaccine is normally a trivalent vaccine, containing two strains of influenza A and one of influenza B. The final strains used are decided, annually, by the WHO and its surveillance teams, to ensure that the most prevalent influenza strains are selected to maximize the vaccine-induced protection.

Live vaccines

Although inactivated influenza vaccines are still recommended by the WHO, they suffer from certain disadvantages, including a poor induction of mucosal IgA antibody and cell-mediated responses, possibly a lower immunogenicity and efficacy in the elderly, and require a painful intramuscular injection – very uncomfortable for young children.

A live attenuated influenza vaccine has now been licensed in the USA and other parts of the world, which can be administered intranasally using a

spray. This influenza vaccine virus strain was developed using the technique of cold-adaptation (the virus was effectively trained to grow optimally at low temperatures (i.e. lower than human body temperature)) to attenuate the virus, so that it cannot replicate efficiently in humans. This resulted in the production of two master strains for influenza A (A/Ann Arbor/6/60-H2N2) and B (B/Ann Arbor/1/66). These master strains possess genes which have been attenuated through cold passage in primary chick kidney cells to grow to a maximum titer at 25°C. The vaccine strain is composed of a genetic reassortment between wild-type virus and these master donor strains, with the genes for hemagglutinin and neuraminidase originating from the wild-type virus, but with the attenuated internal genes coming from these cold-adapted master donor strains. The advantages of a live vaccine include: allowing vaccine virus replication in the areas that are most effective in preventing infection, i.e. the mucosal barriers of the upper respiratory airways, the eliciting of a specific protective immune response as well as producing a longer-lasting and perhaps broader immunity – important, especially in the elderly population.

announces the most appropriate influenza A and B strains to be incorporated into the seasonal influenza vaccine for the coming season. Out of the 10 seasons from 1987 to 1997, a complete match for all three strains was achieved in five seasons.

Influenza vaccination is still the cornerstone of the WHO's international program to reduce the annual influenza mortality and morbidity. For a good match between the vaccine components and the circulating strains, influenza vaccines can offer 70–90% protection against clinical disease in healthy adults, and reduce overall mortality by 39–75% among elderly people (see Further reading). The target groups for vaccination as recommended by the CDC are shown in Box 20.2. Note that the recommendations for the use of the inactivated and live-attenuated vaccines are different. Influenza vaccination during pregnancy is safe and is recommended to protect the mother from the potentially more severe course of influenza illness during pregnancy, as well as for protecting the infant during the first months of life.

Box 20.2 Recommendations for the use of seasonal (inactivated) WHO influenza vaccine (recommendations as of January 22, 2008, adapted from the CDC's website at: http://www.cdc.gov/flu/about/qa/flushot.htm)

Anyone who wants to reduce their chances of getting the flu can be vaccinated. However, certain people should get vaccinated each year. They are either people who are at high risk of having serious flu complications or people who live with or care for those at high risk for serious complications. During flu seasons when vaccine supplies are limited or delayed, the Advisory Committee on Immunization Practices (ACIP) makes recommendations regarding priority groups for vaccination.

People who should get vaccinated each year are those at high risk for complications from the flu, including:

- Children aged 6 months until their 5th birthday
- Pregnant women
- People ≥50 years old
- People of any age with chronic medical conditions (e.g. asthma, diabetes, or heart disease)
- People living in long-stay facilities, e.g. residential and nursing homes
- People who live with or care for those at high risk for complications from flu, including:
  - household contacts of persons at high risk for complications from the flu (see above)
  - household contacts and out-of-home caregivers of children less than 6 months of age (these children are too young to be vaccinated)
- healthcare workers.

Persons who should NOT be vaccinated with the live-attenuated influenza vaccine (recommendations as of January 22, 2008, adapted from the CDC's website at: http://www.cdc.gov/flu/about/qa/nasalspray.htm)

- Children <2 years of age
- People ≥50 years old
- People with a medical condition that places them at high risk for complications from influenza, including:
  - those with chronic heart or lung disease, such as asthma or reactive airways disease
  - those with medical conditions such as diabetes or kidney failure
  - those with illnesses that weaken the immune system
  - those who take medications that can weaken the immune system
- Children <5 years old with a history of recurrent wheezing
- Children or adolescents taking aspirin
- People with a history of Guillain–Barré syndrome (a rare disorder of the nervous system)
- Pregnant women
- People with a severe allergy to chicken eggs or any of the nasal spray vaccine components.

Avian influenza A(H5N1)

Unlike influenza B and C, influenza A viruses have a unique ability to generate new strains with pandemic potential. This phenomenon is mainly due to the unique ecology and genetic composition of influenza A viruses. Whilst influenza A viruses are found in a wide variety of animal species, a tight species barrier exists in nature which usually prevents cross-species transmission. All the 16 H and 9 N subtypes of influenza known to date are found in aquatic and migratory bird species, whereas only a few influenza subtypes (including H1, H2, H3, N1, N2) have successfully established infection and efficient transmission in humans. The natural cross-species barrier protects humans from infection with novel influenza subtypes to which the human immune system is naïve. However, this barrier is not insurmountable.

One possible way for a pre-existing avian influenza strain to cross the species barrier is to acquire the property of human influenza strains through genetic reassortment (Figure 20.4). Provided that the newly reassorted virus can maintain an efficient human-to-human transmission chain, a pandemic may occur. The pandemics that occurred in 1957 and 1968 were the results of such reassortment between pre-existing human and avian viruses, whereas the 1918 H1N1 pandemic is thought to be a result of direct transmission of an avian virus to humans without prior reassortment within an intermediate host.

Until 1997, it was thought that reassortment in an intermediate host is a prerequisite for an avian virus to infect humans. However, direct transmission of influenza A(H5N1) virus infection from chicken to human was documented for the first time in Hong Kong in 1997 (Figure 20.9).

Eighteen people were infected with influenza A(H5N1) virus with six deaths. Subsequent sero-epidemiological studies showed that although human-to-human transmission may have occurred, the efficiency was very low. Subsequently, incidences of direct transmission of purely avian influenza virus to humans continued to occur sporadically. In 2003, a family living in Hong Kong was infected with influenza A(H5N1) and two members died. In 1999 and 2003, three isolated cases of human infection with avian influenza A(H9N2) were identified. All of these infections were mild and self-limiting. In 2003, subsequent to a large poultry outbreak of influenza A(H7N7) in the Netherlands, 89 cases of human infection were identified. Most patients presented with conjunctivitis and some had influenza-like illness. One person died from this influenza A(H7N7) outbreak. In 2004, two cases of human infection with H7N3 were detected in British Columbia, during the surveillance that was performed, following a similar large poultry outbreak.

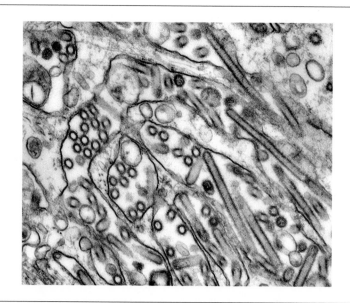

Figure 20.9 A colorized transmission electron micrograph of avian influenza A(H5N1) viruses (gold) grown in MDCK cells (green). Provided by Cynthia Goldsmith, Jacqueline Katz, and Sherif R. Zaki. Courtesy of the Centers for Disease Control and Prevention; from CDC website: http://phil.cdc.gov/phil/details.asp

Table 20.1 Summary of the reported incidences of transmission of an avian influenza virus to humans

Date	Country	Event
1997, May–December	Hong Kong SAR, China	Avian H5N1 (highly pathogenic): caused 18 human infections, six died, no efficient person-to-person transmission, 1.5 million chickens (entire stock) culled in Hong Kong
1999, March	Hong Kong SAR, China	Avian H9N2 (not highly pathogenic): caused mild illness in two children
2003, February	Fujian and Hong Kong SAR, China	Avian H5N1 (highly pathogenic, but different from Hong Kong 1997 strain): caused illness in a family of five travelling between Fujian and Hong Kong SAR in China, two infected, one died, no evidence of person-to-person transmission
2003, February	The Netherlands	Avian H7N7 (highly pathogenic): killed one vet, caused mild illness in 83 people, 30 million birds culled
2003, November	Hong Kong SAR, China	Avian H9N2 (not highly pathogenic): again, caused mild illness in one case
2004, February	British Columbia, Canada	Avian H7N3 (not highly pathogenic): evidence of infection in two human cases
2004, January	Vietnam	Avian H5N1 (highly pathogenic): isolated from severely ill human cases – around the beginning of the multiple H5N1 human cases, continuing to the present day

The infections in humans were again mostly mild with conjunctivitis and an influenza-like illness (see Table 20.1 for a summary of these events and others).

A large series of outbreaks in poultry of highly pathogenic avian influenza A(H5N1) started in late 2003. It soon swept across poultry populations in Asia, and subsequently involved Europe and Africa. The highly pathogenic avian influenza A(H5N1) has now established an ecological niche in Asia and is evolving continuously. Outbreaks continued to recur in many countries despite aggressive control measures and the culling of more than 100 million poultry.

Hundreds of human H5N1 infections have been confirmed since late 2003, with a high mortality rate of around 50%. Most human cases were linked to a contact with infected poultry. Sporadic human-to-human transmission events, probably resulting from close contact, have also been reported. The number of human avian influenza A(H5N1) cases and a timeline of these infections to date, are accessible from this WHO website: http://www.who.int/csr/disease/avian_influenza/country/en/

This series of outbreaks of highly pathogenic avian influenza A(H5N1) in birds and humans represents the largest recorded in history. It is believed by some that another influenza pandemic is imminent, though this may still not necessarily be due to influenza A(H5N1) – it is impossible to predict exactly which virus will cause the next pandemic – if or when it comes. The WHO uses a series of six phases of pandemic alert as a system for informing the world of the seriousness of the threat, and of the need to launch progressively more intense preparedness activities (Table 20.2). The WHO recommends that every country should have a pandemic plan to minimize the disease burden and economic loss should another influenza pandemic occur.

Table 20.2 Phases of pandemic alert used by the World Health Organization (adapted from WHO website: http://www.who.int/csr/disease/avian_influenza/phase/en/index.html)

Phase	Situation		Colour code
1	Interpandemic phase	Low risk of human cases	Green
2	New virus in animals, no human cases	Higher risk of human cases	Green
3	Pandemic alert	No or very limited human-to-human transmission	Yellow
4	New virus causes human cases	Evidence of increased human-to-human transmission	Yellow
4	New virus causes human cases	Evidence of significant human-to-human transmission	Orange
6	Pandemic	Efficient and sustained human-to-human transmission	Red

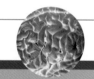

Test yourself

Case study 20.1

Week 1: Mr Li kept a small farm, just outside, south of Guangzhou, the capital of Guangdong province in China. He farmed pigs, ducks, and chickens, which he took to the local live market two to three times a week to sell to feed his family. Despite all the stories about avian H5N1 influenza in the media, his animals were well with no signs of disease.

1. Why has southern China (mainly Guangdong and its surrounding regions) been hypothesized to be the "epicenter of new influenza viruses"?

One day, there was a fierce typhoon which swept far inland, almost reaching the outskirts of Guangzhou itself. The next morning, there were many dead birds – which looked like geese – on his land and that of his neighbors. They thought they had been killed by the typhoon, so they collected them and buried them in a large pit, without much thought. Within a few days, however, some of the ducks and chickens became sick and died, and Mr Li himself was feeling ill. He had a wife and a young son, aged 5 years, who regularly played with the chickens and ducks. His young son also became ill with a high fever and a cough. Within a day or so, his wife became sick, with fever and respiratory problems. Mr Li became concerned about avian influenza – maybe this is what killed the geese, rather than the typhoon? He took his family to the local hospital, where he found many of his neighbors and other local farmers waiting to be seen. There were many other patients there, who had been caught and injured in the typhoon. The doctors and nurses were obviously treating these trauma patients with broken bones and bleeding wounds with a higher priority than the patients with "flu-like" symptoms, not uncommon in the late autumn/early winter season. Very few people were wearing any protective equipment, such as masks, gloves, gowns, or eye protection.

2. What do you think of Mr Li's actions? Do you think he did the right thing in this current climate of heightened, post-SARS (severe acute respiratory syndrome) public awareness of a possible influenza pandemic? Were his actions right in terms of infection control and public health?

Week 2: Over the following few days, it became clear that the healthcare workers at this and other local hospitals in the typhoon-affected areas were becoming sick with some sort of respiratory infection. Their families were also becoming ill. Some of the first patients that attended these hospitals soon after the typhoon had struck were now on the intensive care unit being ventilated as they had developed severe respiratory distress. The same week, there were reports of respiratory illness in clusters of people in Hong Kong, who turned out to be close relatives of some of these farmers. Back-tracing their steps, it was found that fellow passengers on the cross-border train between China and Hong Kong were also some of these people in the Hong Kong clusters now becoming sick with respiratory symptoms.

3. What do you think of the consequences of Mr Li's visit to the hospital now? What would you have done in the same situation? How could this situation have been avoided?

Week 3: It became clear that some of the infected passengers on the cross-border train had been airline staff on the way to Hong Kong International Airport. Some of these staff became ill the next day, having flown to destinations as widespread as India, Australia, Europe, the Americas, and Africa. Having served many of the passengers on these plane flights, it is likely that some of them would have been infected and carried the infection home to their families, and to their work colleagues. However, this was late autumn/early winter in the northern hemisphere and many people were suffering from seasonal coughs and colds.

4. What do you think of the term "influenza-like illness" or "ILI" for short? Is this a helpful term? How many infectious agents can give rise to such an illness (after reading this textbook, you should be able to name at least ten)? What consequences does this have for public health surveillance?

Week 4 and onwards: There were reports of clusters of people dying from a mysterious, severe respiratory illness in Guangdong and Hong Kong, as well as in places as far apart as India, Australia, the UK, Kenya, the USA, and Brazil. ProMed (http://www.promedmail.org), the international email-based alert system, was publishing reports of these clusters and the WHO now realized that this was more than a severe seasonal influenza season. In some case clusters, the mortality had reached 30%, even in the young healthy adults that had been admitted to hospital – and this included a large proportion of healthcare workers, as well as their patients. The emerging pathology was that of a severe, rapidly progressive, hemorrhagic viral pneumonia, with very little accompanying secondary bacterial infection. The WHO pandemic plan was activated and its international network of laboratories began re-examining their influenza A isolates that they had been received over the last 4 weeks. Although influenza A(H1N1) had been the reported identity of this virus, this new virus appeared to be more virulent in humans *in vivo*, despite it giving similar *in vitro* or animal culture, serological and immunofluorescent test results as the less virulent circulating seasonal influenza A(H1N1) strain. Research teams worldwide began to examine the pathogenesis of this new virus (tentatively called "influenza A(H1N1)P" – "P" for "Pandemic") for its unique virulence *in vivo*, in humans. However, this proved extremely difficult, as the mechanisms of the viral pathogenicity could only be examined in patients already infected with the virus, as no obvious virulence factors could be found in *in vitro* or animal experiments. Likewise antiviral and vaccine research was also difficult for the same reason. Existing anti-influenza drugs such as amantadine (of the adamantane family of anti-influenza drugs) and oseltamivir (of the neuraminidase inhibitor anti-influenza drugs) proved to be ineffective, and there was no protective effect from the currently used WHO influenza vaccine from the H1N1 component. Early results from the direct sequencing of the virus obtained from clinical samples seemed to suggest some unique mutations in the internal genes, which could explain its apparent seasonal influenza A(H1N1) identity from the standard diagnostic tests. Such tests could not distinguish the pandemic strain A(H1N1)P from the seasonal strain A(H1N1), nor reveal the devastating virulence of A(H1N1)P in humans, where the reported mortality, worldwide, was now approaching approximately 50% across all age groups.

5. What do you think of this scenario at this stage? Is it realistic? Could it be realistic? If you were a public health official from Guangdong, China, how could you have tried to prevent this spread of this new virus?

Further reading

Seasonal human influenzas

Barnett DJ, Balicer RD, Lucey DR, et al. A systematic analytic approach to pandemic influenza preparedness planning. *PLoS Med* 2005;2:e359

Call SA, Vollenweider MA, Hornung CA, Simel DL, McKinney WP. Does this patient have influenza? *JAMA* 2005;293:987–997

Eccles R. Understanding the symptoms of the common cold and influenza. *Lancet Infect Dis* 2005;5:718–725

Fauci AS. Pandemic influenza threat and preparedness. *Emerg Infect Dis* 2006;12:73–77

Horimoto T, Kawaoka Y. Influenza: lessons from past pandemics, warnings from current incidents. *Nat Rev Microbiol* 2005;3:591–600

Avian influenzas

Beigel JH, Farrar J, Han AM, et al; Writing Committee of the World Health Organization (WHO) Consultation on Human Influenza A/H5. Avian influenza A (H5N1) infection in humans. *N Engl J Med* 2005;353:1374–1385

Chan PK. Outbreak of avian influenza A(H5N1) virus infection in Hong Kong in 1997. *Clin Infect Dis* 2002;34(suppl 2):S58–64

Tran TH, Nguyen TL, Nguyen TD, et al; World Health Organization International Avian Influenza Investigative Team. Avian influenza A (H5N1) in 10 patients in Vietnam. *N Engl J Med* 2004;350(12):1179–1188

Antivirals

Jefferson T, Demicheli V, Rivetti D, Jones M, Di Pietrantonj C, Rivetti A. Antivirals for influenza in healthy adults: systematic review. *Lancet* 2006;367:303–313

Vaccines

Jefferson T, Rivetti D, Rivetti A, Rudin M, Di Pietrantonj C, Demicheli V. Efficacy and effectiveness of influenza vaccines in elderly people: a systematic review. *Lancet* 2005;366:1165–1174

Jordan R, Connock M, Albon E, et al. Universal vaccination of children against influenza: are there indirect benefits to the community? A systematic review of the evidence. *Vaccine* 2006;24:1047–1062

Palese P. Making better influenza virus vaccines? *Emerg Infect Dis* 2006;12:61–65

Useful websites

CDC. Diseases and Conditions. Seasonal Flu. General information on influenza maintained by the CDC. http://www.cdc.gov/flu/

United States Government avian and pandemic flu information managed by the Department of Health and Human Services. http://www.pandemicflu.gov/

WHO. Updates on avian influenza. http://www.wpro.who.int/health_topics/avian_influenza/

WHO. Website on influenza: http://www.who.int/csr/disease/influenza/en/, including influenza vaccine recommendations: http://www.who.int/csr/disease/influenza/vaccinerecommendations/en/index.html

Chapter 21
Infections in the returning traveler

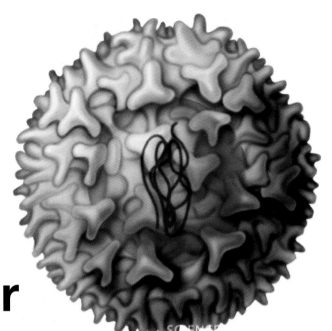

N. Shetty

Foodborne infections
  Traveler's diarrhea
  Typhoid and paratyphoid fever
Vectorborne infections
  Leishmaniasis
  Schistosomiasis (bilharziasis)
  Trypanosomiasis

Rickettsial and related infections
Yellow fever
The zoonoses
  Leptospirosis
  Brucellosis
Airborne infections
  Meningitis

International travel is increasing annually; according to the World Health Organization, tourist arrivals in the year 2005 exceeded 800 million (Figure 21.1). A proportion of these travelers acquire infections in the countries they visit. These might represent diseases indigenous to that country (e.g. malaria in sub-Saharan Africa), or infections that are not unique to a certain place but which are acquired as a result of risk behavior when on vacation (sexually transmitted diseases).

There is a vast spectrum of infectious disease associated with travel; hence it is useful to consider the following question when assessing an unwell individual with a possible travel related infection:

Why did this person, returning from this place, develop these symptoms at this time?

Person
Age: tourist activities often correlate with the age and agility of an individual! Also remember that infectious diseases vary in their presentation and severity with age.
Occupation might offer clues to exposure. A healthcare worker in a refugee camp would have a much higher risk of infection compared to an individual on a work trip to an urban location, or a tourist on holiday (Box 21.1).

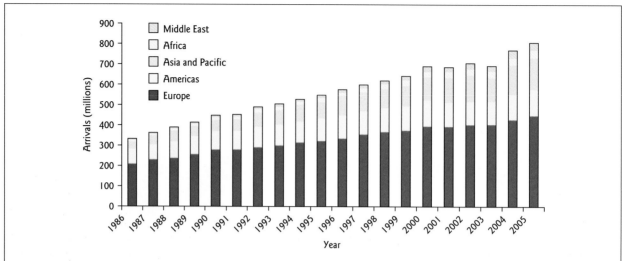

Figure 21.1 International tourist arrivals by region of destination: 1986–2005. Data reproduced from the Health Protection Agency, UK. http://www.hpa.org.uk/infections/topics_az/travel/slides.htm

Box 21.1 Camping by a river in a jungle

A 24-year-old man was referred by his family physician with generalized itching over his hands and feet over the past 2 months. He had visited Cameroon 4 months previously. A routine blood test had revealed an elevated eosinophil count, with all other investigations normal. On enquiry, it was found that he worked as a photographer, and had been filming a documentary about a local tribe

in dense jungle. The film crew had camped out near a river, in an area known to be infested with black flies (figure on left below), the vector for onchocerciasis (figure on right below). A filarial antibody test returned positive, and the patient recovered with a course of diethylcarbamazine (see Chapter 7). See Further reading for information on parasitic infections associated with travel.

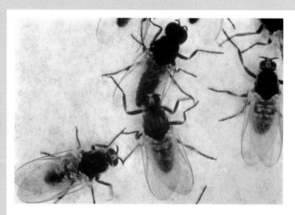

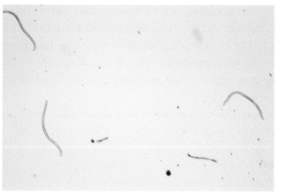

Both figures courtesy of the Centers for Disease Control and Prevention; from CDC website: http://phil.cdc.gov/phil/details.asp

Box 21.2 Activities that could have consequences

- Freshwater exposure (swimming, river rafting): for schistosomiasis, occasionally leptospirosis
- Eating uncooked foods: diarrheal diseases, amoebiasis, typhoid
- Drinking untreated water: cholera, diarrheal disease

- Sleeping in adobe huts in South America: American trypansomiasis
- Safari holidays in Africa: rickettsial infections, occasionally African trypanosomiasis
- Unprotected sex: HIV, syphilis, gonorrhea
- Sleeping without a mosquito net: malaria

Activities

Careful questioning might reveal the mode of infection (Box 21.2). Once a history of travel related activities is documented, potential infection risks can be classified according to mode of acquisition. Broadly they are:

Food- and waterborne diseases are usually acquired by ingestion of food and water that is contaminated. Reduce the risk by taking hygienic precautions with all food and water. Follow the CDC adage that says: "boil it, cook it, peel it or forget it!" Avoid direct contact with polluted, recreational waters. Common diseases transmitted by food and water are: hepatitis A (see Chapter 19); parasitic diarrheas (see Chapter 8), typhoid and traveler's diarrhea including cholera.

Vectorborne diseases: a history of insect bites or a failure to take precautions against bites is the key to diagnosing most travel related infections. Malaria, the most important travel related infection, is dealt with in a separate chapter (see Chapter 17). Other vectorborne parasitic infections include leishmaniasis, trypanosomiasis, and schistosomiasis. Dengue and tickborne encephalitis are dealt with in Chapters 24 and 10 respectively). Chikungunya virus infection is prevalent in many tropical countries (see Chapter 23). Rickettsial infections are prevalent in many forested areas including the USA. Yellow fever is an important and vaccine preventable infection.

Zoonoses are infections that can be transmitted to humans from animals: by contact, bites, or consumption of meat and milk products. Examples are rabies (see Chapter 10), certain viral hemorrhagic fevers (see Chapter 22); anthrax (see Chapter 26) brucellosis, and leptospirosis.

Sexually transmitted diseases are transmitted through unsafe sexual practices, examples are gonorrhea, syphilis (see Chapter 11), hepatitis B (see Chapter 19), and HIV (see Chapter 18).

Bloodborne diseases are acquired through direct contact with infected blood or body fluids, they may also be transmitted through contaminated needles, syringes, or through any other medical or surgical procedures where instruments are not sterilized adequately. Due to burgeoning trade in "medical tourism" cosmetic procedures (including, tattooing or piercing) and other surgical or medical interventions are particularly at risk. Hepatitis B and C, HIV and malaria can be transmitted this way.

Airborne diseases spread from person to person via aerosol and droplets from nose and mouth. Close contact in crowded places favors spread: examples are influenza (see Chapter 20), tuberculosis (see Chapter 16), and infection with *N. meningitides* (also read Chapter 10).

Diseases transmitted from soil infect the skin from cuts and abrasions or as a result of injuries sustained in road traffic accidents. Tetanus is the most important consideration, though rare because of the global emphasis on primary childhood vaccination; others include fungal infections of the skin and soft tissue, collectively known as mycetoma (see Chapter 7).

Place

Up to date facts about disease prevalence for different geographical areas are available from the Centers for Disease Control website. Broad overviews are provided here, but remember that **disease risk can vary by**

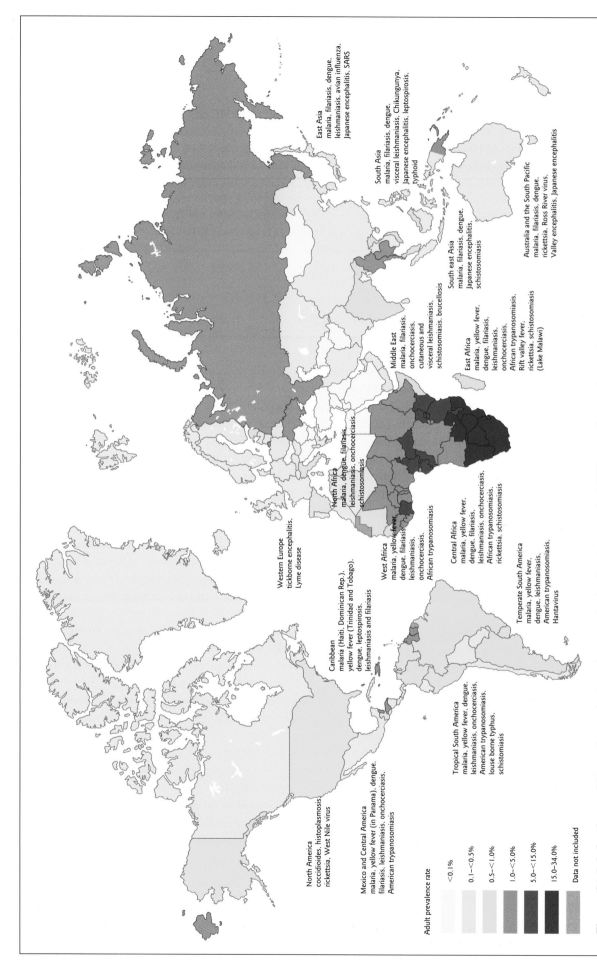

East Asia
malaria, filariasis, dengue,
leishmaniasis, avian influenza,
Japanese encephalitis, SARS

South Asia
malaria, filariasis, dengue,
visceral leishmaniasis, Chikungunya,
Japanese encephalitis, leptospirosis,
typhoid

Australia and the South Pacific
malaria, filariasis, dengue,
rickettsia, Ross River virus,
Valley encephalitis, Japanese encephalitis

South east Asia
malaria, filariasis, dengue,
Japanese encephalitis,
schistosomiasis

Middle East
malaria, filariasis,
onchocerciasis,
visceral leishmaniasis,
cutaneous and
schistosomiasis, brucellosis

East Africa
malaria, yellow fever,
dengue, filariasis,
leishmaniasis,
onchocerciasis,
African trypanosomiasis,
Rift valley fever,
rickettsia, schistosomiasis
(Lake Malawi)

North Africa
malaria, dengue, filariasis,
leishmaniasis, onchocerciasis,
schistosomiasis

West Africa
malaria, yellow fever,
dengue, filariasis,
leishmaniasis,
onchocerciasis,
African trypanosomiasis

Central Africa
malaria, yellow fever,
dengue, filariasis,
leishmaniasis, onchocerciasis,
African trypanosomiasis,
rickettsia, schistosomiasis

Western Europe
tickborne encephalitis,
Lyme disease

Caribbean
malaria (Haiti, Dominican Rep.),
yellow fever (Trinidad and Tobago),
dengue, leptospirosis,
leishmaniasis and filariasis

Temperate South America
malaria, yellow fever,
dengue, leishmaniasis,
American trypanosomiasis,
Hantavirus

North America
coccidioides, histoplasmosis
rickettsia, West Nile virus

Mexico and Central America
malaria, yellow fever (in Panama), dengue,
filariasis, leishmaniasis, onchocerciasis,
American trypanosomiasis

Tropical South America
malaria, yellow fever, dengue,
leishmaniasis, onchocerciasis,
American trypanosomiasis,
louse borne typhus,
schistosomiasis

Adult prevalence rate

<0.1%
0.1–<0.5%
0.5–<1.0%
1.0–<5.0%
5.0–<15.0%
15.0–34.0%
Data not included

Figure 21.2 Infections of importance to travelers against a background of HIV prevalence, by region
Source: WHO 2007

country and region within a country, and can change with time. It is imperative to refer to the most recent data when assessing risk. **Traveler's diarrhea, hepatitis A, and typhoid** can occur in any country where food and water is contaminated by human or animal fecal material.

For the most important travel related infections by World region on a background of HIV prevalence see Figure 21.2.

In the rest of this chapter we will discuss some important travel related infections that have not been covered in the rest of the book; these include the most common examples of travel related infections seen in a typical Travel Medicine clinic. The list is neither exhaustive nor complete, but should serve as a guide to some frequently encountered pathogens. For a complete guide to travel related infections access the CDC website: http://wwwn.cdc.gov/travel/contentDiseases.aspx

Foodborne infections

Hepatitis A is discussed in Chapter 19; parasitic and viral diarrheas are discussed in Chapter 8.

Traveler's diarrhea

The most frequent travel related infection is gastroenteritis; variously and colorfully referred to as "Montezuma's Revenge," "Aztec Two Step," and "Turista" in Mexico, "Delhi Belly" in India, and the "Hong Kong Dog" in the Far East. Traveler's diarrhea is a clinical syndrome that affects visitors from an area where there are high standards of sanitation to those parts of the world where there is poor infrastructure for safe water supply and disposal of human feces. This results in human fecal and therefore microbial contamination of food and water.

Epidemiology

The risk of diarrhea in travelers is linked to the choice of destination: low-risk countries include the USA, Canada, Australia, New Zealand, Japan, and countries in Northern and Western Europe. Intermediate risk countries include those in Eastern Europe, South Africa, and some of the Caribbean islands. High-risk areas include most of Asia, the Middle East, Africa, and Central and South America.

Traveler's diarrhea occurs equally in males and females and is more common in young adults than in older people. In short-term travelers, infection does not appear to protect against further attacks, and more than one episode of diarrhea may occur during a single trip. On average, 30–50% of travelers to high-risk areas will develop traveler's diarrhea during a 1- to 2-week stay. Based on the annual figure of 50 million travelers to developing countries, this estimate translates to approximately 50 000 cases of traveler's diarrhea each day. In more temperate regions, there may be seasonal variations in diarrhea risk. In South Asia, for example, during the hot months preceding the monsoon, much higher traveler's diarrhea attack rates are commonly reported (data from CDC).

Clinical presentation

Clinical symptoms depend on the infecting organism. Bacteria are the most common cause of traveler's diarrhea. In studies of etiological agents at various destinations, bacteria are responsible for approximately 80–85% of cases, parasites about 10% and viruses 5% .

Bacterial causes of traveler's diarrhea are best classified according to their pathogenesis into organisms causing invasive or secretory diarrhea (Table 21.1).

Symptoms of invasive diarrhea include watery or bloody diarrhea associated with abdominal cramps and rectal urgency. Vomiting may occur in up to 15% of those affected and may be accompanied by fever. Secretory diarrhea is characterized by abrupt onset of loose, watery stools with or without vomiting. Viral diarrheas are usually explosive, watery, and may be accompanied by vomiting and fever. Parasitic diarrheas may involve a prodrome of gaseousness and abdominal cramping, and additional symptoms, such as nausea,

Table 21.1 Bacteria associated with traveler's diarrhea

Traveler's diarrhea	
Invasive diarrhea	**Secretory diarrhea**
Shigella	Cholera
Enteroinvasive *E. coli* (EIEC)	Entero-toxigenic *E. coli* (ETEC)
Entero-aggregative *E. coli* (EAEC)*	
Entero-pathogenic *E. coli* (EPEC)*	
Salmonella	
Campylobacter	

Other bacteria that are considered potential pathogens are *Aeromonas hydrophila*, *Plesiomonas shigelloides*, *Yersinia enterocolitica*, and enterotoxigenic *Bacteroides fragilis*.
* Produce no recognizable toxins or invasion factors; however epithelial cell damage is evident.

bloating, and fever, may be associated. Traveler's diarrhea is generally self-limited and lasts 3–4 days even without treatment, but persistent symptoms may occur in a small percentage of travelers. Medical attention should be sought for diarrhea accompanied by a high fever or blood in the stool. Postinfectious sequelae have been described, including reactive arthritis, Guillain–Barré syndrome, and postinfectious irritable bowel syndrome. Postinfectious irritable bowel syndrome may occur in up to 3% of persons who contract traveler's diarrhea.

Etiology and pathogenesis

As mentioned earlier a wide variety of organisms may be implicated in traveler's diarrhea including bacteria, parasites, or viruses. A broad overview of diarrheal disease is presented in Chapter 8. In this Chapter we will discuss the most important organisms associated with traveler's diarrhea.

Diagnostic methods include stool culture and biochemical or serological identification of the organism. Some pathogens like the diarrheagenic *E. coli* are more difficult to diagnose in routine daignostic laboratories and rely on specialized tests in reference faciltites. Being travel related many go undiagnosed.

Invasive diarrhea (bacterial)

Invasive diarrhea is characterized by inflammation and sometimes ulceration of the lining of the gut and may be associated with blood and mucus in the stool with the presence of neutrophils.

Shigella species (dysenteriae, flexneri, boydii, sonnei)

Shigella species are the principal agents of bacillary dysentery. Patients need to ingest a very small infectious dose of these organisms (5–10 organisms) to develop symptoms. Histologically the rectosigmoidal lesions of shigellosis resemble those of ulcerative colitis.

The genus *Shigella* consists of Gram negative, facultative anaerobes. Virulence determinants that code for invasion are encoded by large extrachromosomal elements (plasmids) that are functionally identical in all *Shigella* species and in entero invasive *E. coli* (EIEC). A complex of two plasmid-encoded determinants, designated Invasion Plasmid Antigens (Ipa) B and C, induces the endocytic uptake of shigellae by M cells, epithelial cells, and macrophages. Ipa proteins cause release of the IL-1 cytokine and macrophage apoptosis. Another plasmid-encoded virulence determinant lyses host plasma membranes, resulting in intercellular bacterial spread. A key virulence determinant of shigellae and EIEC is the production of enterotoxins designated ShET1 and ShET2 that are responsible for the diarrheal symptoms.

S. dysenteriae serotype 1 expresses Shiga toxin, an extremely potent, ricin-like, cytotoxin that inhibits protein synthesis in susceptible mammalian cells. This results in rapid cell death and extensive ulceration and inflammation of the colon and recto-sigmoid area. More importantly, Shiga toxin is associated with the hemolytic-uremic syndrome, a complication of infections with *S. dysenteriae* 1. Closely related toxins are expressed by enterohemorrhagic *E. coli* (EHEC) including the potentially lethal, foodborne O157-H7 serotype.

Entero-invasive (EIEC), entero-aggregative (EAEC), and entero-pathogenic *E. coli* (EPEC)

All the diarrheagenic *E. coli* are indistinguishable from commensal *E. coli* with respect to Gram stain and culture characteristics: they are Gram negative facultative anaerobes.

The pathogenesis of EIEC is similar to the *Shigella* species described above.

E. coli strains belonging to the classic EAEC and EPEC serogroups bind intimately to the epithelial surface of the intestine, usually the colon, via an adherence factor or pilus. Even though there is no histological evidence of invasion; the presence of cell damage in the absence of secretory toxins places them potentially in the class of invasive agents

Not much is known about the pathogenesis of EAEC. The formation of a heavy mucus biofilm may contribute to EAEC diarrheagenicity and, perhaps, to its ability to cause persistent colonization and diarrhea. Mucosal damage has also been demonstrated in ileum specimens taken after patients died of EAEC persistent diarrhea in Mexico City. Other workers postulate that toxin secretion may occur, though evidence for this is lacking.

EPEC causes destruction of microvilli. Cell damage occurs in two steps, collectively termed attaching and effacing; attachment occurs initially followed by loss of microvilli. EAEC causes loss of microvilli leading to malabsorption and osmotic diarrhea. Diarrhea is persistent, often chronic, and accompanied by fever. For a summary of diarrheagenic *E. coli* and their main pathogenetic mechanisms see Table 21.2.

Salmonella and *Campylobacter* spp.

Although associated with foodborne outbreaks in industrialized countries, these organisms are important causes of traveler's diarrhea. They have been discussed in detail in Chapter 8.

Secretory diarrhea (bacterial)

Secretory diarrhea is characterized by profuse watery diarrhea, the absence of blood or neutrophils in the stool and, most importantly, the complete lack of any invasion of the gut mucosal surface. The prototype secretory organism is *Vibrio cholerae*, although the most common cause of traveler's diarrhea is an *E. coli* called entero-toxigenic *E. coli* (ETEC) which possesses a similar pathogenetic mechanism to that of *V. cholerae*.

Table 21.2 Diarrheagenic *E. coli* and their main pathogenetic mechanisms

Diarrheagenic *E. coli*	Mechanism
Entero-invasive *E. coli*	Invasive: produces invasion similar to shigellae
Entero-hemorrhagic *E. coli*	Invasive: produces shiga-like entero-cytotoxin
Entero-pathogenic *E. coli**	Causes attachment to and effacement of villous processes
Entero-aggregative *E. coli**	Causes attachment and a (?) mucus biofilm
Entero-toxigenic *E. coli*	Secretory: produces heat labile toxin (LT) increases cyclic AMP and heat stable toxin (ST) increases cyclic GMP

* Not conventionally invasive or toxigenic but with evidence of epithelial cell damage.

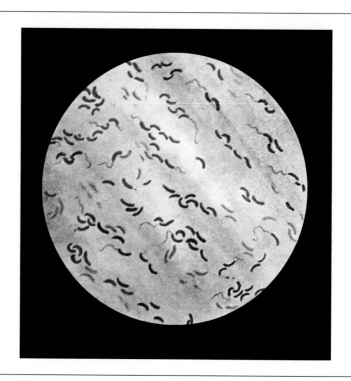

Figure 21.3 *Vibrio cholerae*: Gram stain. Courtesy of the Centers for Disease Control and Prevention; from CDC website: http://phil.cdc.gov/phil/details.asp

V. cholerae

Vibrios are highly motile, Gram negative, curved or comma-shaped rods with a single polar flagellum (Figure 21.3). Of the vibrios that are clinically significant to humans, *Vibrio cholerae* O group 1, the agent of cholera, is the most important. Vibrios are sensitive to low pH and die rapidly in solutions below pH 6 (gastric acid efficiently kills off the cholera vobrio); however, they are quite tolerant of alkaline conditions.

Cholera is a disease of humans exclusively. Infection is acquired by the ingestion of water or food contaminated with the feces of an infected individual. There have been six great pandemics of cholera to date; the disease is still endemic in its ancestral home along the banks of the River Ganges in the Indo-Pakistan river belt. In 1961, the El Tor biotype (based on biochemical react) of *V. cholerae* emerged as the cause of the seventh great cholera pandemic. The pandemic spread from Southeast Asia into Africa. It has also invaded Europe, North America, and Japan. In 1991, a hundred years after this region had last witnessed cholera, the pandemic strain hit Peru with devastating affect and has since spread through most of the Western Hemisphere. In 1992, a new strain of vibrio emerged in South India and rapidly spread across the subcontinent into Bangladesh. It took microbiologists by surprise because it did not belong to the O1 group yet produced disease similar to classical cholera. It was eventually called the O139 strain since there were 138 recognized O groups of vibrio at the time. It was feared that it would replace O1 (both classical and El Tor) as a pandemic strain because of a lack of native immunity to it, however its activity has been restricted to the Indian subcontinent and neighboring countries. Countries where cholera is currently prevalent are described in Figure 21.4.

The Indian subcontinent is endemic for cholera, with epidemics of new cases of cholera occurring every year depending on the amount of rain and degree of flooding. Since humans are the only reservoirs, survival of the cholera vibrios during interepidemic periods probably depends on a relatively constant availability of low-level undiagnosed cases and transiently infected, asymptomatic individuals. Long-term carriers have been reported but are extremely rare. Recent studies, suggest that cholera vibrios can persist for some time in shellfish, algae, or plankton in coastal regions of infected areas where they can exist in "a viable but nonculturable state."

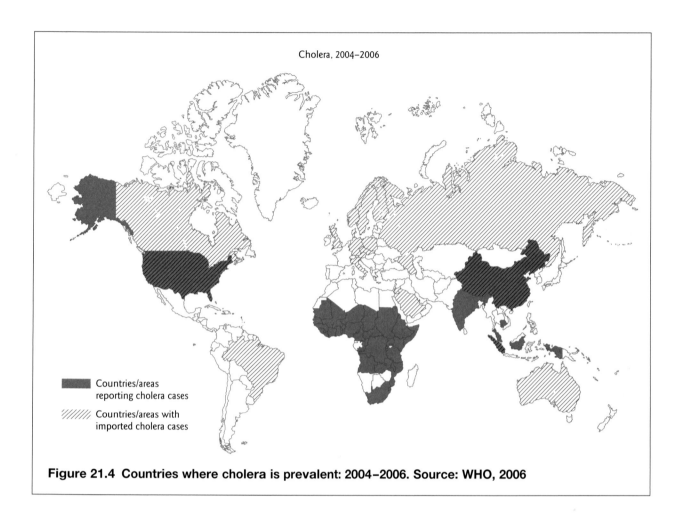

Cholera, 2004–2006

■ Countries/areas reporting cholera cases

/////// Countries/areas with imported cholera cases

Figure 21.4 Countries where cholera is prevalent: 2004–2006. Source: WHO, 2006

Following an incubation period of 6–48 hours, cholera begins with the abrupt onset of profuse watery diarrhea – the characteristic "rice-water stool" (consisting mainly of isotionic body fluid, no fecal matter, and flakes of mucus). Patients may lose a liter of isotonic fluid from the lumen of the gut at a time with several liters of fluid secreted within hours. Vomiting usually accompanies the diarrheal episodes. Muscle cramps occur as water and electrolytes are lost from body tissues. The disease runs its course in 2–7 days; the outcome depends upon the extent of water and electrolyte loss and the timeliness and efficiency of water and electrolyte replacement. Death can occur rapidly due to hypovolemic shock, metabolic acidosis, and uraemia resulting from acute tubular necrosis of the kidney.

The **pathogenesis of cholera** relies on colonization and production of the cholera toxin. To establish residence and multiply in the human small bowel the cholera vibrios have one or more adherence factors that enable them to adhere to intestinal microvilli. Following this the organism mediates diarrhea through the action of the cholera toxin. Cholera toxin **activates the adenylate cyclase enzyme** in cells of the intestinal mucosa leading to increased levels of intracellular cAMP, and the secretion of H_2O, Na^+, K^+, Cl^-, and HCO_3^- into the lumen of the small intestine. The toxin has been characterized and contains **five binding (B) subunits** of 11 500 daltons, an active **(A1) subunit** of 23 500 daltons, and a **bridging piece (A2)** of 5500 daltons that links A1 to the 5B subunits. The B subunits bind to a specific receptor, a glycolipid called GM1 ganglioside, ubiquitous in eukaryotic cells and present on the surface of intestinal mucosal cells. Once binding has occurred the A1 subunit enters the cell; where it enzymatically transfers ADP-ribose from nicotinamide adenine dinucleotide (NAD) to a target protein, the guanosine 5′-triphosphate (GTP)-binding regulatory protein associated with membrane-bound adenylate cyclase. Since GTP hydrolysis is the event that inactivates the adenylate cyclase, the enzyme remains continually activated.

Test yourself

function, and confusion. He needed to be admitted to ICU and dialysed. The peripheral blood smear stained with Geimsa stain is shown here:

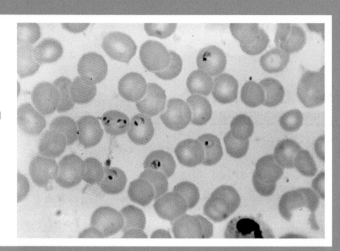

Courtesy of the Centers for Disease Control and Prevention; from CDC website: http://phil.cdc.gov/phil/details.asp

1. What is the likely diagnosis?
2. Name the organism to species level and give your reasons.
3. How could this patient have protected himself?

Further reading

Useful websites

CDC. DPDx. Laboratory Identification of Parasites of Public Health Concern. Parasitic infections associated with travel. http://www.dpd.cdc.gov/dpdx/

CDC. Rocky Mountain Spotted Fever. Prevention and Control. http://www.cdc.gov/ncidod/dvrd/rmsf/prevention.htm

CDC. Traveler's Health: Yellow Book. Prevention of Specific Infectious Diseases. Leptospirosis. http://wwwn.cdc.gov/travel/yellowBookCh4-Leptospirosis.aspx

CDC. Traveler's Health: Yellow Book. Prevention of Specific Infectious Diseases. Traveler's Diarrhea. http://wwwn.cdc.gov/travel/yellowBookCh4-Diarrhea.aspx

CDC. Traveler's Health: Yellow Book. Prevention of Specific Infectious Diseases. Typhoid Fever. http://wwwn.cdc.gov/travel/yellowBookCh4-Typhoid.aspx

CDC. Traveler's Health: Yellow Book. Prevention of Specific Infectious Diseases. Yellow Fever. http://wwwn.cdc.gov/travel/yellowBookCh4-YellowFever.aspx

Part 5
Emerging and resurgent infections

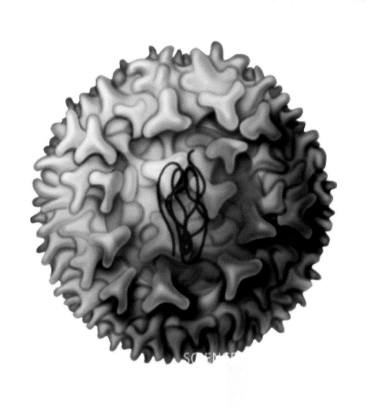

Chapter 22
Viral hemorrhagic fevers

J.W. Tang

Introduction	**Clinical features**
Virology	**Management and treatment**
Epidemiology	**Infection control and containment**
Origins and routes of transmission to humans	**Outcomes of VHF infections**
Diagnosis	**Prevention**

Introduction

Viral hemorrhagic fevers (VHFs) are Biosafety Level 4 (BSL-4) viral infections, which cause profuse bleeding and have a high mortality. They are most often caused by the following families of viruses: filoviruses (Ebola and Marburg viruses), arenaviruses (Lassa, Junin, Machupo, Guanarito, and Sabia viruses), flaviviruses (yellow fever and dengue fever), and bunyaviruses (Crimean-Congo hemorrhagic fever (CCHF) and Rift Valley fever (RVF) viruses, and some hantaviruses). The term "hemorrhagic fever" should not be confused with hemorrhagic manifestations of other viral infections, such as chickenpox (skin), smallpox (skin), and influenza (lung), which can have hemorrhagic presentations in severe forms of these infections. (For dengue hemorrhagic fever (DHF) see Chapter 24.)

Virology

All the VHFs are lipid-enveloped, single-stranded RNA viruses. Filoviruses are negative-sense RNA viruses. The arenavirus are ambi-sense RNA viruses (as they transcribe mRNA in negative and positive directions). Flaviviruses and bunyaviruses are positive- and negative-sense RNA viruses, respectively. The lipid envelope makes the VHF viruses relatively sensitive to detergents and to drying, although it has been reported that Marburg virus can remain infectious after storage at room temperature for up to 5 weeks or after heating at 56°C, for 1 hour. Complete inactivation occurs with ultraviolet irradiation and with 1 hour exposure to formalin, acetone, Chloros, diethlyether, or 60°C temperature.

Epidemiology

The most infamous and lethal of the VHFs are the filoviruses. There are only two members, Ebola and Marburg viruses; both of them have been found mainly in Africa. Ebola virus is named after a river in the Democratic Republic of the Congo (DRC, formerly Zaire), where it was first discovered. It has caused sporadic outbreaks since its discovery in 1976 in both humans and nonhuman primates (monkeys, gorillas, and chimpanzees). There are four recognized subtypes or strains of Ebola that have been named after the countries where they were first recognized, of which three are known to cause human disease: Zaire Ebola (with the highest human mortality), Sudan Ebola, Cote D'Ivoire Ebola. The fourth strain Reston Ebola is named after the town of Reston (Virginia, USA) where there was an outbreak of Ebola in nonhuman primates in a quarantine facility, but without causing significant human disease (now made famous by the book *The Hot Zone* by Richard Preston – see Further Reading). The other member of the filoviruses, Marburg virus, was discovered earlier in 1967 and exists only as a single strain. It also takes its name from that of a town in Germany, where an imported case from Africa caused a local outbreak. However, it also is mainly found in Africa, especially in the gold-mining areas of the DRC and Angola. Like Ebola, Marburg virus can also cause disease in nonhuman primates. Regular updates of new filovirus outbreaks can be found at the websites for the World Health Organization and Centers for Disease Control and Prevention (see Further reading). Outbreaks of new Ebola and Marburg viruses have been occurring more frequently (almost yearly since 2005–2008 as this text goes to press), which may be due to more recent heightened awareness and surveillance for these filoviruses. Most recently, a fifth species of Ebola virus (Bundibugyo ebolavirus) was discovered in 2007 in Uganda. In addition, at the end of 2008, Reston Ebola was discovered in pigs in the Philippines. This virus may be the source of the Reston Ebola virus that infected the monkeys that were imported to the quarantine facility in Virginia, USA.

Lassa fever virus (also known as an Old World arenavirus) comes from the west African countries, around Sierra Leone, extending into western parts of Nigeria. Junin, Machupo, Guanarito, and Sabia viruses (also referred to as the New World arenaviruses) cause Argentine, Bolivian, Venezuelan, and Brazilian hemorrhagic fevers in these South American countries, respectively. Yellow fever virus can be found in countries in both the African and South American continents. Dengue fever can now be found worldwide, reaching 40% of the world's population, and is the most important and widespread human arbovirus infection. Crimean-Congo hemorrhagic fever virus is endemic in many parts of eastern Europe, the Middle East, Asia, and Africa. Rift Valley fever was originally discovered in the Rift Valley area of East Africa but has been since found throughout Africa.

The hantaviruses that typically cause hemorrhagic fever with renal syndrome (HFRS) can be found in parts of Southeast Asia, such as Korea (Seoul virus) and China, and parts of eastern and northern Europe (Dobrava and Puumala viruses). Hantavirus pulmonary syndrome (HPS) caused by Sin Nombre virus was first discovered in the "four corners" area of southwestern USA, but is not normally included as one of the VHFs (the hantaviruses are discussed in the Chapter 23).

Origins and routes of transmission to humans

One of the natural reservoirs for Ebola virus has recently been discovered to be fruit bats, after researchers tested over a thousand small vertebrate animals from Gabon and the DRC between 2001 and 2003 (see Further reading). It is thought that hunting monkeys for "bush meat" by the indigenous population may have initially transmitted filoviruses to humans from infected monkeys. Another alternative is that the viruses are shed in the droppings of bats, thought to be a natural reservoir for some time now, and transmission to humans occurred by the inhalation of dust containing bat feces in caves. The natural host for the arenaviruses is known to be various species of the family of multi-mammate rodent *Mastomys*. The *Mastomys* rodents shed the virus in their urine and droppings, so the virus can be transmitted through direct contact with these excretions, or via touching objects or eating food contaminated with these excretions, or through cuts or sores. Since these rodents often live in and around homes, scavenging human food remains or poorly stored food, transmission of this sort is common in Lassa fever endemic areas. When the urine dries, the viruses are still viable and the dried dust containing live virus can be lifted into the air by air currents and inhaled, causing Lassa fever. Lastly, because *Mastomys* rodents are sometimes consumed as a food source, infection may occur via direct contact when they are caught and prepared for food – a similar mechanism to that suggested for the transmission of filoviruses.

Yellow fever is transmitted to humans from various mammalian hosts, especially livestock animals such as cattle and sheep, by the *Aedes* mosquito, of which *Ae. aegypti* is the primary vector. This mosquito is also the primary vector for dengue fever virus transmission where the virus replicates within the mosquito, which then can transmit it by biting a human host. There is both an urban cycle (between mosquitoes and man) and a jungle cycle (between mosquitoes and other mammals) for both yellow fever and dengue fever viruses. In human infections, the urban cycle is generally more important for human infections for both viruses, but encroachment into forested areas may inadvertently make humans part of the jungle cycle of infection also. Crimean-Congo hemorrhagic fever is transmitted by ticks, again from various livestock species, from which the virus can also be acquired through direct contact with infected blood during slaughtering. With Rift Valley Fever, the natural reservoir is again mainly livestock animals and some studies have shown that sleeping outdoors at night in areas during RVF outbreaks may expose people to bites from RVF-infected vectors, such as mosquitoes. Thus, all people working with animals (herdsmen, abattoir workers, and veterinarians), as well as travellers passing through RVF-endemic areas, are at risk of infection either from direct contact with infected animal tissues and fluids, or RVF-infected mosquito vectors (Figure 22.1).

Generally, therefore, the main mode of person-to-person transmission for most VHFs is by direct (close) contact with infected body fluids: blood, semen, saliva, urine and mucus, though blood will generally contain the highest viral load and pose the highest risk. Infected mosquitoes will transmit vectorborne VHFs between animals and individuals. Contaminated fomites (inanimate objects) can also act as sources of infection, particularly in busy healthcare facilities during an outbreak.

Another source of transmission, which contributed to the original outbreak of Ebola virus in Yambuku in 1976, was iatrogenic. In this outbreak, which was the first appearance of Ebola hemorrhagic fever, poorly sterilized needles were reused and thus responsible for making the local hospital the main source of the subsequent epidemic. Apart from the inhalation of arenavirus virus-infected resuspended dust, aerosol transmission is generally not considered to be a risk, though there was some evidence of this in the Ebola Reston virus outbreak amongst Cynomolgus macaque monkeys (*Macaca fascicularis*) held in quarantine in Reston, Virginia, USA in 1989. In this incident, virtually all the monkeys exposed to this strain died, although no human was clinically affected. See Table 22.1 for a summary of important outbreaks over the years.

Diagnosis

All work with BSL-4 VHF viruses must be carried out using appropriate, authorized high containment laboratories. These are designed to provide total isolation of the operator from the virus. These are either high-level containment cabinets with built-in glove ports (Figure 22.2a), or laboratory personnel wearing biosuits with independent air supplies (Figure 22.2b). These facilities are expensive to construct and maintain and are usually found in developed countries. When outbreaks occur (usually in developing countries) the initial samples require secure transportation to such facilities, such as those at CDC, for testing. Later on, when the outbreak is confirmed, mobile testing units can be transported to the area.

Nowadays, rapid virus detection and identification may be achieved by reverse transcription polymerase chain reaction (RT-PCR) of RNA isolated from infected tissue samples. In addition, electron microscopy (EM – Figures 22.3 and 22.4), immunofluorescence (IF) microscopy, enzyme immunoassays (EIAs), and Western blotting may also be used, where appropriate. Confirmation of virus identity by isolation in cell culture and antigenic analysis may also be the method of choice in some laboratories.

Based on data obtained following an outbreak of Ebola Zaire virus in Gabon in 1996, it seems that asymptomatic infection does occur in some people exposed to the virus. It was suggested that an early, vigorous immune response may have prevented them from developing serious clinical disease. In such cases, a positive serological result may therefore be an indication of exposure, but without clinical disease in these individuals (see Further reading).

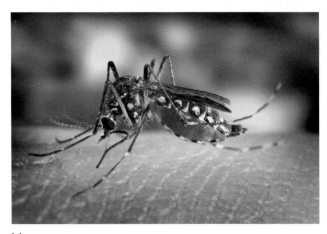

(a)

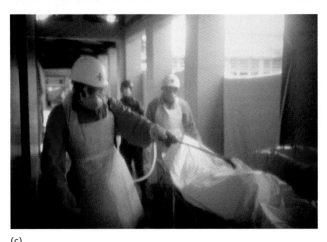

(c)

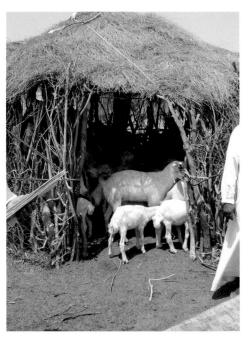

(b)

Figure 22.1 (a) A female *Aedes aegypti* mosquito: the primary vector for the spread of dengue and yellow fevers. Rift Valley fever is also spread by *Aedes* species mosquitos, such as *Ae. vexans arabiensis*. *Ae. aegypti* is a domestic, day-biting mosquito that prefers to feed on humans. Only the female bites and transmits disease. Dengue is spread by the female *Ae. aegypti* only, as the male does not bite.

(b) This photograph was taken during epidemiologic investigations into a Rift Valley Fever (RVF) outbreak in Saudi Arabia. These goats were in a village farm within the area of investigation and may act as a RVF reservoir, transmitting RVF to humans via contact with infected animal blood or other bodily fluids. Humans can also be infected through the bite of an infected *Aedes* mosquito. Therefore, RVF is most commonly associated with mosquito-borne epidemics during years when there is unusually heavy rainfall. (c) Transmission can also occur nosocomially between patients and healthcare workers in healthcare facilities, and also via contact with contaminated fomites. To avoid accidental transmission of Ebola to others, this local Red Cross team is disinfecting the outside of a body bag of an Ebola patient during the outbreak in Kikwit, Democratic Republic of the Congo, 1995. (a) Provided by Professor Frank Hadley Collins. Courtesy of the Centers for Disease Control and Prevention; from CDC website: http://phil.cdc.gov/phil/details.asp. (b) Provided by Abbigail Tumpey. Courtesy of the Centers for Disease Control and Prevention; from CDC website: http://phil.cdc.gov/phil/details.asp. (c) Provided by Ethleen Lloyd. Courtesy of the Centers for Disease Control and Prevention; from CDC website: http://phil.cdc.gov/phil/details.asp

Table 22.1 Details of the outbreaks revealing new strains of the filoviruses. Only the outbreaks showing a new genus or strain of the filoviruses are listed below. New filovirus outbreaks have been occurring with increasing frequency over the last few years. For a comprehensive, up-to-date list of all recent filovirus outbreaks check the CDC Ebola virus website (see Further reading) (adapted from a previous article: Tang JW. Filoviruses: an update. *Postgrad Doct (Africa)* 2001;23(3):54–57)

Year	Country (location)	Virus/subtype	No. of cases/mortality	Transmission source*/ transmission event
1967	Germany/Yugoslavia	Marburg	31/23%	Ugandan monkeys* direct contact/cell cultures
1976	Zaire (Yambuku)	Ebola Zaire	318/88%	Unknown source/close contact, reused needles in hospitals and clinics
1976	Sudan (Nzara and Maridi)	Ebola Sudan	284/53%	Unknown source/close contact, and nosocomial transmission to hospital staff
1989	USA (Pennsylvania, Virginia, Texas)	Ebola Reston	4/0%	Imported monkeys* from Philippines/high monkey mortality, asymptomatic human infection only
1994	Ivory Coast (Tai forest)	Ebola Ivory Coast	1/0%	Wild chimpanzee* in Tai forest/biologist conducted autopsy on monkeys affected by a hemorrhagic disease between 1992 and 1994

* The source of infection in these cases may not be the natural host or reservoir of these filovirus strains.

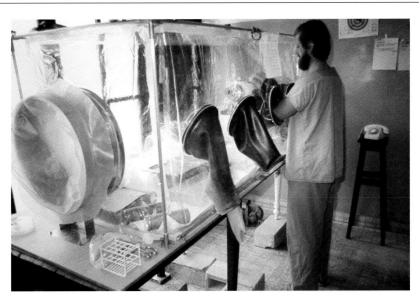
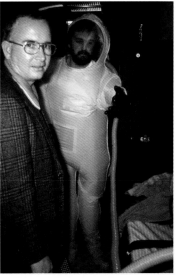

(a)   (b)

Figure 22.2 (a) This isolator was used as a field laboratory in the 1976 Ebola virus outbreak in Zaire (now the DRC) to prepare specimens for further examination at the CDC. (b) This shows one of the CDC's first BSL-4 laboratory containment suits worn by a technician inside the animal laboratory during Lassa fever and Ebola hemorrhagic fever research activities. Clean air is administered through a tube into the air-tight suit and waste air is removed also via this line directly from the suit, keeping the system self-contained and protecting the worker from infection. Provided by Dr Lyle Conrad. Courtesy of the Centers for Disease Control and Prevention; from CDC website: http://phil.cdc.gov/phil/details.asp

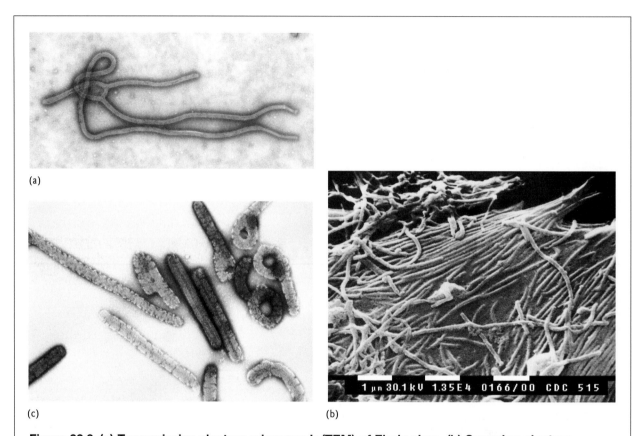

Figure 22.3 (a) Transmission electron micrograph (TEM) of Ebola virus. (b) Scanning electron micrograph (SEM) depicting a number of Ebola virions. (c) Negative stained TEM depicting a number of filamentous Marburg virions. Note the virus's characteristic "Shepherd's Crook" appearance (approximate magnification: 100 000×). (a) Provided by Cynthia Goldsmith. Courtesy of the Centers for Disease Control and Prevention; from CDC website: http://phil.cdc.gov/phil/details.asp. (b) Provided by Cynthia Goldsmith. Courtesy of the Centers for Disease Control and Prevention; from CDC website: http://phil.cdc.gov/phil/details.asp. (c) Provided by Dr Erskine Palmer, Russell Regnery. Courtesy of the Centers for Disease Control and Prevention; from CDC website: http://phil.cdc.gov/phil/details.asp

Clinical features

The main problem with early clinical diagnosis of any of the VHFs is that the early symptoms are very nonspecific, and could easily be mistaken for a "flu-like" illness: headache, fever, a sore or dry throat (making the patient cough), aches and pains, particularly backache. Generally, the incubation periods (the time between infection and onset of symptoms) for the VHFs range from as little as 2 days up to about 3 weeks. This will differ between the various VHFs and different individuals, depending on the inoculating viral load and host immune response. After the incubation period, there may be early, nonspecific symptoms, including headache, high fever, abdominal, muscle and joint pains, with nausea, vomiting and profuse diarrhea, which may become bloody. This state may last from several days up to a week. In some VHF cases there may be an accompanying rash, which starts as small red spots to larger lesions that look like bruises. Eventually, as the disease progresses, there may be bleeding from the nose, mouth, eyes, as well as coughing up blood and bloody diarrhea. Intravenous access and phlebotomy

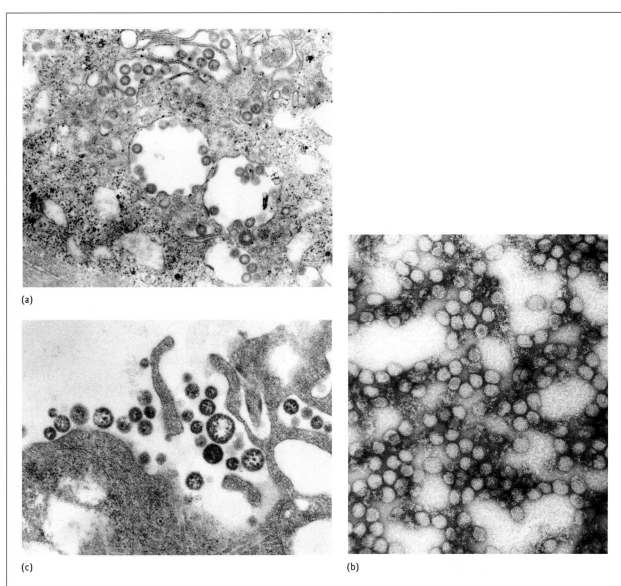

Figure 22.4 (a) TEM depicting a highly magnified view of tissue infected with Rift Valley fever (RVF) virus. **(b)** Multiple virions of the yellow fever virus seen at a magnification of 234 000×. **(c)** TEM showing a number of Lassa virus virions adjacent to some cell debris. **(a)** Provided by F.A. Murphy and J. Dalrymple. Courtesy of the Centers for Disease Control and Prevention; from CDC website: http://phil.cdc.gov/phil/details.asp. **(b)** Courtesy of the Centers for Disease Control and Prevention; fom CDC website: http://phil.cdc.gov/phil/details.asp. **(c)** Provided by C.S. Goldsmith, P. Rollin, M. Bowen. Courtesy of the Centers for Disease Control and Prevention; from CDC website: http://phil.cdc.gov/phil/details.asp

(taking blood samples) often results in prolonged bleeding due to disseminated intravascular coagulation (DIC, where the body's bleeding/clotting system becomes activated inappropriately). The patients with established infection often appear pale, emaciated, dehydrated, lethargic, with death occurring during the end of the first or second week of the disease, due to major blood loss and shock. Many patients recover from Lassa and even the dreaded Ebola fever, although factors that influence survival are not fully understood (Figure 22.5).

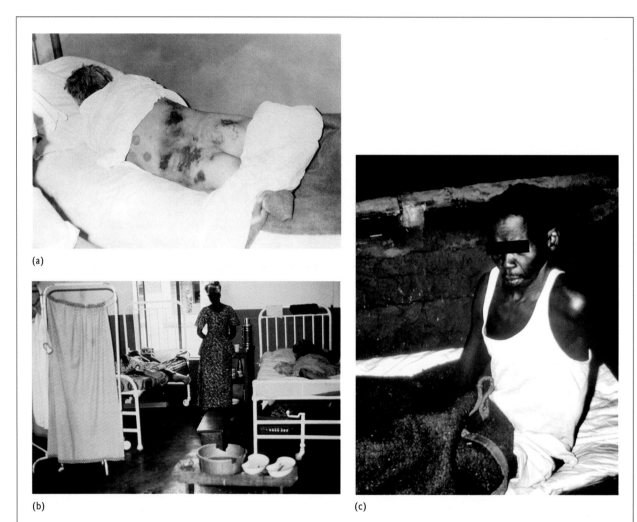

Figure 22.5 (a) A male patient with Crimean-Congo hemorrhagic fever (CCHF). (b) Recovering female Lassa fever patients in a clinic in Segbwema, Sierra Leone in 1977. (c) Recovering Ebola patient sitting up in his bed during one of the Ebola virus outbreaks in 1976. (a) Provided by Dr B.E. Henderson. Courtesy of the Centers for Disease Control and Prevention; from CDC website: http://phil.cdc.gov/phil/details.asp. (b) Courtesy of the Centers for Disease Control and Prevention; from CDC website: http://phil.cdc.gov/phil/details.asp. (c) Provided by Dr Lyle Conrad. Courtesy of the Centers for Disease Control and Prevention; from CDC website: http://phil.cdc.gov/phil/details.asp

Management and treatment

The first major problem with managing patients infected with BSL-4 VHF viruses is that of isolating the patient to protect the healthcare workers, but at the same time, allowing access to the patient to give the appropriate care. A variety of patient isolation units have been developed to manage this seemingly contradictory situation, some more portable than others (Figure 22.6).

In developing countries, where such facilities do not exist and where most outbreaks occur, management focuses primarily on barrier procedures by the medical and nursing personnel. This consists of the use of personal protective equipment (gowns, gloves, masks, eye-glasses, boots, etc.) (Figure 22.7), isolating each patient from noninfected people in the care facility and the community and careful disposal of all potentially

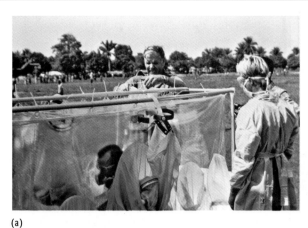

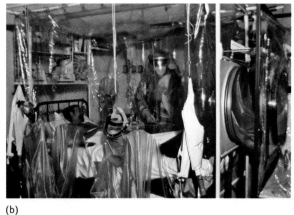

(a)

(b)

Figure 22.6 (a) Photograph taken in 1976 showing a CDC staff member fastening a make-shift bottle anchor to a mobile isolation unit containing a suspected Ebola patient. (b) The same patient in a larger isolation unit at Johannesburg Fever Hospital. The patient became ill with Ebola-like symptoms while working on the Yambuku survey effort during the Zairian Ebola outbreak of 1976. He was evacuated from Yambuku to Johannesburg, South Africa, where he was, luckily, eventually found not to be infected with Ebola virus. (a) Provided by Dr Lyle Conrad. Courtesy of the Centers for Disease Control and Prevention; from CDC website: http://phil.cdc.gov/phil/ details.asp. (b) Provided by Dr Lyle Conrad. Courtesy of the Centers for Disease Control and Prevention; from CDC website: http://phil.cdc.gov/phil/details.asp

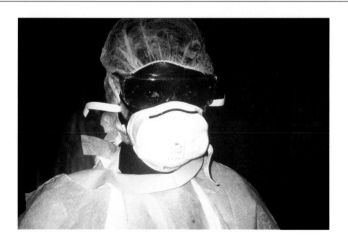

Figure 22.7 A Zairian nurse dressed to enter the Ebola VHF isolation ward during the 1995 outbreak in Kikwit, Zaire. Provided by Ethleen Lloyd. Courtesy of the Centers for Disease Control and Prevention; from CDC website: http://phil.cdc.gov/phil/ details.asp

infectious material. This simple approach also applies to the laboratory testing of specimens from such infected patients in such resource poor areas.

There is currently no specific treatment for any of the VHFs and, generally, supportive management with close monitoring and support of respiratory function, and fluid and possibly blood products replacement are the main approaches. Immunotherapy, using convalescent plasma from a surviving patient, has been tried, but with only limited success. Intravenous ribavirin given within 6 days has been shown to help Lassa fever

---

Box 22.1 The virology of the filoviruses: Ebola and Marburg (adapted from a previous article: Tang JW. Filoviruses: an update. Postgrad Doct (Africa) 2001;23(3):54–57)

These particular VHF viruses, Marburg and Ebola, have inspired many books (see Further reading) and even movies (such as "Outbreak" in 1995). They share similar characteristics:

- Filamentous shapes, sometimes looking like a "shepherd's crook," "6s" or "9s," which vary in length from 130 to 2600 nm . They can be as long as 14 000 nm in some EM preparations, but their diameter is more uniform at around 80–100 nm
- Lipid-enveloped, thus vulnerable to detergents, irradiation and drying (inactivated after 1 hour at 60°C), but can withstand heating to 56°C for 1 hour, or survive for 5 weeks at room temperature
- Single-stranded, negative-sense RNA genome that codes for seven proteins. One of these is a transmembrane glycoprotein which may underlie the pathogenesis of the hemorrhaging by damaging the lining of blood vessel (composed of endothelial cells)
- Transmission is mainly from direct contact with infected body fluids (blood, urine, saliva, feces, semen), and can be from person to person or via contaminated fomites, and presumably via needlestick injuries also. There was some evidence of airborne transmission for Ebola Reston virus in the quarantine facility in Reston, Virginia, USA, when monkeys started to die in rooms connected only by air ducts. However, there was no clinical human disease caused by this Ebola virus strain, which was suspected to have originated from somewhere in the Philippines from where this shipment of monkeys originated

- With modern molecular detection assays, filovirus diagnosis can be very rapid with a combination of reverse-transcriptase polymerase chain reaction (RT-PCR), electronmicroscopy (EM), immunofluorescence (IF), and enzyme immunoassays (EIAs) on infected tissues or blood samples. Virus culture is still useful for result confirmation. All such diagnostic tests must be performed under BSL-4 containment
- A natural reservoir of the filoviruses (for both Ebola and Marburg) has been recently discovered in fruit bats studied in Gabon and the Republic of Congo. This discovery may make it possible to control or even prevent outbreaks of these filoviruses in the future.

---

patients, but there is limited evidence of the effectiveness of ribavirin or other drugs against the other VHFs. However, research is being conducted into the pathogenesis of VHFs, particularly the filoviruses, with the aim of developing new therapies (see Further reading). Patients do survive, particularly those with the nonfilovirus VHF infections, but convalescence is often slow and the debilitating effects of the illness may persist for many weeks to months.

Infection control and containment

In terms of infection control, all known, unprotected human contacts with the patient will need followup and temperature monitoring for the duration of the incubation period of the VHF virus (usually a maximum of about 3 weeks), and where necessary, have their movements restricted or to be in full quarantine. This strategy aims to detect and confine secondary cases as early as possible to contain the outbreak to a limited area or population. As there is no definitive evidence that naturally occurring (as opposed to weaponized) VHFs are easily transmitted between people by the airborne route, such precautions have usually been adequate. The relatively rapid and successful containment of most of the recent Ebola and Marburg outbreaks seem to support this approach. For the vectorborne VHFs (yellow, dengue, Rift Valley

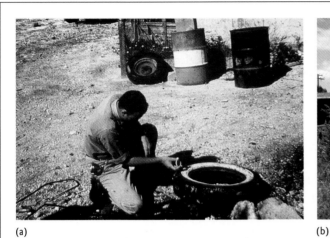

(a)

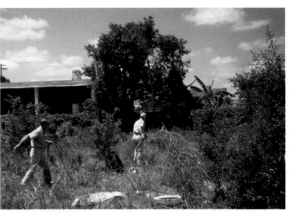

(b)

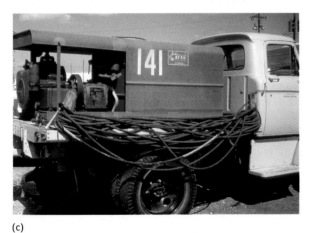

(c)

Figure 22.8 (a) Photograph depicting an entomologic field technician inspecting some discarded automobile tires for the presence of mosquitos, primarily *Aedes aegypti*, the main vector responsible for the transmission of dengue and yellow fever to humans. **(b)** Men spraying mosquito for larvae during the 1965 *Ae. aegypti* eradication program in Miami, Florida. In the 1960s, a major effort was made to eradicate this principal urban mosquito vector of dengue and yellow fever viruses from the southeast USA. **(c)** A mosquito spray truck that was used during this 1965 *Ae. aegypti* eradication program. (a) Courtesy of the Centers for Disease Control and Prevention; from CDC website: http://phil.cdc.gov/phil/details.asp. (b) Courtesy of the Centers for Disease Control and Prevention; from CDC website: http://phil.cdc.gov/phil/details.asp. (c) Courtesy of the Centers for Disease Control and Prevention; from CDC website: http://phil.cdc.gov/phil/details.asp

and Crimean-Congo hemorrhagic fevers), control of the responsible vectors as well as protection of individuals from being bitten, are required (Figure 22.8).

Also read Chapter 24, the sections on West Nile and dengue fever, for more details on vector control.

Outcomes of VHF infections

The filoviruses, Ebola and Marburg, have the highest mortality out of all the VHFs, ranging from 20% to 90%, with Marburg reaching a lethality as high as that of Ebola Zaire in some recent outbreaks in Angola in 2005. With yellow fever, the case-fatality rate can be greater than 20%, but it is usually lower than this and there is an effective live-attenuated vaccine, which is mandatory for entry into many countries where yellow fever is endemic (as shown by the possession of a yellow fever vaccination certificate). These countries are found mainly in the central African belt, and the central and northwestern parts of South America (see the CDC Yellow Book website in Further reading). The case fatality rate for dengue hemorrhagic fever should be <1% with appropriate supportive therapy (see Chapter 24).

Lassa fever is generally mild or asymptomatic in about 80% of people infected with the virus, but the remaining 20% have severe multisystem disease. During epidemics, the case-fatality rate can reach as high as 50%. This may be partly due to the fact that there are so many cases occurring at once that the supportive care of each individual patient is suboptimal as the healthcare services are stretched too thin. In some areas of Sierra Leone and Liberia, where Lassa fever is endemic, it is known that 10–16% of people admitted to hospitals have Lassa fever, which indicates the serious impact of the disease on the population of this region. Crimean-Congo hemorrhagic fever can have a relatively high case-fatality rate of up to 30% and person-to-person transmission through infected body fluids has been documented (see Further reading).

Prevention

Research is being conducted into vaccines against the VHFs. There is already an effective live attenuated yellow fever vaccine that has been in use for many years. A dengue tetravalent vaccine has been progressing through clinical trials in Thailand, but as yet, there are no licensed vaccines for Lassa fever, CCHF, or Rift Valley fever (though there is an unlicensed vaccine for use in staff at high risk from RVF). Some promising results have been obtained with experimental Ebola vaccines in monkeys (see Further reading). Along with drug and vaccine developments, and now that at least one of the natural reservoirs of Ebola virus has been identified, controlling of the sources of these VHFs is a more feasible means of limiting the outbreaks of these serious and frightening diseases.

Test yourself

The following scenario is based on a true case (adapted from Crowcroft NS, Meltzer M, Evans M, et al. The public health response to a case of Lassa fever in London in 2000. *J Infect* 2004;48(3):221–228.)

Case study 22.1
A Peace Corps volunteer worker returned from Sierra Leone, West Africa, well, but developed fever and malaise 1 week later. He attended a local hospital emergency room after 1 day of illness.

❓1. What else would you like to know about this patient?

On further questioning, the patient said that he had been helping the local people in some villages control the number of rodents in the area as part of a local Lassa fever control program. These rodents were of the *Mastomys* species, and he was aware that they may be carrying Lassa fever virus. Also, he had slept in the local village huts on the floor, so he may have been exposed to infected urine from these rodents.

Initially, he was treated as malaria, but multiple malaria screen tests proved negative and he continued to deteriorate and developed bleeding from the nose. Later on the same day the patient started to cough up blood and passed bloody diarrhea stools. Further blood investigations showed deranged hematology and clotting results and a diagnosis of Lassa fever was suspected. CDC was contacted and he was transferred to a high-level containment unit using a mobile patient isolator. Blood was taken for VHF screening and within 12 hours, a positive result by RT-PCR for Lassa fever was obtained from CDC.

Test yourself

?2. What actions are required now?

The patient starts to respond to the ribavirin therapy, but his hematology remains deranged, requiring the infusion of various blood products to replace the volume he has lost through bleeding. During the course of the following 2 weeks, his condition stabilizes and further RT-PCR testing eventually shows no more detectable Lassa fever RNA. None of his contacts report any temperature rises and no further suspicious clinical cases come forward. The patient is allowed to go home after 4 weeks in hospital care, but he has lost several kilograms in weight and feels very weak. His convalescence and return to his previously healthy state takes another 2 months.

This is a fairly typical presentation of a VHF, acquired in an endemic country where malaria is also endemic making it a realistic alternative diagnosis. In this case, the patient was lucky, as the VHF was quickly diagnosed, contained and treated, with a good outcome, not only for the patient, but for public health also.

Further reading

Ahmed AA, McFalls JM, Hoffmann C, Filone CM, Stewart SM, Paragas J, Khodjaev S, Shermukhamedova D, Schmaljohn CS, Doms RW, Bertolotti-Ciarlet A. Presence of broadly reactive and group-specific neutralizing epitopes on newly described isolates of Crimean-Congo hemorrhagic fever virus. *J Gen Virol* 2005;86(Pt 12): 3327–36

Bossi P, Tegnell A, Baka A, et al; Task Force on Biological and Chemical Agent Threats, Public Health Directorate, European Commission, Luxembourg. Bichat guidelines for the clinical management of haemorrhagic fever viruses and bioterrorism-related haemorrhagic fever viruses. *Euro Surveill* 2004;9(12):E11–12

Centers for Disease Control and Prevention (CDC). Outbreak of Marburg virus hemorrhagic fever – Angola, October 1, 2004–March 29, 2005. *MMWR* 2005;54(12):308–309

Crowcroft NS, Meltzer M, Evans M, et al. The public health response to a case of Lassa fever in London in 2000. *J Infect* 2004;48(3):221–228

Ergonul O. Crimean-Congo haemorrhagic fever. *Lancet Infect Dis* 2006;6(4):203–214

Guzman MG, Kouri G. Dengue and dengue hemorrhagic fever in the Americas: lessons and challenges. *J Clin Virol* 2003;27(1):1–13

Jeffs B. A clinical guide to viral haemorrhagic fevers: Ebola, Marburg and Lassa. *Trop Doct* 2006;36(1):1–4

Mahanty S, Bray M. Pathogenesis of filoviral haemorrhagic fevers. *Lancet Infect Dis* 2004;4(8):487–498

McCormick J, Fisher-Hoch S, Horovitz LA. *Level 4: Virus Hunters of the CDC.* Turner Publishing, 1996

A multi-author (including husband and wife team Joe McCormick and Susan Fisher-Hoch) account of encounters with lethal BSL-4 viruses around the world. With similar intentions as CJ Peters' "Virus Hunter"

Miller BR, Godsey MS, Crabtree MB, et al. Isolation and genetic characterization of Rift Valley fever virus from *Aedes vexans* arabiensis, Kingdom of Saudi Arabia. *Emerg Infect Dis* 2002;8(12):1492–1494

Peters CJ. *Virus Hunter: Thirty Years of Battling Hot Viruses Around the World.* Anchor, 1998

An autobiographical account of ex-army colonel CJ Peters and his work with the US Army Medical Research Institute of Infectious Diseases (USAMRIID) dealing with dangerous viruses worldwide

Peterson AT, Bauer JT, Mills JN. Ecologic and geographic distribution of filovirus disease. *Emerg Infect Dis* 2004;10(1):40–47

Preston R. *The Hot Zone.* New York: Random House, 1995

This book is based on real events, but is somewhat dramatized to appeal to the mass market. It describes the first outbreak and recognition of the Reston-Ebola strain of Ebola virus in monkeys in a quarantine facility in the town of Reston, Virginia, USA

Rigau-Perez JG. Severe dengue: the need for new case definitions. *Lancet Infect Dis* 2006;6(5):297–302

Towner JS, Pourrut X, Albariño CG, Nkogue CN, Bird BH, Grard G, Ksiazek TG, Gonzalez JP, Nichol ST, Leroy EM. *Marburg virus infection detected in a common African bat.* PLoS ONE. 2007 Aug 22;2(1):e764

Towner JS, Rollin PE, Bausch DG, et al. Rapid diagnosis of Ebola hemorrhagic fever by reverse transcription-PCR in an outbreak setting and assessment of patient viral load as a predictor of outcome. *J Virol* 2004;78(8):4330–4341

Towner JS, Sealy TK, Khristova ML, Albariño CG, Conlan S, Reeder SA, Quan PL, Lipkin WI, Downing R, Tappero JW, Okware S, Lutwama J, Bakamutumaho B, Kayiwa J, Comer JA, Rollin PE, Ksiazek TG, Nichol ST. *Newly discovered ebola virus associated with hemorrhagic fever outbreak in Uganda.* PLoS Pathog. 2008 Nov;4(11):e1000212. Epub 2008 Nov 21

Useful websites

CDC website. Other VHF information can be located by searching from this page. http://www.cdc.gov/ncidod/dvrd/spb/mnpages/dispages/Ebola.htm

Ebola Reston found in domestic pigs in the Philippines. http://www.who.int/csr/disease/influenza/communications/QAebolareston/en/index.html

WHO. Epidemic and Pandemic Alert and Response. Ebola Virus. Other VHF outbreaks can be located by searching from this page. http://www.who.int/csr/disease/ebola/en/

Chapter 23

Emerging infections I (human monkeypox, hantaviruses, Nipah virus, Japanese encephalitis, chikungunya)

J.W. Tang

Introduction
Human monkeypox
  Epidemiology
  Introduction of monkeypox into the USA
  Virology and diagnosis
  Clinical features
  Treatment and prevention
Hantaviruses

  Epidemiology
  Virology and diagnosis
  Clinical features
  Treatment and prevention
Other emerging infections
  Nipah virus
  Japanese encephalitis
  Chikungunya

Introduction

Emerging infections can be classified into: (i) those which are newly discovered, e.g. as the cause of a previously known disease, like human herpesvirus 8 and Kaposi's sarcoma, or due to a change in the environment, like Ebola virus; (ii) those which are already known but have moved into a new area or into a new population, like West Nile virus and monkeypox in the USA; (iii) those which are already known and have been previously successfully treated but have now developed significant drug resistance or have become widespread for other reasons, e.g. new virulence mutations or routes of transmission like multiple-drug resistant tuberculosis in HIV patients.

Most of the newly emerging infections in the last 20–30 years are viruses. This chapter will cover human monkeypox and hantaviruses (particularly Sin Nombre virus causing hantavirus pulmonary syndrome), both of which are of particular importance in the USA, and briefly touch on other emerging viruses elsewhere in the world, such as Nipah and Japanese encephalitis viruses.

Human monkeypox

After the eradication of smallpox in 1977 (see Chapter 26), monkeypox became a focus for surveillance after the first human case was discovered in 1970 in the Democratic Republic of Congo (DRC), in a 9-month-old infant, initially thought to have smallpox. The virus itself was recognized in 1958 after it caused disease in captive primates (cynomolgus monkeys, *Macaca fascicularis*) held at the State Serum Institute in Copenhagen, Denmark. Since the disappearance of smallpox, it is considered the most important poxvirus infection of humans.

Epidemiology

Previous monkeypox infections in humans were confined to central parts of Africa, particularly the DRC, where there was a particularly large outbreak in 1996–1997 in the Katako-Kombe Health Zone, involving 88 cases. Prior to this, between 1981 and 1986, there were a total of 338 cases identified in the DRC, with a case-fatality rate of 9.8% for those unvaccinated against smallpox (which gives some cross-protection against monkeypox, with about 85% efficacy). The secondary attack rate in smallpox-unvaccinated household members was about 9.3%, though 28% of these secondary cases reported more than one exposure to other monkeypox cases during the incubation period. Unlike smallpox, a transmission chain longer than the secondary cases was unusual, and transmission modeling suggested that sustained human-to-human-transmission was unlikely. Repeated reintroductions of the virus into the human population from the wildlife reservoir would be required to sustain a prolonged epidemic.

Until the recent importation of monkeypox into the USA in 2003, this disease existed nowhere else outside Africa. The natural reservoir still remains uncertain though several candidate species have been postulated including African rope squirrels (genus *Funisciurus*), as well as other primate, rabbit and rodent species that are all susceptible to monkeypox virus infection. The human disease is mainly transmitted via direct animal-to-human contact, but also via respiratory droplets between humans.

Introduction of monkeypox into the USA

On May 24, 2003, the first documented case of human monkeypox was reported in a 3-year old girl from central Wisconsin, when she was hospitalized for fever and cellulitis after being bitten by a prairie dog (Figure 23.1), 11 days earlier, on 13 May. This was not a wild animal, but an animal bought as a pet from a swap meet where animals are traded or bought. The prairie dog itself had become sick on May 13, with papular skin lesions, lymphadenopathy, and discharges from the eye, eventually dying on May 20. Microbiological analysis of a lymph node specimen revealed no obvious causative agent, though plague or tularemia was suspected at the time (see Chapter 26).

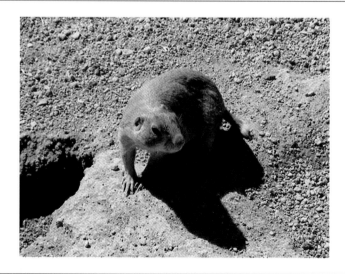

Figure 23.1 Prairie dogs, a member of the genus *Cynomys*, were responsible for many of the first human cases of monkeypox outside Africa, in the USA, during 2003. Most of these people became ill after having contact with pet prairie dogs that were sick with the virus. Provided by Susy Mercado Courtesy of the Centers for Disease Control and Prevention; from CDC website: http://phil.cdc.gov/phil/details.asp

The original importation of the virus into the USA was traced back to a shipment of small animals from Ghana to Texas that contained a sick Gambian giant-pouched rat (*Cricetomys gambianus*). This sick animal was sold to an Illinois animal vendor then was kept close to prairie dogs, which subsequently became infected. The infected prairie dogs were themselves sold to another distributor then two pet shops and at a pet swap meet in Wisconsin. Other animals from the original Ghana–Texas shipment included dormice and rope squirrels that also tested positive for the virus.

Eventually a total of 72 human monkeypox cases were reported in 2003 from six mid-western states (Illinois, Indiana, Kansas, Missouri, Ohio, and Wisconsin), mainly from direct contact with infected animals, though other routes of transmission were possible (see Further reading for detailed accounts of this outbreak).

Virology and diagnosis

Monkeypox is a member of the orthopoxvirus family (Orthopoxviridae) that is genetically distinct from variola (smallpox), vaccinia (the virus in the smallpox vaccine), and cowpox viruses. Like other poxviruses it is a large, lipid-enveloped, double-stranded DNA virus, that can appear as large brick-shaped virions with two distinct forms ("C" capsular and "M" mulberry) under negative stain electron microscopy (EM) (Figure 23.2). In contrast to variola, it has many animal hosts making it unlikely that it will be eradicated by human vaccination. It can be distinguished from variola via different characteristics of pock morphology when cultured on chick embryo chorioallantoic membranes, but cannot be reliably distinguished by neutralization of hemagglutination inhibition assays. However, specific antisera to distinct viral antigens can distinguish between the two viruses, though there has been some difficulty in producing accurate, rapid and reliable diagnostic kits for monkeypox. The genomes of the two viruses are similar at certain points, particularly in the central region coding for structural and enzyme proteins, but the outer ends of the genomes are much less homologous. These regions code for virulence and host-range factors and the larger differences indicate that monkeypox and variola are not ancestors of each other, and it is unlikely for one to mutate into the other. This provides some reassurance that monkeypox will not take the place of smallpox as a worldwide scourge, after the effective eradication of the latter. There are two different genotypes or clades of monkeypox: a milder West African clade (the type imported into the USA) with a lower mortality than the more virulent central African clade (that caused the DRC human monkeypox cases).

The diagnosis of monkeypox requires skin samples from the lesions and blood, though other samples can be requested. Similar to the diagnosis of smallpox, the skin scabs contain a high viral load and can be prepared for EM that will reveal the characteristic poxvirus morphology (Figure 23.2). Specific primers for monkeypox

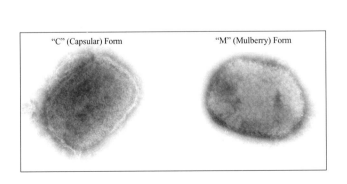

"C" (Capsular) Form   "M" (Mulberry) Form

Figure 23.2 A negative stain electron micrograph demonstrates the two forms of the brick-shaped monkeypox virus from a cell culture. The surface of "M," or "mulberry," virions are covered with short, whorled filaments, while "C," or "capsular," form virions penetrated by stain present as a sharply defined, dense core surrounded by several laminated zones of differing densities. Provided by Cynthia Goldsmith, Inger K. Damon, Sherif R. Zaki. Courtesy of the Centers for Disease Control and Prevention; from CDC website: http://phil.cdc.gov/phil/details.asp

DNA can also be designed and used to detect monkeypox genome from the same skin lesion material, with DNA sequencing to distinguish monkeypox from other pox viruses, if necessary. Culture using chick embryo chorioallantoic membranes is not often available in most diagnostic laboratories, though this can be performed by CDC and other similarly equipped reference laboratories. Serological assays, as stated previously, are generally unreliable for diagnosing monkeypox infection, and indeed, any other poxvirus infections.

Clinical features

There are differences between the well-described monkeypox disease of humans in Africa and the more recent cases in the USA.

The African form of monkeypox has an incubation period of 7–17 days (mean 12 days), with a prodrome of fever, headache, backache, and fatigue. This lasts 2–4 days before the appearance of skin lesions. The disease can be mild to severe, but all cases have marked lymphadenopathy ("swollen glands") in the lower jaw (submandibular), behind the ears (postauricular), neck (cervical), and groin (inguinal) regions. This was an important distinctive feature that separated it from smallpox.

By contrast, the more recent US cases of human monkeypox demonstrate an incubation period of 4–24 days (mean 14.5 days) presenting with rash, fever, chills, sore throat, myalgias, sweats, cough, nausea, vomiting, nasal congestion, back pain, mouth sores, inflammation of the eyes, and gastrointestinal symptoms. Although lymphadenopathy was reported in 71% of 34 confirmed cases, it seemed less marked compared to the previously described African cases.

The most obvious difference in presentation between the African and US forms of the disease lay in the form and development of the skin rash. In particular, the shape, evolution and number of lesions differed between the two forms. In the African form, the skin lesions developed from macules to papules to pustules (see Chapter 7 on skin infections for precise definitions of these terms) that umbilicate (i.e. form a small depression in the center) before drying out and falling off during a period of 14–21 days, often leaving a scar. The lesions are about 0.5 cm in diameter and are usually densest at the extremities (hands and feet) in an "acral" or centrifugal distribution. The lesions also occurred on the palms, soles, and genitals, as well as mucous membranes. In 13% of African cases, there were fewer than 25 lesions, in 38% there were 25–100 lesions, and in 49% there were more than 100 lesions (Figure 23.3).

In the US cases, the skin lesions were much more variable between individuals – even within the same family cluster – and some seemed to originate and spread from the initial bite lesion. Such inoculation lesions were not well described for the African cases. The progression of the lesions also differed from the African cases in that the lesions progressed from red lesions to white vesicles to umbilcated pustules with a

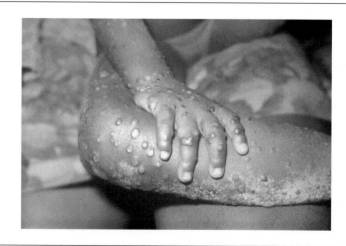

Figure 23.3 Close-up of monkeypox lesions. This is the more typical appearance of monkeypox, the central African genotype, from a female child from the Democratic Republic of Congo. The US cases caused by the milder West African genotype have fewer lesions, surrounded by a red hemorrhagic crust. Courtesy of the Centers for Disease Control and Prevention; from CDC website: http://phil.cdc.gov/phil/details.asp

central hemorrhagic crust and satellite lesions – not seen in the African disease. Erythematous (red) flares accompanied the appearance of the pustules in some cases – again not seen in the African cases. During the final healing stages, these hemorrhagic crusts sloughed off with little or no scarring. In addition, the US cases had a less prominent centrifugal distribution with this being seen in only 48% of cases, with 28% of them having lesions on the palms and 9% on the soles. The distribution of the lesions in the US cases seemed to be linked to spread via the bloodstream after the initial bite inoculation of the virus. There were generally far fewer lesions in the US cases, with 53% of the cases having more than 25 lesions and only 20% having more than 100 lesions.

Several reasons have been suggested as to why these clinical presentations differed so much. Many of the African cases were mainly due to the more virulent central African genotype in contrast to the milder West African genotype imported into the USA. The occurrence of the hemorrhagic lesions in the US cases are thought to be due to a difference in the complement-mediated immune response induced by this West African genotype. In the African cases, the lesions occurred on dark skin that may have hidden the erythematous flare, which was much more obvious in the lighter skin of the Caucasian US cases. The African cases of human monkeypox were not originally described by dermatologists, whereas many of the US cases were, so the language used to describe these two presentations may have differed substantially. In addition, the transmission of human monkeypox in Africa often occurred via the ingestion of infected meat, whereas the US cases occurred after dermal inoculation from the bite of infected animals, which may have altered the presentation of the disease.

Treatment and prevention

No specific antiviral treatment is licensed for human monkeypox, although the drug cidofovir and related agents have been shown to be effective in preventing mortality in an experimentally infected cynomolgus monkey. However, none of the infected patients received this drug in the US cases. The severely ill patients that required hospitalization received supportive therapy including hydration and nutrition, antibiotics (ciprofloxacin and doxycycline), other antivirals (aciclovir and valacyclovir) and/or mechanical ventilation in one case with encephalitis (brain inflammation – usually due to either direct viral damage, or more often the host immune response to the virus infection of the brain).

Prevention of human monkeypox infection can be achieved by smallpox vaccination, and the CDC has recommended this for those at high risk of monkeypox infection, e.g. personnel involved in the investigation or care of animal or human cases of monkeypox. Both pre-exposure and post-exposure (within 2 weeks) of monkeypox have been included in this recommendation, though the evidence for post-exposure smallpox vaccination for monkeypox is less clear. Vaccinia immunoglobulin (VIG) usually used to treat complications of smallpox vaccination (see Chapter 26) has also been considered to treat severe cases of human monkeypox, or as pre-exposure prophylaxis for those at risk of monkeypox exposure in whom smallpox vaccination is contraindicated.

Hantaviruses

Human hantavirus infection can result in two distinct clinical syndromes: respiratory distress and failure – hantavirus pulmonary syndrome (HPS) and a febrile illness with bleeding and renal failure – hemorrhagic fever with renal syndrome (HFRS). The hantaviruses that cause these two distinct clinical presentations are also separated geographically with the Old World (Europe and Asia) hantaviruses, mostly HFRS, and the New World (the Americas) hantaviruses, causing predominantly HPS.

Epidemiology

Hantavirus pulmonary syndrome was first recognized in the USA in 1993 when environmental conditions favored the emergence of this previously unknown disease in the Four Corners region of the USA (New

Mexico, Arizona, Colorado, and Utah). A cluster of fatal cases of HPS resulted in the rapid identification of a new hantavirus, subsequently called Sin Nombre (Spanish for "no name," SN) virus. The virus was also found around the patients' homes in dust and urine excreted by rodents that were trapped around these living areas.

Hemorrhagic fever with renal syndrome is an older disease affecting a far greater number of people in Europe and Asia. The clinical syndrome has been given a number of names, including Korean hemorrhagic fever, epidemic hemorrhagic fever, nephropathia epidemica, and has been described for at least 80 years from Korea, Russia, China, and Sweden. It was finally isolated successfully in cell culture in 1981. The various countries in which HFRS has been reported have also given the virus their own names, e.g. Hantaan (HTN), Seoul (SEO), Puumala (PUU), Dobrava-Belgrade (DOB) viruses, which can all cause the renal failure, hemorrhage, and shock that are all components of HFRS. The epidemiology of the hantaviruses that cause HPS and HFRS are mainly determined by that of their rodent reservoir, as there is very little human-to-human transmission of the hantaviruses.

Table 23.1 summarizes the distribution of the most important hantaviruses that cause disease in man, with two examples of the rodent vectors being shown in Figure 23.4.

Virology and diagnosis

The hantaviruses belong to the family of Bunyaviruses (*Bunyaviridae*) and are zoonoses, with a natural reservoir mainly in rodents with the viruses being transmitted to man as an incidental host. They are lipid-enveloped, single-stranded, negative-sense, segmented RNA viruses (Figure 23.5). There are separate, distinct serotypes of hantavirus (as shown in Table 23.1), though there is significant serological cross-reactivity between the different species.

Hantavirus infection is usually asymptomatic and harmless in the rodent reservoir, and although there seems to be a brisk antibody response to the viral proteins, lifelong infection probably results. Infection between individual rodents occurs by horizontal transmission, with the highest antibody prevalence in the older animals. Most outbreaks of human hantavirus infections occur with large increases in the rodent population that may be a result of changes in the climate, predation, competition, and food supplies. Typical outbreaks of hantavirus infections in Europe and Asia have been associated with the planting and harvesting of field crops when there is the greatest chance of contact with infected rodents. Examples of these have been seen with the Sin Nombre virus HPS outbreak in the Four Corners region of the USA in 1993 due to a massive increase in the rodent population with invasion of human habitats, and the Puumula virus HFRS outbreaks in Scandanavia.

Most of the infections result from inhalation of the aerosolized virus contained in the dried out excreta from infected rodents. Such aerosols can be created by sweeping, the wind, or any other activity that disturbs ground-lying dust. However, human hantavirus have also been documented after bites from infected rodents. Nosocomial transmission of hantavirus between humans is possible as the virus has been isolated from the blood and urine of infected patients. Households tend to exhibit a greater degree of secondary case transmissions, which is also seen in individuals with close personal contact, and there are some cases highly suggestive of person-to-person transmission, but if such cases do occur, they must be considered as extremely rare. Laboratory transmissions of hantavirus to workers have been documented, but these are usually from infected animals to animal handlers. Other possible means of transmission include the consumption of hantavirus-contaminated food or drink, or contact with hantavirus-contaminated objects (fomites) then the touching of mucous membranes (mouth, nose, or eyes).

Laboratory diagnosis usually involves IgM and IgG (a four-fold rise in titer) testing of acute and convalescent sera. Reverse-transcription polymerase chain reaction (RT-PCR) testing of acute sera to detect hantavirus RNA is also useful if such early samples are available. This test can also be designed to detect specific hantavirus species, as required. Culture and electron microscopy (Figure 23.5) are not routinely used to diagnose hantavirus infections in most diagnostic laboratories.

Table 23.1 Human hantavirus infections: their source and geographical distributions

Virus species/ serotypes	Clinical disease type	Main rodent reservoir	Geographical distribution of virus/disease
Sin Nombre (SN)	HPS	Deer mouse (*Peromyscus maniculatus*)	USA, Canada, Mexico
New York (NY)	HPS	White-footed mouse (*Peromyscus leucopus*)	USA
Black Creek Canal (BCC)	HPS	Cotton rat (*Sigmodon hispidus*)	USA
Bayou (BAY)	HPS	Rice rat (*Oryzomys palustris*)	USA
Choclo	HPS	Pygmy rice rat (*Oligoryzomys fulvescens*)	North and South America
Monongahela	HPS	White-footed mouse (*Peromyscus leucopus*)	North America
Muleshoe (MULEV)	HPS	Cotton rat (*Sigmodon hispidus*)	North America
Lechiguanas	HPS	Yellow pygmy rice rats (*Oligoryzomys flavescens*)	South America
Andes (AND)	HPS	Long-tailed pygmy rice rat (*Oligoryzomys longicaudatus*)	South America
Oran	HPS	Long-tailed pygmy rice rat (*Oligoryzomys longicaudatus*)	South America
Central Plata hantavirus	HPS	Yellow pygmy rice rats (*Oligoryzomys flavescens*)	South America
Cano Delgadito	HPS	Cotton rat (*Sigmodon alstoni*)	South America
Laguna Negra (LN)	HPS	Vesper mouse (*Calomys laucha*)	South America
Calabazo virus	HPS	Short-tailed cane mouse (*Zygodontomys brevicauda*)	South America
Araraquara	HPS	Hairy-tailed bolo mouse (*Bolomys lasiurus*)	South America
Hantaan (HTN)	HFRS	Striped field mouse (*Apodemus agrarius*)	China, Russia, Korea
Seoul (SEO)	HFRS	Norway rat (*Rattus norvegicus*)	Worldwide
Puumala (PUU)	HFRS	Bank vole (*Clethrionomys glareolus*)	Europe, Russia, Scandinavia
Dobrava-Belgrade (DOB)	HFRS	Yellow-neck mouse (*Apodemus flavicollis*)	Balkans

HPS, hantavirus pulmonary syndrome; HFRS, hemorrhagic fever with renal syndrome.

Clinical features

The clinical features of HPS and HFRS can greatly overlap. After an incubation period of 1–5 weeks, hantavirus infection in both HPS and HFRS is characterized by an abrupt onset of fever, chills, headache, dizziness, nausea, vomiting, diarrhea, abdominal pain, and muscle aches (myalgia), especially in the large muscle groups (hips, back, and shoulders). More rarely, patients may complain of earache, sore throat, runny nose, and a rash, but these are very uncommon in HPS.

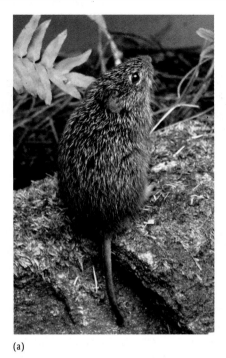
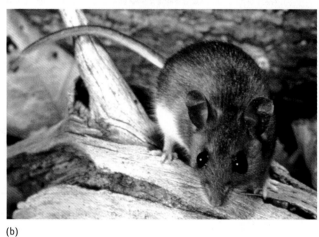

(a)

(b)

Figure 23.4 A cotton rat, *Sigmodon hispidus* (a), the known reservoir for Black Creek Canal virus, one cause of hantavirus pulmonary syndrome (HPS), whose habitat includes southeastern USA, Central and South America. The deer mouse, *Peromyscus maniculatus*, is the main reservoir and transmitter of hantavirus in the USA (b). It is found almost everywhere in North America, including both woodland and desert areas. Dried hantavirus-infected urine and feces from these rodents can be aerosolized by sweeping or other activities and cause hantavirus infection with HPS, when inhaled. Provided by James Gathany. Courtesy of the Centers for Disease Control and Prevention; from CDC website: http://phil.cdc.gov/phil/details.asp

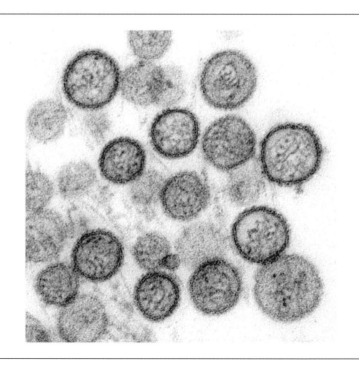

Figure 23.5 Transmission electron micrograph of Sin Nombre virus. Provided by Cynthia Goldsmith and Luanne Elliott. Courtesy of the Centers for Disease Control and Prevention; from CDC website: http://phil.cdc.gov/phil/details.asp

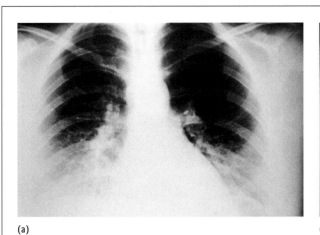
(a)

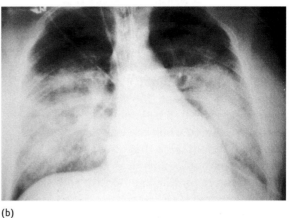
(b)

Figure 23.6 This anterior-posterior (front-to-back) chest X-ray reveals the early (a) and mid-stage (b) bilateral pulmonary edema due to hantavirus pulmonary syndrome (HPS). The radiological evolution of HPS begins with minimal changes of pulmonary edema, progressing to alveolar edema with severe bilateral involvement. Pleural effusions are common and are often large enough to be evident radiographically. Provided by Dr Loren Katai. Courtesy of the Centers for Disease Control and Prevention; from CDC website: http://phil.cdc.gov/phil/details.asp

After this prodromal period that may last 3–5 days, in HPS, coughing and shortness of breath appear, with a rapid increase in the breathing (respiratory) rate. Patients may complain of feeling a "tight band around their chest" or as if "a pillow was put over my face." The main pathology at this point is an acute onset of pulmonary edema (fluid filling the lungs), making it difficult for the lungs to expand and allow air exchange across the alveolar–capillary interfaces. This process can be seen clearly in early and later chest X-rays (Figure 23.6), and upon post-mortem histological examination of the lung tissue (Figure 23.7).

With HFRS, after the prodromal period, there are several further stages with different complications that follow. Five stages are described: febrile (prodromal), hypotensive (low blood pressure), oliguric (little urine output), diuretic (excessive urine output), and convalescent. Not uncommonly, one or more of these stages may be absent. With the prodromal stage, hemorrhage may occur, which may present as facial flushing, reddening or "injection" of the conjunctiva and mucous membranes, and sometimes a petechial (nonblanchable) rash, particularly on the palate and axillary skin folds. Next, a sudden loss of protein into

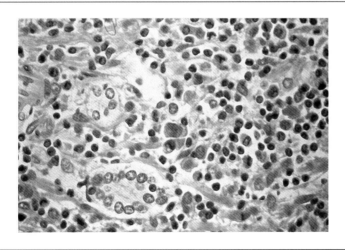

Figure 23.7 Histopathology of lung in hantavirus pulmonary syndrome (HPS). Interstitial pneumonitis and intra-alveolar edema. The disease may be predominated by the host immune response to the virus, resulting in some patients literally "drowning" in their own pulmonary secretions. Provided by Dr Sherif R. Zaki. Courtesy of the Centers for Disease Control and Prevention; from CDC website: http://phil.cdc.gov/phil/details.asp

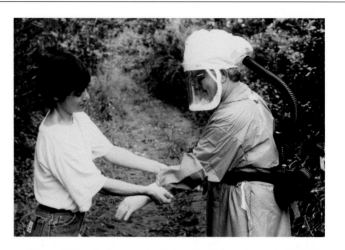

Figure 23.8 Aerosol protection is required when dealing with hantavirus infection. A positive pressure hood and filtered air supply can be seen here, along with the standard personal protective equipment. The virus is typically transmitted by infectious aerosols created when the virus is shed into rodent urine that dries and becomes aerosolized as dust. Courtesy of the Centers for Disease Control and Prevention; from CDC website: http://phil.cdc.gov/phil/details.asp

the urine ("albuminuria") may result in a rapid drop in blood pressure ("hypotension"), which may last for hours to days. Such hypotensive shock can cause nausea and vomiting, and up to 30% of deaths may occur during this hypotensive phase, due to rapid vascular leakage and acute shock. During the next stage ("oliguric"), a lack of urine output causes hypervolemia and fluid overload, during which up to 50% of deaths may occur. If the patient survives this phase, they may still die during the next diuretic phase (excessive urine excretion), again due to hypovolemic shock or other pulmonary complications. The final convalescent stage may last weeks to months before recovery is complete.

Treatment and prevention

When first discovered, HPS with the SN hantavirus in the Four Corners outbreak in 1993 had a case-fatality rate of over 50%. Although, currently, there is no specific hantavirus treatment or vaccine, with early treatment and intensive care support, where patients can be intubated and given oxygen to help them through the period of severe respiratory distress in HPS, their chance of survival is higher. Some hantaviruses causing HPS with additional renal complications may still cause a high mortality, e.g. with BAY, BCC, and AND hantaviruses (Table 23.1). With HFRS, the different viruses have a different mortality rate, though this may be related to the level of healthcare support that the patients receive in those areas. Hantaan HFRS causes the highest mortality of 5–10%, with a lower mortality of 0.1–0.2% for PUU HFRS.

The search for a hantavirus vaccine has been long and, so far, unsuccessful. Even with the advent of modern molecular techniques, developing a safe, effective vaccine that meets all the current stringent health and safety regulations has been problematic. Ribavirin has been shown to be inhibitory for hantaviruses and has been used extensively in the treatment of other viral infections, such as hepatitis B, hepatitis C, respiratory syncytial virus (RSV), and Lassa fever, but randomized controlled trials investigating its efficacy against hantavirus infections are still lacking.

Therefore, at present, prevention relies on the control of the rodent reservoir and vector for hantaviruses. Since anyone who comes into contact with hantavirus-infected rodents is at risk of contracting HPS or HFRS, when working in an area where hantavirus-infected rodents are known to be present, careful use of personal protective equipment against aerosol transmission of the virus is required (Figure 23.8).

Other emerging infections

Many infections can be said to be emerging or re-emerging, but they cannot all be covered here. Some important emerging infections from Asia include Nipah virus, Japanese encephalitis and, most recently, chikungunya virus.

Nipah virus

A mysterious illness broke out in pigs and humans in Malaysia between September 1998 and April 1999, resulting in the deaths of 109 out of 283 infected people, and the destruction of about 1.1 million pigs. The disease was highly contagious in pigs, presenting with fever, respiratory and neurological symptoms. In humans, after an incubation period of 4–18 days, the main clinical feature was encephalitis, rather than respiratory, including fever, headache, myalgia, altered consciousness, disorientation and confusion, progressing to coma within 48 hours in some cases. Nearly all human cases had had direct contact with pigs, rather than via other routes such as mosquitoes or airborne, as close family members of index cases were generally not infected. The disease also spread to Singapore, where an abattoir worker who worked on an infected pig imported from Malaysia also died. Nipah was the name of the Malaysian village from which the first cases were identified.

More recently, in 2005, Nipah virus was reported to be present in Lyle's flying foxes (*Pteropus lylei*) in Cambodia and Thailand, suggesting bats as the possible natural reservoir for this virus. In humans, it appeared again in India in West Bengal as a nosocomial hospital-based outbreak of encephalitis in 2001. It also appeared with similar neurological symptoms in the Tangail district of Bangladesh in 2004–2005, when it was thought to be acquired by the consumption of palm sap that was contaminated by Nipah virus-infected fruit bats (*Pteropus giganteus*).

Molecular analysis of this new virus revealed it to be closely related to Hendra virus, and both of which belong to the genus *Henipah* viruses in the family *Paramyxoviridae* (Figure 23.9). Nipah virus is a lipid-enveloped, single-stranded, negative-sense RNA virus. Diagnosis is usually by serology (IgM and IgG antibody testing) on acute and convalescent sera (taken 10–14 days apart), or by RT-PCR on urine samples, collected from infected patients. Culture and EM are not usually performed for standard diagnostic testing. There is no specific treatment or vaccine for Nipah virus. Treatment remains supportive, e.g. to control the complications of encephalitis, such as seizures. Prevention will rely on the surveillance and control of the apparent bat reservoir, both in their direct contacts with humans and pigs (that may be cross-infected), as well as with food or drink that may be directly consumed by humans.

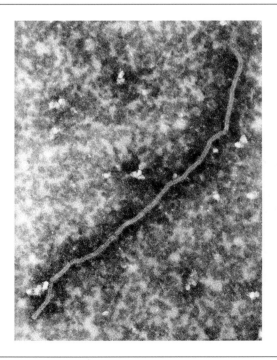

Figure 23.9 A highly magnified (168 000×) transmission electron micrograph of Nipah virus, from the *Henipah* virus genus in the family *Paramyxoviridae*. Courtesy of the Centers for Disease Control and Prevention; from CDC website: http://phil.cdc.gov/phil/details.asp

Japanese encephalitis

Japanese encephalitis (JE) is endemic throughout most of Southeast Asia and infects an estimated 30 000–50 000 people per year, resulting in 10 000–15 000 deaths, but these may be underestimates. It is a mosquito-borne virus, with a lifecycle that does not include man between mosquitoes and birds (particularly wading water birds). Pigs can be infected and act as an amplifier, bringing the virus closer to man. The usual mosquito vectors are of the *Culex* species. Humans become infected from the bite of an infected mosquito, but man is a dead-end host as infected humans do not normally transmit the virus back to the mosquito. Since the virus and its vector are so widespread throughout Asia, most children are normally exposed to the virus prior to adulthood, and in most cases, the infection is subclinical. After an incubation period of 5–15 days, symptomatic infection can be severe, including the various manifestations of encephalitis: a nonspecific febrile illness, followed by altered consciousness, confusion, disorientation, seizures, parkinsonian movements, acute flaccid paralysis, coma and death in up to 20–30% of cases. Half of the survivors will have neurological or psychiatric sequelae. The symptoms are very similar to those described in Nipah virus patients and, initially, JE was thought to be the diagnosis of those cases. However, the epidemiology did not agree with a mosquito-borne route of transmission, as household members of index cases were usually uninfected.

Japanese encephalitis virus is a member of the flavivirus family (*Flaviviridae*), along with dengue, yellow fever, West Nile, and St Louis encephalitis viruses. It is a lipid-enveloped, single-stranded, positive-sense RNA virus. Diagnosis is usually by serological testing on acute and convalescent sera (IgM and IgG antibody testing). If the acute sample is taken early enough (within a few days of onset of illness), RT-PCR testing for JE RNA in the serum may also be useful. Culture and EM are not usually performed for standard diagnostic testing. There is no specific treatment for JE, though there is one report suggesting that intravenous immunoglobulin (IVIg) may be helpful in some cases. Generally, therapy is otherwise supportive, to manage the complications such as seizures, raised intracranial pressure, limb contractures, paralysis, and bed sores. Mechanical ventilation can be given for those with brainstem encephalitis, though the prognosis in such cases may be poor. A live-attenuated JE vaccine produced by serial passage through different cell lines, is currently licensed in China, and has shown excellent safety and efficacy – more than 200 million doses have been given in China. This vaccine has also now been licensed in Nepal, Sri Lanka, South Korea, and India. A new chimeric vaccine based on the 17D yellow fever vaccine is in development and seems promising. However, vector control is still important (Figure 23.10), not just for the control of JE, but other mosquito-borne diseases such as dengue, and more recently chikungunya virus.

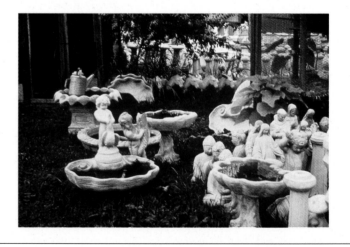

Figure 23.10 Pools of standing water such as in these garden ornaments and in other water containers, are breeding grounds for mosquitoes that can transmit Japanese encephalitis, dengue, and chikungunya viruses. These should be removed or covered to reduce the risk of disease transmission to humans, particularly if they are close to habited areas. Courtesy of the Centers for Disease Control and Prevention; from CDC website: http://phil.cdc.gov/phil/details.asp

Chikungunya

"Chikungunya" is a Swahili (an African dialect) word meaning "that which bends up" and is a description of an infected individual's inability to walk upright because of the joint pains induced by the disease. It is a mosquito-borne virus disease that has been known to be endemic in Southeast Asia and Africa for over 50 years. It has become prominent recently in 2005–2006 due to a large outbreak on islands in the Indian Ocean (Mauritius, Reunion, the Seychelles, and Comoros islands), with subsequent spread of what may be a new strain of the virus to various parts of India with importation into countries worldwide, including Europe, North America, Australia, and Hong Kong. Its usual mosquito vector is of *Aedes* species, with a normal lifecycle involving the mosquito and wild, forest-dwelling primates. Man is an incidental host, but mosquito transmission between man seems to occur. After an incubation period of 3–12 days, infection leads to fever, headache, photophobia (fear of bright lights), sometimes a rash, muscle and joint pains. Usually the illness is mild with few sequeale and almost no mortality, though in the recent outbreak in the Indian Ocean, mortality associated with chikungunya infection was described for the first time. Rarely, severe complications include hemorrhage (e.g. nose bleeds), liver inflammation and failure (fulminant hepatitis), and encephalitis.

Chikungunya virus is member of the *Alphavirus* genus of the Togavirus family (*Togaviridae*). It is a lipid-enveloped, single-stranded, positive-sense RNA virus. Diagnosis is usually by serology (IgM and IgG antibody testing) on acute and convalescent sera. If the acute sample is taken early enough (within 5 days of onset of illness), RT-PCR testing for chikungunya RNA in the serum may also be useful. Culture and EM are not usually performed for standard diagnostic testing. There is no specific treatment or vaccine for chikungunya infection at present and therapy is supportive, though in most cases the disease is mild and self-limiting. As with JE, the main preventative measure is the control of the mosquito vector (Figure 23.10), though this is becoming increasingly difficult with the generally expanding geographical distribution of this insect vector with a globally warmer climate in recent years.

Test yourself

The case study below is based on a true clinical case. The subsequent public health investigation itself and the outcomes discussed are hypothetical, but serve to illustrate the very important public health aspect of investigating emerging infections.

Case study 23.1

Mr Wong is a middle-aged vegetable seller at a local wet market in Hong Kong. He presents to the emergency room with a 2-day history of fever and chills with rigors (shivering), nausea, and vomiting. He states that he has not traveled anywhere outside of Hong Kong recently and has a stable married life. Further questioning revealed that he had visited a local Chinese medicine doctor 10 days earlier for a "flu-like illness," which had not relieved his symptoms. On examination he had a noticeable yellowing of the skin and the whites of his eyes (the "sclera"), a distended abdomen, and dark, tea-colored urine. He also mentioned that his stools were light-colored and foul-smelling and could not be easily flushed away. His circulation and blood pressure appeared to be well-maintained at this point. He remained aware of his surroundings and was able to respond appropriately to all questions.

1. What do you think is going on with this man? Is there anything else you would like to know?

Test yourself

On further questioning, Mr Wong says that he does not drink alcohol regularly and does not give any other history of likely exposure to the waterborne hepatitis viruses A and E (i.e. no drinking of or bathing in contaminated water or the consumption of poorly cooked meat), or the bloodborne hepatitis viruses B and C (i.e. no intravenous drug use or blood product transfusions, or unprotected sexual intercourse with casual partners) (see Chapter 19). He casually mentions that there are lots of rats running around in the wet market and has always worried that he may catch some disease from them.

2. What would you like to ask now?

Although he cannot recall any aerosol-creating actions himself, Mr Wong mentions that a few weeks ago, whilst walking around the back of wet market, he passed close to a cleaning team experimenting with a new water-jet cleaning system for the floor. He thinks he may have inhaled some potentially infected aerosolized particles then. The cleaning crew were wearing protective equipment at the time. Mr Wong is admitted to the hospital for observation. Laboratory testing on paired acute and convalescent sera confirms a progressive rise in the titers of hantavirus IgM and IgG antibodies, and no evidence of any other recent infection by any of the known hepatitis viruses. After the first week, his liver function begins to recover, but he starts to produce large amounts of urine and threatens to go into shock (i.e. a large drop in blood pressure due to loss of circulating fluid volume) during the second week. He is quickly transferred to the ICU where his fluid balance is carefully monitored and maintained, and he eventually makes a complete recovery.

3. If you were the local public health official for this area, what would you do after hearing about this case?

Further reading

AbuBakar S, Sam IC, Wong PF, MatRahim N, Hooi PS, Roslan N. Reemergence of endemic chikungunya, Malaysia. *Emerg Infect Dis* 2007;13(1):147–149

Burfoot D, Reavell S, Tuck C, Wilkinson D. Generation and dispersion of droplets from cleaning equipment used in the chilled food industry. *J Food Eng* 2003;58:343–353

Caramello P, Canta F, Balbiano R, et al. Role of intravenous immunoglobulin administration in Japanese encephalitis. *Clin Infect Dis* 2006;43(12):1620–1621

Chadha MS, Comer JA, Lowe L, et al. Nipah virus-associated encephalitis outbreak, Siliguri, India. *Emerg Infect Dis* 2006;12(2):235–240

Charrel RN, de Lamballerie X, Raoult D. Chikungunya outbreaks – the globalization of vectorborne diseases. *N Engl J Med* 2007;356(8):769–771

Chua KB, Bellini WJ, Rota PA, et al. Nipah virus: a recently emergent deadly paramyxovirus. *Science* 2000;288(5470):1432–1435

Chua KB, Goh KJ, Wong KT, Kamarulzaman A, et al. Fatal encephalitis due to Nipah virus among pig-farmers in Malaysia. *Lancet* 1999;354(9186):1257–1259

Di Giulio DB, Eckburg PB. Human monkeypox: an emerging zoonosis. *Lancet Infect Dis* 2004;4(1):15–25

Goh KJ, Tan CT, Chew NK, et al. Clinical features of Nipah virus encephalitis among pig farmers in Malaysia. *N Engl J Med* 2000;342(17):1229–1235

Hutin YJ, Williams RJ, Malfait P, et al. Outbreak of human monkeypox, Democratic Republic of Congo, 1996 to 1997. *Emerg Infect Dis* 2001;7(3):434–438

Koh YL, Tan BH, Loh JJ, Ooi EE, Su SY, Hsu LY. Japanese encephalitis, Singapore. *Emerg Infect Dis* 2006;12(3):525–526

Kumar R, Tripathi P, Singh S, Bannerji G. Clinical features in children hospitalized during the 2005 epidemic of Japanese encephalitis in Uttar Pradesh, India. *Clin Infect Dis* 2006;43(2):123–131

Laras K, Sukri NC, Larasati RP, et al. Tracking the re-emergence of epidemic chikungunya virus in Indonesia. *Trans R Soc Trop Med Hyg* 2005;99(2):128–141

Lazaro ME, Cantoni GE, Calanni LM, et al. Clusters of hantavirus infection, southern Argentina. *Emerg Infect Dis* 2007;13(1):104–110

Lee N, Wong CK, Lam WY, et al. Chikungunya fever, Hong Kong. *Emerg Infect Dis* 2006;12(11):1790–1792

Luby SP, Rahman M, Hossain MJ, et al. Foodborne transmission of Nipah virus, Bangladesh. *Emerg Infect Dis* 2006;12(12):1888–1894

Mackenzie JS, Chua KB, Daniels PW, et al. Emerging viral diseases of Southeast Asia and the Western Pacific. *Emerg Infect Dis* 2001;7(3 suppl):497–504

Meng G, Lan Y, Nakagawa M, et al. High prevalence of hantavirus infection in a group of Chinese patients with acute hepatitis of unknown aetiology. *J Viral Hepat* 1997;4(4):231–234

Ohrr H, Tandan JB, Sohn YM, Shin SH, Pradhan DP, Halstead SB. Effect of single dose of SA 14-14-2 vaccine 1 year after immunisation in Nepalese children with Japanese encephalitis: a case-control study. *Lancet* 2005;366(9494):1375–1378

Pastorino B, Muyembe-Tamfum JJ, Bessaud M, et al. Epidemic resurgence of chikungunya virus in democratic Republic of the Congo: identification of a new central African strain. *J Med Virol* 2004;74(2):277–282

Reynes JM, Counor D, Ong S, et al. Nipah virus in Lyle's flying foxes, Cambodia. *Emerg Infect Dis* 2005;11(7):1042–1047

Sale TA, Melski JW, Stratman EJ. Monkeypox: an epidemiologic and clinical comparison of African and US disease. *J Am Acad Dermatol* 2006;55(3):478–481

Schmaljohn C, Hjelle B. Hantaviruses: a global disease problem. *Emerg Infect Dis* 1997;3(2):95–104

Schuffenecker I, Iteman I, Michault A, et al. Genome microevolution of chikungunya viruses causing the Indian Ocean outbreak. *PLoS Med* 2006;3(7):e263

Sejvar JJ, Chowdary Y, Schomogyi M, et al. Human monkeypox infection: a family cluster in the midwestern United States. *J Infect Dis* 2004;190(10):1833–1840

Solomon T. Control of Japanese encephalitis – within our grasp? *N Engl J Med* 2006;355(9):869–871

Wacharapluesadee S, Lumlertdacha B, Boongird K, et al. Bat Nipah virus, Thailand. *Emerg Infect Dis* 2005;11(12):1949–1951

Zeier M, Handermann M, Bahr U, et al. New ecological aspects of hantavirus infection: a change of a paradigm and a challenge of prevention – a review. *Virus Genes* 2005;30(2):157–180

Useful websites

CDC. Emerging Infectious Diseases journal. A freely available academic publication covering all emerging/re-emerging infectious diseases. http://www.cdc.gov/ncidod/EID/index.htm

Clinical Medicine and Research journal. http://www.clinmedres.org/cgi/content/full/2/1/1

Marshfield Research Foundation. Photographs of some of the US monkeypox cases. http://www.marshfieldclinic.org/CRC/pages/default.aspx?page=clinical_research_emerg_inf_dis_monk_pox); http://www.marshfieldclinic.org/ldf/MonkeyPox_MarshfieldWI_ClinicalPhotos_v3.ppt; http://www.marshfieldclinic.org/ldf/MonkeyPox_MarshfieldWI_ClinicalPhotos_v3.pdf

National Institute of Allergy and Infectious Diseases. National Institutes of Health website on emerging/re-emerging infections. http://www3.niaid.nih.gov/research/topics/emerging/default.htm (including a disease-by-disease hyperlink index page, though the number of diseases covered is quite limited at the time of writing); http://www3.niaid.nih.gov/healthscience/healthtopics/emerging/default.htm

Chapter 24

Emerging infections II (West Nile virus, dengue, severe acute respiratory syndrome-associated coronavirus)

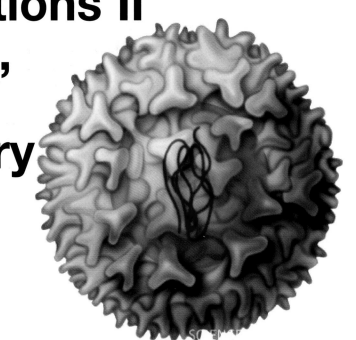

J.W. Tang, P.K.S. Chan*

Introduction
West Nile Virus
Dengue fever
  Virology
  Clinical features and diagnosis
  Diagnostic virological investigations
  Management
  Control
  Vaccine development

Severe acute respiratory syndrome-associated coronavirus (SARS-CoV)
  The virus
  Origin and transmission
  Clinical features
  Laboratory diagnosis
  Treatment
  Summary

Introduction

This chapter continues the theme of emerging viruses as introduced in the previous chapter. All of these new, emerging viruses have at least one thing in common: that they have all emerged from identifiable animal sources, i.e. that they are all zoonoses. Very often, in such cases, human infections are accidental and a "dead-end," such that further onward transmission back to other human or animal hosts may be inefficient.

West Nile Virus

West Nile virus (WNV) is a mosquito-borne arbovirus that is a relatively new pathogen in the USA, but it was first discovered in 1937 in a patient from the West Nile district in northern Uganda. Since the discovery of WNV in the North-Eastern USA in the late summer of 1999 (Box 24.1), it has spread steadily west across the country with the reported number of human cases (number of deaths) being reported each year being 62 (7) in 1999, 21 (2) in 2000, 66 (9) in 2001, 4156 (284) in 2002, 9862 (264) in 2003, 2539 (100) in 2004, and 3000 (119) in 2005, with an average case-fatality of 7–8%.

* Paul K.S. Chan is the main author of the section "Severe acute respiratory syndrome-associated coronavirus (SARS-CoV)," with contributions from Julian W. Tang.

Box 24.1 The US West Nile virus probably originated from a virus found in a dead goose in Israel in 1998

With modern molecular techniques, such as reverse-transcription polymerase chain reaction (RT-PCR) and DNA sequencing, it was possible to trace the origin of the US WNV. The WNV genome consists of single-stranded, positive-sense RNA, meaning that it acts as its own messenger RNA (mRNA) that codes directly for WNV proteins. There are several WNV-encoded proteins that can be generally divided into nonstructural proteins (mainly enzymes that do not form the actual structure of the virus) and structural proteins (that form the viral capsid, envelope, and membrane proteins). It is important to choose the right protein coding region or gene to sequence when one is searching for the possible geographic origin of a particular virus strain within the same species (WNV). The gene chosen for sequencing must not be too conserved, otherwise it will just appear the same as other viruses of the same species isolated from all over the world. Typically, such conserved genes are found in the nonstructural enzyme genes, as these are essential to viral replication and cannot vary too much, otherwise they will not function. Therefore, often the structural genes are chosen, particularly the genes coding for "external" structures, such as the envelope or membrane protein-coding genes. These are the most exposed to the external host environment and may change between different hosts in response to the local immune response or drugs, for example.

For WNV, the US investigators, in 1999, chose the envelope or E gene to sequence. This was still recognizable as a WNV-specific protein, but had just enough variation between different strains obtained from all over the world, to show from where the US strain may have originated. Once they had this sequence of this E gene, they compared this sequence with other WNV E gene sequences from all over the world by applying a technique called "phylogenetic analysis" using various computer software programs. The comparison WNV E sequences from other countries worldwide had been deposited by investigators into various public sequence databases accessible via the internet, with one of the most popular being "Genbank," which is maintained at the US National Center for Biotechnology Information (NCBI, at: http://www.ncbi.nlm.nih.gov/entrez/query.fcgi?db= Nucleotide). Using these techniques, the US investigators constructed a "phylogenetic tree" that showed that the US WNV E gene sequence was most closely related to that obtained from a dead goose in Israel in 1998. It is uncertain how this virus reached the USA from the Middle East, but it is likely to have been via an infected bird that may have flown near or been blown off course in passing close to the USA during its migration. *Culex* mosquitoes from the USA may then have fed on this bird, become infected with WNV, and transmitted WNV to local US birds as well as humans.

Culex mosquitoes are the main vector of WNV transmission to humans, with *Cx. pipiens* being the main vector in the northeast, *Cx. quinquefasciatus* in the south, and *Cx. tarsalis* (Figure 24.1) in the west. Birds are the main amplifying host for WNV, and the level of viremia in birds can infect feeding mosquitoes (Figure 24.1). Not all birds are well adapted and immune to WNV infection; in particular, WNV causes a high mortality in crows and jays (from the bird family *Corvidae*) and such bird deaths have been used to monitor the spread of WNV across the USA. Humans are an incidental, dead-end host, with the levels of WNV in the blood of infected patients unlikely to be high enough to infect mosquitoes.

Most WNV human infections are asymptomatic. After being bitten by an infected mosquito, there is an incubation period range of about 2–14 days (typically 2–6 days), with a variety of nonspecific complaints in symptomatic cases: sudden onset of high fever (usually >39°C), headache, myalgia (muscle pains), and weakness with gastrointestinal symptoms. These acute symptoms often resolve after a week, but prolonged fatigue is common. Occasionally, there is also a transient macular (flat, red) rash on the trunk and limbs. In some individuals, persisting neck pain or stiffness with muscle weakness and fatigue lasted up to 1 month after onset. In more severe cases, specific organ damage is evident, including damage to the liver (hepatitis), pancreas (pancreatitis), heart (myocarditis), muscles (rhabdomyolysis), testicles (orchitis), and eyes (ocular

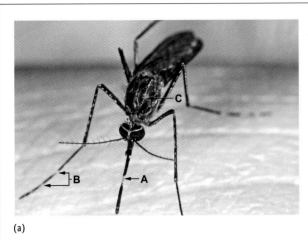

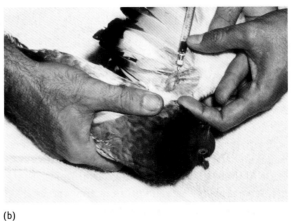

(a)   (b)

Figure 24.1 (a) A close-up view of a *Culex tarsalis* mosquito as it is about to begin feeding on the skin of a human host. Note the light-colored band wrapped around its dark-scaled proboscis (A), and the multiple similarly light-colored bands wrapped around the tibia and femur, of its forelegs and middle legs (B), identifying this as *C. tarsalis*. Other identifying characteristics include the presence of two silver dots on its dorsal scutum; however, in this particular image, only one of the two bilateral silver scutal marks is visible (C). (b) Blood being extracted from the wing vein of a pigeon to be tested for arboviruses. Birds are the natural reservoir and part of the transmission cycle of numerous arboviruses, including West Nile virus. Provided by James Gathany. Courtesy of the Centers for Disease Control and Prevention; from CDC website: http://phil.cdc.gov/phil/details.asp

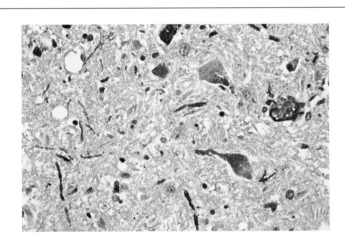

Figure 24.2 Brain tissue from a West Nile encephalitis patient, showing antigen-positive neurons and neuronal processes (in red). Provided by J. Shieh and S. Zaki. Courtesy of the Centers for Disease Control and Prevention; from CDC website: http://phil.cdc.gov/phil/details.asp

disease). The most serious form of WNV disease, fortunately involving less than 1% of cases, affects the central nervous system (CNS) in the form of meningitis, encephalitis, and paralysis. Encephalitis patients can range in severity from mild confusion, to coma and death (Figure 24.2). Patients with other CNS disease develop severe tremors, incoordination, movement disorders, and Parkinsons disease-like symptoms. (See Box 24.2 for a case study of an unusual manifestation of WNV.)

West Nile fever and/or encephalitis is caused by a WNV, a member of the flavivirus family. It is a lipid-enveloped, single-stranded, positive-sense RNA virus, with a genome of about 11 000 nucleotides (11 kb), and a diameter of approximately 50 nm. Diagnosis of WNV infection usually relies on serological testing, i.e. detection of WNV IgM antibodies in a single sample of blood or cerebral spinal fluid (CSF – the fluid

Box 24.2 An unusual manifestation of human West Nile Virus infection

In most cases, WNV infection is asymptomatic. In symptomatic cases, most suffer nonspecific symptoms such as fever, headache and malaise, some nausea and vomiting, and muscle aches. More serious cases involve neurological symptoms which may not resolve fully, even when the patient has "recovered" from the acute infection. However, very occasionally, a rare manifestation may occur and be confused with other possible infections, with the true cause of illness being diagnosed only at post-mortem.

A 35-year-old landscape gardener, previously fit and well, had just returned home to Florida after a 2-week safari in South Africa. He remained well on the flight home and for the first week after returning home. At the beginning of the second week, he started to feel ill, with a fever, chills, and a headache. He told his boss that he wouldn't be coming into work that day, that it was probably just "flu" and he would take some pain-killers and go to sleep. The next morning, he felt worse and noticed what looked like blood in his urine and stools. His wife was concerned and insisted that he go with her to the local hospital.

At the local hospital, he was rapidly triaged (i.e. prioritized for physician consultation based on his clinical history and presentation) into an isolation room, and was soon seen by a senior member of the ER staff. The initial concern was that he had contracted a viral hemorrhagic fever (VHF – see Chapter 22), such as Crimean-Congo, Ebola or Marburg hemorrhagic fevers. Various blood samples were taken from the patient for testing using strict universal precautions and he was admitted to the hospital's only negative-pressure isolation room for further observation. The wife was also considered to be infected and incubating the organism, and was also quarantined in another isolation room (though without negative pressure facilities), near to her husband. All blood samples were treated under Biosafety Level 4 (BSL-4) containment and CDC was contacted about a possible imported VHF case.

On admission, clinical examination revealed multiple small bruises ("petechiae") all over his arms and legs with some larger bruises ("ecchymoses") on his abdomen and thighs. He had a low blood pressure of 90/50 mm Hg, was febrile at 39°C, a fast pulse rate (130 beats per minute – "tachycardia"), and a rapid breathing rate (26 breaths per minute – "tachypnoea"). The main findings on his blood investigations were that his platelet levels were low – presumably used up in trying to stop internal bleeding – and his clotting factors were deranged. His doctors were concerned that he was developing a blood clotting disorder, sometimes seen in severe infection, called "disseminated intravascular coagulation" (DIC). This occurs when the infection triggers inappropriate blood clotting in the blood vessels, and at the same time the body reacts by trying to remove these clots. The result is that all the body's blood clotting factors are used up, and eventually the patient may bleed to death, internally, as can be seen in VHFs. Blood samples were couriered urgently to CDC BSL-4 laboratories for VHF testing. Later that night, CDC contacted the physician on-call to say that none of the tests detected any VHFs, however further samples were required to make sure of this. No other pathogens, bacterial (e.g. rickettsial species), parasitic (e.g. malaria), or otherwise, had been detected so far, but he had been started on broad-spectrum antibiotics since admission.

The next day, the patient deteriorated. He had developed more bruising and extremely low, life-threatening hypotension (low blood pressure), a condition known as "septic shock." He now needed intensive care level support to monitor his heart function in response to intravenous fluids and drugs given to support his failing circulation. This equipment was brought into and set up in the isolation unit with great difficulty. Later that day, he developed multi-organ failure including renal, liver and respiratory requiring ventilation, but in spite of all the support, he died that evening.

His wife remained well throughout this 24-hour period, but she was required to stay in quarantine for longer, at least until they could identify the organism, and if not for possibly up to 3 weeks. This was longer than the incubation period of most organisms that could cause a hemorrhagic fever, similar to that seen in her husband. The wife consented for a post-mortem to be performed to this end. Almost as an after thought, the wife mentioned that he had complained of mosquito bites, both during his time in Africa, as well as after returning home to Florida.

At post-mortem, various tissue biopsies were taken from all the major organs including heart, lung, liver, kidney, skin, and brain, and sent to CDC for further VHF testing. In response to the wife's mention of mosquito bites, they were also tested for mosquito-borne diseases, such as dengue, St Louis and Japanese encephalitis viruses, yellow and Rift Valley fever, as well as WNV. The next day, CDC called back saying that virtually all the samples that they had received were positive for WNV by RT-PCR and IF testing, so the most likely diagnosis was fatal hemorrhagic fever due to disseminated WNV infection. Further sequencing and phylogenetic analysis revealed that this WNV strain was a local US strain, commonly found in Florida.

In summary then, this patient died of a rare manifestation of an otherwise well-recognized disease. The alternative that was considered, which ultimately turned out to be a red-herring, was a common manifestation of an otherwise rare disease, such as certain VHFs, though some like Crimean-Congo hemorrhagic fever are not uncommon in southern African countries.

In medicine, the correct diagnosis often hinges on that diagnosis having being thought of in the first place, and being included in the differential diagnoses that are correctly investigated and interpreted.

surrounding the brain and spinal cord). Normally, such WNV IgM antibodies will be detectable about 8 days after onset of symptoms (in symptomatic patients), with IgG antibodies becoming detectable about 4 days later. A pair of blood samples taken 10–14 days apart showing a fourfold rise in WNV IgG antibody titers is also diagnostic of recent WNV infection. Interestingly, the presence of WNV IgM antibodies may be detectable for at least a year in some patients, so a positive result may not necessarily mean a recent infection with WNV. Nowadays, molecular techniques allow WNV infection to be diagnosed earlier, before antibodies appear, by detecting the WNV genome or RNA by reverse-transcription polymerase chain reaction (RT-PCR) in blood or CSF or other tissues, such as brain tissue in post-mortem investigations. The only problem with this is that samples taken for these molecular tests must be taken early, soon after infection, as the viremia is transient and starts to drop around the time that antibody starts appearing. The virus can also be grown in cell culture with identification by immunofluorescence testing (IF). The virus can also be seen using electron microscopy (EM, Figure 24.3), though this is not the normal diagnostic test of choice, as it

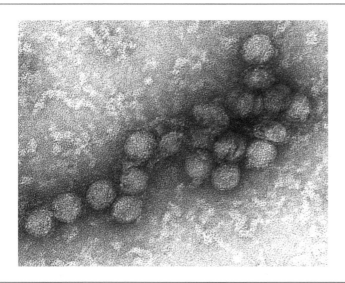

Figure 24.3 An electron micrograph of the West Nile virus. West Nile virus is a flavivirus commonly found in Africa, West Asia, and the Middle East. It is closely related to St Louis encephalitis virus found in the USA. The virus can infect humans, birds, mosquitoes, horses, and some other mammals. Provided by Cynthia Goldsmith. Courtesy of the Centers for Disease Control and Prevention; from CDC website: http://phil.cdc.gov/phil/details.asp

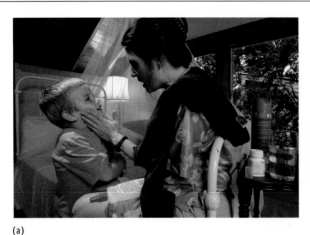
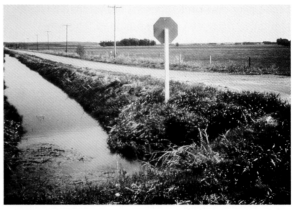

(a)   (b)

Figure 24.4 (a) A mother applying mosquito repellent to her child's skin, in order to prevent mosquitoes from biting, thereby preventing many arboviral, infections such as West Nile virus. (b) Roadside drainage ditches like this are breeding sites for *Culex tarsalis* mosquitoes that can carry and transmit West Nile virus. Courtesy of the Centers for Disease Control and Prevention; from CDC website: http://phil.cdc.gov/phil/details.asp

does not distinguish WNV from other flaviviruses, such as dengue and St Louis encephalitis viruses. There is also cross-reactivity between the antibody tests of these various flaviviruses, and specific IF and RT-PCR testing may be required to distinguish these different flavivirus species.

Management of WNV infection is generally supportive, as there is no specific antiviral therapy. Headaches, meningitis, nausea and vomiting, muscle aches and pains are treated with analgesic and antiemetic (antivomiting) medication. Patients presenting with serious CNS disease with fits can be given anticonvulsives and may need sedation and ventilation. The prognosis is variable, generally related to the severity of clinical illness. Patients with CNS disease tend to require hospitalization and generally have worse outcomes, with persisting neurological deficits (either physical or cognitive impairment), for months or years later.

Prevention is still based on the avoidance of mosquito bites, and the removal of breeding sites for mosquito larvae (Figure 24.4). Although there has been a recent live, attenuated vaccine developed and tested in healthy adult human volunteers, it is still at an early stage.

Dengue fever

Dengue virus causing dengue fever is the most ubiquitous of the vector-borne arboviruses. It is estimated that dengue fever is endemic in over 100 countries and that 40% (approximately 2.5 billion people) of the world's population are at risk, with about 50–100 million cases of infection occurring each year. This includes 250 000–500 000 (0.5%) cases of severe dengue hemorrhagic fever (DHF), with an untreated mortality of as high as 12–44%. However, with treatment, the mortality of DHF can be as low as 0.2%. Increasing levels of international travel, effects of global warming, lack of piped water supplies, and the increase of standing water storage in poorer areas all contribute to the increased survival and spread of the mosquito vectors responsible for dengue infection of humans. The main vector for the transmission of dengue virus to humans is the *Aedes (Ae.)* mosquito, *Ae. aegypti* in particular, but also other species, particularly *Ae. albopictus* and *Ae. polynesiensis*, *Ae. scutellaris* and, possibly, *Ae. cooki* and *Ae. hebrideus* (Figure 24.5).

Climate conditions limit the scope of these vectors to approximate latitudes 35°N and 35°S, though temperature changes associated with global warming may alter these boundaries in the future. One example

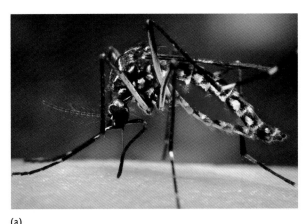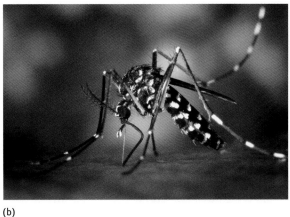

(a)   (b)

Figure 24.5 *Aedes aegypti* (a) and *Aedes albopictus* (b) female mosquitoes feeding on a human host. © James Gathany. Courtesy of the Centers for Disease Control and Prevention; from CDC website: http://phil.cdc.gov/phil/details.asp

of this is the expanding range of *Ae. albopictus*, which can now be found not just in Asia, but also North and South America, Southern Europe, and the Pacific Islands.

Virology

Dengue virus is a Flavivirus: an enveloped, single-stranded, positive-sense RNA virus, about 50 nm in diameter. It has a 11-kb genome coding for 10 proteins (three structural and seven nonstructural), and is classified into four serotypes (dengue 1–4). It shares extensive serological cross-reactivity with other flaviviruses, such as yellow fever, West Nile fever, Japanese encephalitis, and St Louis encephalitis viruses. Infection with one dengue serotype produces lifelong immunity to that serotype, but only partial and temporary protection to the other serotypes. Such cross-reacting antibody may give rise to more serious dengue disease (such as dengue hemorrhagic fever and dengue shock syndrome) in patients previously infected with one serotype and subsequently infected with another, different serotype – a mechanism referred to as antibody-dependent enhancement (ADE). Dengue virus is transmitted by the bite of mosquitoes of the *Aedes* genus, in which the virus replicates and the mosquitoes remain infected for life.

Clinical features and diagnosis

Dengue virus infection can result in a range of clinical outcomes, ranging from asymptomatic to fatal disease. A general classification of severity is used by most clinicians: classic dengue fever, dengue hemorrhagic fever and dengue shock syndrome. The severity of disease can be determined by the degree of hemoconcentration (indicating vascular permeability and leakage), thrombocytopenia (low platelet count), and clotting derangement.

Classic dengue fever (DF) is the most common manifestation of dengue virus infection, affecting mainly older children and young adults. It has an abrupt onset and can be very incapacitating. The usual incubation period after getting bitten by an infected mosquito is 4–7 (range 3–14) days. There may be a prodromal period of 6–12 hours when the patient may experience headache, malaise, backache, chills, fatigue, anorexia, and sometimes a rash. With fever onset, these symptoms may worsen, and other symptoms like retro-orbital pain, more severe headaches, conjunctival congestion, severe myalgia, and backache contribute to the typical features of dengue "breakbone fever." Normally, the fever subsides after 5–7 days, but may reach a peak of 40°C and may follow a biphasic course before defervescence. During this period, a rash may be present, usually patchy and maculopapular, with areas of erythema surrounding normal skin.

Dengue hemorrhagic fever (DHF) and dengue shock syndrome (DSS) are more severe forms of dengue fever distinguished from classic DF by more extreme disturbances in the hematocrit, platelet count. and clotting factors. Initially, patients with DHF may present as for DF, although the maculopapular rash and arthralgia are less frequently seen. The patient may show signs of circulatory problems with restlessness, sweating, cold, clammy skin, tachycardia (high heart rate), and low blood pressure due to loss of intravascular circulating volume. The hematocrit rises, the platelet count falls and disturbances develop in the clotting cascade, with prolongation of prothrombin time (PT) and partial thromboplastin time (PTT). With appropriate supportive therapy (fluid replacement, correction of platelet and coagulation defects), the patient generally recovers. If the disease progresses, then DSS may develop, manifest by a rapid weak pulse, narrowing of the pulse pressure (the difference between systolic and diastolic blood pressures), and hypotension with ascites and pleural effusions due to leakage of fluid from the vascular system. Further deterioration is indicated by disseminated intravascular coagulation (DIC), metabolic acidosis, profound shock, and multi-organ failure.

The following features are consistent with a diagnosis of DHF: fever lasting 2–7 days; hemorrhagic diathesis (as shown by a positive tourniquet test (Box 24.3), or petechiae/ecchymoses/purpura, or bleeding from mucosa/gastrointestinal tract/injection sites/other locations, or hematemesis or melaena); thrombocytopenia ($\leq$100 000 mm^3); evidence of plasma leakage (as evidenced by a hematocrit $\geq$20% above average, or a fall in hematocrit $\geq$20% of baseline following fluid replacement, or a rise in hematocrit $\geq$20% during the course of the illness). In addition, WHO guidelines give an additional sign of plasma leakage as the presence of pleural effusions, ascites, or hypoproteinemia. These signs can be used for confirming the diagnosis of DHF when the hematocrit cannot be easily measured.

Features of DHF together with signs of circulatory failure signify a further deterioration to DSS. The WHO guidelines list the following signs as indications of circulatory failure: either tachycardia together with narrowed pulse pressure ($\leq$20 mmHg), or hypotension for age (defined as BP <80 mmHg for those less than 5 years of age, and <90 mmHg for those aged 5 years or older), together with cold, clammy skin and restlessness.

Box 24.3 Tourniquet test (source: Pan American Health Organization. Dengue and Dengue Hemorrhagic Fever: Guidelines for Prevention and Control. Washington, DC: PAHO. 1994;12.)

The tourniquet test assesses capillary fragility. You inflate the blood pressure cuff to a point midway between the systolic and diastolic blood pressures for 5 minutes. After deflating the cuff, wait for the skin to return to its normal color, and then count the number of petechiae visible in a one-inch-square (2.5 × 2.5 cm) area on the ventral surface of the forearm. Twenty or more petechiae in the one-inch-square patch constitutes a positive test.

This slide demonstrates what a typical positive result from a tourniquet test may look like. This patient has more than 20 petechiae per square inch.

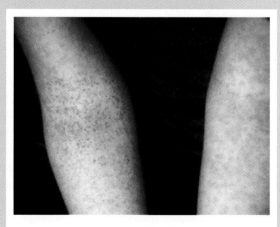

Courtesy Centers for Disease Control
http://www.cdc.gov/ncidod/dvbid/dengue/
slideset/set1/vi/slide10.htm

There are four grades of severity of DHF/DSS used by the WHO: Grade I: fever with nonspecific symptoms and minor bleeding or easy bruising; Grade II: Grade I features with, in addition, spontaneous bleeding from the skin or other sites; Grade III: Grade I and II features with signs of circulatory failure; Grade IV: profound shock with undetectable pulse or blood pressure.

Diagnostic virological investigations

The most common diagnostic test for suspected dengue infection is serology. On a single sample, a dengue-specific IgM response may be detected 5–7 days after fever onset. This IgM response peaks after about 2 weeks, then becomes undetectable 2–3 months later. Alternatively, acute infection can be demonstrated by a fourfold rise in dengue-specific IgG titers on paired acute and convalescent sera (taken 2–4 weeks later) using complement fixation, hemagglutination inhibition, or type-specific plaque-reduction assays. Commercial kits are available to detect both dengue IgM and IgG, though the IgG kits are not quantitative and seroconversion for IgG on acute and convalescent sera, rather than a fourfold rise in titers, will confirm a recent dengue infection.

Culture of dengue virus can be performed in live mosquitoes or mosquito cell lines such as C6/36. Serum samples collected within 5 days of illness (before the appearance of antibody), inoculated into C6/36 cells or live mosquitoes and incubated for 10–14 days, may reveal virus antigen by immunofluorescence detection or enzyme immunoassay (EIA). Not all dengue viruses will produce a visible cytopathic effect (CPE). Sensitivity of this approach is variable, between 36% and 80%, depending on the experience and expertise of the laboratory and the quality of the clinical specimens. Generally, molecular techniques are more sensitive.

Dengue RNA detection by reverse-transcriptase polymerase chain reaction (RT-PCR) offers an early diagnosis, within 5 days of illness onset, before an antibody response is detectable. In addition to being highly sensitive, viable virus is unnecessary, as long as sufficient viral RNA is present in the specimen (usually serum). If specific typing primers are used, then the dengue serotype can also be rapidly reported, without the need for time-consuming serotype-specific neutralization assays. Molecular detection of dengue RNA can even be performed later on in the disease, when antibodies and immune complexes are present, as the RNA extraction process will remove this excess protein, enhancing the sensitivity of this diagnostic approach. More recently, some studies have demonstrated that patients with more severe dengue disease tend to exhibit a higher dengue RNA viral load, although it is uncertain exactly what level of viral load is predictive of more severe dengue disease.

Management

The pathogenesis of dengue infection involves increased vascular permeability due to the activation of various cytokine cascades. This leads to the leakage of plasma from blood vessels into the extravascular spaces leading to fluid collections such as ascites and pleural effusions, and hypotension and shock in severe, untreated disease. In addition, disturbances of the clotting system occur in severe disease, including capillary fragility, thrombocytopenia, and clotting factor derangement. Presently, no specific antiviral drug exists for treating dengue, and supportive therapy consists of careful monitoring and replacement of fluids and clotting factors as required.

Control

The control of dengue infection in humans relies on two complementary approaches. Controlling the mosquito population (vector control) is difficult but includes the use of insecticides and the removal of standing water where mosquito larvae can breed. Countries such as Singapore, where dengue is endemic, may also use indoor spraying during dengue epidemics, to control the adult mosquito population. Individuals may reduce their risk of contracting dengue fever by reducing the number of mosquito bites by the use of protective clothing and/or nontoxic insecticides applied to the skin. In addition to this, surveillance of both the mosquito vector and human dengue cases may give warning of a possible approaching dengue outbreak and allow healthcare services time to prepare.

Vaccine development

At present there is no licensed vaccine for dengue fever, though several are in development. The main problem to overcome is the possible unintentional risk of more severe dengue disease due to vaccine-induced antibody-dependent enhancement. One way to overcome this is to make a tetravalent vaccine to induce, simultaneously, protective antibodies to all four dengue serotypes. However, the difficulty then lies in ensuring that each serotype component of the vaccine induces an adequate protective immune response: this is the subject of ongoing studies and trials.

Severe acute respiratory syndrome-associated coronavirus (SARS-CoV)

"Severe acute respiratory syndrome (SARS)" refers to an emerging infectious disease first recognized in late 2002/early 2003. The disease appeared initially as an outbreak of atypical pneumonia of unknown etiology in November 2002 in Foshan, Guangdong Province in southern China. The disease soon spread to neighboring cities, and escalated in February 2003 to involve Vietnam, Hong Kong, Canada, and more than 30 countries subsequently worldwide. The global outbreak ended in July 2003, with a total of 8098 probable cases and at least 774 deaths. After a period of quiescence, a cluster of infection was detected again in December 2003 and January 2004 in Guangdong Province. Since then, no more human cases have been reported. SARS is due to infection with a newly identified coronavirus named as SARS-associated coronavirus (SARS-CoV).

The virus

SARS-CoV is member of the family *Coronaviridae*. Coronaviruses have a wide range of host tropism causing acute respiratory, enteric and central nervous system diseases in pigs, cats, dogs, cattle and avian species. Two human coronaviruses (HuCoV-229E and HuCoV-OC43) were identified in the mid-1960s. Both cause mild upper respiratory tract infections and therefore have not received much medical attention. In additional to SARS-CoV, two other coronaviruses, HCoV-NL63 and HCoV-HKU1, were recently found to cause respiratory tract illnesses in humans.

Coronaviruses are classified into three genera, usually referred as groups, based on their antigenicity. Group 1 comprises HuCoV-229E, HuCoV-NL63, porcine diarrhea epidemic virus, transmissible gastroenteritis virus, feline infectious peritonitis virus, and canine coronaviruses. Group 2 contains HuCoV-OC43, HuCoV-HKU1, mouse hepatitis virus, hemagglutinating encephalomyelitis virus, and bovine coronavirus. Group 3 are exclusively found in birds including avian infectious bronchitis virus and turkey coronavirus. The newly identified SARS-CoV is antigenically distinct from the previously recognized three groups.

Coronaviruses contain the largest genome among RNA viruses known today. The 30-kb positive-sense, single-stranded, polyadenylated RNA is organized into ~15 open reading frames. The RNA molecule is complexed with nucleocapsid proteins (N). Inserted on the surface of the viral envelope are spike glycoproteins (S) that are responsible for receptor-binding and initiation of infection cycle (Figure 24.6). The name "corona" means "crown" in Latin, which describes the characteristic appearance of the round or elliptical virion that is surrounded by multiple, regularly inserted, long petal-shaped spikes (Figure 24.7). The overall size of the virion ranges from 60 to 220 nm.

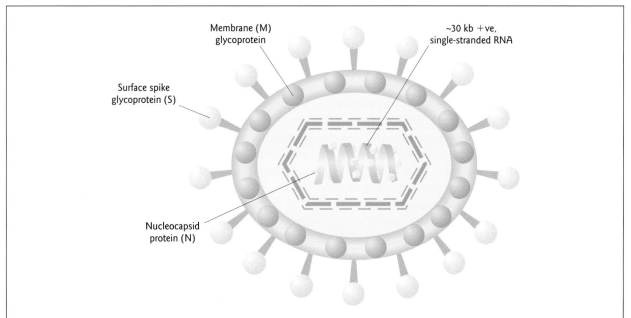

Figure 24.6 Structure of coronavirus. Figure kindly provided by Professor Paul K.S. Chan, Department of Microbiology, The Chinese University of Hong Kong, Hong Kong SAR

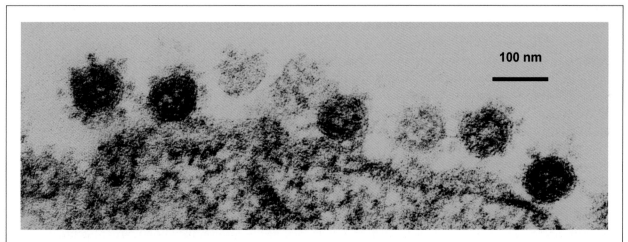

Figure 24.7 Electron micrograph of coronavirus. Thin section of a Vero cell showing budding of coronaviruses through the plasma membrane. The characteristic morphology of "crown" (corona in Latin) is demonstrated. Image courtesy of the Department of Microbiology, The Chinese University of Hong Kong, kindly provided by Professor Paul KS Chan

Origin and transmission

Before November 2002, no human infection with SARS-CoV had been previously documented. Analysis of the viral genome sequences did not reveal any evidence of recent recombination with human coronaviruses. The source of infection is likely to be a direct cross-species transmission from an animal reservoir. This is supported by the fact that the early SARS cases in Guangdong Province had some history of exposure to live wild animals in markets serving the restaurant trade (Box 24.4). Animal traders working with animals

Box 24.4 Animal and human coronaviruses mixing in live animal markets

Severe acute respiratory syndrome (SARS)-like coronaviruses have been found in several animals, in particular the Himalayan palm civet (*Paguma larvata*) and the raccoon dog (*Nyctereutes procyonoides*). More recently, coronaviruses have been found in several species of bats, including horseshoe bats (*Rhinolphus* spp.), large-winged and bent-winged bats (*Miniopterus* spp.), and pipistrelle bats (*Pipistrellus* spp.). Some scientists are therefore convinced that the bat is the natural animal reservoir for the SARS-CoV. However, these bat coronaviruses are quite dissimilar to SARS-CoV, particularly in the part of their genomes that code for receptor binding to host cells. So, there may be yet another intermediate animal host within which these bat coronaviruses further mutate to emerge as SARS-CoV that can infect civets and humans. The mixing of coronaviruses from different animal species may occur in the traditional live animal markets found in southern China, in Guangdong province, where live bats and civets were sold as food. Since the 2003 SARS outbreaks, the Chinese government authorities are restricting the types of animals that can be sold in these live markets, in particular, the sale of civets has now been banned. It may be necessary to also restrict or ban the sales of live bats for the same reasons.

in these markets had higher seroprevalence for SARS coronavirus, though they did not report any illness compatible with SARS. More importantly, SARS-CoV-like virus detected from some animal species had more than a 99% homology with human SARS-CoV. Subsequent phylogenetic analysis performed on a large number of full-genome sequences indicated that the Himalayan palm civet cat (*Paguma larvata*) was likely to be at least one of the sources of these early human SARS-CoV infections.

SARS-CoV can spread in humans in several ways. Like other respiratory viruses, it is spread mainly by droplets generated by upper respiratory tract symptoms, e.g. coughing and sneezing. One unique feature of SARS-CoV is that the virus shedding, and thus the infectivity, peaks at the second week of illness rather than during the initial few days as seen in other respiratory viruses, like influenza. A few so-called "super-spreading" events of SARS-CoV have been documented. One of these was thought to be the result of the use of a nebulizer (a respiratory assist device that supplies high-flow oxygen and bronchodilating drugs in a vapor form) on an unrecognized case of SARS in an overcrowded, poorly ventilated ward.

There is also evidence to suggest that SARS-CoV might have spread by the airborne route during a major outbreak in a private residential complex, Amoy Gardens, in Hong Kong. In addition to the respiratory tract, a high viral load was also found from stool samples during the second and third weeks of illness. Although SARS-CoV is an enveloped virus, it survives well in the environment. The virus is stable in stool at room temperature for at least 1–2 days and up to 4 days in higher pH stool, such as that found in patients with diarrhea. Direct contact with objects contaminated with infected respiratory secretions or feces is another possible direct contact route of infection.

Clinical features

SARS has an incubation period of 2–10 days. The clinical presentation is quite pronounced and is typical of acute systemic viral infections. Fever, chills, and malaise are the most frequent symptoms in adult, but are less obvious in young children and the elderly. Although, SARS-CoV primarily attacks the respiratory tract, respiratory symptoms including cough, sputum, runny nose ("rhinorrhea"), and sore throat are relatively uncommon at presentation. About 10–15% of patients experienced watery diarrhea during the second week of illness (Table 24.1).

The clinical course of SARS varies from a mild upper respiratory tract illness, usually seen in young children, to respiratory failure which occurred in around 20–25% of mainly adult patients. As the disease

Table 24.1 Presenting symptoms of 1312 laboratory confirmed SARS patients in Hong Kong (data from Chan JCK, Sung JJY, Yam LYC. Clinical course of SARS. In: Chan JCK, Taam Wong VCW (eds) *Challenges of Severe Acute Respiratory Syndrome.* Singapore: Elsevier, 2006;254–276)

Presenting symptom	% of cases
Fever	93
Chills	61
Malaise	58
Myalgia	46
Rigor	38
Cough	41
Sputum	19
Shortness of breath	12
Diarrhea	17
Nausea	12
Vomiting	10

progresses, patients start to develop shortness of breath. From the second week onwards, patients progress to respiratory failure and acute respiratory distress syndrome, often requiring intensive care.

The predominant radiographic abnormality of SARS is airspace opacification at the lower zones and the periphery of the lung field. About half of the patients had multifocal involvement. Computed tomography (CT) is more sensitive than radiography to detect pulmonary lesions. Common CT findings of SARS include ground-glass opacification with or without consolidation, interlobular septal and intralobular interstitial thickening. Some patients also develop pneumothorax and pneumomediastinum. However, none of the imaging characteristics alone are specific enough for a diagnosis of SARS. Extrapulmonary manifestations of SARS include diarrhea, lymphopenia, reactive hepatitis, low-grade disseminated intravascular coagulation, and more rarely, status epilepticus.

The overall mortality rate of SARS as reported by WHO was 11%, and the reported rate from various countries ranged from 7% to 17%. Elderly persons, aged >65 years, and those with comorbidity suffered a more severe course of illness with a mortality as high as 50%. A high presenting and peak serum lactate dehydrogenase (LDH) level and a high presenting peripheral blood neutrophil count were found to be associated with a poor outcome. Some degree of long-term pulmonary function impairment was observed in around 25% of survivors in a cohort of Hong Kong patients. Infection in children is much milder and no deaths were reported.

Asymptomatic infection of SARS-CoV in adults is very rare, but data on children and elderly is less comprehensive.

Laboratory diagnosis

Infection with SARS-CoV can be confirmed by virus isolation, serology, or molecular amplification of the viral RNA. Unlike other human coronaviruses, SARS-CoV grows readily in Vero cells, a monkey kidney derived cell line commonly used in diagnostic laboratories. Characteristic cytopathic effects appear around 3–4 days following the inoculation of the virus (Figure 24.8). The yield from virus isolation is generally higher for deep respiratory specimens, low for stool, and very poor for urine. A major concern when

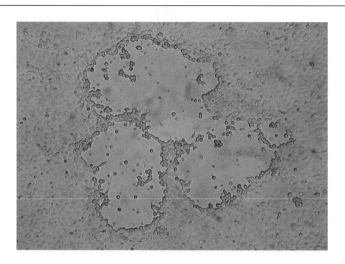

Figure 24.8 Cytopathic effect of SARS-CoV. A Vero cell monolayer infected SARS-CoV. Infected cells are round and refractile, and become detached from the surface. Image courtesy of the Department of Microbiology, The Chinese University of Hong Kong, by Professor Paul K.S. Chan

performing virus isolation for SARS-CoV is the requirement for a physical containment level 3 facility that is not always available.

Serological diagnosis can be established by demonstrating seroconversion (from undetectable to any level of specific SARS-CoV antibody), or a fourfold or greater increase in antibody level between acute and convalescent blood samples. SARS-CoV-specific IgM is a reliable marker for diagnosing current SARS-CoV infection. Antibody avidity (a measure of the maturity of the antibody, or how well it "fits" and therefore how strongly it binds to the antigen) is also useful in estimating when the exposure to SARS-CoV occurred, as antibodies mature over time.

Molecular amplification of viral RNA provides a sensitive and rapid means to diagnose SARS-CoV infection. This approach provides a high diagnostic yield for both respiratory and stool specimens, with the best chances of detecting the presence of the virus in these samples taken within the first 5 days of illness. When a sensitive molecular technique is used, viral RNA can be detected from blood samples taken within first few days after the onset of illness.

Treatment

To date, no antiviral agents have proved to be effective for treating SARS. Ribavirin, a nucleoside analog that has activity against a number of viruses *in vitro*, was widely used in the early phase of the 2003 epidemic. Protease inhibitors, a combination of lopinavir and ritonavir, were used by some centers in the later phase of the outbreak. However, the available data are not sufficient to assess the efficacy of these antiviral compounds.

During the second and the third week of illness, despite a fall in systemic viral load and a rise in SARS-specific IgG antibody, clinical deterioration continued to occur in some patients. This lead to the hypothesis that the deterioration was immune-mediated. Furthermore, the pathological findings of bronchiolitis obliterans organizing pneumonia (BOOP) and acute respiratory distress syndrome are in line with immune hyperactivity resulting from cytokine dysregulation (or a so-called "cytokine storm"). Systemic steroids were therefore the mainstay of treatment for cases with signs of deterioration. In general, steroid treatment was associated with radiographic improvement, fever defervescence, and improved oxygenation.

Summary

SARS arrived as the first emerging infection in the 21st century. It swept through many cities within a few months. The infection proved to be highly infectious under certain environmental conditions. Infection is almost always symptomatic in adults, severe with respiratory failure in around 20% of cases. Elderly patients and those with comorbidity had a poorer prognosis, whereas children tended to run a mild clinical course. Sensitive, specific and rapid diagnostic methods are now available. Systemic steroid therapy for those with signs of deterioration improved the outcome of infection in some cases. The global outbreak of SARS was stopped by a rigorous case finding and isolation policy. Since the second outbreak in late 2003/early 2004, no further natural human infection has been recorded. Early detection, prompt isolation, and contact tracing are essential to prevent another outbreak of this devastating infection.

Test yourself

Case study 24.1

This example case study was adapted from: Auyeung TW, Que TL, Lam KS, Ng HL, Szeto ML. The first patient with locally acquired dengue fever in Hong Kong. *Hong Kong Med J* 2003;9(2):127–129.

A 30-year-old man presented to his local family doctor, 2 days after returning home to London, from a trip to Thailand. He complained of a 2-day history of fever, chills, headache, sore throat, backache, myalgia, and retro-orbital pain. He was sent to the local hospital for further investigation. On arrival, his examination revealed a generalized maculopapular rash, but no petechiae present. His face was flushed, tonsils enlarged, and pharynx congested. A 1-cm diameter firm lymph node was present on the left side of his neck. Clinical examination of all other systems was unremarkable. His temperature was 38°C, blood pressure (BP) 115/50 mm Hg with no tachycardia. His admission hemoglobin (Hb) was 149 g/L (normal: 140–175 g/L), white cell count (WCC) 3.9×10^9/L (normal: $4.5–11.0 \times 10^9$/L), platelet (Plt) count 100×10^9/L (normal: $150–450 \times 10^9$/L), renal and liver function tests were normal.

1. What is the typical incubation period for dengue fever? Does this patient's history, therefore, make dengue fever a possibility?
2. What diagnostic test could you do to quickly determine a diagnosis of dengue fever at this stage?
3. How would you manage the patient at this stage?

The patient's fever rose to 40°C the next day (fourth day of illness), his WCC was 1.9×10^9/L and his Plt 49×10^9/L. His Hb rose from 149 g/L to 168 g/L, with corresponding hematocrit rises of 43% to 49%, respectively (both within normal limits). The prothrombin time (PT) was normal but the activated partial thromboplastin time (APTT) was prolonged at 42.1 seconds (normal: 25–40 seconds). His alanine transferase had increased from normal to 305 U/L (normal: 10–40 U/L). His BP had dropped to 95/45 mm Hg. The clinical virologist calls the ward saying that the tests on the patient's samples show that he has a dengue serotype 1 infection.

4. What is happening to the patient now? What should be done?

The next day (fifth day of illness) the patient's temperature normalized and his general condition improved. His laboratory parameters normalized by the following day (sixth day of illness) and he was discharged home with a followup outpatient appointment 1 week later. He remained well at followup and consented to having a convalescent serum sample taken. Paired testing of the acute and convalescent sera showed a seroconversion for dengue-specific IgM and IgG antibodies. Dengue virus neutralization studies on the convalescent sera at the local reference laboratory confirmed a dengue serotype 1 infection.

Further reading

Chan JCK (ed). *The Challenges of Severe Acute Respiratory Syndrome*. Hong Kong: Hospital Authority of Hong Kong, 2006

Gibbons RV, Vaughn DW. Dengue: an escalating problem. *BMJ* 2002;324:1563–1566

Groneberg DA, Poutanen SM, Low DE, Lode H, Welte T, Zabel P. Treatment and vaccines for severe acute respiratory syndrome. *Lancet Infect Dis* 2005;5:147–155

Hayes EB, Gubler DJ. West Nile virus: epidemiology and clinical features of an emerging epidemic in the United States. *Annu Rev Med* 2006;57:181–194 [review]

Hayes EB, Komar N, Nasci RS, Montgomery SP, O'Leary DR, Campbell GL. Epidemiology and transmission dynamics of West Nile virus disease. *Emerg Infect Dis* 2005;11(8):1167–1173 [review]

Hayes EB, Sejvar JJ, Zaki SR, Lanciotti RS, Bode AV, Campbell GL. Virology, pathology, and clinical manifestations of West Nile virus disease. *Emerg Infect Dis* 2005;11(8):1174–1179 [review]

Jiang S, He Y, Liu S. SARS vaccine development. *Emerg Infect Dis* 2005;11:1016–1120

Lanciotti RS, Roehrig JT, Deubel V, et al. Origin of the West Nile virus responsible for an outbreak of encephalitis in the northeastern United States. *Science* 1999;286(5448):2333–2337

Mahony JB, Richardson S. Molecular diagnosis of severe acute respiratory syndrome: the state of the art. *J Mol Diagn* 2005;7:551–559

Sung JYY (ed). *Severe Acute Respiratory Syndrome. From Benchtop to Bedside*. London: World Scientific, 2004

World Health Organization. *Dengue Haemorrhagic Fever: Diagnosis, Treatment, Prevention and Control*, 2nd edition. Geneva: WHO, 1997

Useful websites

CDC. Division of Vector-Borne Infectious Diseases. West Nile Virus. http://www.cdc.gov/ncidod/dvbid/westnile/index.htm

Chapter 25
Diphtheria

N. Shetty

Public health impact of diphtheria: past and present
Clinical manifestation of diphtheria

Pathogenesis of *Corynebacterium diphtheriae*
Microbiology
Virulence mechanisms: mode of action of diphtheria toxin

Known as the "deadly scourge of childhood," diphtheria struck fear in the hearts of many and claimed the lives of innumerable children in the 19th and early 20th centuries. As far back as 1890, Emil von Behring, a German physician and scientist, found that certain diseases were the expression of the action of toxins which could be neutralized by antitoxins. Behring and his assistant Kitasato, a Japanese scientist, inoculated animals with modified, noninfectious (attenuated) forms of the infectious agents of diphtheria and tetanus, the animals produced neutralizing antitoxin serum. Serum from these animals was injected into nonimmunized animals that were previously infected with the fully virulent bacteria. The ill animals could be cured through the administration of the serum. They thus introduced passive immunization into modern medicine and for this, von Behring was awarded the French legion of honour and the Nobel Prize in 1901 (http://nobelprize.org/nobel_prizes/medicine/articles/behring/index.html).

Despite this, physicians and public health experts viewed diphtheria as one of the most difficult to treat and control of all childhood diseases. It was only in 1930, after the successful immunization of thousands of preschool- and school-aged children in the USA, that the power of immunization to control this most deadly infectious disease was apparent.

Public health impact of diphtheria: past and present
In the 1920s, before the introduction of an effective vaccine in the USA, a total of 206 939 cases of diphtheria were reported in the USA (incidence rate: 190 cases per 100 000 population), including 15 520 deaths (case-fatality rate: 7.5%).

A rapid decrease in disease incidence was apparent with the widespread use of toxoid in the late 1920s. In the 1980s and 1990s diphtheria was seen most frequently in Native Americans and persons in lower

---

Box 25.1 Toxigenic *Corynebacterium diphtheriae* – Northern Plains Indian Community, August–October 1996 (report from *MMWR* June 6, 1997/46(22);506 – 510)

On June 1, 1996, a 62-year-old American Indian woman with a history of alcoholism and severe necrotizing skin ulcers on both legs was admitted to an Indian Health Service (IHS) hospital in South Dakota for treatment of alcohol intoxication and infected leg ulcers. A blood culture obtained from the patient on June 1 was sent to a regional reference laboratory, and *C. diphtheriae*, was identified. At CDC's Diphtheria Laboratory, this isolate demonstrated weak toxigenicity. On admission, the patient's skin ulcers and throat were not swabbed.

In response to isolation of this organism, the South Dakota Department of Health (SDDOH), the Aberdeen Area Office of the IHS, and CDC initiated enhanced surveillance to evaluate the possibility of *C. diphtheriae* infections among other persons in the community where the patient lived. During August 1 to October 7, all persons presenting to the IHS hospital and three satellite clinics for evaluation of pharyngitis, draining middle-ear infections, or skin ulcers were cultured for *C. diphtheriae* as part of their routine clinical care. Specimens were obtained from 133 patients. *C. diphtheriae* was isolated from the swabs from six (5%) of the 133 patients; their ages ranged from 3 to 60 years; four were school-aged children (aged 6–15 years). Five of the six patients reported sore

throat, and one patient presented with otitis media. Local public health nurses and SDDOH staff investigated the household contacts of all these patients. Of the 14 household contacts from whom cultures were obtained, *C. diphtheriae* was isolated from four (29%). Household contacts received postexposure prophylaxis with penicillin and a dose of diphtheria toxoid.

Eight of the ten isolates demonstrated toxigenicity by the immunoprecipitation test and by polymerase chain reaction testing (PCR), which can detect both A and B subunits of the diphtheria toxin gene, (see action of the toxin in Box 25.2 below). Molecular typing methods indicated that the isolates from this area were genetically closely related to each other but differed from *C. diphtheriae* strains isolated either from other regions of the USA or from countries of the former Soviet Union affected by the ongoing diphtheria epidemic (see below).

Editorial note: Molecular analysis suggests continuous presence of the organism in this community despite the absence of reported cases since 1976. The presence of toxigenic *C. diphtheriae* in this community underscores the need to reemphasize the importance of timely vaccination against diphtheria among persons of all ages in the USA.

---

socioeconomic strata. Read about an interesting epidemiological investigation in Box 25.1. From 1980 through 2004, 57 cases of diphtheria were reported in the USA and only five cases since 2000, all of them adults. The current age distribution of cases corroborates the finding that there are inadequate levels of circulating antitoxin in many adults.

Since the introduction and widespread use of diphtheria toxoid (diphtheria toxin that has been treated to destroy its toxic properties without eliminating its capacity to stimulate the production of antitoxins by the immune system) beginning in the 1920s, respiratory diphtheria has been well controlled in the USA. However, diphtheria remained endemic in some states through the 1970s, with reported incidence rates of greater than 1.0 per million population in six states (Alaska, Arizona, Montana, New Mexico, South Dakota, and Washington).

In recent years diphtheria has re-emerged as an important threat to health in many parts of the world. In the 1990s, a massive epidemic throughout the Newly Independent States of the former Soviet Union marked the re-emergence of epidemic diphtheria in industrialized countries. There were approximately 140 000 cases and more than 4000 deaths reported since 1990. This epidemic, primarily affecting adults of the former Soviet Union, demonstrated that, in a modern society, diphtheria can still spread explosively and cause extensive illness and death. Factors contributing to the epidemic included a large population of susceptible adults; decreased childhood immunization due to breakdown of the public health infrastructure, and high population movement. The epidemic also demonstrated that a concerted worldwide public health effort to vaccinate both children and adults could bring the epidemic under control within a few years.

The fact remains that parts of Eastern Europe, the Indian subcontinent, and many countries in Southeast Asia are still endemic for diphtheria. With increasing tourist travel diphtheria continues to be a potential health hazard in travelers returning from these areas. Many reports have documented cases of cutaneous diphtheria in returning travelers (see Chapter 7 and Further reading).

Widespread uptake of the vaccination has yielded interesting changes in the clinical and epidemiological presentation of the disease. A preponderance of nontoxigenic strains has been noticed, as has the broadening spectrum of disease caused by these strains (see Further reading). Development of severe and sometimes recurrent sore throat is the primary presentation of infection with nontoxigenic strains. An interesting report from London (see Further reading) described a cluster of throat infections caused by the same strain of nontoxigenic *Corynebacterium diphtheriae* in a population of inner London men who had sex with men, reflecting transmission within a small community sharing similar lifestyle and behavioral patterns.

In the following sections we will limit our discussions to classical diphtheria as a result of an upper airways infection. Cutaneous diphtheria is discussed in Chapter 7.

Clinical manifestation of diphtheria

Classically, diphtheria is an infection that can be attributed to the effects of the potent exotoxin produced by toxigenic strains of *Corynebacterium diphtheriae*. The organism enters the body through inhaled aerosols and infects the upper airways. The incubation period is between 2 and 5 days. The patient complains of fever, malaise, headache, enlarged lymph nodes, and a sore throat. The exotoxin released by the organism causes local necrosis of the respiratory epithelium, resulting in the formation of a typical pseudomembrane accompanied by inflammation of the pharynx, larynx, and tonsils. The pseudomembrane is generally a firmly adherent, thick, fibrinous, gray-brown membrane (a necrotic coagulum of fibrin, leukocytes, erythrocytes, dead respiratory epithelial cells, and organisms). The membrane typically bleeds if touched. Respiratory distress may occur if the membrane occludes the airways.

Another characteristic of respiratory diphtheria is the gross swelling (edema) of the tonsils, uvula and anterior neck, producing the characteristic bull-neck appearance (Figure 25.1). Difficulty in breathing (stridor) and large anterior cervical (neck) lymph nodes and small hemorrhages may also be noted. Occasionally inflamed or ulcerative lesions may also be seen in the eyes, nose, and vagina.

As the exotoxin enters the bloodstream, systemic manifestations are apparent if the patient is untreated. Toxicity to the cardiovascular system is evident 1–2 weeks after the illness begins. Inflammation of the cardiac muscle (myocarditis), circulatory collapse, heart failure, and disturbances in cardiac rhythm have been reported. Almost 75% of patients also have neurological disease. Neuritis (inflammation of nerves) and motor paralysis may occur several weeks after the primary infection. Necrosis of the kidneys, liver and adrenal glands may be observed.

Diagnosis is confirmed by culturing the organism from a throat swab. Toxigenic strains are identified by testing for toxin production with specific antibody or by detection of the toxin gene using molecular methods.

Diphtheria is a clinical emergency; prompt administration of antitoxin is essential. Systemic toxicity is directly related to the amount of time that has elapsed before giving antitoxin. Diphtheria antitoxin is a hyperimmune antiserum produced in horses that neutralizes toxin before entry into cells.

Antibiotics (erythromycin is the drug of choice) have a secondary role in the management of diphtheria, they eradicate throat carriage, limit toxin production, and prevent spread of organisms.

All close contacts should be screened for throat carriage, their immunization status reviewed and if at risk, they should be given prophylactic antibiotics and booster doses of the vaccine. Diphtheria is a vaccine preventable illness; worldwide, a childhood death due to diphtheria is a travesty to modern medicine. See Further reading for the current recommendations for the prevention and treatment of diphtheria.

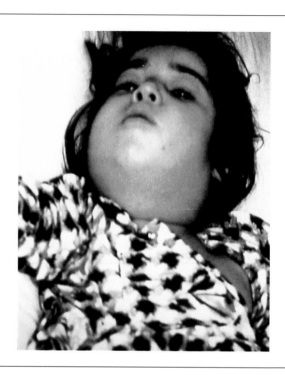

Figure 25.1 Gross swelling (edema) of the tonsils, uvula and anterior neck in respiratory diphtheria producing the characteristic bull-neck appearance. Courtesy of the Centers for Disease Control and Prevention; from CDC website: http://phil.cdc.gov/phil/details.asp

Pathogenesis of *Corynebacterium diphtheriae*

Microbiology

C. diphtheriae is an aerobic, club-shaped, Gram positive, nonmotile, nonencapsulated, pleomorphic (different shapes) bacillus with terminal swellings (Figure 25.2).

When Albert's stain is used, the bacilli are often found in clusters that form sharp angles with each other and resemble Chinese letters; dark staining metachromatic granules are also visible (Figure 25.3). The granules contain inorganic phosphates and act as energy reserves.

C. diphtheriae reduces tellurite to tellurium and produces characteristic black colored colonies when grown on tellurite containing media. Classically three strain types of *C. diphtheriae* are described: gravis, intermedius, and mitis. They are differentiated by colonial morphology (Figure 25.4). All are capable of

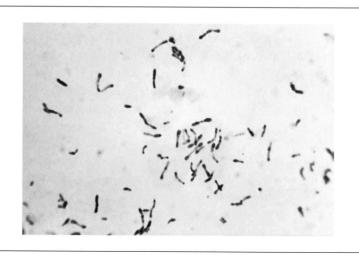

Figure 25.2 Gram stain of *C. diphtheriae* showing pleomorphic Gram positive rods. Provided by Dr P.B. Smith. Courtesy of the Centers for Disease Control and Prevention; from CDC website: http://phil.cdc.gov/phil/details.asp

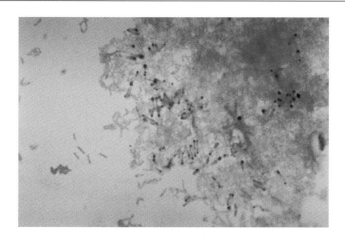

Figure 25.3 Albert's stain of *C. diphtheriae* showing "Chinese letter" arrangement and metachromatic (purple) granules (1000×).

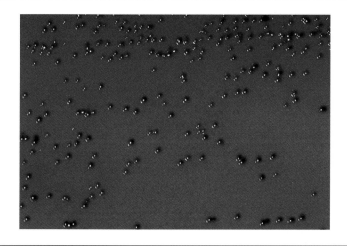

Figure 25.4 *Corynebacterium diphtheriae* growing on blood tellurite agar showing characteristic black colonies. Provided by Dr W.A. Clark. Courtesy of the Centers for Disease Control and Prevention; from CDC website: http://phil.cdc.gov/phil/ details.asp

producing toxin and causing the same spectrum of disease. Recent studies suggest no differences in virulence between strains.

Virulence mechanisms: mode of action of diphtheria toxin

The diphtheria toxin is the main virulence determinant of *C. diphtheriae*. It is also the substance that is chemically modified (toxoided) to yield a highly immunogenic and successful vaccine.

For *C. diphtheriae* to produce disease it needs to colonize the upper respiratory tract and produce toxin. Toxin production is dependent on two important factors: (i) the presence of low extracellular concentrations of iron and (ii) infection by a virus, also called a bacteriophage.

- **The role of iron.** The gene that encodes toxin production is carried on the phage but a bacterial repressor protein controls the expression of this gene. The active repressor binds to the tox gene operator and prevents transcription. When iron is removed from the surrounding medium, derepression occurs, the repressor is inactivated, and transcription of the tox genes can occur. The repressor is activated by iron, which is why iron influences toxin production. High yields of toxin are synthesized only by lysogenic bacteria under conditions of iron deficiency. This has been demonstrated *in vitro* and is presumed to be the same *in vivo*.

- **The role of bacteriophage.** A phage that infects a bacterium and does not lyse it, but endows it with other properties such as toxin production, is called a lysogenic phage. Only those strains of *C. diphtheriae* that are lysogenized by a specific bacteriophage produce diphtheria toxin. The phage contains the structural gene for the toxin molecule.

Mechanism of action of diphtheria toxin

Diphtheria toxin is a potent protein exotoxin (see Chapter 3) and is composed of two important components: A (active) and B (binding) units. The B subunit helps the toxin molecule to bind to specific receptors on target cells; the toxin is then internalized by receptor-mediated endocytosis. Following this acidification of the endocytic vesicle occurs by a membrane-associated, ATP-driven proton pump. This releases the enzymatically active A fragment. Once this has happened, the A subunit is able to exert its toxin activity (Figure 25.5). The A subunit catalyzes the transfer of ADP-ribose from NAD to the eukaryotic elongation factor 2 (EF-2). This inhibits protein synthesis and ultimately leads to cell death.

See Box 25.2 for other *Corynebacterium* species that harbor the diphtheria toxin.

Prevention

Diphtheria is a vaccine preventable infection. Acquired immunity to diphtheria is due to production of toxin-neutralizing antibody (antitoxin) as a result of immunization with the toxoid. Passive immunity *in utero* is acquired transplacentally and can last for a few months after birth.

Immunization with diphtheria toxoid in combination with tetanus toxoid and acellular pertussis vaccine (DTaP) during infancy is the protocol recommended by the World Health Organization as part of Universal Immunization Of Childhood; it is also recommended by the CDC for children in the USA. Combination vaccines contain diphtheria and tetanus toxoids and either whole-cell pertussis antigens (DTwP) or acellular pertussis antigens (DTaP). DTwP vaccine is no longer available in the USA but is used in other countries.

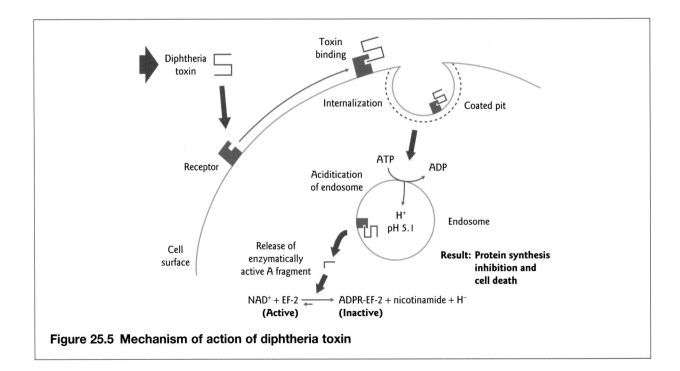

Figure 25.5 Mechanism of action of diphtheria toxin

Box 25.2 Respiratory diphtheria caused by *Corynebacterium ulcerans* – Terre Haute, Indiana, 1996 (report from *MMWR*, April 18, 1997/46(15);330–332)

On October 24, 1996, a 54-year-old woman residing in Terre Haute, Indiana, had onset of fever, sore throat, and difficulty swallowing and breathing. On physical examination, her temperature was normal, but she had marked swelling of the soft palate with a membranous exudate covering both tonsils and bilateral cervical (neck) lymph nodes. The patient reported never having received any vaccinations. Based on the history and physical findings, a preliminary diagnosis of respiratory diphtheria was made. She was treated with equine diphtheria antitoxin and 2 g of erythromycin intravenously per day. On October 28, her symptoms began to improve, and by October 29, the membrane and neck swelling had begun to recede.

The patient worked as a telephone sales operator, had not traveled outside the state during the previous month, and had no known contact with any international travelers, although she had attended a large rural folk arts festival on October 20.

A polymerase chain reaction (PCR) assay for the toxin gene performed directly on the clinical specimens at CDC on October 31 was positive. A strain of *Corynebacterium ulcerans* was subsequently isolated from the culture specimen at CDC, and toxin production by this strain was confirmed.

Editorial note: Most cases of diphtheria result from infection with toxin-producing strains of *C. diphtheriae*; however *C. ulcerans*, a related species found more commonly in cattle than other animals, can carry the same bacteriophage that codes for the toxin elaborated by toxigenic strains of *C. diphtheriae*. Sporadic cases of diphtheria caused by *C. ulcerans* have been reported in humans, and at least two of these cases have been fatal. *C. ulcerans* infection in humans frequently has been associated with antecedent contact with farm animals or with consumption of unpasteurized dairy products.

Immunization for infants and children up to the seventh birthday consists of five doses of DTaP vaccine. The first three doses are usually given at ages 2, 4 and 6 months, the fourth dose at ages 15–18 months, and the fifth dose at ages 4–6 years.

Immunity after childhood vaccination against diphtheria may gradually wane; travelers and laboratory workers are encouraged to take booster doses before commencing travel or taking up a laboratory post.

Test yourself

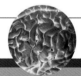

Case study 25.1
A Croatian family (parents, two children) emigrated from Zagreb in 1993. They returned in 2006 to visit family, were not advised of any infectious disease risks, and consequently did not take prophylaxis. Two weeks after they returned to the USA, the younger child developed a painful sore throat, fever, and difficulty in swallowing. A review of her immunizations revealed that primary immunizations were interrupted due to civil unrest in her country. On examination, she was unwell, febrile, tachycardic, with large tender cervical lymph nodes. Culture of her throat yielded *C. diphtheriae*. The pathogenesis of *C. diphtheriae* is mainly through production of a potent exotoxin which acts as an ADP-ribosylator.

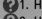1. How does the diphtheria toxin exert its action?

2. How do the toxins of *C. botulinum*, *C. tetani*, *Pseudomonas*, and *Shigella dysenteriae* exert their action? Compare their mode of action and end results. Are the effects permanent or reversible?

Further reading

de Benoist A, White JM, Efstratious E, et al. Imported cutaneous diphtheria, United Kingdom. *Emerg Infect Dis* 2004;10:511–513

Reacher M, Ramsay M, White J, et al. Nontoxigenic *Corynebacterium diphtheriae*: an emerging pathogen in England and Wales? *Emerg Infect Dis* 2000;6:640–645

Successful control of epidemic diphtheria in the states of the Former Union of Soviet Socialist Republics: lessons learned. *J Infect Dis* 2000;181(suppl 1):S10–22

Wilson AP, Efstratiou A, Weaver E, et al. Unusual nontoxigenic *Corynebacterium diphtheriae* in homosexual men. *Lancet* 1992;339:998

Useful websites

CDC. Disease Listing. Diphtheria. http://www.cdc.gov/ncidod/dbmd/diseaseinfo/diptheria_t.htm

Chapter 26
Agents of bioterrorism

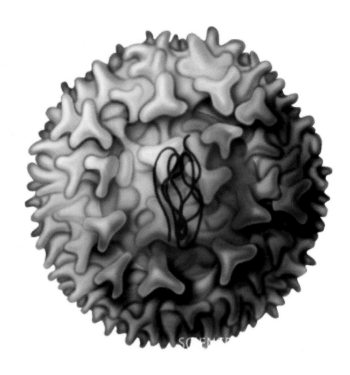

J.W. Tang

History of biological agents used in warfare
Definitions
    Category A Diseases/Agents: high priority agents that
      pose a risk to national security, and are rarely seen
      in the USA
    Category B Diseases/Agents: second highest priority
      agents

Category C Diseases/Agents: emerging infections
    diseases
Anthrax (*Bacillus anthracis*)
Botulism (*Clostridium botulinum* toxin)
Plague (*Yersinia pestis*)
Tularemia (*Francisella tularensis*)
Smallpox (Variola major)

History of biological agents used in warfare

There is a long history of the use of microorganisms as weapons in human conflicts, whether intentionally or unintentionally. Records show that the Romans used dead animals to foul enemy water supplies, and that during medieval times, the Tartars catapulted the bodies of plague victims over the walls into the city of Kaffa. In the 1500s, during their conquest of the Aztecs, the Spanish explorers Diego Velasquez and Hernan Cortes with their men carried measles, chickenpox, smallpox, and possibly other infectious diseases that may have killed more of the Aztecs than they did with their weapons. Later, during the French and Indian war (1754–1763), smallpox-contaminated blankets were given to native Indians by the British army under the command of Lord Jeffrey Amherst. More recently during the wars of the early 20th century (1918–1942), the notorious Japanese army Unit 731 released plague in China by spraying it from planes, dropping it in bombs, and releasing plague-infected rats. The British also experimented with anthrax as a bioweapon in 1943 on Gruinard Island, off the Scottish coast. The island remained in quarantine for almost 50 years since these experiments, and has only recently been cleaned up and declared free of anthrax. Between 1942 and 1969, the US bioweapons program based at Fort Detrick demonstrated in 1966 that a release of a harmless bacterium, *Bacillus subtilis*, at one subway station could infect the whole subway system within a few hours (Box 26.1).

    As a result of all these high-risk experiments being conducted in the name of national war and defence, an agreement being made between the world superpowers at that time (the USA, Soviet Union, and UK),

Box 26.1 Deliberate release of biological agents on underground train transport systems

A clandestine experiment on the New York subway in 1966 involved the dropping of light bulbs filled with harmless bacteria, *Bacillus subtilis* (variant Niger), to test how far and how fast this organism would be disseminated by the "piston" action of the underground trains. The conclusions were that such a release of a biological agent would be extremely effective in killing thousands of the millions of passengers using the underground system each day. Such underground train systems exist in all the major capital cities of the world (London, Paris, Tokyo, Moscow, Beijing, Shanghai, Hong Kong, Singapore, just to name a few). The other outcome of such a release event is that due to the variable incubation times of the different biological weapons agents and the rapidity of modern travel, those infected may travel across the country or even worldwide, before becoming ill and transmitting their infection to others (with those agents that are directly transmissible between people). In this sense, the easy mechanism of release, with the potential widespread fallout from secondary, perhaps even tertiary, cases has given the biological weapon an alternative name: the "poor man's atomic bomb." In recent years, a popular US TV series surrounding the activities of a Los Angeles-based US government counter-terrorism unit (CTU) "24" in its season 3 storyline, graphically depicts the possible consequences (both for the public and the government) of a terrorist attack in the USA using a genetically engineered biological agent.

the "Convention on the Prohibition of the Development, Production and Stockpiling of Bacteriological (Biological) and Toxin Weapons and on Their Destruction," more commonly known as the "Biological and Toxin Weapons Convention (BTWC)". This was simultaneously opened for signature in Moscow, Washington, and London on April 10, 1972 and entered into force on March 26, 1975. The BTWC bans the development, production, stockpiling, acquisition and retention of microbial or other biological agents or toxins, in types and in quantities that have no justification for prophylactic, protective, or other peaceful purposes. It also bans weapons, equipment or means of delivery designed to use such agents or toxins for hostile purposes or in armed conflict. As of November 2001, 162 states had signed the BTWC and 144 of these had ratified it. However, the BTWC lacked teeth and legal force, so some countries continued their biological weapons programs in secret. The defection of a high level scientist, Ken Alibek in 1992 (see Further reading), who was involved in the Russian Biopreparat biological weapons research and development program in laboratories at Novosibirsk, confirmed that the Soviet Union was, indeed, effectively ignoring the BTWC agreement that it had signed. An accident at one of their bioweapons facilities in Sverdlovsk (see Further reading) resulted in the release of anthrax spores and 66 deaths in the local population downwind of the factory.

More recently in 1984, a religious cult called the Rajneeshee, deliberately contaminated salad bars with *Salmonella typhimurium* in the state of Oregon (USA), in order to incapacitate voters to win a local election. About 750 people were affected though there were no deaths. Serious concerns that Iraq under the leadership of Saddam Hussein (1988–1990), was involved in producing bioweapons, were confirmed when a factory at Al-hakam was found producing anthrax and botulinum toxin, despite numerous inspections by the United Nations Special Commission (UNSCOM). The factory was eventually demolished in 1996 under the supervision of UNSCOM. From 1990 to 1995, another religious cult, this time from Japan, the Aum Shinrikyo, mounted several failed projects to collect and release biological agents in Tokyo. This included failed attempts to obtain Ebola virus from Zaire, and failed attempts to release botulinum toxin and anthrax within the city. They were, however, eventually successful in releasing sarin nerve gas on the Tokyo underground train system, killing about 20 people and incapacitating several thousand. Soon after these events, the Centers for Disease Control and Prevention (CDC) began their Bioterrorism Preparedness and Response Program.

Definitions

Since the September 11, 2001 terrorist attacks in the USA, the "anthrax letters," and former concerns about the possible existence of biological warfare agents in Iraq, the threat of future attacks with biological agents has been taken seriously. The CDC have defined and categorized the most serious of these into three categories (A, B, and C), though this chapter will only review the Category A agents. The characteristics of some of these agents is shown in Table 26.1.

Table 26.1 Characteristics of some potential biological warfare agents

Agent	Infective dose (by aerosol)	Incubation period	Diagnostic samples (BSL)	Diagnostic assay
CDC Category A agents				
Anthrax (*Bacillus anthracis*)	8000–50 000 spores	1–5 days	Blood (BSL-2), tissue	Culture, Gram stain, Ag and Ab detection, PCR
Botulinum toxin	0.001 mg/kg (type A)	1–5 days	Nasal swab (possibly BSL-2)	Ag detection, mouse bioassay, PCR
Plague (*Yersinia pestis*)	100–500 organisms	2–3 days	Blood, sputum, tissue, lymph node aspirate (BSL-2/3)	Culture, Gram or Wright-Giemsa stain, Ag and Ab detection, PCR
Tularemia (*Francisella tularensis*)	10–50 organisms	2–10 days	Blood/serum, sputum, tissue (BSL-2/3)	Culture, Ab detection, PCR, EM of tissue
Smallpox (*Variola major*)	Assumed to be low (10–100 organisms)	7–17 days	Pharyngeal swab, scab material (BSL-4)	Culture, Ab detection, PCR, EM of scab material
Viral hemorrhagic fevers	1–10 organisms	4–21 days (species-dependent)	Blood/serum (BSL-3/4, species dependent)	Culture, Ag and Ab detection, PCR, EM of tissue or serum in some cases
CDC Category B agents				
Brucellosis (*Brucella* spp.)	10–100 organisms	5–60 days (months sometimes)	Blood (paired acute/convalescent sera), bone marrow (BSL-3)	Culture, Ab detection, PCR
Q fever (*Coxiella burnetii*)	1–10 organisms	10–40 days	Serum (BSL-2/3)	Ab detection, PCR
Staphylococcal enterotoxin B	30 ng/person (to incapacitate); 1.7 mg/person (lethal)	1–6 hours	Nasal swab, serum, urine (BSL-2)	Ag and Ab detection, PCR
Viral encephalitides	10–100 organisms	2–14 days (species-dependent)	Serum (BSL-2/3, species dependent)	Culture, Ab detection, PCR

Incubation periods quoted here may vary slightly from those described in the text, due to the different reference sources used. Antigen (Ag) and antibody (Ab) detection can be performed using enzyme immunoassay (EIA), immunofluoresence (IF), or agglutination test formats. Nowadays, molecular tests (PCR) can be designed to detect most organisms by targeting specific conserved gene regions in their genomes. Other abbreviations: CDC, Centers for Disease Prevention and Control; PCR, polymerase chain reaction; EM, electronmicroscopy; BSL, biosafety level.

Category A Diseases/Agents: high priority agents that pose a risk to national security, and are rarely seen in the USA

- that can be easily disseminated or transmitted from person to person
- that can result in high mortality rates with the potential for major public health impact
- that may cause public panic and social disruption
- that require special action for public health preparedness.

The agents in this category are:

- anthrax (*Bacillus anthracis*)
- botulism (*Clostridium botulinum* toxin)
- plague (*Yersinia pestis*)
- smallpox (Variola major)
- tularemia (*Francisella tularensis*)
- viral hemorrhagic fevers (filoviruses, e.g. Ebola and Marburg; arenaviruses, e.g. Lassa, Machupo).

Category B Diseases/Agents: second highest priority agents

- that are moderately easy to disseminate
- that result in moderate morbidity rates and low mortality rates
- that require special enhancements of CDC's diagnostic capacity and enhanced disease surveillance.

The agents in this category are:

- brucellosis (*Brucella* species)
- epsilon toxin of *Clostridium perfringens*
- food safety threats, e.g. *Salmonella* species, *Escherichia coli* O157:H7, *Shigella*
- glanders (*Burkholderia mallei*)
- melioidosis (*Burkholderia pseudomallei*)
- psittacosis (*Chlamydia psittaci*)
- Q fever (*Coxiella burnetii*)
- ricin toxin from *Ricinus communis* (castor beans)
- staphylococcal enterotoxin B
- typhus fever (*Rickettsia prowazekii*)
- viral encephalitis, e.g. alphaviruses: Venezuelan equine encephalitis, eastern equine encephalitis, western equine encephalitis
- water safety threats, e.g. *Vibrio cholerae, Cryptosporidium parvum*.

Category C Diseases/Agents: emerging infections diseases

Examples of agents in this category are:

- Nipah virus, hantavirus, severe acute respiratory syndrome-associated coronavirus (SARS-CoV).

Anthrax (*Bacillus anthracis*)

Anthrax is so named due to the black, coal-like skin lesions caused by the disease (Figure 26.1). Anthrax spores are very hardy and may remain dormant in the environment for many years, and it is thought by

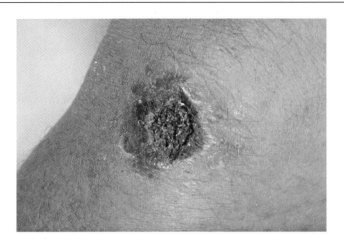

Figure 26.1 Anthrax lesion on the skin of the forearm caused by the bacterium _Bacillus anthracis_. Here the disease has manifested itself as a cutaneous ulceration, which has begun to turn black, hence the origin of the name "anthrax," after the Greek name for coal. Provided by James H. Steele. Courtesy of the Centers for Disease Control and Prevention; from CDC website: http://phil.cdc.gov/phil/details.asp

many to be the bioterrorists' agent of first choice. This has already been seen in 2001 in the USA, where letters containing anthrax powder were sent through the postal system causing 22 cases of anthrax (see Further reading). However, a large number of anthrax spores (8000–50 000) have been estimated to be required to cause fatal disease in an individual, and it is not know to transmit from person to person.

Anthrax has been used previously as an agent of warfare in the First and Second World Wars by Germany and Japan, respectively, as well as playing a major role in the biological weapons programs of the former Soviet Union, Iraq, and the USA. Previous models by the WHO (1970) have estimated that 50 kg of anthrax spores released upwind of a city of population 500 000, in a 2-km-long line, would result in 95 000 deaths (almost a 20% mortality rate). In the USA (1993) another estimate predicted that between 130 000 and 3 million deaths might result from 100 kg of anthrax spores released upwind of Washington DC. An accidental release of an aerosol of anthrax spores from a biological weapons factory in Sverdlovsk in the former Soviet Union resulted in 68 deaths in 1979 (see Further reading).

Anthrax has three different clinical disease manifestations in humans: cutaneous, gastrointestinal, and inhalational. Cutaneous and gastrointestinal forms can be acquired from handling, or eating, poorly cooked meat from anthrax-infected animals, respectively. The first symptoms to occur in cutaneous anthrax are a small sore that first develops into a blister, then an ulcer with a black central area, all of which are painless. In gastrointestinal anthrax, the first symptoms are nausea, loss of appetite, bloody diarrhea, fever, and severe stomach pains. Inhalational anthrax used to be seen in workers in slaughterhouses and the textile and tanning industries, where anthrax spores were inhaled during the handling of contaminated wool, hair, meat, and hides. Nowadays, inhalational anthrax is the most likely form of bioterrorist attack using anthrax, as the spores have a diameter of 2–6 μm, which can be easily inhaled into the lower respiratory tract. Once there, macrophage phagocytosis of the spores results in germination into anthrax bacilli, which produces a rapid-onset, necrotizing hemorrhagic mediastinitis. From the Sverdlovsk (1979) cases, the incubation can be very variable, from 2 to 43 days, though within 7 days is more typical. The disease progresses very rapidly after germination, so without early clinical suspicion the patient may already be severely ill before the diagnosis is made.

Clinical features are initially very nonspecific, and include fever, dry cough, malaise, fatigue, and myalgia, very similar to an atypical bacteria or viral pneumonia. However, shortly afterwards, respiratory distress and failure follow, with shock and death within 24 hours, if the infection has not been suspected, rapidly diagnosed, and treated appropriately. A widened mediastinum on the chest X-ray (Figure 26.2), together with a rapidly progressing, severe pneumonic illness, is almost pathognomonic of inhalational anthrax in a previously healthy individual.

Laboratory diagnosis involves the identification of _Bacillus anthracis_ bacteria using culture, serology or molecular techniques. It is a Biosafety Level (BSL) 2 agent and should be handled in appropriate containment

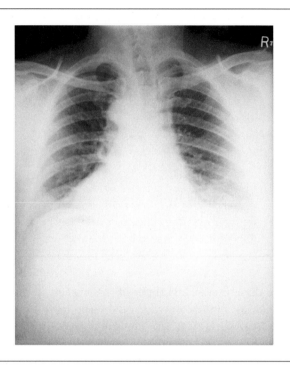

Figure 26.2 Chest radiograph showing widened mediastinum due to inhalation anthrax. This posteroanterior (PA) chest X-ray was taken 4 months after the onset of anthrax in a 46-year-old male. This patient, had worked for 2 years as a card tender in a goat hair processing mill and contracted anthrax. X-ray revealed bilateral pulmonary effusion, and a widened mediastinum, which are hallmarks of the disease process. Provided by Arthur E. Kaye. Courtesy of the Centers for Disease Control and Prevention; from CDC website: http://phil.cdc.gov/phil/details.asp

facilities. It is an aerobic, Gram positive, sporing, nonmotile rod that can be grown on selective media (polymixin-lysozyme-EDTA-thallous acetate agar) if other contaminants are present. *B. anthracis* grows on sheep blood agar with rough, gray-white colonies, with characteristic "comet-tail" projections (Figure 26.3). Growth in such culture should occur within 24 hours, though it may take another 24 hours from blood culture samples, and the laboratory needs to be specifically requested to look for *B. anthracis*.

Enzyme-linked immunoassays (EIAs) can measure antibody titers to one of the exotoxins (protective antigen, PA) or capsule proteins. Molecular tests include polymerase chain reaction (PCR)-based detection of *B. anthracis* DNA, of which there are several kits on the market, including hand-held, rapid detection instruments for use in the field. Antigen detection is also possible using an electrochemiluminescence (ECL)

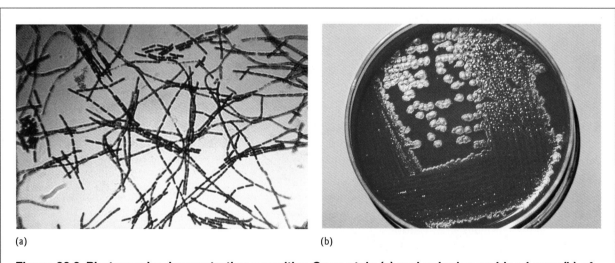

(a)

(b)

Figure 26.3 Photographs demonstrating a positive Gram stain (a) and colonies on blood agar (b) of *Bacillus anthracis*. (a) and (b) courtesy of the Centers for Disease Control and Prevention; from CDC website: http://phil.cdc.gov/phil/details.asp

technique where magnetic beads carrying capture antibodies can bind to the PA antigen in patient samples and another, ruthenium-labeled detector antibody, binds to the captured antigen, forming a sandwich that can be detected by the presence of the resulting ECL signal.

The treatment of choice is ciprofloxacin or doxycycline (both given orally) initially, with penicillin (intravenously) given later if the organism is sensitive. There is always the possibility of genetically engineered antibiotic-resistant strains being present, and at least one example of a tetracycline/penicillin-resistant strain has been previously reported. Vaccines against anthrax do exist and have been targeted at the PA antigen. However, they are mainly used for military personnel and those working specifically with anthrax in laboratories or elsewhere.

Botulism (*Clostridium botulinum* toxin)

The toxins produced by *Clostridium botulinum* are some of the most toxic compounds known. It is 100 000 times more toxic than sarin and as a biological weapon it can be aerosolized or used to poison food. Three types of botulism are usually recognized. Foodborne botulism is caused by preformed toxin that causes illness within hours to days, and very occasionally, weeks later. It is a public health emergency because the food may still be available and consumed by others. Infant botulism (Figure 26.4) occurs in a few infants each year who have *C. botlinum* in their gastrointestinal tract. Wound botulism occurs when *C. botulinum* contaminates or infects a wound, in anaerobic conditions (often deep-penetrating wounds), and secretes the toxin to cause disease. Botulinum toxin is not transmitted from person to person.

The bacteria produces seven toxins (A–G), all of which are neurotoxins that block the release of the neurotransmitter, acetylcholine. Inhalation of the toxin causes the same effects as ingestion, though the time to disease may differ. Onset of symptoms usually occurs within 12–36 hours of exposure, including cranial nerve palsies such as: blurred or double vision, drooping of the eyelid, photophobia, a hoarse voice, and difficulties swallowing. A symmetrical, descending, progressive paralysis of voluntary muscles follows, with sudden onset respiratory failure requiring urgent ventilation, possible at any time. For more detail regarding the mechanism of action of botulinum toxin see Chapter 3.

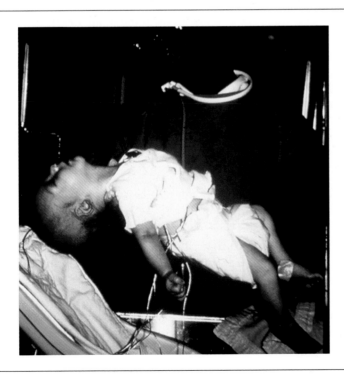

Figure 26.4 Six-week-old infant with botulism, which is evident as a marked loss of muscle tone, especially in the region of the head and neck. Courtesy of the Centers for Disease Control and Prevention; from CDC website: http://phil.cdc.gov/phil/details.asp

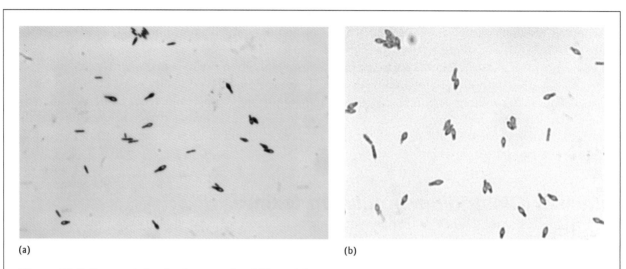

(a)   (b)

Figure 26.5 Gram-stained micrograph of *Clostridium botulinum* Type-A in thioglycolate broth was incubated for 48 hours at 35°C (a). *C. botulinum* endospores stained with Malachite Green Stain, appearing as green spheres, while the bacilli themselves appear purple (b). (a) Provided by Dr George Lombard. Courtesy of the Centers for Disease Control and Prevention; from CDC website: http://phil.cdc.gov/phil/details.asp. (b) Provided by Larry Stauffer. Courtesy of the Centers for Disease Control and Prevention; from CDC website: http://phil.cdc.gov/phil/details.asp

Clostridium botulinum is a Gram positive, anaerobic, sporing, nonmotile bacterium (Figure 26.5). It can be considered as a BSL-2 agent and should be handled in appropriate containment facilities. Diagnosis can be made on clinical grounds, though rapid confirmatory laboratory testing using molecular techniques, such as PCR assays targeting one of the toxin genes or the toxin-encoding messenger RNA, are rapid and sensitive. To diagnose the presence of pre-formed botulinum toxin as is the case in many food-poisoning incidents, these molecular methods cannot be used, and the classic, slower, mouse bioassay may be required.

Antitoxins are available for botulinum toxin and early administration neutralizes the toxin and halts symptom progression. Three antitoxins are available in the USA: a trivalent equine (covering toxins A, B, and E) from CDC, a monovalent human antiserum (covering toxin A) from the California Department of Health Services, and a "despeciated" equine heptavalent antitoxin (covering all seven toxins A–G) developed by the US Army Medical Research Institute for Infectious Diseases (USAMRIID). There is no licensed vaccine presently available. The usual respiratory supportive therapy (intubation and ventilation) should also be given or be at hand, in case of sudden respiratory failure in such patients.

Plague (*Yersinia pestis*)

Plague has caused the death of millions over the centuries, most notably the plague pandemic starting in 1346, also known as the "black death," that killed 20–30 million Europeans. It is a zoonosis, being enzootic in rodent species such as rats, ground squirrels, and prairie dogs (Figure 26.6), with human disease occurring after being bitten by infected fleas causing the "bubonic" form of plague. Recently, another model of this ancient disease has postulated that the soil is a significant reservoir for this organism, with burrowing rodents as the first link, then human ectoparasites (e.g. fleas) as the main force behind human plague epidemics (see Further reading).

This form of plague is characterized by "buboes" or swollen, tender lymph glands (Figure 26.7), which are not present in the pneumonic form of plague. However, untreated bubonic plague will disseminate throughout the body via the bloodstream, eventually reaching the lungs when a secondary form of pneumonic plague can be produced, where *Y. pestis* can be spread via aerosols produced by coughing or sneezing, for example.

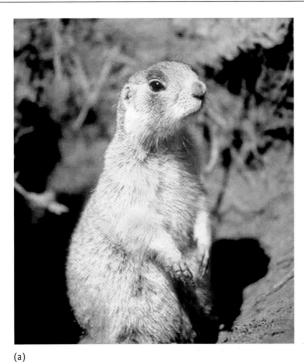
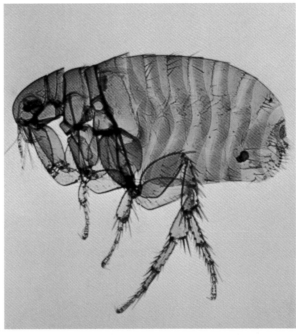

(a) (b)

Figure 26.6 (a) Prairie dog. This burrowing rodent of the genus *Cynomys* can harbor fleas infected with *Yersinia pestis*, the bacterium that causes plague. (b) This is an enlargement of a female *Xenopsylla cheopis* flea, also known as the "oriental rat flea," one of the insect vectors responsible for transmitting *Y. pestis*. (a) Courtesy of the Centers for Disease Control and Prevention; from CDC website: http://phil.cdc.gov/phil/details.asp. (b) Provided by the World Health Organization. Courtesy of the Centers for Disease Control and Prevention; from CDC website: http://phil.cdc.gov/phil/details.asp

About 1000–3000 cases of plague occur worldwide each year, of these about 5–15 are reported from the rural and semi-rural areas in the western USA. In North America, plague is found in certain animals and their fleas from the Pacific Coast to the Great Plains, and from southwestern Canada to Mexico. Most human cases in the United States occur in two regions: (i) northern New Mexico, northern Arizona, and

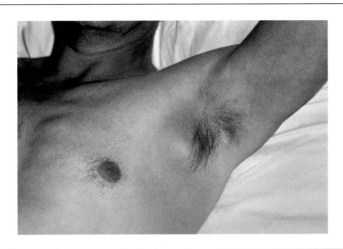

Figure 26.7 An axillary bubo and edema exhibited by a plague patient. Provided by Margaret Parsons and Dr Karl F. Meyer. Courtesy of the Centers for Disease Control and Prevention; from CDC website: http://phil.cdc.gov/phil/details.asp

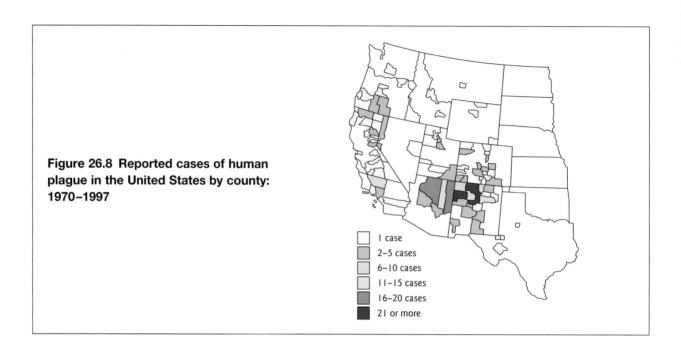

Figure 26.8 Reported cases of human plague in the United States by county: 1970–1997

☐	I case
▨	2–5 cases
▨	6–10 cases
▨	11–15 cases
▨	16–20 cases
■	21 or more

southern Colorado; and (ii) California, southern Oregon, and far western Nevada (Figure 26.8). These are usually cases of bubonic plague, and cases of naturally occurring pneumonic plague are relatively rare. The bubonic form of plague has been used as a bioweapon previously by the Japanese (their notorious unit 731), who dropped plague-infected fleas in China during the Second World War. The bubonic form of plague cannot be transmitted from person to person, but once in the lungs, the secondary pneumonic form can transmit aerosolized *Y. pestis* between people.

Both the USA and the Soviet Union, during former previous biological weapons programs, developed means of aerosolizing plague to allow it to be inhaled to cause the pneumonic form of plague (Figure 26.9). This is thought to be the most likely form of bioterrorist attack using this agent. As it is easily found in nature, it is difficult to control access to this organism, though a certain level of knowledge and technology is required before it could be effectively weaponized. The pneumonic form of plague can be transmitted between people, though relatively close contact (within 6 feet) is needed. A few hundred organisms may be

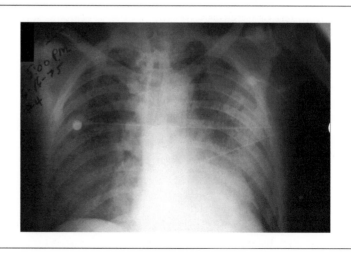

Figure 26.9 Anteroposterior X-ray revealing a bilaterally progressive plague infection involving both lung fields. Provided by Dr Jack Poland. Courtesy of the Centers for Disease Control and Prevention; from CDC website: http://phil.cdc.gov/phil/ details.asp

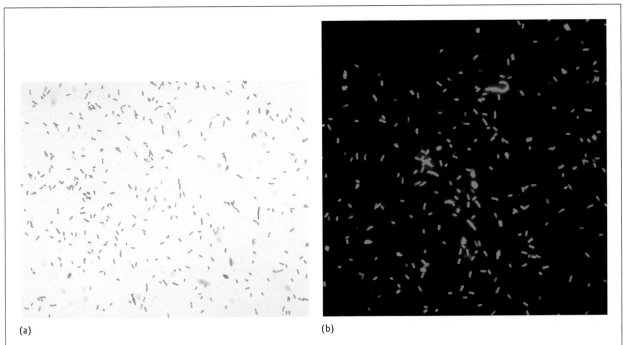

(a)   (b)

Figure 26.10 (a) *Yersinia pestis*, a small (0.5 × 1.0 µM) Gram negative bacillus. Bipolar staining occurs when using Wayson, Wright, Giemsa, or methylene blue stain, and may occasionally be seen in Gram-stained preparations. **(b)** To identify the antigens present in animal tissues, and appropriate cultures, a direct fluorescent antibody staining technique (DFA) can be used that targets the specific conjugated antiserum to the *Y. pestis* capsular antigen. (a) and (b) provided by Larry Stauffer. Courtesy of the Centers for Disease Control and Prevention; from CDC website: http://phil.cdc.gov/phil/details.asp

sufficient to cause pneumonic plague by inhalation and the organism may survive up to 1 hour depending on environmental conditions, though the natural form of the bacillus is easily destroyed by sunlight and drying. The incubation period is 1–6 days for pneumonic plague, after inhalation, with symptoms of high fever, chills, rigors, headache, malaise, cough (with blood), vomiting, abdominal pain, with rapid progression to respiratory failure and death, if untreated. Pneumonic plague should be suspected whenever there are large numbers of previously healthy people developing severe Gram negative pneumonia, particularly if they start coughing up blood. Outbreaks do occur naturally, but they are rare enough to raise suspicion of possible bioterrorist activity.

Y. pestis is a Gram negative rod that shows bipolar ("safety pin") morphology when stained with Wright, Giemsa, or Wayson stains (Figure 26.10). It is a BSL-2/3 agent and should be handled in appropriate containment facilities. Culture on blood or MacConkey agar usually takes 48 hours, and the colonies may appear smaller than other Enterobacteriaceae. Its identification can be confirmed by biochemical tests (a lactose nonfermenter, urease and indole negative).

Antigen detection immunoassays can detect the *Y. pestis* F1-antigen in patient sera, and PCR assays have been developed to detect specific genes of *Y. pestis*, such as the plasminogen activator gene.

Without early treatment, pneumonic plague is normally fatal, especially if treatment has been delayed for more than 24 hours after the onset of symptoms. Recommended therapy can be intravenous (streptomycin, gentamicin) or oral (ciprofloxacin, doxycycline) given for at least 7 days, preferably 10–14 days. Post-exposure prophylaxis in those who have been exposed to plague consists of doxycycline, ciprofloxacin, tetracycline, or chloramphenicol. Currently, there is no licensed vaccine against pneumonic plague, though there are some candidates in the experimental phases of testing.

Tularemia (*Francisella tularensis*)

Tularemia (also known as rabbit or deer fly fever) is a zoonotic disease most often acquired by humans through contact with infected animals or via bites of infected insects (e.g. deer flies, mosquitoes, or ticks). Occasionally, inhalation of infected dust or ingestion of infected food may be the cause. It is endemic in much of North America, Europe, and Asia. In the USA, cases have been reported from every state except Hawaii, with the majority from south-central and western states. The natural reservoir is diverse, including water, soil, vegetation, and a variety of small animals (e.g. voles, mice, water rats, squirrels, rabbits, hares). Most cases in the USA occur from June to September when the insect vectors are most active, and cases in winter tend to occur in hunters and trappers who handle infected animal carcasses. The worldwide incidence of tularemia is not known for certain, but it is likely that the numbers are underreported. In the USA, there were 1409 cases and 20 deaths reported during 1985–1992, with a case fatality rate of 1.4%.

Aerosolization of this organism leading to typhoidal or pneumonic forms of tularemia is thought to be the most likely approach by bioterrorists. Untreated, the bacilli multiply and disseminate via the lymph nodes then throughout the body. Major target organs are the lymph nodes, lungs, spleen, liver, and kidney. The infectious dose of the agent is very low, about 10–50 organisms may cause disease. Exposure to aerosols of the agent results in severe respiratory disease, life-threatening pneumonia and generalized infection. It is not known to spread between people, directly, and is endemic in many parts of the USA. However, weaponization of the organism would require a sophisticated level of knowledge and technology.

Clinical disease in humans can take six different forms: glandular and ulceroglandular (arising from infection via broken skin, Figure 26.11), oculoglandular (via eye contamination), oropharyngeal (via oral inoculation, with accompanying cervical lymph node involvement), typhoidal (severe systemic illness), and pneumonic (severe respiratory illness). Clinical symptoms occur after an incubation period of 1–5 (range 1–21) days, including a sudden onset of fever (38–40°C), rigors, chills, headaches, nausea, vomiting, diarrhea, muscle and joints pains, with a dry cough and general weakness. The exact clinical syndrome depends on how the individual was exposed to the organism. Generally, tularemia is expected to have a

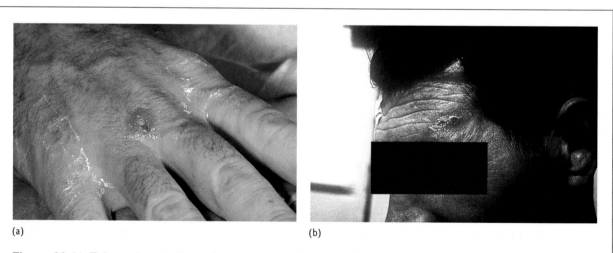

(a)   (b)

Figure 26.11 Tularemia, manifested as cutaneous lesions on the hand and the forehead. (a) Provided by Dr Brachman. Courtesy of the Centers for Disease Control and Prevention; from CDC website: http://phil.cdc.gov/phil/details.asp. (b) Provided by Dr Roger A. Feldman. Courtesy of the Centers for Disease Control and Prevention; from CDC website: http://phil.cdc.gov/phil/details.asp

slower disease progression and a less fatal outcome than either anthrax or pneumonic plague. Mild forms of tularemia may resemble Q fever and laboratory diagnosis is required to distinguish the two.

F. tularensis is a small, nonmotile, aerobic, nonsporing, hardy Gram negative coccobacillus that can survive for weeks at low temperature in water, moist soil, hay, and decaying animal carcasses. It is a BSL-2/3 agent and should be handled in appropriate containment facilities. Suspected cases of tularemia should have respiratory secretions, tissue, body fluids, and blood samples collected for laboratory diagnosis. Direct Gram staining or specific fluorescent antibody staining of secretions and tissues can identify the organism within several hours of receipt of the specimens. Culture of *F. tularensis* from respiratory specimens, fasting gastric aspirates and occasionally blood, provides a definitive diagnosis of tularemia. Specific antigen and antibody testing are also used as well as PCR testing directed against specific *F. tularensis* genes (e.g. the outer membrane protein or *tul 4* genes) (Figure 26.12).

Therapy includes ciprofloxacin (orally), gentamicin, or streptomycin (intravenously) – the latter being the preferred choice. However, sensitivities should be rapidly determined if a bioterrorist release is suspected, as the organism may have been selected or designed to be antibiotic resistant. A live, attenuated vaccine is available (using the avirulent *F. tularensis* biovar palaeartica, type B) that is normally given to laboratory staff routinely working with the organism.

Smallpox (variola major)

Smallpox can exist in two clinical forms: **variola major**, which has a high mortality (about 30%) and **variola minor**, a less common presentation, with a much lower mortality of about 1%. The last case of naturally occurring variola major occurred in Bangladesh in 1975 (Figure 26.13) and that of variola minor in Somalia in 1977, this being the last case of naturally occurring smallpox in the world. The World Health Organization (WHO) declared smallpox to be officially eradicated in 1980. All laboratory smallpox stocks were to be destroyed or transferred to two WHO-approved laboratories (CDC, Atlanta, USA and Institute of Virus Preparations, Koltsovo, Novosivirsk, Russia), with final destruction of the virus scheduled by June 1999, i.e. the final eradication of smallpox from the planet. However, this was postponed to the end of 2002 by a decision in December 1999. This delay may have been partly due to rumours of large smallpox stockpiles in the former Soviet Union, created as a result of their cold war biological weapons program. Such rumours were later confirmed by a scientist who was the Deputy Director of this program, Ken Alibek, who defected to the USA in 1992 (see Further reading). Since then, smallpox has been maintained in the WHO-approved laboratories for further study. The gradual discontinuation of smallpox vaccination after its "official" eradication has left the younger generations vulnerable to this disease, making it an ideal biological weapon, as it is also aerosol transmitted, relatively stable, and transmitted from person to person.

Clinically, there are four types of variola major smallpox: "ordinary," the most frequent type, occurring in about 90% of unvaccinated cases, with a mortality from 10% in patients with discrete lesions, up to 60% in those with confluent lesions; "modified," which occurred in both unvaccinated (1–2%) and previously vaccinated persons (25% of cases) was relatively mild; "flat" and "hemorrhagic" forms, occurring in about 7% and 1–2% of unvaccinated cases, respectively. Pregnant women seemed particularly susceptible to the hemorrhagic form. The mortality of these latter two forms was very high, 93–100%. Hemorrhagic smallpox was particularly difficult to recognize unless there was a known contact history. This difficulty lead to an outbreak of smallpox in Europe, arising from an unsuspected imported case, after it had been eradicated from that region.

After exposure, and an incubation period of 10–14 days (can be as short as 7 or as long as 19 days), illness begins with an abrupt onset of high fever (38–40°C), headache, backache, chills, abdominal pain, vomiting, during which patients are severely unwell and generally stay in bed. This severely incapacitating prodrome, ironically, reduces the potential effectiveness of natural smallpox as a biological weapon. The characteristic rash follows 1–4 days later. The rash starts with lesions on the mucous membranes (the mouth, tongue, oropharynx) before spreading approximately 24 hours later to the skin. Commonly, the rash starts on the face and spreads throughout the body over the next 24–48 hours, in a "centrifugal" distribution (more lesions on the extremities than on the trunk – the opposite distribution of chickenpox). Lesions are initially

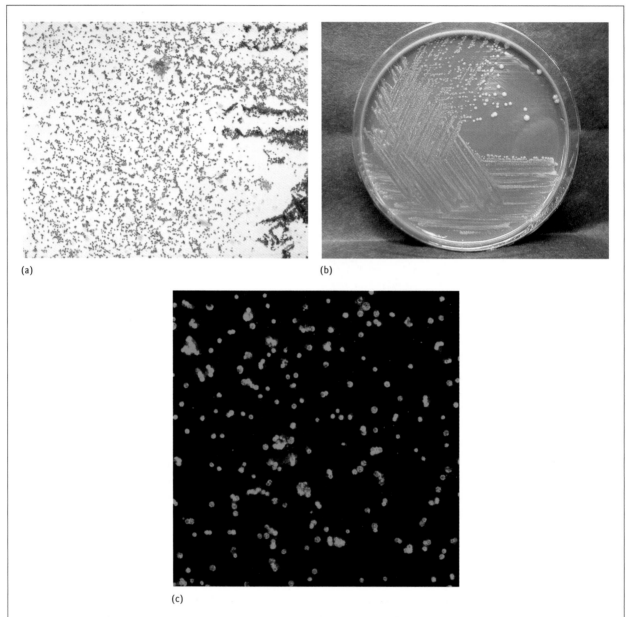

(a)

(b)

(c)

Figure 26.12 *Francisella tularensis* is Gram negative in its staining morphology. It is a poorly staining, very tiny Gram negative coccobacillus (0.2–0.7 μm), seen mostly as single cells. Bipolar staining is not a distinctive feature. (a) *F. tularensis*. (b) Colony characteristics when grown on Chocolate, Martin Lewis, or Thayer-Martin medium include colony size of 1–3 mm, gray-white at 48–72 hours. (c) *F. tularensis* as seen with Direct Fluorescent Antibody Stain (DFA, 1000×), which can be performed directly in tissue, sputum, or culture. (a)–(c) provided by Larry Stauffer. Courtesy of the Centers for Disease Control and Prevention; from CDC website: http://phil.cdc.gov/phil/details.asp

macular and evolve into papules (by the second day) then vesicles (fourth to fifth days) then pustules (seventh day). Rash lesions are about 7–10 mm in diameter, and all are in the same stage of development on all parts of the body (unlike chickenpox), and the lesions are dermal and relatively difficult to break (again unlike chickenpox, where the rash is epidermal). The number of pustules can vary between several to several thousand and can be discrete (generally indicating less serious disease) to confluent (more serious disease).

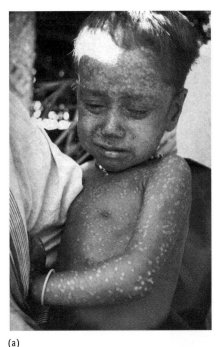
(a)

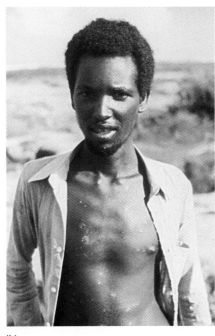
(b)

Figure 26.13 (a) Photograph taken in 1975 depicting a 2-year-old female by the name of Rahima Banu, who was actually the last known case of naturally occurring smallpox, or variola major, in the world. The case occurred in the Bangladesh district of Barisal, in a village named Kuralia, on Bhola Island, October 16, 1975. Note the distribution of the pustules, for their greatest density was found on her face and extremities, which is characteristic of the smallpox maculopapular rash. The last case of smallpox in the USA was in 1949. (b) A photograph of the last known person in the world to have smallpox of any kind: variola minor in a 23-year-old, Ali Maow Maalin, from Merka, Somalia, in 1977. Provided by World Health Organization; Stanley O. Foster. Courtesy of the Centers for Disease Control and Prevention; from CDC website: http://phil.cdc.gov/phil/details.asp

The pustules begin to form a crust, and then scab over. By the end of the second week after the onset of the rash, most of the pustules have scabbed over. When the scabs fall off they leave marks on the skin that eventually become pitted scars. Most of the scabs will have fallen off 3 weeks after the onset of the rash. Until all the scabs have fallen off, the individual is contagious. Younger survivors of smallpox have a reduced risk of severe skin scarring.

Complications of the disease include corneal ulcers and keratitis with blindness, arthritis and limb deformities, pneumonitis, and encephalitis (about 1 : 500 cases of variola major). Related complications include secondary bacterial infections of the skin lesions, joints, bones, and other organs, including generalized sepsis. The most obvious complication in survivors is the skin scarring and facial pockmarks (65–80% of survivors).

Variola is a double-stranded DNA virus in the genus *Orthopoxvirus*. It is a BSL-4 agent and should be handled in appropriate containment facilities. The virus enters the body via the oropharynx, or respiratory mucosa, spreads systemically, and eventually localizes in small blood vessels of the dermis, which is the layer of skin located below the more superficial epidermis. It can be detected by electronmicroscopy (EM) from vesicle or pustule fluid or scrapings and identified by its characteristic orthopoxvirus morphology (Figure 26.14). It has to be distinguished from other members of this family (cowpox, vaccine, and monkeypox) by the patient's clinical and epidemiological history and other laboratory tests. Variola major used to be identified, specifically, using culture on chorioallantoic membranes of chicken embryos (Figure 26.14).

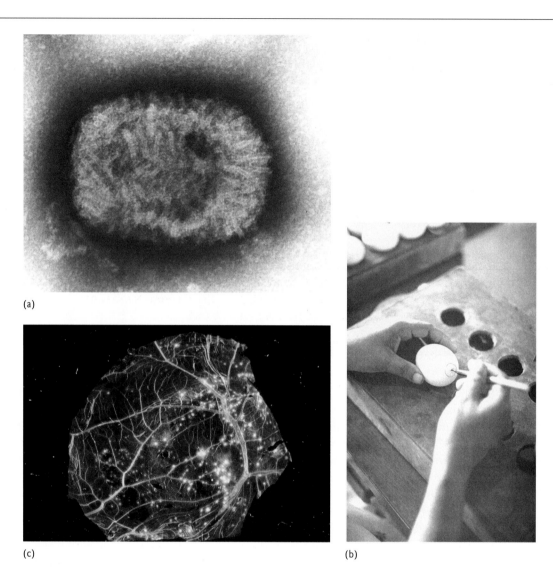

(a)

(c)   (b)

Figure 26.14 (a) Highly magnified at 310 000×, this negative-stained transmission electron micrograph (TEM) depicts a smallpox (variola) virus particle, or a single "virion". (b) This image shows the process of preparing an embryonated chicken egg to be inoculated with vaccinia virus. (c) Poxviruses are very easy to isolate, and will grow in a variety of cell cultures, producing characteristic hemorrhagic pocks on the embryonic chicken chorioallantoic membrane. (a) Provided by J. Nakano. Courtesy of the Centers for Disease Control and Prevention; from CDC website: http://phil.cdc.gov/phil/details.asp. (b) Provided by Stanley O. Foster. Courtesy of the Centers for Disease Control and Prevention; from CDC website: http://phil.cdc.gov/phil/details.asp. (c) Provided by John Noble. Courtesy of the Centers for Disease Control and Prevention; from CDC website: http://phil.cdc.gov/phil/details.asp

However, nowadays, with modern technology and to reduce the risk of laboratory-acquired disease, molecular tests using PCR or restriction fragment length polymorphisms (RFLP) will give specific species identification. Like EM, serological test cannot distinguish between different species of orthopox viruses.

There is no proven specific antiviral treatment for smallpox, though cidofovir (a nucleotide analog) has been most studied recently, as it is known to inhibit the poxvirus DNA polymerase. The traditional smallpox vaccine, based on inoculation with live vaccinia virus (from which the term "vaccination" is derived), has a high complication rate, some of which can be fatal. The original vaccine against smallpox, created by

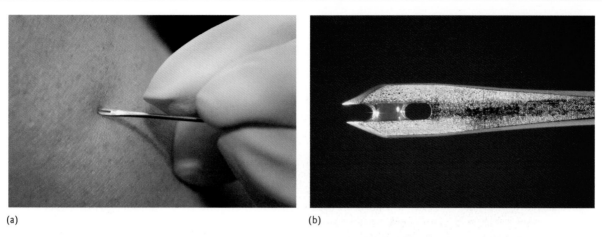

(a)   (b)

Figure 26.15 A close-up of the application to the skin of the bifurcated needle used for smallpox vaccination (a) and how the correct amount of vaccinia virus vaccine fluid is held between the two tines (b). (a) and (b) provided by James Gathany. Courtesy of the Centers for Disease Control and Prevention; from CDC website: http://phil.cdc.gov/phil/details.asp

Edward Jenner in 1796 from human cowpox lesions, was eventually replaced by vaccinia (grown on the skin of live animals), which was eventually used for the WHO smallpox eradication campaign (1966–1980). Several strains of vaccinia virus were used during this campaign, including the "Lister-Elstree" and "New York City Board of Health" strains. The vaccine is usually administered using a two-pronged or bifurcated needle that held the correct amount of vaccine between its tines (Figure 26.15), by rapid repeated jabbing (15 times) with just enough pressure to draw blood after waiting for 15–20 seconds. Successful vaccination ("a take") leads to the formation of a papule then vesicle and eventually a pustule between days 3 and 8 after vaccination. Inflammation is obvious from days 5 to 10 after vaccination, with the pustule reaching maximum size at around day 8. If there is no lesion after 7 days, then revaccination should be performed.

Complications with the vaccine (Figures 26.16 and 26.17) have been categorized as follows: postvaccinial encephalitis, progressive vaccinia, eczema vaccinatum, generalized vaccinia, accidental self-innoculations or transmission to other unvaccinated contacts, nonspecific rashes, and fatal vaccinia. Most of these complications are due to the infection with the live vaccinia virus itself, but some complications are related to specific groups of individuals. Postvaccinal encephalitis occurs at a rate of 3 per million primary vaccines, of which 40% of the cases are fatal, with some patients being left with permanent neurologic damage. Progressive vaccinia occurs among those who are immunosuppressed (e.g. due to a congenital defect, malignancy, radiation therapy, or AIDS), when the vaccinia virus simply continues to multiply. Unless these patients are treated with vaccinia immune globulin, they may not recover. Patients with eczema or atopic dermatitis can develop a serious disseminated cutaneous vaccinia infection that can be fatal. Pustular material from the vaccination site may also be transferred to other parts of the body or to other unvaccinated contacts, sometimes with serious results, including the complications outlined above. More recently, myopericarditis has been identified as a new complication related to smallpox vaccination, during the 2002 military and civilian (mainly adult) smallpox vaccination programs in the USA. Such complications are one of the reasons (apart from the cost of manufacture and administration) for the discontinuation of smallpox vaccination once smallpox was declared eradicated – the vaccine became more dangerous than the pathogen, which was no longer a threat. Vaccinia immunoglobulin (VIG) composed of was serum collected from post-vaccinated individuals has been shown to be relatively effective in treating some of these complications. However, stocks of VIG are becoming scarce since the discontinuation of routine smallpox vaccination.

With the recent focus on bioterrorist threats, new, safer forms of smallpox vaccine, based on non-animal-cultured vaccine virus sources are in development. Second generation smallpox vaccines using tissue culture

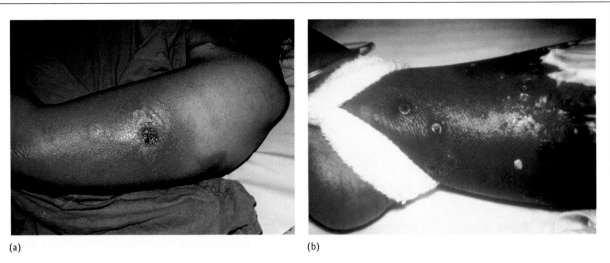

(a)   (b)

Figure 26.16 (a) Female patient with chronic myelogenous leukemia who presented with vaccinia gangrenosum 1 month after a smallpox vaccination, now referred to as progressive vaccinia. This is one of the most severe complications of smallpox vaccination, and is almost always life threatening. Those who are most susceptible to this condition are the immunosuppressed. This patient presented with complications around her smallpox vaccination site. (b) Such complications can be seen in people who have eczema or atopic dermatitis – eczema vaccinatum. (a) Provided by Allen W. Mathies, MD, John Leedom, MD. Courtesy of the Centers for Disease Control and Prevention; from CDC website: http://phil.cdc.gov/phil/details.asp. (b) Provided by Arthur E. Kaye. Courtesy of the Centers for Disease Control and Prevention; from CDC website: http://phil.cdc.gov/phil/details.asp

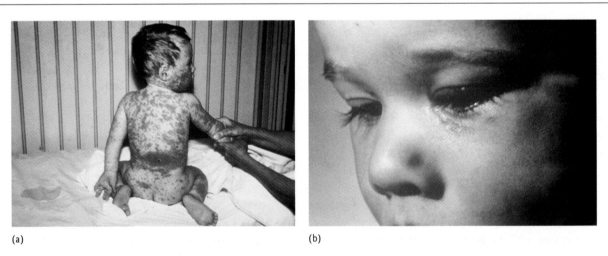

(a)   (b)

Figure 26.17 (a) Child manifesting a generally distributed maculopapular rash after receiving a primary smallpox vaccination. Generalized vaccinia is the result of the systemic spread of smallpox virions from the vaccination site. Despite the lesions, it is usually a benign complication of a primary vaccination that is self-limited, except in some immunosuppressed individuals. (b) The periorbital lesions around this baby's left eye are due to post-smallpox vaccination autoinoculation of vaccine virus transferred from the site of vaccination. The most common sites involved are the face, eyelid, nose, mouth, genitalia, and rectum. Most lesions heal without specific therapy. (a) Provided by Arthur E. Kaye and J. Michael Lane. Courtesy of the Centers for Disease Control and Prevention; from CDC website: http://phil.cdc.gov/phil/details.asp. (b) Provided by Dr Michael Lane. Courtesy of the Centers for Disease Control and Prevention; from CDC website: http://phil.cdc.gov/phil/details.asp

rather than live animal skin cultures of vaccinia virus are free of the animal bacterial and viral contaminants, and also allows a more efficient means of vaccine production. Clinical trials using immunological surrogate markers of protection (since testing in humans against direct smallpox challenge is ethically impossible) have suggested that they are, at least, immunologically equivalent to the original (first generation) animal-derived smallpox vaccinia vaccines. Third generation smallpox vaccines use attenuated vaccinia strains that have been either passaged through nonhuman cell lines or genetically altered. However, these vaccines are still in early stages of human trials. First and probably second generation smallpox vaccines will have more complications than third generation vaccines, but the effectiveness of the latter against smallpox will be difficult to demonstrate. They may have a role as a "pre-vaccination vaccine" to reduce the adverse effects of the first or second generation vaccines. Subunit vaccines that consist of only the immunogenic vaccinia proteins would have even fewer adverse effects, and there has been some protection demonstrated in mice and nonhuman primates, but human trials have not been performed yet.

The last group of potential biological warfare agents in Category A, the **viral hemorrhagic fevers**, is covered in Chapter 22.

Test yourself

Case study 26.1

A 30-year-old male presents to the local hospital in Atlanta (Georgia, USA) with a 2-day history of fever and general malaise, and has now developed a maculopapular rash on his face. He is triaged quickly and admitted to an isolation room in the emergency room (ER) within minutes of entering.

? 1. You are part of a team of microbiologists and infection control personnel attending. You see the patient with a surgical mask and wearing gloves. What is your initial differential diagnosis from this limited history? What else would you like to ask him?

He tells you that he has not been outside the USA for several years but has traveled around the US on holiday and visiting friends in the last month, some of whom live in rural areas where he may have had some insect bites. He is single but has a girlfriend and is very definitely heterosexual. He believes that his girlfriend is faithful. He says that he has definitely had a few mosquito bites when sitting in his garden at home in the evenings eating and drinking with friends in the last week. He does not complain of any myalgia or arthralgia and his previous health has been good. He works in a local garden center.

? 2. You recommend admission to an isolation ward for further observation and investigation. What investigations will you request now?

The next day, whilst waiting on laboratory investigations, you get an urgent call from the isolation ward. The patient is now unrousable and the maculopapular rash has become generalized and now hemorrhagic, in the space of just 18 hours. You take your team to see this patient urgently. When you arrive, you can see that the patient is obviously comatose, and not only is the rash hemorrhagic, but he is bleeding from nose and intravenous cannula site.

Your team is now considering some sort of viral hemorrhagic fever (VHF), such as Ebola, Marburg or Lassa, but since these viruses are found in Africa, other more likely candidates are Bolivian (Machupo) or Argentine (Junin) from South America. However, he has had no history of travel there. Later that morning, you receive calls from colleagues working in infectious diseases from hospitals nearby reporting similar cases, all within the last week: patients admitted with fever, general malaise, and rash, all of whom have deteriorated to a VHF-like presentation, virtually overnight.

Test yourself

After some urgent meetings, your team decides to call in the CDC to coordinate the isolation and investigation of all these cases. If it is some sort of VHF, your local hospitals do not have the Biosafety Level 4 (BSL-4) containment wards or laboratories to deal with such cases. The patients are cohorted together in a secure isolation unit by the CDC, and are now effectively out of your hands.

After further investigations, the pathogen turns out not to be one of the VHFs but a weaponized strain of variola major that invariably results in the highly lethal hemorrhagic form of the disease. The CDC informs your team that all the patients had been infected with this weaponized hemorrhagic smallpox strain, which has somehow been genetically altered to be transmitted by mosquitoes. Further investigation into the origin of this virus, many months later, show that it is has been modified from a smallpox strain that has been stored at CDC. In addition, although not yet confirmed, there is a rumor that three CDC scientists are under investigation. Each of them were working on different projects, one on orthopoxvirus pathogenesis, one on mosquito-borne viral infections, and the other the genetic modification of viruses to be used as live attenuated vaccines.

Further reading

Alibek K, Handelman S. *Biohazard: The Chilling True Story of the Largest Covert Biological Weapons Program in the World – Told from Inside by the Man Who Ran It*. New York: Dell Publishing, Random House, 1999

Beeching NJ, Dance DA, Miller AR, Spencer RC. Biological warfare and bioterrorism. *BMJ* 2002;324(7333):336–339 [review]

Broussard LA. Biological agents: weapons of warfare and bioterrorism. *Mol Diagn* 2001;6(4):323–333

Christopher GW, Cieslak TJ, Pavlin JA, Eitzen EM Jr. Biological warfare. A historical perspective. *JAMA* 1997;278(5):412–417

Drancourt M, Houhamdi L, Raoult D. *Yersinia pestis* as a telluric, human ectoparasite-borne organism. *Lancet Infect Dis* 2006;6(4):234–241

Henderson DA. Smallpox: clinical and epidemiologic features. *Emerg Infect Dis* 1999;5(4):537–539 [special issue of EID devoted to bioterrorism]

Henderson DA, Thomas V, O'Toole T (eds). *Bioterrorism: Guidelines for Medical and Public Health Management*. Chicago, IL: American Medical Association, 2002

Moore ZS, Seward JF, Lane JM. Smallpox. *Lancet* 2006;367(9508):425–435 [review]

Preston R. *The Cobra Event*, reprint edition. New York: Ballantine Books, 1998 [fiction]

This book is **fiction**, but not outside the limits of possibility with the current levels of modern technology.

Useful websites

American Society for Microbiology. Bioterrorism Threats to Our Future: The Role of the Clinical Microbiology Laboratory in Detection, Identification, and Confirmation of Biological Agents. Prepared by James W Snyder, PhD and William Check, PhD. 2001. http://www.asm.org/Academy/index.asp?bid=2159

CDC. Emergency Preparedness and Response. Bioterrorism Agents/Diseases. http://www.bt.cdc.gov/agent/agentlist-category.asp#catdef

Fenner F, Henderson DA, Arita I, Jezek Z, Ladnyi ID. Smallpox and its Eradication. Geneva: World Health Organization, 1988. http://whqlibdoc.who.int/smallpox/9241561106.pdf

Answers to test yourself questions

Chapter 4

Case study 4.1

1 Numerous polymorphs Gram positive cocci in clusters.
2 Large beta-hemolytic colonies seen.
3 Methicillin resistant *Staphylococcus aureus* (MRSA).

Case study 4.2

1 Numerous Gram positive cocci in pairs.
2 Heavy growth of mucoid alpha haemolytic colonies.
3 *Streptococcus pneumoniae.*

Case study 4.3

1 Numerous polymorphs and numerous Gram negative bacilli seen.
2 Heavy growth of lactose fermenting colonies seen.
3 *Escherichia coli.*

Chapter 6

Case study 6.1

1 C Number of susceptible people exposed to infection – **denominator**

D Minimum incubation period
E Maximum incubation period } *Time period of secondary cases – the numerator*

Note: The maximum infectious period is not necessary here as no child attended school once symptomatic.
2 2/19 = 10.5%. The three assumptions: (i) that each secondary case is derived from a single primary case; (ii) all cases of successful transmission are symptomatic; (iii) all individuals in the denominator are equally susceptible.
3 False. Co-primary cases are excluded from numerator and denominator as they are neither secondary cases nor are they part of the susceptible and exposed pool that forms the denominator. Tertiary cases form part of the denominator as they were part of the exposed susceptible pool but not the numerator as they are not secondary cases.
4 The basic reproduction number (R_0) is the average number of infective secondary cases produced by each infective case in a totally susceptible population. Net reproduction number (R) is the average number of secondary infective cases produced by each primary case in a population where some of the individuals are not susceptible. If all individuals mix together at random, so that infectious cases are likely to make contact with susceptible as well as immune individuals, then R is the product of R_0 times the proportion of the population that are susceptible (x).

In this nursery, at the start of the epidemic, these two are the same because none of the children had any previous exposure to chickenpox and childhood vaccination was not offered.

5 The SAR would be larger only if the numerator stayed the same; as the denominator would now be smaller, i.e. it would only include the susceptible nonvaccinated individuals. However due to vaccinated individuals in the pool, transmission would be lower, so if the numerator was reduced the SAR would also be reduced.

Net reproduction number (R) would need to be used – as all individuals mixed together at random, and infectious cases made contact with susceptible as well as immune individuals, then R is calculated as the product of R_o times the proportion of the population that are susceptible (x). In this case R would be lower than R_o due to the pool of vaccinated cases.

6 The formula is:

$$R_o = c \times p \times d$$

$c = 16$, $p = 0.3$ (0.7 for the duration of infectivity, i.e. 7 days, but here the child was sent home on the day of illness, the child was a potential infection risk for only 3 days), $d = 3$

$$16 \times 0.3 \times 3 = 14.4$$

We would expect 14 children to contract the infection.

Case study 6.2

1 Point source outbreak: here the cases are clustered tightly around a single peak. There is a sharp upslope and a trailing downslope. This indicates that they were probably infected from the same source at the same time. The spread of cases around the peak reflects the variation in incubation periods between cases.

2 Minimum incubation period: 12–18 hours. Median incubation period: 12–36 hours. Maximum incubation period: 12–28 hours.

Case study 6.3

1 Living in a mud hut and collecting firewood were the most likely risk factors based on the data provided.

Activity	Risk (attack rate) (%)	Relative risk
Working in fields	68/658 = 10.33	(68/658) ÷ (12/142) = 1.22
Owning pigs	10/147 = 6.80	(10/147) ÷ (70/653) = 0.63
Washing clothes in the river	15/110 = 13.64	(15/110) ÷ (65/690) = 1.45
Collecting firewood	41/220 = 18.64	(41/220) ÷ (39/580) = 2.77
Owning cattle	24/207 = 11.59	(24/207) ÷ (56/593) = 1.23
Living in a mud hut	27/78 = 34.62	(27/78) ÷ (53/722) = 4.72

2

		Gold Standard test (microscopy)		
		Positive	Negative	Total
New test	Positive	a 60	b 36	96
	Negative	c 20	d 684	704
Total		80	720	800

Positive predictive value: a/(a + b) = 62.5%. Negative predictive value: d/(c + d) = 97.2%.

3 As the new test has 75% sensitivity, it follows that 25% of the patients tested would not be detected or treated if the new test was used instead of microscopy. The new test is not recommended as a replacement for microscopy.

Case study 6.4

1

Food eaten	Guests with diarrhea (total = 111)	Guests without diarrhea (total = 188)	Total = 299	Risk (%)	Relative risk
Prawns	65	72	137	65/137 = 47.45	(65/137) ÷ (46/162) = 1.67
Liver pâté	37	44	81	37/81 = 45.68	(37/81) ÷ (74/218) = 1.35
Pasta and cheese salad	51	79	130	51/130 = 39.23	(51/130) ÷ (60/169) = 1.11
Chicken and rice	93	162	255	93/255 = 36.47	(93/255) ÷ (18/44) = 0.89
Green salad	95	37	132	95/132 = 71.97	(95/132) ÷ (16/167) = 7.51
Chocolate cake	37	82	119	37/119 = 31.09	(37/119) ÷ (74/180) = 0.76
Mango mousse	8	5	13	8/13 = 61.54	(8/13) ÷ (103/286) = 1.71

The green salad was the most likely food stuff to have caused the outbreak on the basis of these results. Calculations are tabulated above.

Try the case studies from the CDC website for further insight into epidemiologic investigations. See Further reading for details.

Chapter 7

Case study 7.1

1 Erysepilas.
2 *Streptococcus pyogenes.*
3 Scarlet fever or streptococcal toxic shock.
4 Necrotizing fasciitis or puerperal fever.

Case study 7.2

1 Carbuncle.
2 *Staphylococcus aureus.*
2 Scalded skin syndrome and staphylococcal toxic shock syndrome.
4 Amoxicillin is inactivated by β-lactamase, an enzyme produced by about 80% of staphylococci making them resistant to amoxicillin. β-lactamase stable penicillins such as nafcillin or flucloxacillin are the agents of choice here.

Case study 7.3

1 Osteomyelitis.
2 *Staphylococcus aureus.*
3 Blood cultures.

4 Spread of organisms from a distant focus into the bone occurs via two main routes: (a) via the bloodstream, where infection is caused by bacterial seeding into bone from the blood. The clinical picture varies with age. In children through the age of puberty the long bones of the extremities are most often involved with the metaphysis as the initial infected site. The apparent slowing and turbulence of blood flow as the vessels make sharp angles at the distal metaphyseal end of bone are increased risks for the formation of clots and the subsequent seeding of bacteria. This results in inflammation and necrosis of bone.

In adults, hematogenous osteomyelitis most often affects the spine. The vertebral bodies become more vascular with age and bacteremia may result in bacterial seeding of vertebral bodies, preferentially at the more vascular anterior vertebral end plates. In addition, many large lumbar veins communicate freely with pelvic veins; retrograde flow from pelvic tissues (urethra, prostate, bladder) to lumbar vertebrae is a possible route for the spread of pelvic infections to the lumbar vertebrae.

(b) In about 25% of patients with osteomyelitis, the predisposing factor is trauma to the bone at or near the site of infection (direct or contiguous osteomyelitis). Bacteria seed directly into bony tissues from a contiguous site of infection or as a result of sepsis after surgery.

Chapter 9

Case study 9.1

1 Splinter haemorrhages under the nail bed, Janeway lesions in the palms and Osler's nodes in the pulp of finger.
2 Infective endocarditis.
3 Inflammation of the small blood vessels and microemboli can manifest as splinter hemorrhages under the nail bed and immune complex deposition occurs in the skin and subcutaneous tissues resulting in Janeway lesions and Osler's nodes.
4 Viridans group streptococci.

Case study 9.2

1 *Streptococcus pneumoniae.*
2 The polysaccharide capsule is the major virulence factor since it interferes with phagocytosis by neutrophils.
3 Splenectomized individuals or those lacking a functioning spleen.
4 Resistance is mediated by the synthesis of a novel penicillin binding protein (PBP 2a) by the organism, this has reduced affinity for penicillin. Since penicillin cannot bind, it is unable to act on the cell wall.

Case study 9.3

1 Whether childhood immunizations are up to date for her age.
2 *Bordetella pertussis.*
3 The bacteria attach to the respiratory tract and release a toxin that causes inflammation and paralyzes the cilia. This prevents the removal of respiratory secretions.
4 Immunity is waning in the adult population because of immunization in early childhood and absence of a booster effect as immunization of children has greatly decreased the circulation of the organism in the childhood population. This causes the adult pool of susceptible individuals to expand and if one infected individual enters this pool transmission of infection is greatly facilitated.

Case study 9.4

1 *Legionella pneumophila.*
2 Working with highly aerosolized water.

3 Urine for *Legionella pneumophila* serogroup 1 antigen test; and antibody detection methods on patients' serum.

4 Infection with *Legionella* species can be avoided by maintenance of air conditioning systems including regular hyperchlorination treatment and ensuring that hot water supplies are above 45°C to prevent bacterial multiplication.

Case study 9.5

1 *Chlamydia psittaci.*
2 Inhalation of dust containing bird droppings.
3 By serological methods.
4 No.

Chapter 10

Case study 10.1

1 *Haemophilus influenzae* type B. (a) Age of child and incomplete childhood vaccinations. (b) 500 polymorphs (very high), high CSF protein and low CSF glucose compared to blood glucose. CSF Gram: few polymorphs, very scanty Gram negative coccoid bacteria, some are more rod shaped.
2 Hib vaccine. Childhood vaccination against *Haemophilus influenzae* type B has been the single most important development in the prevention of this infection: the widespread use of childhood Hib vaccination has decreased the incidence of Hib meningitis in children in many countries by more than 90%.

Case study 10.2

1 *Neisseria meningitidis.*
2 Living in dormitory accommodation, prodrome of a flu-like illness.
3 *Neisseria meningitidis* serogroup B; the freshman year would have received the meningococcal conjugate vaccine (MCV4) against serogroups A,C,Y,W135 that was introduced in 2005.
4 The other residents of the "dorm" would have been given antibiotic prophylaxis according to the guidelines from CDC. Rifampin for 2 days or ciprofloxacin single dose.

Case study 10.3

1 The stain shows Gram positive cocci predominantly in pairs. Probably *Streptococcus pneumoniae.*
2 Pneumonia.
3 Development of penicillin resistance mediated by altered penicillin binding proteins (PBPs).
4 Pneumococcal vaccine. Read further on: http://www.cdc.gov/vaccines/vpd-vac/pneumo/default.htm
5 Presence of a functioning spleen, i.e. rule out sickle cell disease.

Case study 10.4

1 Viral meningitis. Justification: child with nonblanching rash, acute onset, predominantly lymphocytes in the CSF, borderline protein and normal glucose levels in the CSF.
2 Name the agents most commonly implicated in this type of infection:
Enteroviruses: echoviruses; coxsackie viruses A and B; poliovirus.
Herpes viruses: herpes simplex virus 1 and 2.
Paramyxovirus: as a complication of mumps.
3 HSV-2 is a more common cause of viral meningitis than HSV-1, and first-time attacks are often associated with primary genital infection; hence HSV-2 infection causing meningitis is unlikely in a child.
4 No.

Case study 10.5

1 Frontal lobe brain abscess.
2 Chronic sinusitis and poor teeth.
3 *Streptococcus milleri*
Staphylococcus aureus, and other alpha and beta-hemolytic streptococci
Anaerobic Gram positive and negative organisms (i.e. *Bacteroides* species, *Fusobacterium* spp., anaerobic streptococci).

Chapter 11

Case study 11.1

1 Candidal infection with *C. albicans* is the commonest cause.
2 She may be pregnant.

Case study 11.2

1 *Trichomonas vaginalis.*
2 Treat her partner.

Case study 11.3

1 Normal vaginal smear showing epithelial cells and Gram positive lactobacilli.
2 Reassure her.

Case study 11.4

1 Herpes simplex virus.
2 Primary infection.
3 The source of infection is likely to be her new male partner with asymptomatic infection. The virus can be spread to other parts of her own body causing oral or disseminated lesions, and can also be spread to other people by either direct contact or sexually. She should consider treatment for herself and her partner, good hand hygiene, and contraception such as a condom.

Case study 11.5

1 Other possible symptoms could be joint pains and/or arthritis.
2 *Chlamydia trachomatis.* He would not have been infected by his baby daughter. The chain of transmission is likely to be from him to his partner sexually, then from partner to the child during vaginal delivery.
3 Possible reactive disease in the eye, Reiter's syndrome.
4 Swab the urethra and order nucleic acid amplification tests (NAATs) for *C. trachomatis*, and refer to a sexual health clinic for a complete workup.
5 For a neonate aquiring this infection via a vaginal delivery, lipopolysaccharide is thought to be the predominant antigen responsible for inducing proinflammatory cytokines. The possible complications are severe neonatal conjunctivitis and risk of pneumonia. Treatment options: macrolide; hospital referral.
6 Investigate the partner. Take specimens by urine or cervical swab. Order NAAT for *C. trachomatis* and refer to a sexual health clinic for a complete workup.
7 Yes. Macrolide is suitable for taking while breastfeeding.

Case study 11.6

1 Numerous polymorphs, Gram negative intracellular diplococci suggestive of *N. gonorrheae*.
2 See pathogenesis of organism in this chapter.
3 Development of resistance to several antibiotics.
4 Epididymitis, orchitis, urethral stricture.

Case study 11.7

1 Syphilis.
2 *Treponema pallidum*.
3 Serological tests for syphilis.
4 Secondary stage. Ask the patient if he noticed a painless ulcer (chancre) in his penis up to 12 weeks ago that resolved spontaneously.
5 Cardiac or neurological complications, gumma.

Case study 11.8

1 Epithelial cells studded with Gram positive cocco-bacilli = clue cells.
2 Bacterial vaginosis.
3 KOH whiff test.
4 Sexual partner/s, condoms, vaginal douches.

Case study 11.9

1 Dipstick, detects leukocyte esterases and nitrites produced by bacteria which utilize nitrates.
2 Clean the area, collect a midstream sample of urine (MSU).
3 First stream washes away colonizing bacteria in the lower end of the urethra removing potentially contaminating bacteria, hence culture result will reflect organism that may be causing infection in the bladder.

Case study 11.10

1 Yes.
2 It was a suprapubic aspirate, so all counts would be significant.
3 Lactose fermenter, pink colonies.
4 Risk of developing reflux and renal scarring, complete urological investigation of the urinary tract and specialist referral, early and rigorous antibiotic treatment.

Chapter 12

Case study 12.1

1 Ophthalmia neonatorum.
2 During vaginal delivery, through an infected birth canal.
3 Infection with *Neisseria gonorrhoeae*.

Case study 12.2

1 Asymptomatic bacteriuria during pregnancy is common because of stasis of urine in the bladder and incomplete emptying of the bladder during pregnancy.

2 Yes because bacteria have a greater to tendency to ascend into the upper renal tract in pregnancy, due in part to the pressure of the fetus on the bladder and in part due to lax sphincter tone associated with hormonal changes in pregnancy.

3 An increased risk of pyelonephritis can cause intrauterine growth retardation, premature labor, and all its associated complications

Case study 12.3

1 Neonatal sepsis probably due to Group B beta hemolytic streptococci (GBS).

2 Early onset as it has occurred in less than 7 days after delivery.

3 Early onset sepsis is associated with organisms that are acquired during passage through the maternal birth canal, while late onset sepsis is associated with person-to-person transmission and therefore represents hospital or environmentally acquired organisms.

4 Long labor and difficult delivery eventually needing the use of forceps. Premature rupture of membranes, maternal fever of 38.5°C during labor.

5 (a) Screening-based approach: Women who are at high risk are identified by detection of GBS carriers through collection of recto-vaginal cultures at 35−37 weeks of gestation.

(b) Risk-based approach: recognition of certain obstetrical risk factors, such as having a threatened premature delivery or prolonged rupture of the membranes irrespective of vaginal colonization. These women are given intrapartum antibiotics (penicillin).

Chapter 13

Case study 13.1

1 During the initial month following hematopoietic stem cell transplantation (HSCT) patients are profoundly neutropenic. The chemotherapeutic regimens used to facilitate hematopoietic stem cell transplantation give rise to profound and sometimes prolonged immunosuppression particularly cell-mediated immunity.

2 Prophylactic antifungal drugs and maintenance of the environment to deliver clean air are the most important. See Further reading to this chapter.

Case study 13.2

1 *Pneumocystis jirovecii* (previously classified as *Pneumocystis carinii*) was previously classified as a protozoa. Currently, it is considered a fungus based on nucleic acid and biochemical analysis. Yes it is an AIDS defining condition

2 *Pneumocystis* pneumonia (PCP), which is caused by *Pneumocystis jirovecii*, is frequently the first serious illness encountered by HIV-infected persons. During the early years of the AIDS epidemic, PCP was the AIDS-defining illness for as many as two-thirds of patients in the USA. Although a decline in incidence of PCP occurred during the era of highly active antiretroviral therapy (HAART), PCP remains the most common serious opportunistic illness in HIV-infected persons. Patients in the developing world without access to PCP prophylaxis or antiretroviral drugs remain at high risk, and PCP continues to develop in certain groups in industrialized countries.

Case study 13.3

1 HIV test.

2 A capsulated yeast fungus.

3 Pigeon droppings.

Case study 13.4

1 All capsulated organisms, notably: *S. pneumoniae, N. meningitidis, H. influenzae.*
2 The spleen is the major organ responsible for producing opsonizing IgM antibodies and for generating phagocytic macrophages that ingest the opsonized organism.
3 *S. pneumoniae* Gram positive cocci in pairs.
4 Pneumococcal vaccine and prophylactic oral penicillin for life.

Case study 13.5

1 Defective T cell-mediated immunity.
2 It is a filamentous, branching Gram positive organism. It causes a chronic, granulomatous, progressive inflammatory disease, particularly in patients who are immunosuppressed.

Case study 13.6

1 *Toxoplasma gondii.*
2 Yes.
3 Cats are the definitive hosts and shed the infective form in the feces.
4 Consumption of undercooked infected meat containing sporulated oocysts, ingestion of the oocyst from fecally contaminated hands, i.e. while gardening or changing cat litter.
5 Cats are the definitive hosts for the sexual stages of *T. gondii* and thus are the main reservoirs of infection. After tissue cysts or oocysts are ingested by the cat, viable organisms are released and invade epithelial cells of the small intestine. Here they undergo an asexual followed by a sexual cycle and then form oocysts, which are excreted. The unsporulated oocyst takes 1–5 days after excretion to sporulate (become infective).

Case study 13.7

1 The enzyme-linked immunosorbent assay (ELISA) test detects the release of interferon gamma (IFN-γ) in fresh heparinized whole blood from persons who have been exposed to *Mycobacterium tuberculosis*. The presence of IFN-γ therefore indicates that the patient has been exposed to *M. tuberculosis* at some time. Because the test does not cross-react with antigens from the Bacille Calmette–Guérin (BCG) vaccine strains and from commonly encountered nontuberculous mycobacteria (NTM) except *M. kansasii, M. szulgai,* and *M. marinum*, QFT-G is expected to be more specific for *M. tuberculosis* than tests that use tuberculin purified protein derivative (PPD) as the antigen.
2 Treatment of latent TB infection (LTBI) is essential to controlling and eliminating TB in the USA. Treatment of LTBI substantially reduces the risk that TB infection will progress to disease. Certain groups are at very high risk of developing TB disease once infected, and every effort should be made to begin appropriate treatment and to ensure those persons complete the entire course of treatment for LTBI. For more information see Further reading.
3 These products work by blocking tumor necrosis factor alpha (TNF-α), an inflammatory cytokine, and are approved for treating rheumatoid arthritis and other selected autoimmune diseases. TNF-α is associated with the immunology and pathophysiology of certain infectious diseases, notably TB; blocking TNF-α can allow TB disease to emerge from latent *M. tuberculosis* infection.

Case study 13.8

1 Poorly functioning neutrophils.
2 *Rhizopus* have nonseptate or sparsely septate broad hyphae (branches), rhizoids (root-like hyphae), sporangia or spore containing bodies, and sporangiospores. *Mucor* are similar but have no roots as in the figure in the question. See Further reading.

Case study 13.9

1 Profound granulocytopenia and mucosal damage usually develop about a week after the start of chemotherapy. Fever develops around a week later, and, if there is bacteremia, it mostly occurs at this time. See Figure 13.2.
2 Bacteria: predominantly Gram positive
Enterobacteriacae, *Pseudomonas* species
Candida species and *Aspergillus* species.
3 Embolic deposits of *Pseudomonas* species in the blood vessels leading to vasculitis, causes them to rupture leading to necrosis of the skin and soft tissue supplied by those vessels.

Case study 13.10

1 Chronic granulomatous disease (CGD) is caused by defects in the pathway for the production of hydrogen peroxide in the phagosomes of phagocytic cells. This results in a defective respiratory burst and an impaired response to certain microorganisms.
2 Fungi such as *Aspergillus* species.

Case study 13.11

1 Strongyloidiasis should always be considered in the differential diagnosis of patients from endemic communities who present with moderate to severe signs suggestive of respiratory, gastrointestinal and cutaneous infection because these regions are endemic for the parasite.
2 *S. stercoralis* is able to cause autoinfection giving rise to chronic infestations in the immunocompetent. Chemotherapy, for example with corticosteroids, impairs the containment of the autoinfection cycle leading to the hyperinfection syndrome.
3 Gram negative sepsis arises from the larval stages that carry Gram negative organisms while migrating from gastrointestinal tract.

Case study 13.12

1 Because the child had chickenpox in the past, reactivation with the virus lying dormant in his dorsal root ganglia has occurred as he is now neutropenic and immunosuppressed (treatment related).
2 Shingles.
3 Yes, the lesions contain live virus.

Chapter 14

Case study 14.1

1 *Clostridium difficile.*
2 Yes it is widespread in hospitals because of broad-spectrum antibiotic use, acquisition in the community is known but uncommon.
3 Age and previous hospital admission and having taken amoxicillin.
4 Attention to handwashing, isolation in a single room, use of protective clothing by healthcare staff such as gown/apron and gloves. Masks are not necessary.

Case study 14.2

1 Exogenous because he came into hospital free of MRSA, admission screen results were negative.
2 Hands of healthcare staff.
3 Venous cannula and surgical wound.
4 Overweight, diabetic.

5 Infection as it also grew from blood culture and he had symptoms of fever and redness around the cannula site.

6 Attention to handwashing, isolation in a single room, use of protective clothing by healthcare staff such as gown/apron and gloves. Masks are not necessary.

Case study 14.3

1 Age, smoker, limited mobility, previous hospitalization, and exposure to antibiotics (therefore presumed colonization with resistant organisms).

2 In this case, it is probably exogenous as typing of the organism revealed that it was indistinguishable from other strains prevalent in the ICU in the same bay and over the same time period.

3 Yes as the organisms are indistinguishable from each other and they came from patients in the same bay and over the same time period (overlaps in person, place, and time).

4 Respiratory care of the intubated and ventilated patient, manipulation of the central venous catheter and urinary catheter.

5 Attention to handwashing before touching the patient, isolating infected patients in a side room. Training and education of healthcare staff and constant surveillance with regard to emergence of resistance, rational antibiotic prescribing.

Chapter 15

Case study 15.1

1 Childhood fever with a rash has many causes, some of which are so characteristic that they have been given numbers sequentially: "first disease" ("rubeola," measles virus), "second disease" ("scarlet fever," Group A betahemolytic *Streptococcus*), "third disease" ("German measles," rubella virus), "fifth disease" ("slapped cheek" disease, parvovirus B19, PVB19), and "sixth disease" ("exanthem subitum" or "roseola infantum," human herpesvirus 6, HHV6). As well as the relative timing of onset of the fever and the rash (including where the rash started), you would want to know: (i) the distribution of the rash, e.g. mainly central like chickenpox, more peripherally distributed like smallpox (see Chapter 26) or patchy like PVB19 "slapped cheek" disease and shingles?; (ii) the character of the rash, e.g. flat "macular" like rubella sometimes, raised "papular" like rubella and measles, red "erythematous" like rubella and measles or vesicular like chickenpox?; (iii) other related features, e.g. itchy like chickenpox, blanchable (disappears when you press on it) like some rubella lesions, painful on pressure like hand-foot-and-mouth and shingles?; (iv) other associated systemic features, e.g. red eyes like measles, red tongue like scarlet fever, or bleeding like dengue hemorrhagic fever (see Chapter 24). Other rashes caused by infectious agents commonly seen in this age group include herpes virus simplex type 1 (HSV-1, individual or small clusters of vesicular lesions in and around the mouth) (see Chapter 7).

2 You should know the specific types of diagnostic tests available at your local laboratory for the common childhood rash illness described in A1. For measles, rubella and PVB19, serology testing for IgM (testing for recent, acute infection) and IgG (testing for immunity or past infection) antibodies are usually performed (taking about 2–4 hours, depending on the kit used). There is also VZV IgM and IgG testing, but some laboratories may not have VZV IgM testing available. For VZV (including both chickenpox and shingles cases), often a skin scraping to obtain virus from the skin lesions directly for immunofluorescent staining (which can be completed within 2–3 hours) is preferred and may be quicker (this is also the case for suspected HSV-1 lesions). Scarlet fever can be diagnosed using a throat swab and performing bacterial culture for *S. pyogenes*. For HHV6 diagnosis, serology is more difficult and the polymerase chain reaction (PCR) assay can be used to detect HHV6 DNA directly, though this must be performed on a serum sample collected as soon as possible after the illness begins, as the viral DNA is soon cleared by the body's immune system. This also applies to the other viruses, i.e. their RNA or DNA can be detected by PCR if the blood sample is taken early enough and if the laboratory has the assay available. However, for many of these viruses (as described above) usually, serological testing is sufficient and well established and few laboratories will have these PCR tests for this reason.

3 Occasionally, childhood rash illness may lead to complications such as encephalitis and pneumonitis, but this is rare. It is difficult and impractical to keep all such children in hospital for observation for the duration of their illness or to wait for the results of all their blood tests. Clinical judgment based on knowledge and experience is required to make such decisions on a case-by-case basis. If allowed home, the mother should be advised of other considerations, as her child is potentially infectious until he has fully recovered and has developed antibodies to the presumed infecting agent. For example, the mother needs to keep her child away from other potentially susceptible children, pregnant women, and immunocompromised patients. In the latter case, this may occasionally be another family member sharing the same household. Finally, if the child does develop any complications or seems to get worse rather than better, the mother should bring the child back to hospital as soon as possible for re-evaluation. In this case, the child turned out to have HHV6 (sixth disease or exanthema subitum or roseola infantum), which is only transmissible by direct contact (usually via infected saliva), which rarely develops complications in otherwise healthy children (though encephalitis is a recognized complication of HHV6 sixth disease and can be severe).

Chapter 16

Case study 16.1

1 Yes as she is sputum smear positive and can disseminate organisms into the air while coughing.

2 She can re-attend after completing a 2-week course of anti-TB therapy (usually supervised therapy).

3 If she is not systemically unwell and is compliant with taking medication she can be treated at home; if hospitalization is needed it is recommended that she stay for 2 weeks; this period is crucial because actively multiplying organisms are targeted in this period of therapy and most patients convert to sputum smear negative during this period.

4 They need to be investigated in a credited TB clinic for latent TB infection and appropriately managed. For more information see the Further reading.

5 See: http://www.cdc.gov/mmwr/preview/mmwrhtml/rr5415a1.htm. The plan includes:
Interview contacts by trained personnel; maintain confidentiality
Perform TST and/or IGRA tests
Evaluate results: physicians must ensure that active disease is not present.
Accepted treatment regimens are available at: http://www.cdc.gov/mmwr/preview/mmwrhtml/rr5415a1.htm

6 The tuberculin skin test (**TST**) is widely used to test for LTBI in close contacts. Below is the interpretation of a TST:

Induration of ≥5 mm is considered positive in:	Induration of ≥10 mm is considered positive in:	Induration of ≥15 mm is considered positive in:
HIV positive persons **Recent contacts of TB case patients** **Persons with chest X-ray evidence of prior TB** **Patients with organ transplants and other immunosuppressed patients**	Recent immigrants from high-prevalence countries Injection drug users Residents and employees of high-risk congregate settings, i.e. prisons, nursing homes/elderly care homes, all healthcare facilities, residential facilities for AIDS patients, homeless shelters Mycobacteriology laboratory personnel Persons with silicosis, diabetes mellitus, chronic renal failure, cancer patients, weight loss of 10% of ideal body weight, gastrectomy, and jejunoileal bypass Children <4 years of age, or infants, children, and adolescents exposed to adults at high risk	Persons with no known risk factors for TB

At the present time, the Interferon Gamma Release Assay (**IGRA**) method may be used in all circumstances in which the TST is currently used. According to the most recent published US Centers for Disease Control and Prevention (CDC) TB infection control guidelines, the sensitivity of the IGRA method for LTBI might be less than the TST, and IGRAs should be used with caution in immunocompromised patients as it has not been used extensively in this group. In direct comparisons, the sensitivity of the IGRAs is similar to that of the TST in infected persons with culture positive TB. The IGRAs are expected to be more specific than the TST as they will not react to BCG vaccine or to many commonly encountered nontuberculous mycobacteria. Currently, the CDC supports the use of IGRAs as an acceptable alternative to TSTs, but does not advocate using it as a confirmatory test for persons with a positive TST. It should be noted that some other countries are utilizing the IGRAs as confirmatory tests for positive TST results.

Chapter 17

Case study 17.1

1 This man's immunity to local strains of malaria is likely to have waned if he has lived in the USA for several years. The combination of artemether and lumefantrine should be highly effective against *P. falciparum* from Nigeria; however the tablets he bought in the street may have been counterfeit, and contained no active drugs. Urgent blood films for malaria parasites are needed. If they reveal *P. falciparum* infection, he needs urgent admission and prompt therapy. Oral doxycycline and intravenous quinidine with electrocardiographic monitoring are the agents of choice.

Case study 17.2

1 This patient requires urgent expert examination of a blood film for malaria parasites, or an urgent rapid diagnostic test for malaria. The most common species of malaria in Afghanistan is *P. vivax* although *P. falciparum* causes a small proportion of infections so this patient is at risk of severe *P. falciparum* disease. If a blood film reveals *P. vivax* parasites, Malarone tablets would have killed the circulating *P. vivax* parasites but the hepatic hypnozoites would not have been eradicated by this treatment. Reactivation of these hypnozoites has caused a relapse of her symptoms. She should be treated with oral chloroquine followed by oral primaquine (after pregnancy is excluded). If she were planning further travel to Afghanistan, prophylaxis with atovaquone/proguanil, doxycycline, or mefloquine would be appropriate, as chloroquine resistance in *P. falciparum* has been reported in Afghanistan.

Case study 17.3

1 Chloroquine would be inappropriate in view of local resistance patterns. The resistance of local malaria strains to Fansidar may be masked by the local population's partial immunity to local *P. falciparum* strains. The refugee population may experience higher rates of clinical disease and failure of Fansidar treatment than the local population. The use of an artemisinin combination therapy for empirical treatment in the refugee camp is likely to be more effective, though more costly than Fansidar.

Chapter 18

Case study 18.1

1 In a man of this age, it is still possible that this may be a late presentation of epilepsy and a detailed account of the events leading up to the seizure should be obtained from any witnesses, as routine. It could also be a drug reaction or some other type of allergy or a "space-occupying lesion" (i.e. a tumor – benign or malignant). Even some types of video games and movies with stroboscopic, high-frequency flashing light effects may trigger a seizure in susceptible individuals. However, in the current context, an infectious cause is more likely, such as tuberculosis, toxoplasmosis, or some sort of viral encephalitis (see Chapter 10).

2 As always, additional history from a close relative is often the key to making the diagnosis, especially when the patient is incapacitated as in this scenario. The history given seems to suggest an infectious cause with the coughing and shortness of breath over the past 2 weeks, but the longer 6-month history suggests something more sinister is going on. This could be compatible with tuberculosis or an underlying malignancy (cancer). Both cause long-term weight loss, and most types of cancer may predispose to frequent infections as the immune system becomes suppressed due to the spreading malignancy. The information about the patient's family life also seems reassuring, as does the relative absence of any foreign travel or exposure to bites from possible vectors that may transmit one of the local viral encephalitides, i.e. mosquitoes carrying West Nile virus (see Chapter 24).

3 Low lymphocyte counts and PCP immediately suggest an immunocompromised state (see Chapter 13). Given the 6-month history of weight loss and the recent chest infection, a possible diagnosis should now be emerging. HIV testing is indicated.

4 In many countries (if not all), doctors are allowed to act in the patient's best interest, even though explicit consent is not always given. Given the pattern of illness described above, the ICU team is working within this realm of "patient's best interest" to test for HIV, which can present in this way (weight loss, chest infection, seizure, respiratory failure). Note that the diagnosis of HIV may be unexpected given his apparently stable family life – however, histories can be sometimes deceiving.

5 In many countries, for HIV testing, the explicit (often written and signed) consent of the patient is required. This is because, occasionally, relatives or other third parties (who may consent for other procedures if the patient is incapacitated, like surgery), may exploit HIV testing for their own ends. However, in this situation, the ICU team has taken this initiative without the patient's explicit consent. If they tell the wife of the HIV diagnosis before the patient has recovered, when the patient awakens, he may consider it inappropriate that the ICU team tested him then revealed his HIV status to his wife without his formal consent, and take legal action against the hospital. This is an issue of preserving an individual patient's confidentiality, which should be a priority in all patient–doctor relationships. However, if they do not tell the wife of his HIV diagnosis, she may be infected and not only require diagnosis and treatment for her own health, but she may also transmit the virus to others, if she has other partners. So, this is also an issue of public health (see further discussion that follows).

Chapter 19

Case study 19.1

1 This is a difficult case. The woman seems to have multiple causes for her condition, but the cause of the jaundice (yellow skin and eyes) could be either alcohol or viral or both. She smells strongly of alcohol, and she has obvious needle track marks on her arms and in her groin – strong risk factors for transmission of blood-borne viruses (particularly HBV and HCV). Indications of sexual trauma make us concerned about HIV, and her general condition suggests a life on the street, making this concern even higher. The fact that she is pregnant further complicates things, as now we need to consider the effects of the alcohol and the drugs, as well as the possible viral infections, on the fetus.

2 The mother has evidence of alcohol and drug abuse, as well as a rough life on the streets as a prostitute (commercial sex worker). Thus, the baby is at risk of harm from both chemical (alcohol and heroine) as well as viral (HIV, HBV, and HCV) causes. The baby is already showing signs of a losing battle in the womb and is delivered by cesarean and requires detoxification for the alcohol and heroine. Furthermore, the baby requires treatment for HBV and HIV exposure, by giving HBV accelerated immunization

(0, 1, 2 and 12 months after birth) and HBIG (200 international units by intramuscular injection within 12 hours of birth), and HIV PEP, respectively. In resource rich countries like the USA, HIV PEP in such situations can involve single agent (AZT) or triple agent (containing drugs from at least two classes) ART, i.e. highly active ART (HAART), depending on the severity of the mother's HIV/AIDS condition. With a CD4 count of 50 and an HIV load of 100 000 copies/ml, she and her baby would meet the criteria for HAART treatment that will continue postnatally, until the baby's HIV infection status is established. Delivery by cesarean section and avoidance of breast feeding are both standard precautions in HIV-infected women to reduce the risk of HIV transmission to their babies.

3 The accepted risk of acquiring HIV, HCV, or HBV from a needlestick injury from a hollow needle is approximately 0.3%, 3%, and 30%, respectively. This doctor was already immune to HBV (though there is always the possibility of the patient carrying a mutant HBsAg virus), and had taken PEP for HIV. There is literature suggesting that the wiping effect of wearing gloves may remove 50–80% of surface blood from a penetrating sharps injury as it passes through the gloves, but scalpel injuries are generally more serious as the wounds are often larger and deeper. The HCV load is relatively high in this patient, and although the HIV PEP probably prevented her from contracting HIV (as high as 90% effectiveness), there was no recommended PEP for HCV. The literature does suggest, however, that intense treatment with high-dose interferon alone may clear the infection after 24 weeks, if started in the acute phase of infection (within the first 3–6 months after infection). The main problem then becomes one of compliance – i.e. will the doctor finish the treatment in spite of the side-effects? Luckily, in this scenario, the doctor finished the therapy and cleared the HCV infection without long-term complications.

Chapter 20

Case study 20.1

1 Professor Ken Shortridge, an avian influenza specialist, postulated in the early 1980s that southern China could be an origin for new influenza viruses. This is mainly because of its unique traditional combined pig, duck (and chicken) farming that has existed there for hundreds if not thousands of years. These domesticated animals live in close proximity to their human farmers – sometimes even sleeping in the same room as them. This would allow both human and animal influenza viruses to co-infect and possibly exchange gene segments among these different human and animal hosts. Specifically, the pig has receptors for both the human, duck and chicken (i.e. avian) influenza viruses. This could result in the generation of a new, unique human pandemic influenza A virus, to which no one has been previously exposed, making all individuals susceptible to infection with this new virus. This is one possible origin of a new influenza pandemic (see Further reading).

2 This is a difficult question and may not have a definitive right and wrong answer. It is natural to bring your family to hospital once they start to fall sick. In this way, he may also act as a sentinel case, alerting the health authorities to the presence of a new pathogen. However, this action may also have the potential to spread the illness to others who are also unwell with other diseases. During the SARS outbreaks in Southeast Asia in 2003, people became more and more afraid of going to hospital as many of the outbreaks started there (see Chapter 24).

3 At the beginning of an outbreak with a new infectious agent, there is a lack of awareness and knowledge about the disease and how it behaves, so it is difficult to instruct the general public on how to behave until the disease and its agent are characterized further. This, unfortunately, almost inevitably means that more cases need to present themselves and be studied – as was seen with the severe acute respiratory syndrome (SARS) outbreaks of 2003. In the context of another disaster (a typhoon in this case – referred to as hurricanes in the USA), such impending outbreaks, especially from a new infectious agent, may be virtually impossible to identify or distinguish from other diseases, injuries, fatigue and exhaustion related to such disaster scenarios. Eventually, in cases such as Mr Li's, once the new agent and disease has been characterized, he may be able to call specific healthcare hotlines who may advise him to stay at home (home-quarantine) and not come to hospital (to limit cross-infection), and await a special unit to visit him at home to deal with his disease cluster. Of course, in the typhoon scenario given here, all communications lines may be down, leaving him no choice but to travel to the nearest hospital to seek healthcare for his sick family and himself.

4 Seasonal "coughs and colds" can be a great confounder when trying to identify serious emerging infections. Patients presenting with characteristic skin rashes, such as smallpox, chickenpox, and measles, are much easier to identify and isolate or quarantine as required. However, "influenza-like illness" can be caused by: influenza A or B, parainfluenza types 1–4, respiratory syncytial virus (RSV), adenovirus, rhinoviruses, enteroviruses, as well as various species of bacteria (see Chapter 9). For infectious respiratory disease surveillance in the general population, individuals presenting to family doctors (rather than those that are seen in or admitted to hospitals), for relatively mild respiratory symptoms (e.g. coughing, sneezing, sore throat, runny nose, headache, etc.), who do not often perform laboratory testing to diagnose the infectious agent (due to a lack of time or funding or both), influenza-like illnesses caused by newly emerging and potentially severe pathogens cannot be easily distinguished from the usual seasonal infections that are normally mild and self-limiting.

5 Given the answers to questions 3 and 4 above, this is probably an unfair question, but it is a question that the World Health Organization and national government public health institutions are struggling with presently, regarding the potential (some still say inevitable) emergence of a new pandemic influenza virus strain. One tool that has been used extensively, recently, in an attempt to predict the possible behavior of any future pandemic virus, is the mathematical model. These models involve characterizing an infectious agent using mathematical symbols (e.g. incubation period, infectiousness – how many cases can be produced from a single case, mortality rate, recovery period, period of infectivity, etc.), then inserting values for such parameters into a mathematical expression governing how these terms interact. From this, the predicted number of infected, dead, recovered and immune individuals can be determined for any given set of parameters. They can also take into account any public health interventions proposed, such as vaccination, various levels of immunity and responses to treatment, social-distancing, isolation and quarantine, etc. The problem is that the initial assumptions may be incorrect, resulting in inaccurate advice being given to public health officials in planning for the next pandemic. The behavior of the next pandemic virus may bear little resemblance to the previous pandemic viruses on which these model parameters were based, which may be likely since, by definition, the new virus must be sufficiently different from previous viruses in order to produce a pandemic. Unfortunately, like the stock market, past behavior may not govern the future behavior of pandemic viruses, but this may be the only guidance that we have for public health planning at present.

Chapter 21

Case study 21.1

1 *V. cholerae* and entero-toxigenic *E. coli*.

2 *V. cholerae*: **Cholera toxin activates the adenylate cyclase enzyme** in cells of the intestinal mucosa leading to increased levels of intracellular cAMP, and the secretion of H_2O, Na^+, K^+, Cl^-, and HCO_3^- into the lumen of the small intestine. The toxin has been characterized and contains **five binding (B) subunits** of 11 500 daltons, an active **(A1) subunit** of 23 500 daltons, and a **bridging piece (A2)** of 5500 daltons that links A1 to the 5B subunits. The B subunits bind to specific receptor, a glycolipid called GM1 ganglioside, ubiquitous in eukaryotic cells and present on the surface of intestinal mucosal cells. Once binding has occurred the A1 subunit enters the cell, where it enzymatically transfers ADP-ribose from nicotinamide adenine dinucleotide (NAD) to a target protein, the guanosine 5′-triphosphate (GTP)-binding regulatory protein associated with membrane-bound adenylate cyclase. Since GTP hydrolysis is the event that inactivates the adenylate cyclase, the enzyme remains continually activated.

Thus, the ADP-riboxylation reaction essentially locks adenylate cyclase in its "on mode" and leads to excessive production of cyclic adenosine monophosphate (cAMP) which stimulates mucosal cells to pump large amounts of Cl^- into the intestinal contents. H_2O, Na^+, and other electrolytes follow due to the osmotic and electrical gradients caused by the loss of Cl^-. The lost H_2O and electrolytes in mucosal cells are replaced from the blood. The toxin-damaged cells become pumps for water and electrolytes causing the diarrhea, loss of electrolytes, and dehydration characteristic of cholera.

E. coli: Enterotoxins produced by ETEC include the LT (heat-labile) toxin and/or the ST (heat-stable) toxin, the genes for which may occur on the same or separate plasmids. The **LT enterotoxin** is very similar to cholera toxin both structurally and immunologically, and like cholera toxin exerts its action by activating cyclic AMP Like the cholera toxin, it is an 86-kDa protein composed of an enzymatically active (A) subunit surrounded by five identical binding (B) subunits. It binds to the same enterocyte receptors that are recognized by the cholera toxin (i.e. GM1 ganglioside), resulting in the same outpouring of electrolytes and water into the lumen of the intestine that constitutes the characteristic watery diarrhea.

The **ST enterotoxin** is a composite of many small molecular weight heat stable peptides of about 2000 daltons. Two major functional components have been described: STa and STb. STa stimulates intestinal guanylate cyclase, the enzyme that converts guanosine 5′-triphosphate (GTP) to cyclic guanosine 5′-monophosphate (cGMP). Increased intracellular cGMP inhibits intestinal fluid uptake, resulting in net fluid secretion. The role of STb in causing diarrhea has not been fully understood.

3 Fecal contamination of water. The Ganges belt is endemic for cholera and ETEC is the commonest cause of traveller's diarrhea in endemic areas.

Case study 21.2

1 Hepatitis A, hepatitis E, leptospirosis, dengue, malaria.
2 Leptospirosis due to waters being contaminated with rat urine; highly prevalent in caves and rivers. The risk is much higher if there has been recent flooding when surface contaminants from rat holes run into water reservoirs.

Case study 21.3

1 *Salmonella* Paratyphi.
2 Taken care to eat and drink with caution: avoided uncooked foods and salads, drunk only bottled water, not accepted ice in drinks.
3 No. *S.* Typhi vaccine does not protect against *S.* Paratyphi.

Case study 21.4

1 Malaria.
2 *P. falciparum*: only ring forms seen, more than one ring per erythrocyte, erythrocytes that are infected are the same size as uninfected ones.
3 Appropriate chemoprophylaxis (Chapter 17). Wearing insect repellent at all times, particularly in the evenings. Sleeping under an insecticide treated bed-net.

Chapter 22

Case study 22.1

1 You should ask questions related to possible exposure to various infectious disease agents, including VHFs, as you know that Sierra Leone is endemic for Lassa fever. Malaria is also endemic in this area and can present in a similar way. Hence, information on the patient's occupation and travel history, mosquito bites, living conditions, any contact with animals or people ill and dead from unknown causes, should be obtained. Also, the timing of the onset of illness should be checked. If the patient remained well for at least 3 weeks after returning home, then it is more likely that the illness was acquired in the USA, rather than from abroad, as the incubation period would be too long then.

2 For the patient, intravenous ribavirin should be given, as there is some evidence that this is effective treatment when given within 6 days of onset of illness. He should be isolated, but closely monitored by appropriately trained healthcare staff. For infection control, a list of the patient's contacts needs to be obtained and these people (including family and friends) need to be contacted to monitor their temperature on a daily basis for at least 21 days (3 weeks) and to report to a member of the infection control team if it rises significantly (e.g. >37.5°C). In addition, all clinical samples obtained from this patient should be traced from the various diagnostic laboratories and archived together in a high-level, secure (BSL-4 if possible) containment laboratory for either further testing or destruction. Finally, all other possibly infected waste/fomites need to be traced and collected for destruction to prevent other members of the public from becoming infected with Lassa fever. This may include items of clothing, cutlery, tissues, food containers in garbage, etc.

Chapter 23

Case study 23.1

1 This man appears to have developed "flu-like" symptoms about 10 days before admission, for which he tried traditional Chinese remedies, all to no avail. Later on, his condition deteriorated and he was forced to come to the hospital ER. Interestingly, the initial "flu-like" symptoms have not progressed to a serious chest infection, but to an acute hepatitis. Abdominal distension ("ascites") with dark-colored urine and pale smelly stools usually implies liver disease. It would be worthwhile checking his drinking habits and any other potential exposure to water- or blood-borne hepatitis viruses.

2 To really understand the environment of a wet market in Hong Kong, it is useful to view some images, such as those at: http://en.wikipedia.org/wiki/Wet_market or under a Google Images (available at: http://images.google.com/imghp?hl=en&tab=wi) search using the terms "wet markets Hong Kong" or similar. It is immediately obvious why there might be many rats running around the floor in such wet markets, as a lot of food (raw, cooked, or half-eaten) is dropped or discarded on the floors. Ask if he has been sweeping or cleaning the floor around his stall recently, or if there has been any other event that may have aerosolized floor debris and dust. Such dust may be potentially contaminated with rat urine infected with a hantavirus (shed in the urine of an infected rat). Hantavirus may cause an acute hepatitis though this not usually the main presenting feature of the infection.

3 This is a difficult question. Since the incubation period for hantaviruses is long and variable (1–5 weeks), Mr Wong could have contracted his hantavirus infection from elsewhere and not from the wet market area at all. Alternatively, if he did contract the hantavirus infection from the wet market vicinity, why were there not more cases appearing throughout the year? Perhaps Mr Wong was just unlucky or unusually susceptible to this particular infection? Maybe the rat index case carrying the hantavirus was only passing through and the majority of rats living in and around the wet market are not infected with hantavirus? To fully investigate this case, the wet market would need to be closed down, and samples of floor debris and dust would need to be collected for further analysis to test whether hantavirus was indeed present and how widespread the problem was. Even if it was found all over the wet market area, it still begs the question why more cases were not being diagnosed and reported. Closing down the wet market will be expensive to the vendors and inconvenient to the customers. If hantavirus is found, there is a duty to report these findings for public health reasons, but it seems that its presence may not be harming the vast majority of the people. The investigation will also be lengthy and costly to the public purse, so such decisions need to be carefully considered.

Chapter 24

Case study 24.1

1 Typical incubation period 4–7 days. Yes, dengue fever is a possibility, as the patient could have been infected just prior to leaving Thailand and incubated his dengue fever infection during his journey home.

2 A dengue virus reverse-transcriptase polymerase chain reaction (RT-PCR) on a serum sample, which can also determine the dengue serotype. It is probably too early to detect a dengue IgM response, as the patient has presented within 5 days of onset of illness. Some serum could also be put into culture for dengue virus if the laboratory has the appropriate facilities. This would confirm any positive RT-PCR result, but it will take 10–14 days to grow. An aliquot of this acute serum can also be kept and tested together with a convalescent serum taken from the patient 10–14 days later for both dengue-specific IgM and IgG. The first acute sample is likely to be negative for both IgM and IgG and the convalescent sample positive for both antibodies, if the patient has dengue fever. This would demonstrate a seroconversion, also confirming a positive RT-PCR result. The convalescent serum can also be used for serotyping the dengue virus, thereby confirming the RT-PCR dengue serotype result, if necessary.

3 Probably just symptomatic treatment, observation and monitoring with further hematological/biochemical blood tests. At present there are no overt signs of vascular leakage or clotting derangement to warrant any more invasive interventions.

4 The patient now has an initial diagnosis of dengue fever and may be proceeding towards DHF/DSS. However, this is by no means certain, though fluid supplements should be given to maintain his BP. Although his platelet count is low, this is not dangerously low and there is no overt bleeding, so a platelet infusion is not required at this point. Further close observation and monitoring is warranted.

Chapter 25

Case study 25.1

1 The A subunit of diphtheria toxin possesses ADP-ribosyltransferase activity. The substrate of the reaction is human elongation factor 2 (EF2), an essential part of the protein biosynthetic machinery.

ADP-ribosyl transferases are enzymes that promote the breakdown of nicotinamide adenine dinucleotide (NAD) into nicotinamide and adenine diphosphate ribose (ADPR). The covalent binding of the ADPR to various proteins inactivates the bound protein:

$$\text{EF2} + \text{NAD} \xrightarrow{\quad\text{diphtheria toxin}\quad} \text{ADPR-EF2} + \text{nicotinamide} + \text{H}^+$$

The end result of this reaction is inhibition of protein synthesis and cell death.

2 Botulinum toxin is a potent neurotoxin that acts on motor neurons by preventing the release of acetylcholine at neuromuscular junctions, preventing muscle excitation and resulting in flaccid paralysis. Recovery occurs through proximal axonal sprouting and muscle re-innervation by formation of a new neuromuscular junction. De Paiva and colleagues, 1999, suggest that eventually the original neuromuscular junction regenerates.

Tetanus toxin acts in a different manner; it is taken up at neuromuscular junctions, transported along axons to synapses; here it acts by inactivating neurons that play a part in inhibiting muscle contraction, resulting in prolonged contraction and a rigid paralysis. Once the toxin becomes fixed to neurons, it cannot be neutralized with antitoxin. Recovery of nerve function from tetanus toxins requires sprouting of new nerve terminals and formation of new synapses.

Pseudomonas: The toxin has two functional subunits: the B unit binds to target cells, while the A unit has the toxic activity. It inhibits protein synthesis in many cell types by inhibiting elongation factor 2 (EF 2) in ribosomes, inhibiting peptide chain elongation, and eventually causing cessation of protein synthesis. Inhibition of protein synthesis in a cell eventually leads to cell death (necrosis). Effects are irreversible on the cells affected.

Shigella dysenteriae, the shiga toxin, inhibits protein biosynthesis at the ribosome leading to cell death. Effects are irreversible on the cells affected.

Chapter 26

Case study 26.1

1 You might consider any of the rash illnesses: measles, rubella, parvovirus, chickenpox (prevesicular), glandular fever (Epstein–Barr virus, EBV) if the patient has taken ampicillin or amoxicillin, HIV seroconversion illness. You should ask him about any recent travel history, especially in the last 2–3 weeks, recent and past sexual activity – as HIV has a very variable incubation period. Also, ask if he has had any insect or other animal bites in the last few weeks. It would be useful to know his occupation.

2 As well as the routine blood test, you could consider tests for the rash illnesses, IgM antibodies for measles, rubella, parvovirus, EBV, chickenpox, and total antibodies for HIV. You could also request tests for mosquito-borne diseases such as West Nile fever, as well as the tick-borne rickettsial diseases like Rocky Mountain Spotted Fever.

Index

Page numbers in *italics* refer to figures; page numbers in **bold** refer to tables or boxes.

abacavir 152
abscesses
  brain 282–3, 377
  breast 184, 336
  skin 182–4
Acanthamoeba infections 276, 277
aciclovir 151
  adult chickenpox 341
  immunocompromised host 374
  neonates 346
  in pregnancy 344, 346, 358
acid-fast bacteria 21–3, 89, **90**
acid-fast staining 21, *22*, **90**, 452
Acinetobacter infections 405
acquired immunodeficiency syndrome *see* AIDS
Act A 340
actinomycetomas 203, **204**
actinomycosis **204**
acute phase proteins 51
acute respiratory distress syndrome (ARDS) 75
adaptive immunity 53–9, 363
  defects **365**, 366–7
adefovir 153
adenovirus(es) 230
  derived vaccines 66
  diagnostic testing **235**, **376**
  enteric **223**, 224, 230
  immune avoidance mechanisms 80
  myocarditis 244, 245
  pericarditis 247
  pneumonia 263
  upper respiratory tract infections 252, 254
  vaccine **64**
  virology *9*, 230, *231*
adjuvants 65
ADP-ribosyl transferases *72*, 194, 529–30, **605**
Aedes (including *A. aegypti*) mosquitoes *556*, *589*
  chikungunya virus 579
  control measures *563*
  dengue fever 588–9
  yellow fever 542, 555
aflatoxins 68
African meningitis belt 547, *548*
African tickbite fever **536**
African trypanosomiasis 35, 535
agar 92–3, *94*, *95*
age, disease susceptibility and 43
agglutination tests
  direct 102
  indirect or passive 102
AIDS 480, 481

opportunist infections **368**, 373, 481, *482*
  see also human immunodeficiency virus (HIV)
airborne transmission 162
  travel related 523, 547
  see also droplet transmission
alanine amino transferase (ALT) 493–4, 501, 502–3
albendazole **149**
Albert's stain *194*, 602, *603*
alcohol abuse **368**
alcohol hand rubs 407, *408*
aldolase tests, *Plasmodium* 470
alemtuzumab 372
Alibek, Ken 608, 619
allyamine antifungals 146
α_1 antitrypsin 51
α hemolysis 93, *94*
alpha toxin 193
amantadine 28, 154, 511–12, 513
amastigotes 35, *37*, 532–3
amebae 33
amebiasis 233–4
amebic meningitis, primary 276–7
amebicides 148
American trypanosomiasis 35, 534–5
amikacin 139, 140, 141, **145**
aminoglycosides 139–41, **145**
  mechanism of action *136*, 138
  resistance 139, **140**, 141
amniocentesis 343, 349
amoxicillin 130, **131**, **144**
amoxicillin-clavulanic acid (co-amoxiclav) 130, **144**
amphotericin B 146, 149
ampicillin 130, 131, **144**
ampicillin-sulbactam 130
amprenavir 153
Amsel's diagnostic criteria, bacterial vaginosis 301
anaerobes
  biochemical detection 101
  culture 94, 96
  normal flora 47
  postpartum infections 336
anaplasmosis **537**
Ancylostoma braziliense 206
Ancylostoma caninum 206
Ancylostoma duodenalis **13**, **149**
Andes hantavirus **573**, 576
anemia
  malaria 464, **465**
  parvovirus B19-induced 347
aneruptive fever **536**
Anopheles mosquitoes 458, 461, 463–4

anthrax 610–13
  as biological weapon 607, 608, **609**, 610–11
  clinical features 611, *612*
  cutaneous 189, 611
  laboratory diagnosis 611–13
  treatment 613
  vaccine **64**, 613
  see also Bacillus anthracis
antibacterial agents 126–44, **144–5**
  see also antibiotics
antibiotic associated diarrhea (AAD) 47, 402
antibiotics 124–44, **144–5**
  bactericidal 127
  bacteriostatic 127
  broad-spectrum 372
  choice of agent **125**, 126
  effects on normal flora 44, 47
  empirical treatment 379
  mechanisms of action 17, 19, 20, *126*, *136*
  minimum inhibitory concentrations (MIC) 114, 115
  pregnancy and childbirth 336
  resistance *see* antimicrobial resistance
  susceptibility tests 113–15
  urinary tract infections 324
  see also antifungal agents
antibodies 55
  detection using ELISA 102, **104**, *104*
  maternal transfer 61–2
  to normal flora 46
antibody-dependent cellular cytotoxicity (ADCC) 57
anti-folate agents 471
antifungal agents 145–7
  empirical treatment 379
  mechanisms of action 146–7
  spectrum of activity **146**
antigen
  detection using ELISA 102, *103*, **104**
  presentation 54
  processing 54
antigen–antibody reactions, diagnostic use 101–8
antigenic drift 82, 507–9
antigenic shift 82, 507–8, 509
antigenic variation 84
antigen presenting cells (APCs) 53–4, *56*
antihelminth medications 149–50
anti-idiotype vaccines 66
anti-influenza virus compounds 154–5, 511–13
antimalarial agents 470–1
antimicrobial chemotherapy 124–56
  healthcare associated infections and 394
  see also antibiotics; antifungal agents; antiviral drugs
antimicrobial resistance
  genetic exchange mechanisms 76–8
  laboratory diagnosis 113–15
  mechanisms 127–8
antimicrobial susceptibility tests 113–16
  automated 115
  bacterial (and some fungal) 113–15
  manual disc methods 114
  viral 115–16

antimony compounds 149
antiprotozoal drugs 147–9
anti-retroviral drugs 152–4, 484
  mechanisms of action 27, 28, 29
  postexposure prophylaxis **486**
  in pregnancy 357
  see also highly active antiretroviral therapy
antistreptolysin O antibodies 190
antitoxins 62, 68–9, 599
anti-tuberculosis drugs 438
  resistance 439–41
antiviral drugs 150–6
  mechanisms of action 28, 29, **150**
  susceptibility and resistance testing 115–16
API rapid identification system 97, *98*
aplastic crisis **428**
aprons, protective 409
arabinogalactan *22*
Araraquara virus **573**
arboviruses 10, *585*, 588
  encephalitis 279, 287–8
  see also specific viruses
arenaviruses 553, 554
artemisinin combination therapy (ACT) 471
artemisinins 471
arthralgia, rubella associated 423
arthritis
  parvovirus B19 associated **428**, 429
  septic 187–8
  sexually acquired reactive (SARA) 298
Ascaris lumbricoides **13**, 84, **149**
aspergillosis, invasive 406
Aspergillus 12
  antifungal drug activity **146**
  diagnostic testing **375**
  healthcare associated infections 406
  immunocompromised host 373
Aspergillus flavus 406
Aspergillus fumigatus 406
assembly, viruses 29
Astrakhan spotted fever **537**
astroviruses 231
  diagnostic testing **235**
  gastroenteritis **223**, 224
atazanavir 153
athlete's foot **203**, *205*
atovaquone 471
attack rate 171
  secondary (SAR) 163–4
Aum Shinrikyo religious cult 608
auramine-rhodamine staining **90**, 452
Australian spotted fever **536**
autoimmunity 80
autolysins, endogenous 128–9
automation, laboratory 113, 115
avian influenza 506–7, 509, 516–17
axial filaments 23
azidothymidine (AZT) 152
azithromycin 135, 136
azlocillin 130

azole antifungals 146
aztreonam 134, **144**

Bacille Calmette–Guérin (BCG) 453
bacilli 5, 7
Bacillus 16
Bacillus anthracis
    as biological weapon **609**, 610–13
    escape mechanisms 67
    host defences 42
    see also anthrax
Bacillus cereus 226–7
    food poisoning **215**, 216–17
    identification **235**
    pathogenesis of disease 227
Bacillus subtilis, release on subway 607, **608**
bacteremia, infective endocarditis 241
bacteria 4–8
    antimicrobial susceptibility tests 113–15
    attachment 66–7
    capsule 24, 286
    cell membrane 17
    cell wall 18–23
    cell wall-less forms 21
    culture 92–6
    detection of products 101
    diagnostic identification 97–8, **375**
    drug resistance 76–8
    fimbriae 23–4
    flagella 23
    genetic basis of virulence 76–8
    growth phases 8
    intracellular 24–5, 67
    normal flora 44–8
    nuclear equivalent 15–16
    sizes, shapes and arrangement 4–5, *6–8*
    slime production 24
    structure and function 15–24
    virulence mechanisms 66–78, 284–6
    vs. eukaryotic cells **4**
bacterial infections
    congenital 338–41
    diarrheas 214–21, 224–8, 235
    healthcare associated 402–5
    immunocompromised host 364, **365**, 373
    lower respiratory tract 254, 259–64
    meningitis 274–6, 277, **278**, 283–6
    neonatal/perinatal 352–5
    pericarditis 246, 247
    secondary to common cold 251, 252
    skin, soft tissues, bone and joint 180–94
    traveler's diarrhea 526–30
    upper respiratory tract 248–9
    urinary tract 319–24
    see also specific infections
bacterial vaginosis (BV) 48, 300–1
bactericidal agents 127
bactericidal factors, soluble 48, 51–2
bacteriophages 76
    diphtheria toxin production 603–4

bacteriostatic agents 127
Bactrim *see* co-trimoxazole
Balantidium coli 33, 39
    diagnosis **235**
    gastroenteritis 233
Baltimore classification of viruses 28
band forms 467, *469*
barriers to infection, physical 43–4
    defects 364, **365**, 394
Bartonella **537**
basic reproductive rate (R_o) 164–5
bats **279**, 554, 577, **594**
Bayou (BAY) virus **573**, 576
B cells 53, 367
BCG (Bacille Calmette–Guérin) 453
Behring, Emil von 599
β hemolysis 93, *94*
β-lactam antibiotics 128–34
    chemical structure *128*
    mechanisms of action 19, 20
    mechanisms of resistance 127–8
    see also penicillin(s)
β-lactamase inhibitors 130
β-lactamases 127–8, **127**
    extended spectrum (ESBLs) 128, 405
    resistant penicillins 130
    susceptible broad spectrum penicillins 130
bifidobacteria 47
bilharziasis *see* schistosomiasis
biochemical identification methods, bacteria 97–8
biofilms 24, 192, 243, 403
Biological and Toxin Weapons Convention (BTWC) 608
biological warfare agents 607–26
    definitions and categories 609–10
    history 607–8
biopsy samples 87–8, 117
Biosafety Level 3 (BSL-3) organisms 266, 545
Biosafety Level 4 (BSL-4) organisms 200, 553, 555, *557*
biosafety levels, biological warfare agents **609**
bioterrorism, agents of 607–26
bird flu *see* avian influenza
birds 287, 584, *585*
Black Creek Canal (BCC) virus **573**, *574*, 576
Black Death 157, 614
black disease 533
blackflies **522**
blackwater fever 464, **465**
Blastomyces dermatidis 204
blastomycosis 204
bleeding problems *see* hemorrhagic problems
blood agar 92–3, *94*
blood and blood product transfusions
    hepatitis C transmission 498, **499**
    HIV transmission 476–7
bloodborne diseases, travel related 523
bloodborne viruses (BBVs) 11
    healthcare settings **486**, **496**
    neonatal/perinatal infections 356–7
    see also hepatitis B virus; hepatitis C virus; human
        immunodeficiency virus

blood–brain barrier (BBB) 271–2, *273*
blood cultures 87, 113
   infective endocarditis 243
blood samples 88, 117
blood smears 117, *118*
   malaria diagnosis 467–9
bloodstream infections, healthcare associated 400
boils (furuncles) 182–4
bone infections 186–8
   hospital acquired 188
   tuberculosis 446
bone marrow transplantation *see* hematopoietic stem cell
     transplantation
Bordetella parapertussis 249
Bordetella pertussis 249, **250**, 254, 261
   see also pertussis
Bornholm disease 246
Borrelia burgdorferi **280**, 281
botfly, human 206
BOTOX® **70**
botulinum toxin 69–70, 613–14
   as biological weapon **609**, 613
botulism
   antitoxins 62, 614
   as biological weapon 613–14
   foodborne **221**, 613
   infant 613
   wound **70**, 613
Boutonneuse fever **537**
bovine spongiform encephalopathy (BSE) **9**
bradyzoites 352
brain 271
   abscess 282–3, 377
branched DNA hybridization assay (bDNA) 111
Brazilian spotted fever **537**
breakbone fever 589
breast abscesses 184, 336
breast milk
   antibodies 61–2
   transmission of viruses 356, 357
bronchiectasis 254
bronchiolitis, viral 254
bronchitis 254
bronchopneumonia 256, *257*
Brucella abortus 545, 547
Brucella melitensis 545, 547
brucellosis 545–7, **609**
BSE (bovine spongiform encephalopathy) **9**
bubo 309
bunyaviruses 553, 572
Burkholderia cepacia 254, 264
Burkholderia pseudomallei 264
bystander damage 80

Calabar swellings 206
Calabazo virus **573**
calcofluor white stain **91**
caliciviruses, human 228–9
   gastroenteritis **215**, 222, **223**

pathogenesis and virulence 229
   transmission 10
Calymmatobacterium granulomatis 309, 319
Campylobacter
   appearance 5, 7
   gastroenteritis **215**, 216, 226
   identification **235**
Campylobacter jejuni 216, 225–6
cancer chemotherapy 364, *366*, 370–1
Candida 299
   diagnostic testing **375**
   immunocompromised host 373, 378
   neonatal infections 355
Candida albicans 11, 12, 315–16
   antifungal drug activity **146**
   reproduction 32
   urine cultures 323
   vaginal infections 300
candidiasis
   disseminated, HIV infection/AIDS 481, *482*
   vulvovaginal 300
Cano Delgadito virus **573**
capsid, viral 25–6
capsomeres 25
capsule, bacterial 24, 286
carbapenems 130–1, **144**
carbenicillin 130
carbolfuschin stain **90**, 452
carboxypeptidases 19, 20
carbuncles 182–4
cardiac murmurs **239**, 241
cardiovascular syphilis 306–7
cardiovascular system infections 239–48
case control studies 171–2
case definition 167
caspofungin 147
catalase **50**, 51
catalase peroxidase 448
cat flea rickettsiosis **536**, 540–1
cathepsin G **50**, 51
catheter-associated infections
   indwelling central venous access 370, 379
   urinary tract 322, 324, 399–400
cat-scratch disease **537**
CD4+ T cell counts, HIV infection 480–1
CD4+ T cells 54, 55
   HIV infection 478, 480
   see also helper T cells
CD8+ T cells 54, 55
   see also cytotoxic T lymphocytes
CDC *see* Centers for Disease Control and
     Prevention
cefepime 133
cefotaximases 405
cefotaxime 133
cefoxitin 133
ceftazidime 133
ceftriaxone **132**, 133
cefuroxime 133

cell(s)
  bacterial *vs.* eukaryotic 4
  transformation by viruses 79
  viral attachment 26–7
  viral penetration (entry) 27, *28*
cell-mediated immunity 53, 56–9
  dysfunction **365**, 366
  tuberculosis 449–50
cell membrane
  bacterial 17
  fungal 31, 146
  fusion of viruses with 27
cellulitis 181, *182*
  anaerobic 188
cell walls
  bacteria 18–23
  fungi 31–2, 147
Centers for Disease Control and Prevention (CDC)
  biological warfare agents 608, 609–10
  group B streptococcus guidance 353
central nervous system (CNS) 271–3
central nervous system (CNS) infections 271–93
  immunocompromised host 377–8
  neonatal/perinatal 359
Central Plata hantavirus **573**
central venous access catheters, indwelling 370, 379
cephalosporinases 128, 405
cephalosporins 132–3
  allergy 131
  chemical structure *128*
  first generation **132**, 133, **144**
  second generation **132**, 133, **144**
  third generation **132**, 133, **144**
  fourth generation **132**, 133, **144**
cercariae 534
cerebrospinal fluid (CSF) 87, 271, **278**
ceruloplasmin 51
cervical cancer 201, 202, 303
cervicitis 299
cesarean section 336, 357
cestodes **13**, 14
Chagas disease 35, 534–5
chancre, syphilitic 301, 304, *305*, 317
chancroid 309, 318–19
chemokines 58
chemotherapy, cancer 364, *366*, 370–1
chest X-rays
  inhalational anthrax 611, *612*
  lower respiratory tract infections 256, *257*, 266
  tuberculosis *444*, *447*
chickenpox (varicella) **416**, 423–7
  childhood illness 415, 424–7
  close contact in pregnancy 344–6
  complications 423–4, 426
  congenital 344–6
  diagnosis 197–200, 426
  immunocompromised host 374, 424
  neonatal 346, 356, 424
  pneumonitis 263, 341, 344, 426

  in pregnancy 344
  primary infection in adults 341–2
  rash 196–7, 424–6
  transmissibility 194–5
  treatment 427
  vaccine 344, **426**
  virus *see* varicella zoster virus
Chiclero ulcer 205–6
chikungunya virus 523, 579
childbirth 335–6
childhood rash illnesses 414–34
  characteristic features 414–15, **416–17**
  contact with pregnant women **345**
  naming 415
  transmissibility 194–5
  see also specific diseases
children
  diarrheal disease 212–13, 235, 236
  genital herpes **199**
  malaria 459, 464, 466
  urinary tract infections **321**, 321–2
chitin 31
chlamydiae 24–5, 263
chlamydial infections
  asymptomatic 296
  clinical presentation 298–9
  public health impact 296–7
Chlamydia pneumoniae 25, 263
Chlamydia psittaci 263
Chlamydia trachomatis 312–14
  clinical manifestations 24–5, 298–9
  microbiology 312, *313*, 355
  ophthalmia neonatorum 354–5
  pneumonitis 355
  virulence mechanisms 313–14, 355
chloramphenicol *136*, 142, **145**
chloroquine 470, 472
Choclo virus **573**
cholera 528–30
  pandemics 528
  pathogenesis 529–30
  vaccine **64**
cholera toxin 71, *72*, 529–30
chromogens 93
chromosome, bacterial 15–16
chronic granulomatous disease (CGD) **368**, 369
chronic granulomatous reaction 67
chronic lymphocytic leukemia **368**, 369–70
chronic wasting disease (CWD) **9**
ciclosporin 372
cidofovir 151, 200, 571
cilastatin 130
cilia 33
ciliates **13**, 39
cinchona bark 470
ciprofloxacin 137, 138, **139**, **145**
cirrhosis of liver 491, 495
civet cat, Himalayan palm 594
clarithromycin 135, 136, **144**

clathrin-coated pits 27, *28*
clavulanic acid 130
clevudine 495
clindamycin 135, 136, **144**
    malaria 471
    toxoplasmosis 148
Clinical and Laboratory Standards Institute (CLSI) 114
Clonorchis sinensis **13**
Clostridium 16, 193–4
    gas gangrene/anaerobic cellulitis 188, 193
    microbiology 193
    toxins 69–70, 193–4
    virulence mechanisms 193–4
Clostridium botulinum 69, **221**, 614
    toxin *see* botulinum toxin
Clostridium difficile 45, 378, 405
    antibiotic associated colitis 47, 402
    virulence mechanisms 405
Clostridium perfringens 227–8
    enterotoxin 227–8
    food poisoning **215**, 218, **219**
    gas gangrene 193, 194
    identification **235**
    microbiology 227
Clostridium tetani 69
clothing, protective *see* personal protective equipment
clotrimazole 146
clue cells 301
CMV *see* cytomegalovirus
CNS *see* central nervous system
coagulase 72, 98
coagulase negative staphylococci 192, 243
    healthcare associated infections 400, 403
    see also Staphylococcus epidermidis
co-amoxiclav (amoxicillin-clavulanic acid) 130, **144**
cocci 5, *6*
Coccidioides immitis 11–12, 204, 264
    diagnostic identification 266
coccidioidomycosis 204, 264, **265**
cohort studies 171
cohorting of patients 408
cold sores 196, 197, *287*
    see also herpes simplex virus 1
collagenase 71
colonization 44–5
    mechanisms 66–7
    resistance 44, 45
common cold 248, 251–3
    agents causing 252
    economic burden **251**
community acquired pneumonia (CAP) 255–6, *257, 258*
    microbiology and pathogenesis 259–66
complement 52
    activation **52**
    opsonization by 52, *53*, 67
concomitant immunity 83
concurrent illness 373
condyloma lata 304, *306*
condylomata acuminata (genital warts) *201*, 303–4

congenital infections 337–52
    bacterial 338–41
    causes **338**
    definition **337**
    parasitic 349–52
    viral 341–9
congenital rubella syndrome (CRS) 342–3
congenital varicella syndrome (CVS) 344
conjugation 77–8
conjunctiva, normal flora 48
conjunctivitis
    measles 418
    neonatal 354–5
constitutional factors, innate immunity 42–3
contact transmission, healthcare settings 396
control measures, outbreak 172
co-primary cases 163–4
cordocentesis 343, 349
core polysaccharide 20, *21*
corneal scrapings 87
coronary care unit 400
coronaviruses 592, *593*
    non-SARS 251, 252, 592
    see also severe acute respiratory syndrome-associated
        coronavirus
corticosteroid therapy 366, 372
Corynebacterium diphtheriae 194, 249, 602–4
    identification 266
    inclusion bodies 16
    microbiology 194, 602–3
    Native American community **600**
    nontoxigenic strains 601
    virulence mechanisms 194, 603–4
    see also diphtheria; diphtheria toxin
Corynebacterium ulcerans **605**
co-trimoxazole (trimethoprim-sulfamethoxazole) 142,
    145
    immunocompromised host 378
    urinary tract infections 324
cotton rat *574*
cough reflex 259
cowpox viruses 569
Coxiella 535
Coxiella burnetii 263–4, 266, **537**
    as biological weapon **609**
    endocarditis 243
coxsackie B4 enterovirus *200*
coxsackieviruses
    hand-foot-and-mouth disease 432
    meningitis 286
    myocarditis 244
    pericarditis 246
"crabs" (pubic lice) **310**
C-reactive protein (CRP) **49**, 51–2
Crimean-Congo hemorrhagic fever (CCHF) 555, *560*, 563,
    564
Crimean-Congo hemorrhagic fever (CCHF) virus 553, 554
croup 253–4
cryoglobulinemia 500

Cryptococcus neoformans 12
    antifungal drug activity **146**
    diagnostic testing **375**
    escape mechanisms 67
cryptosporidiosis 233, **234**
Cryptosporidium parvum 12, 33, 233
    diagnostic testing 116, 118, **235**
    life cycle 38, *39*
Culex mosquitoes 578, 584, *585*
culture 92–100
    bacteria 92–6
    fungal 98–9
    mycobacterial 453
    protozoa and helminths 116
    routine and selective 93–4
    sites with normal resident flora 96
    sterile body sites 96
    tissue 100
    viral 100
culture media 92–3
    chromogenic 93, *95*
    liquid 93
    selective 93, 94
Cyclospora cayetanensis 39, 233, **235**
Cynomys rodents (prairie dogs) 568–9, *615*
cystic fibrosis 254, 264
cysts, protozoan 33–4, 39
    detection methods 116, *117*
    tissue *see* oocysts
cytokines **54**, 57–9
    immunoassays 106–8
    mediating SIRS 74, 75
    mediating viral disease 79
cytomegalovirus (CMV or HCMV) 348–9
    childhood rash illness 432
    congenital 348–9
    diagnostic testing **375**
    drug treatment 151, 152, 349
    HIV infection/AIDS 481
    immune avoidance mechanisms 80, 81
    immunocompromised host 348, 371, 377, 378
    immunosuppressive effects 373
    preemptive treatment 379
    primary infection in pregnancy 348, 349
    prophylaxis 378
    vaccine **64**
cytopathic effect (CPE) 78–9, 100
cytotoxic T lymphocytes (CTLs or Tc cells) 53, **54**, 55, 56
cytotoxins 70–1

Dane particles *494*
daptomycin 137, **145**
DDT 473
deafness
    congenital cytomegalovirus 348, 349
    congenital rubella 343
deer fly fever *see* tularemia
deer mouse *574*
α-defensins **50**, 51

β-defensins 51
delavirdine 153
delayed-type hypersensitivity (DTH) 450
delta virus *see* hepatitis D virus
dengue fever 554, 588–92
    clinical features 589
    control measures 562–3, 591–2
    diagnosis 591
    management 591
    transmission 555, *556*
dengue hemorrhagic fever (DHF)
    clinical features 590–1
    mortality 564, 588
dengue shock syndrome (DSS) 590–1
dengue vaccine 564, 592
dengue virus 589, 591
dental caries 24, 46, 66
dental treatment **239**, 240, 243
deoxyribonucleases 191
Dermacentor-borne necrosis and lymphadenopathy (DEBONEL) **537**
Dermacentor ticks 538
Dermatobia hominis 206
dermatophytes 11, 202, *203*, *205*
    antifungal drug activity **146**
    identification 98
    microscopic appearance *203*
descriptive epidemiology 168–71
diabetes mellitus **368**
    osteomyelitis 186
    skin and soft tissue infections 183
    urinary tract infections 322
diagnosis 85–123
    antigen–antibody reactions 101–8
    assessing a new test 119
    automated methods 113
    culture-based methods 92–100
    non-culture-based methods 101–12
    nucleic acid-based 108–12
    protozoal and helminth infections 116–19
    see also laboratories, diagnostic
diarrhea/diarrheal disease 212–37
    agents causing **213**
    antibiotic associated (AAD) 47, 402
    bacterial 214–21, 224–8, 235
    diagnostic tests 234–5
    food and waterborne 212–21
    immunocompromised host 378
    management principles 235–6
    parasitic 231–4, 236
    pathophysiology 224–31
    travelers 525–31
    viral 222–4, 228–31, 236
didanosine (DDI) 152
diethylcarbamazine (DEC) **149**
diloxanide furonate 148
dimorphic fungi 11, 32
    antifungal drug activity **146**
    identification 89, 99

diphtheria 599–606
  cutaneous 189, 194
  pathogenesis 602–4
  prevention 604–5
  public health impact 599–601
  respiratory 249, 601, *602*, **605**
  see also *Corynebacterium diphtheriae*
diphtheria antitoxin 62, 601, 604
diphtheria, tetanus and acellular pertussis vaccine (DTaP)
      604–5
diphtheria toxin 70–1, 603–4
  clinical effects 601
  mechanism of action 604, **605**
  production 76, 603–4
diphtheria toxoid 600, 604–5
Diphyllobothrium latum **13**
diplococcus 5
direct agglutination test 102
directly observed treatment, short course (DOTS) 440–1
disc diffusion methods 114
disseminated intravascular coagulation (DIC) 75, 559, **586**
DNA
  bacterial 15–16
  branched (bDNA) 111
DNA gyrase 16
DNA polymerase 29, 81–2
DNA vaccines 66
DNA viruses
  classification **30**
  immune escape mechanisms 81–2
  replication 29
  transcription 28
Dobrava–Belgrade (DOB) virus 572, **573**
Dobrava virus 554
Donovan bodies 319
donovanosis 309, *310*, 319
doxycycline 141, **145**, 471
droplet transmission
  healthcare settings 397–9
  influenza 509
  see also airborne transmission
drug treatment
  increasing infection risk 394
  see also antimicrobial chemotherapy
Duffy blood group antigens 42, 462
dysentery
  amebic 233–4
  bacillary 71, 526–7

ear infections see otitis media
Eastern equine encephalitis 288
Ebola fever 559, *560*
  infection control/containment *561*, 562
  outcome 563
Ebola virus 553, 554, **562**
  diagnostic testing 555, *557*, *558*
  immune avoidance mechanisms 81
  source of transmission 554, 555, *556*, **557**
ecchymoses 195–6

echinocandins 147
Echinococcus granulosus **13**, **149**
echocardiography 243
echovirus type 9 *200*
Eco-Challenge vacation, Borneo **544**
ecthyma 181
ecthyma gangrenosum 376
ectoplasm 32
eczema vaccinatum 623, *624*
edema
  respiratory diphtheria 601, *602*
  slapped cheek disease 429
education 409–11
efavirenz 153
efflux pumps, antibiotic 127
eggs
  helminth, detection 116, 117, 118, *119*
  hen's, *Salmonella* 214
ehrlichiosis 24, **537**
elastases 73
elderly
  healthcare associated infections 394
  urinary tract infections **321**, 322
electron microscopy (EM) 89, *91*, *92*
elementary bodies (EB) 24, 312, *313*, 355
ELISA 102–4
emboli, infected 240, *241*, 242
emerging and resurgent infectious diseases 158, 567–82, 583–98
  factors influencing 158, **159**, *160*
  neonatal/perinatal 359
  see also specific diseases
empirical treatment, immunocompromised host 379–80, **380**
empyema 257, *258*
emtricitabine 152, 495
encephalitis 278–82
  postvaccinial 623
  viral see viral encephalitis
encystation 33
endarteritis obliterans 306–7, 317
endemic 161
endemic disease, basic reproductive rate 165
endocarditis, infective see infective endocarditis
endocytosis, receptor-mediated 27, *28*
endoplasm 32
endospores 16
endotoxemia 73–4
endotoxin 19, 21, **69**
  role in SIRS 73, 74–5
enfuvirtide/T-20 154, 484
Entamoeba histolytica 12, 233–4
  diagnostic methods 116, 118, **235**
  drug treatment 148
  immune escape mechanisms 84
  intestinal infections (amebiasis) 233–4
  life cycle 33
  structure 32, 33
entecavir 495
enteric fever 531–2
Enterobius vermicularis **13**, 117, 150

Enterococcus spp.
  infective endocarditis **242**, 243
  urinary tract infections **320**
  see also vancomycin resistant enterococci
Enterocytozoon bieneusi 233
entero-mammary axis 62
enterotoxins 71
enteroviruses 286, 287
  hand-foot-and-mouth disease 200–1, 432–3
  meningitis 276, 277, *278*
  myocarditis 244, 245, 246
  neonatal/perinatal infections 359, 433
  pericarditis 247
  skin lesions 200–1
envelope, viral 25–6
environmental factors, disease susceptibility 43
enzyme-linked immunosorbent assay (ELISA or EIA) 102–4
enzyme-linked oligonucleotide assay (ELONA) 111
enzymes
  antimicrobial resistance 127, 128
  microbial 68, 71–3
eosinophils 51, 57
epidemic 161
epidemic curve 168–70
epidemic hemorrhagic fever *see* hemorrhagic fever with renal
    syndrome
epidemiology 157–75
  analytical 171–2
  definition 160
  descriptive 168–71
  natural history of disease 161–2
  outbreak investigation 166–73
  terminology 161
  transmission 162–5
  triad 160
  vaccination and herd immunity 165
Epidermophyton 99, 202, *203*
epiglottitis, acute 248, 249, 266
Epstein–Barr virus (EBV) infections 371, 432
  diagnosis **375**
  HIV infection/AIDS 481, *482*
ergosterol 31, 146
ertapenem 131
erysipelas 184
erythema infectiosum *see* slapped cheek disease
erythema migrans **280**
erythema multiforme 429
erythematous rash 415
erythrocytes *see* red blood cells
erythrogenic toxin 184, 191
erythromycin 135–6, **144**
ESBL *see* extended spectrum β-lactamase
escape mechanisms, microbial 66–84
Escherichia coli 7
  attachment 67
  cell wall 19, *20*
  diagnostic methods *88, 95*
  diarrheagenic strains 527
  entero-aggregative (EAEC) 527

entero-hemorrhagic (EHEC) 228, 527
entero-invasive (EIEC) 527
entero-pathogenic (EPEC) 527
entero-toxigenic (ETEC) 23, 71, 527, 530
ESBL producing 405
flagella (H antigen) 23
F or sex pilus 24, 77–8
LT enterotoxin 71, 530
neonatal sepsis 354
normal flora 47
outer membrane 21
postpartum infections 336
shiga-like toxin 71
ST enterotoxin 530
uropathogenic strains 320–1
virulence factors 76, 354
Escherichia coli O157 228
  diagnostic testing **235**
  illness caused by **215**, 218–19
  large outbreaks **220**
espundia 205–6, 533
etanercept 372
E-tests 114, *115*
etiology of infectious disease 3–14
eukaryotes 4, 11, 32
exanthema subitum *see* "sixth disease"
exfoliatin toxin (ET) 192
exotoxins 68–71
exposure-prone procedures (EPPs) **496**
extended spectrum β-lactamase (ESBL) producing organisms
    128, 405
extensively drug resistant tuberculosis (XDR-TB) 440, **441**
eye swabs 87

famciclovir 151
Fansidar 471
Far Eastern spotted fever **536**
Fasciola hepatica **13**
feces, specimens 87, 116
fetal blood sampling 343, 347, 349
fetal hydrops 347, 430
fever
  childhood rashes with *see* childhood rash illnesses
  immunocompromised host **377**, **379**
  malaria 464
  postpartum 336
F factors 78
fibrinogen 51
fibronectin 191
fibronectin-binding proteins 190, 191
"fifth disease" *see* slapped cheek disease
filoviruses 553, 554, **557**, **562**
fimbriae 23–4
"first disease" *see* measles
Fitz–Hugh–Curtis syndrome 299
flagella 23, 33
flagellates **13**, 33–5
flaviviruses 503, 542, 553, 578
flesh-eating bacteria **183**, 191

Flinders Island spotted fever **536**
flora, normal *see* normal microbial flora
flu *see* influenza
flucloxacillin 130, **144**
fluconazole 146
flucytosine **146**, 147
fluid mosaic model, cell membrane 17
fluid specimens 87
flukes **13**, 14
fluorescence polarization assay (FPA) 104, **105**
fluorochrome stains **90**, 452
fluoroquinolones 137–9
    urinary tract infections 324
folliculitis 182–4
fomites 10
fomivirsen 152
foodborne infections 212–21
    healthcare settings 399
    travel related 523, 525–32
    see also specific infections
foscarnet 152
"fourth disease" 415
fowlpox 66
F pilus 24, 77–8
Francisella tularensis **609**, 618–19, *620*
fungal infections
    healthcare associated **403**, 406
    hematopoietic stem cell transplant recipients 370
    HIV infection/AIDS 481
    immunocompromised host **11**, 12, 204, 364, **365**, 373–4
    respiratory tract 264–6
    skin and soft tissues 11, 202–4
    systemic 11–12, 204
    see also specific infections
fungi 11–12
    antimicrobial susceptibility tests 113–15
    classification **11**
    culture 98–9
    detection of products 101
    diagnostic identification 98, **375**
    dimorphic *see* dimorphic fungi
    of medical importance 12
    microscopy 89, **91**
    pathogenesis of disease 66–78
    pathogenic 11–12
    specimens 88
    structure and function 31–2
    toxins 68
furuncles 182–4
Fusarium **375**
fusidic acid 143–4, **145**
fusion inhibitors, HIV 484

gametocytes *461*, 462, 463, *469*
gamma globulins, human 62
    see also intravenous immunoglobulin
ganciclovir 151, 349
gangrene
    gas (clostridial) 188, 193, 194

meningococcal disease 277
    streptococcal *see* necrotizing fasciitis
Gardnerella vaginalis 299, 301
gastroenteritis 212–37
    classification **213**
    healthcare associated 402
    see also diarrhea/diarrheal disease
gastrointestinal infections, immunocompromised host 378
gastrointestinal (GI) tract
    barriers to infection *43*, 44
    normal flora 47
    tuberculosis 446
GBS *see* group B streptococci
gene probes, *Mycobacterium tuberculosis* 452
general paralysis of the insane 307
genetic factors, disease susceptibility 42
genetic reassortment 82
gene transfer, bacterial 76–8
genital herpes 301, 302–3
    in children **199**
    partner infidelity and **198**
    pathogenesis 317–18
    in pregnancy 303, 357, 358
    skin lesions 196, 197
    see also herpes simplex virus 2
genital lesions 301–9
genital warts (condylomata acuminata) *201*, 303–4
genitourinary tract
    host defences 296, 299, 319–20
    infections 294–331
    normal flora 47–8
    tuberculosis 446
genomes
    sizes 10
    viral 25, 82
gentamicin 139, 141, **145**
German measles *see* rubella
Giardia lamblia 12, 232
    diagnostic testing *117*, **235**
    drug treatment 148
    life cycle 33–4
    structure 32
giardiasis 232
glandular fever 432
gloves 409
    incorrect use 396, *398*
glucan polymers 31
glucose-6-phosphate dehydrogenase deficiency 472, 539
glycocalyx 33, 243
glycolipids, mycobacterial cell wall 22–3
glycopeptide-resistant enterococci (GRE) 45, 134
glycopeptides 134–5
Gohn focus 442–3
gonococcus *see* Neisseria gonorrheae
gonorrhea (gonococcal infection) 296
    asymptomatic 296
    clinical presentation 298–9
    host defences 42
    public health impact 297

gowns 409
graft versus host disease (GVHD) 371
Gram negative bacteria 5, 7
  cell wall *18*, 19–20
  drug resistance 77, 127–8, **127**
  empirical treatment 379
  healthcare associated infections 405
  immunocompromised host 364, **365**, 373
  outer membrane 19, 20–1
  systemic inflammatory response syndrome 73–5
  vaccine **64**
Gram positive bacteria 5, *6*
  cell wall 18–19
  drug resistance 77, 127–8, **127**
  empirical treatment 379
  immunocompromised host 364, **365**
Gram stain 4–5, *6*, **89**
granulocyte colony stimulating factor (G-CSF) 380
granuloma inguinale (or venereum) *see* donovanosis
granulomas, tuberculosis 450
gray baby syndrome 142
griseofulvin 147
group A β-hemolytic streptococcus *see Streptococcus pyogenes*
group B streptococci (GBS) 352–4
  early onset neonatal sepsis 352–3
  late onset neonatal sepsis 355
  normal flora 48
growth
  bacterial 8
  factors, bacterial 92, **93**
Guanarito virus 553, 554
gummatous syphilis 307

HAART *see* highly active antiretroviral therapy
HACEK group of organisms **242**, 243
Haemophilus ducreyi 309, 318–19
Haemophilus influenzae 260
  bronchitis and bronchiectasis 254
  colonization 47
  genome 10
  identification 266
  microbiology 260, *261*, 284, *285*
  pneumonia 256
  splenic dysfunction 367
  virulence mechanism 260
Haemophilus influenzae type b (Hib) 260, 284
  epiglottitis 248, 249
  meningitis 274, 275
  vaccine 63, 267, 275, 378
Hajj pilgrims 547
hand-foot-and-mouth disease (HFMD) 200–1, 432–3
hands, transmission of infection *395*, 396, *397*
handwashing 407, **410**
hanging groin 206
Hantaan virus 572, **573**, 576
hantaviruses 554, 571–6
  epidemiology 571–2, **573**
  virology and diagnosis 572, *574*

hantavirus pulmonary syndrome (HPS) 554, 571–2
  clinical features 573–5
  treatment and prevention 576
H antigen 23
healthcare associated infections (HAI) 393–413
  common types 399–402
  definition 393
  infection control measures 407–11
  microbiology 402–6
  risk factors 393–5
  skin, soft tissue, bone and joint 188
  source 45, 396
  transmission 396–9
  viral hemorrhagic fevers 555, *557*
  viral hepatitis **496**, 498, **499**
healthcare workers (HCWs) 393
  handwashing 407
  hepatitis B prophylaxis 497, 498
  hepatitis B risks 495, **496**
  HIV exposure **486**
  personal protective equipment 409, 560–1
  transmission of infection 394–5, **496**
heart transplant recipients 371
Helicobacter pylori 47
helminth infections
  diagnosis 116–19
  drug treatment 149–50
  see also specific infections
helminths 12–14
  host defence 51, **54**
  pathogenic and escape mechanisms 82–4
helper T cells 53, **54**, 55
hemagglutinin (H) 507
  genetic reassortment 82, 509, *510*
  mutations 82, 508–9
hematological conditions, parvovirus B19 infection **428**
hematological malignancies **368**, 369–70
hematopoietic stem cell transplantation (HSCT) **368**, 370–1, 378
  management of infections **380**
hemazoin 462
hemochromatosis **368**
hemodialysis **368**
hemoflagellates 34–5
hemolysins 71
  SH-activated 340
hemolysis
  blood agar 93, *94*
  enzymes causing 71
  intravascular, in malaria 464
hemolytic uremic syndrome (HUS) 219, 527
hemorrhagic fever with renal syndrome (HFRS) 554, 571, 572
  clinical features 573, 575–6
  treatment and prevention 576
hemorrhagic problems
  complicating rubella 423
  viral hemorrhagic fevers 558–9
Hendra virus 577

hepatitis
   chronic 491
   fulminant 491, 493
   immunocompromised host 378
   viral *see* viral hepatitis
hepatitis A (virus) (HAV) 493–4, 525
hepatitis B 494–8
   chronic/carriers 494, 495
   diagnosis 495
   drug therapy 152–3, 156, 495, **497**
   neonatal/perinatal 356–7
   postexposure prophylaxis (PEP) 498
   transmission **486**, 494–5, **496**
hepatitis B immune globulin (HBIG) 62, 356, 498
hepatitis B vaccine 65, 495–8
   newborn babies 356
   testing response 497–8
hepatitis B virus (HBV) 9, 494
   antenatal screening 356
   disease pathogenesis 80
   hepatitis D virus coinfection 501
   immune avoidance mechanisms 81
   immune escape mechanisms 82
   mutant **496**
   replication 29
hepatitis C 498–500
   chronic 500
   clinical features *492*, 500
   diagnosis 500
   drug therapy 155, 156, **497**, 500
   neonatal/perinatal 356–7
hepatitis C virus (HCV) 498–9
   immune avoidance mechanisms 81
   transmission in healthcare settings **486**, 498, **499**
hepatitis D virus (HDV) 10, 500–1
hepatitis E (HEV) 501–3
hepatitis F 503
hepatitis G (HGV; GBV) 503
hepatocellular carcinoma 491, 495
herd immunity (HI) 165
herd immunity threshold (HIT) 165, **166**
herpes
   genital *see* genital herpes
   neonatal 303, 357–8
   oro-facial *see* cold sores
herpes simplex virus (HSV) 317–18
   diagnosis of infections 197–200
   drug treatment 151, 152
   genital lesions 301, 302–3
   immune avoidance mechanisms 80
   immunocompromised host 378
   meningitis/encephalitis 276, 277, 287
   microscopy *91*, *92*
   skin and soft tissue infections 197–200
herpes simplex virus 1 (HSV-1) 194–5, 287
   genital lesions 302, 303
   meningitis/encephalitis 276, 287
   neonatal/perinatal infection 357–8
   oral lesions (cold sores) 196, 197, *287*

herpes simplex virus 2 (HSV-2) 194–5, 287
   childhood infection **199**
   genital lesions 196, 197, 302, 303
   meningitis/encephalitis 276, 287
   partner infidelity and **198**
   see also genital herpes
herpes viruses *9*
   drug treatment 151–2
   immunocompromised host 374
herpes zoster *see* shingles
highly active antiretroviral therapy (HAART) 152, 480
   monitoring of therapy 483–4
Histoplasma capsulatum 11–12, 265–6
   diagnostic testing 266, **375**
histoplasmosis 265–6
HIV *see* human immunodeficiency virus
homeless people, tuberculosis **441**
homosexual men *see* men who have sex with men
hospital acquired infections *see* healthcare associated
      infections
host defence 41–66, 363
   see also immunity
host range, viruses 10
host-specificity, viruses 10
HPV *see* human papilloma viruses
HSV *see* herpes simplex virus
Hugh and Leifson medium 97
human bocavirus (HBoV) 251
human cytomegalovirus *see* cytomegalovirus
human endogenous retroviruses (HERVs) 30–1
human herpes virus 6 (HHV6) 430–1
   childhood illness *see* "sixth disease"
   diagnosis of infection **376**, 432
human herpes virus 7 (HHV7) 430–1
human herpes virus 8 (HHV8) 481, *482*
human immune globulin (HIG) 62
human immunodeficiency virus (HIV) 10, 476–90
   antibodies (Ab) 480, 482–3
   chancroid interaction 318–19
   classification 477
   drug resistance 484
   entry into target cells 27, 478
   immune avoidance mechanisms 80, 81
   immune escape mechanisms 82
   laboratory diagnosis 482–4
   p24 antigen (Ag) 480, 482–3
   postexposure prophylaxis **486**
   quasispecies 485
   RNA load 480, 482–3
   type 1 (HIV-1) 476, 477, *479*
   type 2 (HIV-2) 476, 477
   vaccines **64**, 484–5
   virology 477–9
human immunodeficiency virus (HIV) infection 476–90
   antenatal screening 356
   clinical features 480–1
   drug treatment *see* anti-retroviral drugs
   epidemiology 476–7
   fungal infections 12, 481

legal/ethical aspects 485, **486**
natural history 480, *481*
neonatal/perinatal 356–7
opportunist infections **368**, 373, 481, *482*
pericarditis 246, 247
Pneumocystis carinii pneumonia (PCP) **383**
primary (PHI) 480
protozoal infections 12
seroconversion illness 480
treatment **380**, 484
tuberculosis coinfection 439, 442, 447, 450–1
see also AIDS
human papilloma viruses (HPV) 201–2, 303, 318
mechanism of carcinogenesis 318
vaccine 202, 303–4
humoral immunity 53, 55
defects **365**, 367
Hutchinson's teeth 341
hyaluronidase 71, 191
hydradenitis 181
hydrops fetalis 347, 430
Hymenolepis nana **13**
hyperplastic skin lesions 201–2
hyphae 11, 32
hypnozoites *461*, 462
hypogammaglobulinemia **368**
hypoglycemia, severe malaria 464, **465**, 472
hyposplenism, functional 367

iatrogenic transmission
hepatitis C 498, **499**
viral hemorrhagic fevers 555
see also healthcare associated infections
IgA **55**
bacterial proteases 260, 315
secretory 61–2, 67
IgD **55**
IgE **54**, 55, 67
parasitic infections 84
IgG 55, 61
passive immunization 62
IgM 55, 61
imidazole antifungals 146
imipenem 130–1
immune response
mediating disease pathogenesis 66, 79–80
microbial escape mechanisms 66–84
primary 60–1
secondary 61
immune therapy 380
immunity 363
adaptive 53–9, 363
cell-mediated 53, 56–9
cell types involved **42**
humoral 53, 55
innate 42–52, 363
immunization 60–6
active 62–5
historical milestones **60**

new approaches 65–6
passive 61–2, 599
immunoassays 102–4
automation 113
cytokine 106–8
fluorescence-based 104, **105**
protozoal and helminth infections 118
radio-immunoassays 104
sandwich 102
immunoblotting 105–6, *107*
immunocard tests 105
immunochromatography 105, *106*
immunocompromised host 363–92
brain abscesses 282, 377
clinical approach to diagnosis 374–6
clinical presentations 376–8
clinical syndromes 367–73
cytomegalovirus infection 348, 371, 377, 378
fungal infections **11**, 12, 204, 364, **365**, 373–4
infecting organisms 44, 373–4
Norwegian scabies **208**
parvovirus B19 infection **428**, 430
pathophysiology 364–7
prevention and treatment of infections 378–80
smallpox vaccination complications 623, *624*
vaccination 64, 378
viral skin infections 197, 200
immunodeficiency syndromes
primary 367–9
secondary 367, **368**
immunofluorescence 106, **108**
direct 106, *107*
indirect 106, *107*
microscopy 89, *91*
immunoglobulins 55
passive immunization 62
see also IgA; IgE; IgG; intravenous immunoglobulin
immunohistological techniques 106
immunosuppressive medications 371–2
immunosuppressive viral proteins 81
impetigo 180–1
incidence 161
inclusion bodies, virus-infected cells 29
inclusions, bacterial 16
incubation period 161
determination 170
Indian tick typhus **537**
indinavir 153
indwelling devices 394
infant mortality rate 161
infection
natural history 161–2
vs. colonization 44–5
infection control measures 407–11
viral hemorrhagic fevers 562–3
infectious disease(s)
definition 157
epidemiology 157–75
global burden 158, *159*

infectious disease(s) (*cont'd*)
    natural history 161–2
    surveillance 409–11
    transmission 162–5
infectious mononucleosis 432
infectious period 161–2
infective endocarditis (IE) 239–44
    blood culture negative **242**, 243
    clinical presentation 241–2
    diagnosis 243
    microbiology 242–3
    pathophysiology 240, *241*
    predisposing factors 239, **240**
    prevention 244
    treatment 243–4
infertility, female 299
inflammatory response, cytokines 57–8
infliximab 372
influenza 263, 506–20
    avian 506–7, 509, 516–17
    clinical features 510
    croup 254
    drug treatment 154–5, 253, 511–13
    epidemics 506, 507
    epidemiology 506–7
    laboratory diagnosis 511, *512, 513*
    pandemic alert system 517, **518**
    pandemics 507–8, 509
    transmission 509–10
influenza A virus 507
    avian H5N1 strain 516–17
    strains causing pandemics 509
influenza B virus 507
influenza C virus 507
influenza-like illnesses 250–1, 511
influenza vaccines 267, 506, 514–15
    recommendations for use **515**
    types available **514**
influenza viruses 11, 252, 507–9
    antigenic variation 82, 507–9, *510*
    release from cells 29
    virology 507, *508, 509*
injecting drug users *see* intravenous drug users
injection practices, safe 409
innate immunity 42–52, 363
    dysfunction/defects 364–6
insect bites, infected **180**
insecticide-treated nets (ITNs) 473
intensive care unit (ICU) **395**, 400
interferon(s) (IFN) 52
    antiviral therapy 155–6, 495, **497**, 500
    type I 58, **497**
    type II 59, **497**
interferon-α (IFN-α) 58, **497**
interferon-β (IFN-β) 58, **497**
interferon-γ (IFN-γ) 57, 59, **497**
    release assay, tuberculosis 108, 454–5
interleukin 1 (IL-1) 51, 58
interleukin 2 (IL-2) 57, 58

interleukin 6 (IL-6) 58
interleukin 8 (IL-8) 58
interleukin 11 (IL-11) 58
intestinal specimens 116–17
intracellular microorganisms
    immune escape mechanisms 67
    obligate 24–5
intravascular device/catheter associated infections 400, *401*
intravenous drug users (IVDUs) **368**
    hepatitis C 498
    HIV infection 476
    skin and soft tissue infections 184
    wound botulism **70**
intravenous immunoglobulin (IVIG) 62
    neonatal enterovirus infections 359
    parvovirus B19 infection **428**, 430
    viral myocarditis 246
Invasion Plasmid Antigens (Ipa) 526
iodine staining 116
Iraq 608
iron
    diphtheria toxin production and 604
    overload **368**
    requirements of bacteria 67–8, 92
irritable bowel syndrome, postinfectious 526
isolation (of patients) 408–9
    protective 408–9
    source 408
    viral hemorrhagic fevers 560, *561*
isoniazid resistance, tuberculosis 439–40, **441**
Isospora belli
    diagnostic testing 116, **235**
    gastroenteritis 233
    life cycle 38
Israeli tick typhus **537**
itraconazole 146
ivermectin **149**
IVIG *see* intravenous immunoglobulin

Janeway lesions 242
Japanese encephalitis (JE) 578
    vaccine **64**, 578
Jarisch–Herxheimer reaction 317
jaundice
    malaria 464
    viral hepatitis 491, *492*
Jenner, Edward 60, 623
jock-itch **203**
joint infections 187–8
    hospital acquired 188
    tuberculosis 446
Junin virus 553, 554

Kabat, E.A. 55
kala azar 533
kanamycin 139, **140**, 141
Kaposi's sarcoma 481, *482*
Kaposi's sarcoma herpes virus (KSHV) 481, *482*
kappa toxin 194

Katayama fever 534
keratitis
  Acanthamoeba 277
  congenital syphilis 307, *308*
killer (K) cells 57
Kirby-Bauer disc diffusion method 114
Klebsiella 405
Koch, Robert 85, 433
Koch's postulates 85, **86**
Koplik's spots 418
Korean hemorrhagic fever *see* hemorrhagic fever with renal
    syndrome
Kyasanur Forest disease vaccine **64**

laboratories, diagnostic
  automation 113
  high-level containment 555, *557*
  quality control/assurance 120
  see also diagnosis
La Crosse encephalitis 288
lactobacilli 46, 47–8, 296, 299, *300*
lactoferrin **50**, 51, 68
Laguna Negra (LN) virus **573**
lamivudine (3TC) 152, 495
Lancefield grouping of streptococci 98, 189
large bowel, normal flora 47
larva currens 206
larva migrans 206
laryngeal papillomatosis 202
laryngeal tuberculosis 447
laryngitis 248
laryngo-tracheo-bronchitis 253
Lassa fever 559, *560*, 561–2, 564
Lassa fever virus 553, 554, *559*
latent period, infection 161
latent virus infections 30
Lechiguanas virus **573**
lecithinases 71, 193
Leeuwenhoek, Antony van 3
Legionella pneumophila 261–2
  diagnostic testing 266, **375**
  pneumonia 256, *257*, 261
  prevention of infections 267
Legionnaire's disease (LD) 261, **262**
  healthcare associated 400, **401**
Leishman–Donovan bodies *see* amastigotes
Leishmania 12
  detection methods 117, *118*
  drug treatment 149
  life cycle 35, *37*
Leishmania braziliensis 205–6, 533
Leishmania chagasi 533
leishmaniacides 149
Leishmania donovani 33, 533
Leishmania infantum 533
Leishmania major 533
Leishmania mexicana 205–6
leishmaniasis 532–3
  cutaneous 205–6, 533

immunocompromised host 374
  visceral 149, 533
Leishmania tropica 37, 205–6, 533
leprosy vaccine **64**
Leptospira 5, *8*, 545
Leptospira biflexa 545
Leptospira interrogans 545
leptospirosis 543–5
leucolysis, enzymes causing 71
leukemia **368**, 369–70
leukocidins 72
leukoplakia, oral hairy 481
levamisole **149**
levofloxacin 137, 138–9, **145**
lice
  body 540, 541
  pubic **310**
lichen planus *492*
lincosamides 135–6
linezolid 136–7, **145**
Lipid A 20–1
lipoarabinomannan *22*
lipopolysaccharide (LPS) 19, 20–1
  complement activation 67
  role in SIRS 73, 74–5
lipopolysaccharide (LPS)-binding protein 74, 75
lipoteichoic acids (LTA) 190
Listeria monocytogenes 274, 338–40
listeriolysin O (LLO) 340
listeriosis 338–40
liver disease, severe **368**
liver transplant recipients 371
loaiasis 206
Loa loa 13, **149**, 206
lopinavir 153
louse *see* lice
Löwenstein–Jensen culture medium 453
lower respiratory tract, host defence 259
lower respiratory tract infections (LRTIs) 254–67
  bacterial 254, 259–64
  diagnosis 266
  microbiology and pathogenesis 259–66
  viral 250–1, **252**, 253–4
  see also pneumonia
LPS *see* lipopolysaccharide
lumbar puncture 87
lung transplant recipients 371
Lyell disease (scalded skin syndrome) 185–6, 192
Lyme disease **280**, 281
lymphangitis associated rickettsiosis **536**
lymph nodes, tuberculosis 444–5
lymphocytes **42**, 53
  large granular 51, 57
  see also B cells; T cells
lymphogranuloma venereum (LGV) 297, 309,
    312
lymphoma 369–70, 371
lysis, virus-infected cells 29
lysozyme 20, 44, **50**, 51

MacConkey agar 93, *95*
McFarland standard 114
Machupo virus 553, 554
macroconidia *99, 203*
macrolides 135–6
macrophage inflammatory proteins (MIP) 58
macrophages 48, 53–4
    activation 56–7, 59
    Mycobacterium tuberculosis infection 442, 443, 448, 449
    resistance to 67
macular rashes 195–6, 415
maculatum infection **536**
maculopapular rashes 195–6, 415
Madura foot 202
maggot therapy **207**
major histocompatibility (MHC) antigen 54–5
malaria 35–6, 458–75
    cerebral 465, 472
    clinical features 464–7
    diagnosis 119, 467–70
    epidemiology and burden 458–60
    global control 474
    parasite *see Plasmodium*
    pathogenesis 83, 84
    in pregnancy 464–5, **466**, 472
    prevention 472–3
    quartan 466–7
    rapid diagnostic tests (RDTs) 468–70
    tertian 466
    treatment 470–2
    vaccines **64**, 473–4
    vector control 473
Malarone 471
Malassezia 11
Mallon, Mary ("Typhoid Mary") 531
mannose-binding lectin (MBL) deficiency 373
mannose-binding protein 51
M antigen (M-protein) 23, 66–7, 190
Mantoux test 450, 453
Marburg fever 562, 563
Marburg virus 553, 554, **562**
    electron microscopy *558*
    source of transmission **557**
masks 409
mastitis 184, 336
mastoiditis 282
Mastomys rodents 554
measles (rubeola) **416**, 418–20
    complications 419
    encephalitis 64, 419
    prophylaxis 420
    rash *195*, 195–6, 415, 419
    respiratory tract disease 254, 263, 419
    transmissibility 194–5, 418
measles-mumps-rubella (MMR) vaccine 420
measles virus *196*, 418
    immune avoidance mechanisms 80, 81
mebendazole **149**, 150
mec A gene 402

Mediterranean spotted fever **536**
Mediterranean tick fever **537**
mefloquine 470
melioidosis 264
memory, immunologic 61
meninges 271
meningitis 273–8
    bacterial 274–6, 277, **278**, 283–6
    causes **274**
    clinical presentation 277–8
    diagnosis 278
    immunocompromised host 377
    media interest 271, *272*
    microbiology and pathogenesis 283–7
    primary amebic 276–7
    public health impact 274–7
    travel related 547, *548*
    tuberculous **278**, 446
    vaccines 63
    viral (aseptic) 201, 276, 277, **278**, 286–7
meningococcal disease 274, 277
    travel related 547
meningococcal vaccines 63, 275–6, 547
meningococcus *see Neisseria meningitidis*
mental retardation, congenital cytomegalovirus 348, 349
men who have sex with men (MSM)
    HIV infection 476
    lymphogranuloma venereum 297
    nontoxigenic *Corynebacterium diphtheriae* 601
    syphilis 297, 340
meropenem 130–1
merozoites 38, *461, 462, 469*
mesosomes 17
metabolic factors, disease susceptibility 43
metapneumovirus, human (hMPV) 251
methicillin 130
methicillin resistant *Staphylococcus aureus* (MRSA) 45, 402–3
    community acquired **404**
    skin and soft tissue infections 180
methotrexate 372
metronidazole 142–3, **145**, 148
micafungin 147
microarrays 112
microbes 3–12
    discovery 3
    host defence against invasion 41–66
    normal flora *see* normal microbial flora
    pathogenesis and escape mechanisms 66–84
    structure and function 15–40
microconidia *99, 203*
microfilaria, detection 117, *118*
micronutrients 92, **93**
microscopy 88–90, *91*
microsporidia 233
Microsporum 11, *99*, 202, *203*
mid-stream urine (MSU) 322–3
mimivirus 9
Minas Gerais exanthematic typhus **537**
minimum inhibitory concentrations (MIC) 114, 115

miracidia 534
MLS group of antibiotics 135–6
Mobiluncus 301
molds 11
molecular diagnosis 90, 108–12, 113, 119
  see also nucleic acid-based diagnosis
molecular mimicry 80
Mollaret's meningitis (syndrome) 277
molluscum contagiosum 200
monkeypox 567–71
  clinical features 200, 570–1
  epidemiology 568
  introduction to USA 568–9
  treatment and prevention 571
  virology and diagnosis 569–70
monobactams 134
monoclonal antibodies 372
monocyte chemoattractant proteins (MCP-1, MCP-2,
    MCP-3) 58
Monongahela virus **573**
Moraxella catarrhalis 249, 256, 261
morbidity rate 161
mosquitoes 36
  bite prevention 472, *588*
  chikungunya virus 579
  control measures 472, *563*, *578*, 588, 591–2
  dengue fever 588–9
  encephalitis transmission 287–8
  Japanese encephalitis 578
  malaria 458, 461, 463–4
  viral hemorrhagic fevers 555, *556*
  West Nile virus 584, *585*
  yellow fever 541–2, 555, *556*
mother-to-child transmission (MTCT) 11
  hepatitis B 497, 498
  see also neonatal infections; perinatal infections
mouth, normal flora 46–7
moxifloxacin 137, 138–9, **145**
MRSA *see* methicillin resistant *Staphylococcus aureus*
mucociliary escalator, respiratory tract 259
mucormycosis, cerebral 378
mucosal associated lymphoid tissue (MALT) 62
mucositis, oral *366*, 370, 373, 378
mucus-secreting surfaces (mucous membranes) 44, 67–8
Muleshoe virus (MULEV) **573**
multi-drug resistant tuberculosis (MDR-TB) 439–40, **441**, 442
mumps virus 276, 287
mutations, virus 81–2, 115–16
mycetoma 202–3, **204**
mycobacteria
  culture 453
  diagnostic methods **90**
mycobacteria, atypical/nontuberculosis **445**
  diagnostic tests **375**
  pericarditis 246
Mycobacterium africanum 442, 448
Mycobacterium avium-intracellulare complex 22, 138, **445**
Mycobacterium bovis 442, 446, 448
Mycobacterium kansasii **445**

Mycobacterium leprae 22, 42, 67
Mycobacterium marinum **445**
Mycobacterium microti 442, 448
Mycobacterium scrofulaceum **445**
Mycobacterium tuberculosis 447–50
  cell wall 22
  diagnostic testing **375**, 451–5
  genetic variability 451
  immune response 67, 448–50
  microbiology 447–8
  pathogenesis of infection 442–3
  urine cultures 323, 446
  virulence mechanisms 448
  see also tuberculosis
Mycobacterium ulcerans **445**
mycolic acids 22–3, **90**
Mycoplasma genitalium 299
Mycoplasma pneumoniae 21, 262–3
  respiratory infections 254, *257*
mycoplasmas 21, 101
mycoses **11**, 204
myelitis 279
myeloma **368**, 370
myeloperoxidase **50**, 51
myiasis 206
myocarditis 244–6

N-acetylglucosamine (NAG) 18, 19
N-acetylmuramic acid (NAM) 18, 19
Naegleria fowleri 276
nafcillin 130, **144**
Nagayama spots 431
nasal swabs 86
nasopharyngeal aspirate (NPA) 87, 252
natural history of disease 161–2
natural killer (NK) cells 51, 57
  tuberculosis 449
Necator americanus **13**, **149**
necrotizing fasciitis 182, 191
needlestick injuries (NSI) **486**
  hepatitis B transmission **496**
  prevention 396, *398*, 409, *411*
negative predictive value (NPV) 119
Negri bodies 289
Neisseria gonorrheae (gonococcus) 314–15
  antibiotic resistance 315
  ophthalmia neonatorum 354–5
  septic arthritis 187
  virulence mechanisms 23, 314–15, 355
  see also gonorrhea
Neisseria meningitidis (meningococcus)
  colonization 44–5, 47
  meningitis 274
  microbiology 283, *284*
  travel related infection 547, *548*
  see also meningococcal disease; meningococcal vaccines
nelfinavir 153
nematodes **13**, 14
neomycin 139, **140**, 141

neonatal infections 337, 352–9
  bacterial 352–5
  case **337**
  causes **338**
  chickenpox 346
  definitions **337**
  disseminated herpes 303
  early onset 337, **338**, 352–5
  emerging diseases 359
  late onset 337, **338**, 355
  listeriosis 339
  urinary tract **321**
  viral 356–9
neonates, antibodies 61–2
Neorickettsia sennetsu **537**
nephropathia epidemica *see* hemorrhagic fever with renal
    syndrome
netilmicin 139, 140, 141
net reproductive rate *(R)* 164–5
neuraminidase (N) 71, 507, *508*
  genetic reassortment 82, 509, *510*
  inhibitors 29, 154–5, 512–13
  mutations 82, 508–9
neuroendocrine factors, disease susceptibility 43
neurological infections *see* central nervous system (CNS)
    infections
neurosyphilis 307
neurotoxins 69–70
neutropenia 364, **365**, *365*
  causes 369–70
  infecting organisms 373
  management of infections 379, **380**
  pneumonia 400
  sequence of events *366*
nevirapine 153
New York virus **573**
niclosamide **149**
Nightingale wards 396, *397*
Nipah virus 577
nitric oxide 51
nitrofurantoin 143, **145**
Nocardia **375**
nongonococcal urethritis (NGU) 24–5, 299
non-nucleoside reverse transcriptase inhibitors (NNRTIs) 153
non-steroidal anti-inflammatory drugs (NSAIDs), viral
    myocarditis 245
norfloxacin 137
normal microbial flora 44–8
  beneficial effects 45–6
  constituents 46–8
  culture of sites with 96
  as source of infection 364
noroviruses
  diagnostic testing 224, **235**
  gastroenteritis **215**, 222, **223**, 224
  healthcare associated infections 402
  pathogenesis and virulence 229
  transmission 10
  travel related 531

North Asian tick typhus **536**
Norwalk-like viruses *see* noroviruses
nosocomial infections *see* healthcare associated infections
nucleic acid-based diagnosis 108–12
  automation 113
  HIV infection 483–4
  malaria 470
  signal amplification methods 108, 111–12
  target amplification methods 108, 109–11, *112*
  tuberculosis 452
nucleic acid sequence-based amplification (NASBA) 111, *112*
nucleocapsid 25
nucleoside reverse transcriptase inhibitors (NRTIs) 152–3, 484
nucleotide reverse transcriptase inhibitors 153, 484
nutrients, bacterial 92, **93**
nystatin 146

obligate intracellular microorganisms 24–5
obstetric infections 335–6
odds ratio 172
ofloxacin 137, 138
omp proteins 21
Onchocerca volvulus **13**, **149**, 206
onchocerciasis 206, **522**
oncogenes 79
onychomycosis **203**, *205*
oocysts (tissue cysts)
  Cryptosporidium parvum 38, *39*, 233
  malaria *461*, 463
  toxoplasmosis 36–8, 352
  see also cysts, protozoan
ookinetes *461*, 463
ophthalmia neonatorum 354–5
opportunist infections 44, 368, 373–4
  diagnostic tests **375–6**
  HIV infection/AIDS **368**, 373, 481, *482*
  prevention and treatment 378–80
opsonins 48, **49**, 53–4
opsonization 52, *53*, 67
optochin sensitivity 98
oral cavity, normal flora 46–7
oral hairy leukoplakia 481
Oran virus **573**
organ transplantation, solid 368, 371, **380**
Oriental sore 205–6, 533
Oriental spotted fever **536**
Orienta tsutsugamushi **537**
Oroya fever **537**
orthopoxviruses 569
oseltamivir 29, 154–5, 512–13
Osler's nodes 242
O-specific polysaccharide (O antigen) 20, 21
osteomyelitis 186–7, *188*
otitis media, acute 249, *250*, 252
  measles 419
  spread to CNS 282
outbreaks
  continuing or extended common source 168–9
  establishing existence 167

interventions/control measures 172
investigation 166–73
point source 168, *169*
point source with secondary cases 168, *169*
propagated 169, *170*
outer membrane, Gram negative bacteria 19, 20–1
oxacillin 130
oxazolidinones 136–7
oxidative burst *see* respiratory burst

palivizumab **64**
pandemic 161
Panton-Valentine (PV) leukocidin 180, 192
Paracoccidioides braziliensis 11–12, 204
paracoccidioidomycosis 204
Paragonimus westermani **13**, 118, **149**
parainfluenza (PIF) viruses 251, 252, 254, 263
parasites
    identification 90, 116–19, **376**
    pathogenic and escape mechanisms 82–4
parasitic infections
    congenital 349–52
    diarrheas 231–4, 236
    drug treatment 147–50
    immunocompromised host **365**, 374, 378
    skin and subcutaneous tissues 205–7
    travel related **522**
    see also specific infections
paratyphoid fever 531–2
parvovirus B19 (PVB19) *196*, 427
    childhood illness *see* slapped cheek disease
    close contact in pregnancy **345**
    complications of infection **428**, 430
    congenital 346–7, 430
    diagnosis of infections 430
    myocarditis 244
    primary infection in adults 341–2
    transmissibility 194–5
pathogen associated molecular patterns (PAMPs) 48–50
pathogenesis, disease 66–84
pattern-recognition receptors (PRRs) 48–50
PCR *see* polymerase chain reaction
pediculosis pubis **310**
pelvic inflammatory disease (PID) 299
penciclovir 151
penicillin(s) 127–31, **144**
    allergy 131
    β-lactamase inhibitor combinations 130
    β-lactamase resistant 130
    β-lactamase susceptible broad spectrum 130
    classification **129**
    extended spectrum 130
    mechanisms of action 128–9
    resistance 127, 129
    side-effects and tolerability 131
    tolerance 129
penicillin binding protein 2a 127, 402
penicillin binding proteins (PBPs) 19, 128
penicillin G 129–30, 131, **144**

penicillin V 129, **144**
pentamidine isetionate 149
peptidoglycan 18–19, 20, 22
perforin 51
pericarditis **245**, 246–8
    tuberculous 246, 247, 446
perinatal infections 352–9
    definition **337**
    viral 356–9
    see also neonatal infections
peritonitis, tuberculous 446
Peromyscus maniculatus 574
person, outbreak characterization by 166, 170–1
personal protective equipment
    hantaviruses 576
    healthcare workers 409, 560–1
    laboratory workers 555, *557*
pertussis (whooping cough) 249, **250**
    vaccine 267
    see also Bordetella pertussis
pertussis toxin 261
petechiae 195–6, 277, 415
phagocytic cells **42**, 48–51
phagocytosis 48–51
    microbial resistance 67
    opsonization facilitating 52, *53*
phagolysosomes 50
pharyngitis (sore throat) 248–9
    diagnosis of cause 266
    diphtheria 249, 601
    nontoxigenic *Corynebacterium diphtheriae* 601
    streptococcal 248–9, 420–1
phenoxymethyl penicillin (penicillin V) 129, **144**
phosphatidylinositol mannosides (PIM) *22*
phospholipases 71
Phthirus pubis **310**
pigs 577
pili 23–4
pinworms *see Enterobius vermicularis*
piperacillin 130
piperacillin-tazobactam (piptazobactam) 130, **144**
piperazine **149**, 150
place, outbreak characterization by 166, 170
placenta 337
plague 157, 614–18
    as biological weapon 607, **609**, 616–17
    bubonic 614, *615*
    pneumonic 614, 616–17
    treatment 617–18
plasmids 16, 78
Plasmodium (malaria parasite) 12, 458, 460–4
    immune escape mechanisms 83, 84
    life cycle 35–6, 461–4
    microscopy 467–9
Plasmodium aldolase tests 470
Plasmodium falciparum 458, **463**
    clinical features 464–5
    diagnosis *468–9*, 468–70
    drug resistance 470, 471

Plasmodium falciparum (*cont'd*)
  epidemiology 459, 460
  immunity to 466
  immunization 473–4
  life cycle *461*, 462
  in pregnancy 464–5
  recrudescence 467
  severe infections 464, *465*, 472
  treatment 470–1, 472
Plasmodium falciparum erythrocyte membrane protein 1
    (*Pf* EMP1) 462, 466
Plasmodium falciparum histidine-rich protein 2 (HRP-2)
    468
Plasmodium lactate dehydrogenase (PLDH) tests 470
Plasmodium malariae 458, **463**
  diagnosis 467, *469*
  epidemiology 459
  infections 464, 466–7
  life cycle 462
Plasmodium ovale 458, **463**
  diagnosis 467
  epidemiology 459
  infections 464, 466, 467
  life cycle *461*, 462
  treatment 471, 472
Plasmodium vivax 458, **463**
  diagnosis 467, *468–9*
  drug resistance 470
  epidemiology 459, 460
  immunization 473
  infections 464, 466, 467
  life cycle *461*, 462
  treatment 471, 472
pleconaril 28
  hand-foot-and-mouth disease 201, 432–3
  neonatal infections 359
  viral myocarditis 246
pleurodynia, epidemic 246
pneumococcal vaccine 63, 267, 275, 284
  immunocompromised host 378
pneumococcus *see Streptococcus pneumoniae*
Pneumocystis pneumonia (PCP)
  HIV infection/AIDS **383**
  immunocompromised host 371, 374, 377
Pneumocystis jiroveci (formerly *carinii*) 12, 374
  diagnostic testing **375**
pneumolysin 260, 286
pneumonia 255
  aspiration 256
  atypical 255–6
  community acquired (CAP) 255–6, *257*, *258*
  complicating influenza 510
  diagnostic testing 266
  healthcare associated 400, **401**
  immunocompromised host 376–7
  interstitial 256, *257*
  lobar 256
  microbiology and pathogenesis 259–66
  ventilator associated (VAP) 400
  viral 253, 263

point of care tests (POCT) 105
polio vaccine 64
poliovirus *28*
polyene antifungals 146
polymerase chain reaction (PCR) 109–11, 119
  influenza virus 511, *512*, *513*
  Mycobacterium tuberculosis 452, **453**
  real time 110–11, *513*
polymorphonuclear neutrophils (PMN) 48
porins 21, 127, 315
positive predictive value (PPV) 119
postherpetic neuralgia **425**
postpartum sepsis 336
postsplenectomy sepsis (PSS) 367
post-transplant lymphoproliferative disease (PTLD) 371
postvaccinial encephalitis 623
poxviruses 9, 10
  skin lesions 200, 570–1
  transcription 28
  vector vaccines 65–6
  see also monkeypox; smallpox; vaccinia virus
prairie dogs 568–9, *615*
praziquantel **149**
preemptive treatment, immunocompromised host 379
pregnancy 335–6, **368**
  antenatal screening 341, 342, 356
  close chickenpox contacts 344–6
  cytomegalovirus infection 348, 349
  emerging infections 359
  genital herpes 303, 357, 358
  hepatitis E 502
  listeriosis 338–9
  malaria 464–5, **466**, 472
  parvovirus B19 346–7
  postpartum infections 336
  primary viral infections 341–2
  rubella 342, 343
  syphilis 341
  termination 343, 351
  toxoplasmosis 350
  Treponema pallidum screening 341
  urinary tract infections 322, 336
  VZV infections 344, 346
  see also congenital infections
premature infants
  healthcare associated infections **394**
  VZV prophylaxis 346
premunition 84, 466
prenatal diagnosis 342
  congenital cytomegalovirus 349
  congenital rubella 343
  congenital varicella 344
  fetal parvovirus B19 347
prevalence 161
primaquine 471, 472
primary cases 163
prions **9**
proguanil 471, 472
prokaryotes 4
promastigotes 35, *37*

prosthetic devices, staphylococcal infections 192
prosthetic heart valves 239, *241*
prosthetic joint implants, infection 187–8
protease, viral 29, 153
protease inhibitors (PIs) 29, 153, 596
protective equipment, personal *see* personal protective
    equipment
protein A, staphylococcal 192
Proteus (*mirabilis*) **320**, 321
protozoa 12, 32–9
    classification 12, **13**
    life cycles 33–9
    pathogenic and escape mechanisms 82–4
    structure 32–3
protozoal infections
    diagnosis 116–19
    drug treatment 147–9
    traveler's diarrhea 531
    see also specific infections
pseudohyphae 32
pseudomembrane, diphtheria 601
pseudomembranous colitis 378, 402
Pseudomonas, healthcare associated infections 405
Pseudomonas aeruginosa 73, 254
Pseudomonas exotoxin A 71
psittacosis 263
pubic lice **310**
puerperal sepsis 336
pulmonary edema
    hantavirus pulmonary syndrome 575
    malaria 464, 465, 472
purified protein derivative (PPD) 450, 453
pus 87, 96
putsi fly 206
Puumala (PUU) virus 554, 572, **573**, 576
pyelonephritis 322, 324
    in pregnancy 336
pyrimethamine 141
    malaria 471, 472
    toxoplasmosis 148, 350–1
pyuria, sterile 323

Q fever 263–4, 266, **537**
    as biological weapon **609**
    see also Coxiella burnetii
qinghaosu 471
quality assurance (QA) 120
quality control (QC) 120
QuantiFERON-TB Gold (QFT-G) 454–5
Queensland tick typhus **536**
quinidine 471
quinine 470, 471, 472
quinoline-like antimalarial compounds 470–1
quinolones 137–9
quinupristin–dalfopristin 135, 136

rabbit fly fever *see* tularemia
rabies **279**, 281–2
    pathogenesis 288–9
    vaccination 282

rabies immune globulin 62
rabies virus 288–9
racial differences, disease susceptibility 42
radio-immunoassays (RIA) 104
rashes
    blanchable 195–6, 415
    childhood *see* childhood rash illnesses
    distribution 415
    erythematous 415
    hyperplastic 201–2
    macular 195–6, 415
    maculopapular 195–6, 415
    meningitis 277, *278*
    nonblanchable 196, 277, 415
    parasitic 206, 207
    Rocky Mountain spotted fever 538, *539*
    secondary syphilis 304, *305*
    vesicular 196–201, 415
    viral 194–202
    viral hepatitis 491, *492*
reassortment, genetic 82
receptors, viral cellular 27
recombinant immunoblot assay (RIBA) 106
recombination, viral 82
rectal swabs 87
red blood cells
    parvovirus B19 infection **428**
    Plasmodium life cycle *461*, 462
red man syndrome 134
reduviid bugs 534, 535
rehydration 235, 236
Reiter's syndrome 298
relative risk 171
Relenza *see* zanamivir
religious cults 608
renal failure
    leptospirosis 544–5
    malaria 464, **465**
replication, viral 29
reproduction, fungi 32
reproductive rates
    basic (R_o) 164–5
    net (R) 164–5
research 409–11
resolvase 78
respiratory (oxidative) burst **50**, 51, *369*
respiratory syncytial virus (RSV) 251, 252, 254, 255, 263
    palivizumab **64**
respiratory system
    barriers to infection *43*, 44
    host defence 259
respiratory tract infections 248–67
    diagnosis 266
    healthcare associated 400
    microbiology and pathogenesis 259–66
    prevention 267
    treatment 266
    see also lower respiratory tract infections; upper respiratory
        tract infections
reticulate bodies (RB) 24, 312, 355

retroviruses 477
    cell transformation 79
    endogenous 30–1
    see also human immunodeficiency virus
reverse transcriptase (RT) 28
    inhibitors 28, 29, 152–3
    mutations 82, 115–16, 152, 153
reverse transcriptase polymerase chain reaction (RT-PCR)
        109–10, 553
Reye's syndrome 510
R factors 78
rheumatic fever, acute 80
rhinoviruses 252
ribavirin 155
    hantavirus infections 576
    hepatitis C 500
    SARS 596
    viral hemorrhagic fevers 561–2
ribosomes, bacterial 16
rickettsiae 24, 535–8
    detection 101
    spotted fever **536–7**, 538
    typhus fever **536**
Rickettsia felis **536**, 540–1
rickettsial infections 523, 535–41
rickettsialpox **536**
Rickettsia prowazekii 24, **536**, 540
Rickettsia rickettsii 24, **537**, 538
Rickettsia typhi 24, **536**, 540–1
rifampicin (rifampin) 143, **145**
    resistance, gene probes 452
    resistant TB 439–40, **441**
Rift Valley fever (RVF) 562–3
    source of transmission 555, *556*
Rift Valley fever (RVF) virus 553, 554, *559*
rimantadine 154, 511–12, 513
ring forms, *Plasmodium* 462, *468*
ringworm (tinea) 11, 202, **203**, *205*
    see also dermatophytes
risk
    concept of 166
    relative 171
ritonavir 153
Ritter disease (scalded skin syndrome) 185–6, 192
RNA:DNA hybrids, capture 111
RNA polymerases 81–2
RNA viruses
    classification **30**
    immune escape mechanisms 81–2
    replication 29
    transcription 28
Rocky Mountain spotted fever (RMSF) 24, **537**, 538–40
rodent reservoirs
    hantaviruses 572, **573**, *574*
    leptospirosis 543
    plague 615–16
    rickettsiae **536**, **537**
    viral hemorrhagic fevers 554
rose gardener's disease 204

roseola infantum *see* "sixth disease"
rotaviruses 229–30
    diagnostic testing **235**
    gastroenteritis 222–4, 229–30
    genetic reassortment 82
    pathogenesis and virulence 230
    transmission 11
    vaccines **236**
    virology *91*, 229–30
Roth's spots 242
roundworms **13**, 14
rubella **416**, 421–3
    antenatal screening 342, 356
    childhood illness 195, 196, 415, 422–3
    close contact in pregnancy **345**
    complications 423
    congenital 342–3
    diagnosis 423
    primary infection in adults 341–2
    prophylaxis 423
    transmissibility 194–5, 421
rubella virus *196*, 421, *422*
rubeola *see* measles

Sabia virus 553, 554
St. Louis encephalitis 288
Salmonella 224–5
    gastroenteritis 214–16, 225
    identification **235**
    microbiology 224, *225*
    pathogenesis and virulence 224–5
Salmonella enterica serotype Paratyphi (*S.* Paratyphi)
        531–2
Salmonella enterica serotype Typhi (*S.* Typhi) 531–2
Salmonella typhimurium 608
samples, microbiological 86–8
sanatorium movement 437–8
sandflies 35, *37*, 532
sanitation 213, **214**
Sao Paulo exanthematic typhus **537**
sapoviruses 222, 224
saquinavir 153
Sarcoptes scabiei 207, *208*, **311**
sarin nerve gas 608
SARS *see* severe acute respiratory syndrome
scabies 207, *208*
    Norwegian or crusted **208**
    sexually transmitted **311**
scalded skin syndrome 185–6, 192
scarlet fever 249, **416**, 420–1
    clinical features 184, *185*, 420–1
    pathogenesis 191
Scedosporium **375**
Schistosoma **13**, 83
Schistosoma haematobium 118, *119*, 533, 534
Schistosoma japonicum 533, 534
Schistosoma mansoni 533, 534
schistosomiasis 533–4
    diagnosis 118, *119*, 534

drug treatment **149**
therapy associated HCV transmission **499**
schistosomula 534
schizogony
  erythrocytic *461*, 462
  exo-erythrocytic *461*, 462
schizonts *461*, 462, *469*
Schüffner's dots 462, 467, *469*
scombroid poisoning **221**
scrapie **9**
scrub typhus **537**
seasonal variation 166
secondary attack rate (SAR) 163–4
secondary cases 163, 168, *169*
"second disease" *see* scarlet fever
Sennetsu fever **537**
sensitivity, diagnostic 119
Seoul virus 554, 572, **573**
sepsis 74
  induced immunosuppression 372
  neonatal *see* neonatal infections
septic arthritis 187–8
septicemia, Gram negative 73–4
serological tests
  automation 113
  ELISA/EIA 102, **104**, *104*
seroprevalence **164**, 165
serum amyloid A 51
severe acute respiratory syndrome (SARS) 592–7
  clinical features 263, 594–5
  treatment 595–6
severe acute respiratory syndrome-associated coronavirus
    (SARS-CoV) 592, *593*
  laboratory diagnosis 595–6
  origin/transmission 158, 399, 593–4
severe combined immunodeficiency (SCID) 368–9
sex pilus 24, 77–8
sexual abuse, child **199**
sexual history 297–8
sexually transmitted diseases (STDs) 294–319
  clinical presentation 298–309
  diagnosis 310
  history taking 297–8
  management 311, *312*
  microbiology and pathogenesis 312–19
  public health impact 296–7
  public health messages 294, **295**, *295*, *312*
  returning travelers 523
sexually transmitted infections (STIs) 295–6
sharps disposal 396, *398*, 409, *411*
sharps injuries *see* needlestick injuries
shellfish poisoning **221**
shiga like toxins (SLT) 228
shiga toxin 71, 76, 228, 526–7
Shigella 228, 526–7
  identification **235**
  infections (shigellosis) 220–1, 526–7
  pathogenesis and virulence 228, *229*, 526–7
Shigella boydii 220, 526

Shigella dysenteriae 228, 526–7
Shigella flexneri 220, 526
Shigella sonnei 220, 526
shingles (herpes zoster) 196, 197, **425**
  contact during pregnancy **345**, 346
  fetal 344
  immunocompromised host 374, **425**
  during pregnancy 344, 346
  varicelliform or disseminated **425**
  VZV vaccination and **426**
siderophores 68, 92
Sigmodon hispidus 574
simian immunodeficiency viruses (SIVs) 476
Sin Nombre virus **573**, 576
  electron microscopy *574*
  epidemiology 554, 572
  see also hantavirus pulmonary syndrome
sinusitis 249, 282
SIRS *see* systemic inflammatory response syndrome
"sixth disease" (roseola infantum; HHV6 infection) 415,
    416, 430–2
  see also human herpes virus 6
skin
  barrier to infection 43–4
  breaches 394
  normal flora 46
  scales, transmission via 399
skin infections 179–211
  bacterial 180–94
  fungal 11, 202–4
  hospital acquired 188
  parasitic 205–7
  viral 194–202
skin rashes *see* rashes
slapped cheek disease ("fifth disease"; erythema infectiosum)
    417, 427–30
  complications **428**, 430
  rash 195, 196, 415, 429
  transmissibility 195
  see also parvovirus B19
sleeping sickness, African 35, 535
slime layer, bacterial 24, 192
smallpox (variola) 619–25
  as biological weapon 607, **609**, 619
  clinical features 619–21
  laboratory diagnosis 200, 621–2
  last known cases 619, *621*
  major and minor forms 619, *621*
  monkeypox and 568, 569
  rash 196–7, 426, 619–21
  virus 621–2
smallpox vaccines/vaccination 622–5
  administration 623
  complications 623, *624*
  monkeypox prevention 571
smears, stained
  bacterial and fungal infections 88–9, *90*
  protozoal and helminth infections 116, 117, *118*
snails 534

sodium stibogluconate 149
soft tissue infections 179–211
  hospital acquired 188
soil, diseases transmitted from 523, 614
somatic recombination 55
sore throat *see* pharyngitis
Soviet Union, former 608, 611, 619
species specificity 42
specificity, diagnostic 119
specimen collection and transport 86–8, 116–18
spheroplasts 21
spinal cord 271
spiral bacteria 5, *8*
spiramycin 148, 350–1
Spirillum 5
spirochaetes 5, 23
  see also Treponema pallidum
splenectomy 367, **368**
  management of infections **380**
splenic dysfunction **365**, 367
  bacterial meningitis and 286
splinter hemorrhages 242
spongiform encephalopathies **9**
spores
  bacterial 16
  fungal 32
sporogonic cycle *461*
sporotrichosis 203–4
sporozoa **13**, 35–9
sporozoites 35–6, 38
  Plasmodium 461, 462
sporulation 38
spotted fever rickettsiae **536–7**, 538
spreading factors 71
sputum 87, 118, 266
standard precautions **410**, *410*
staphylococcal chromosome cassette (SCC) *mec* gene 402
staphylococcal enterotoxin B, as biological weapon **609**
staphylococcal enterotoxins (SE) 192
staphylococcal scalded skin syndrome (SSSS) 185–6, 192
staphylococcal toxic shock syndrome (TSS) 184–5, 192
staphylococci 5, *6*, 191–2
  coagulase negative *see* coagulase negative staphylococci
  transmission on skin scales *399*
Staphylococcus aureus 191–2
  bronchiectasis 254
  cell wall 18–19
  coagulase 72, 98
  colonization 46, 48, 180
  diagnostic methods *88*, 98, **235**
  enterotoxin 227
  food poisoning **215**, 218, 227
  immune escape mechanisms 67
  infective endocarditis 240, 241, **242**, 243
  methicillin resistant *see* methicillin resistant *Staphylococcus aureus*
  microbiology *6*, 191, 227
  neonatal sepsis 355
  osteomyelitis 186
  pericarditis 246

  pneumonia 256
  septic arthritis 187
  skin and soft tissue infections 180, 182–4
  toxin-associated conditions 184–6
  toxins *191*, 192
  urinary tract infections 321
  vancomycin intermediate (VISA) 403, **404**
  vancomycin resistant (VRSA) 403, **404**, 405
  virulence mechanisms 191–2
Staphylococcus epidermidis 192
  bone and joint infections 186, 188
  healthcare associated infections 400, 403
  infective endocarditis **242**, 243
Staphylococcus saprophyticus **320**, 321, 323
staphylokinase 71
stavudine (D4T) 152
stem cell transplantation, hematopoietic *see* hematopoietic stem cell transplantation
steroid therapy 366, 372
sterols 31
stibogluconate, sodium 149
strawberry tongue 184, *185*, 249, 420
streptococcal pharyngitis (strep sore throat) 248–9, 420–1
streptococcal pyrogenic exotoxins (SPE) (erythrogenic toxin) 184, 191
streptococcal toxic shock 184, 191
streptococci 5, *6*
  alpha-hemolytic 98
  beta-hemolytic 98, 189
  enzymes 72
  group A β-hemolytic *see Streptococcus pyogenes*
  group B hemolytic *see* group B streptococci
  infective endocarditis **242**
  Lancefield groups 98, 189
  oral 46–7
  spheroplasts 21
  viridans *see* viridans streptococci
Streptococcus agalactiae see group B streptococci
Streptococcus milleri 46–7
Streptococcus mutans 24, 46, 66
Streptococcus pneumoniae (pneumococcus) *6*, 259–60
  bronchitis 254
  colonization 47
  diagnostic identification 98, 266
  escape mechanisms 67
  meningitis 274–5
  microbiology 259–60, 284
  pneumonia 138, 255, 256
  splenic dysfunction 367
  vaccine *see* pneumococcal vaccine
  virulence mechanisms 260, 286
Streptococcus pyogenes (group A β hemolytic streptococcus; GABHS) 189–91
  attachment 23, 66–7, 190
  colonization 47
  diagnostic identification 266, 421
  microbiology 189–90
  postpartum sepsis 336
  rheumatogenic M-types 190

scarlet fever *see* scarlet fever
skin and soft tissue infections 182, **183**
sore throat (pharyngitis) 248–9, 420–1
streptococcal toxic shock 184
virulence mechanisms 190–1
streptogramins 135–6
streptokinase 71, 190–1
streptolysins 72, 190
streptomycin *136*, 139, 140–1, 438
Strongyloides stercoralis **13**, 84
diagnosis 116, 118, **376**
drug treatment **149**
immunocompromised host 374
larva currens 206
subacute sclerosing panencephalitis (SSPE) **416**, 419
sulbactam 130
sulfadiazine 148, 350–1
sulfadoxine-pyrimethamine (SP) 471
sulfasalazine 141
sulfonamides 141–2
superantigens 73
staphylococcal 192
Streptococcus pyogenes 191
viral 80
superoxide dismutase **50**, 51, 448
surgical site infections (SSI) 400
surveillance, disease 409–11
swabs 86–7
syphilis 304–7
congenital 307, *308*, 340–1
diagnosis 310, 341
late 296, 306–7
latent 304, 317
pathogenesis 316–17
primary 301, 304, *305*, 317
public health impact 297
secondary 304, *305*, **306**, *306*, 317
systemic inflammatory response syndrome (SIRS) 21, 73–5

T-20/enfuvirtide 154, 484
tabes dorsalis **307**
tachyzoites *38*, 352
Taenia saginata **13**
Taenia solium **13**, **149**
Tamiflu *see* oseltamivir
tamponade, cardiac 247
tapeworms **13**, 14
tazobactam 130
T cells 53, 366
subsets **54**
teicoplanin 134–5, **144**, 405
telbuvidine 495
tellurite staining 602–3
tenofovir 153
terbinafine 146
termination of pregnancy 343, 351
tertiary cases 164
tetanus 523
tetanus antitoxin 62

tetanus toxin **69**, 70
tetracyclines *136*, 141
Th1 cells 53, **54**, 56
Th1-type response
HIV–TB coinfection 451
tuberculosis 450
Th2 cells 53, **54**
Th2-type response
HIV–TB coinfection 451
tuberculosis 450
Thai tick typhus **536**
thalassemia **368**
theta toxin 193
thiabendazole **149**
"third disease" *see* rubella
threadworms *see Enterobius vermicularis*
throat swabs 87
thrombocytopenia
malaria 464
rubella associated 423
thrombotic thrombocytopenic purpura (TTP) 219
thymidine kinase (TK) 151
ticarcillin 130
tick-borne lymphadenopathy (TIBOLA) **537**
ticks 280, **536–7**, 538, 540, 555
time
of exposure, determination 170
outbreak characterization by 166, 168–70
time resolved fluorescence assays (TRFA) 104, **105**
tinea 11, 202, **203**, *205*
see also dermatophytes
tinidazole 148
Tiselius, A. 55
tissue culture 100
tissue tropism, viruses 10
tobramycin 139, 140, 141
toll-like receptors 48–50
topoisomerases 16
tourniquet test, dengue **590**
toxic shock syndrome (TSS) 73, **74**, 184–5, 192
toxic shock syndrome toxin-1 (TSST-1) 185, 192
toxins, microbial 68–71
conditions caused by 184–6
detection 101
Toxocara canis **13**
toxoids 62–3
Toxoplasma gondii 12, 349–50
diagnostic tests 350, **376**
immune escape mechanisms 83, 84
life cycle 36–8, 351–2
virulence 351–2
toxoplasmosis 349–52
clinical features 281, 350
congenital 350, 351
diagnosis 350
drug treatment 148, 350–1
immunocompromised host 374, 377–8
organ transplant recipients 371
trachoma 24–5, 312

transcription, viral 28
transcription mediated amplification (TMA) 111, *112*
transduction, bacterial 76
transformation
    bacterial 76, 77
    viral 79
transfusion-transmitted virus (TTV) 503
transglycosylases 19, 20
translation, viral proteins 29
transmissible mink encephalopathy (TME) **9**
transmission 162–5
    direct 162
    healthcare associated infections 396–9
    indirect 162
    probability 162–5
    viral 10–11
transpeptidases 19, 20
transposase 78
transposition 78
transposons 78
trauma, physical 394
travelers, returning 521–50
    airborne infections 547
    diphtheria 601
    foodborne infections 525–32
    malaria 467, 472
    questions to ask 521–5
    vectorborne infections 532–43
    zoonoses 543–7
traveler's diarrhea 525–31
    clinical presentation 525–6
    epidemiology 525
    etiology and pathogenesis 526–31
    invasive (bacterial) 525, 526–7
    parasitic protozoal 525–6, 531
    secretory (bacterial) 525, 527–30
    viral infections 531
trematodes **13**, 14
trench fever **537**
Treponema pallidum 304, 316–17
    diagnostic tests 341
    see also syphilis
Triatoma infestans 35, *36*, 534
triazole antifungals 146
Trichinella spiralis **13**
trichomonacides 148
Trichomonas vaginalis 12, 315
    detection 118
    life cycle 33, 34
    microbiology 315, *316*
    vulvovaginitis 300
Trichophyton 11, *99*, 202, *203, 205*
trichrome staining 116, *117*
Trichuris trichuria **13**, 149
trimethoprim 142, **145**
trimethoprim-sulfamethoxazole (TMP-SMX) *see* co-trimoxazole
trophozoites 33, 34
    detection methods 116
    Plasmodium 461, 462, *469*

tropical ulcer 189
Trypanosoma 12
Trypanosoma brucei 35, *36*, 535
    antigenic variation 84
    life cycle *35*
Trypanosoma cruzi 35, 534, *535*
    immune escape mechanisms 83, 84
trypanosomiasis 35, 534–5
trypomastigotes 35
tsetse flies 35, 535
tuberculin skin test (TST) 453–4, 455
    booster effect 454, 455
    interpretation **454**
    pathophysiology 450
tuberculosis (TB) 437–57
    bronchiectasis 254
    clinical features 444–7
    clinical presentation 442–3
    diagnosis **375**, 451–5
    directly observed treatment, short course (DOTS) 440–1
    disease, defined 442
    drugs for *see* anti-tuberculosis drugs
    epidemiology in USA 442
    extensively drug resistant (XDR-TB) 440, **441**
    extrapulmonary 444–7
    genitourinary 446
    global trends 438–41
    HIV coinfection 439, 442, 447, 450–1
    infection, defined 442
    interferon gamma release assay 108, 454–5
    latent infection (LTBI) 443
    management 455
    meningitis **278**, 446
    miliary 442, *443*
    multi-drug resistant (MDR-TB) 439–40, **441**, 442
    pathogenesis and virulence 447–51
    primary 442–3, 444
    pulmonary 444
    reactivation/post-primary 443, 444–7
    see also Mycobacterium tuberculosis
tularemia **609**, 618–19
tumbu fly 206
tumor necrosis factor (TNF) 58
    antagonists 372, 443
tumor necrosis factor alpha (TNF-α) 74, 75, 451
turtles, pet **216**
typhoid fever 525, 531–2
typhoid vaccines 531, 532
typhus fever **536**, 540–1
    epidemic (louse-borne) **536**, 540
    murine (endemic; flea-borne) 24, **536**, 540–1
    scrub **537**
    tick **536**

ultrasound scanning 347
uncoating, viruses 28
undulant fever 546
universal (standard) precautions **410**, *410*
upper respiratory tract, normal flora 46–7

upper respiratory tract infections (URTIs) 248–53
  CNS spread 277, 282
  diagnosis 266
  viral 250–3
Ureaplasma urealyticum 299
uremia **368**
urethra, normal flora 48
urethritis 298–9
urinalysis
  automated 113
  sticks (dipsticks) 323
urinary tract, defence mechanisms 319–20
urinary tract infections (UTIs) 319–24
  bacterial pathogenesis 320–1
  catheter-associated 322, 324, 399–400
  classification 321–2
  clinical presentation 322
  diagnosis 322–3
  healthcare associated 399–400
  management 324
  predisposing factors 319–20, **321**
  in pregnancy 322, 336
urine
  cultures 323, *324*
  detection of parasites 118, *119*
  microscopy 323
  mid-stream (MSU) 322
  specimens 87, 322–3
urogenital tract *see* genitourinary tract

vaccination 62–6
  immunocompromised host 64, 378
  programs and herd immunity 165
vaccines 62–6
  DNA 66
  experimental and restricted use **64**
  killed 62, 63
  live attenuated 62, 63, 64
  mucosally delivered 65
  new approaches 65–6
  novel adjuvants 65
  polysaccharide conjugated 63
  recent developments 64–5
  recombinant 63, 65
  subunit 65
  synthetic peptide 65
  toxoid 62–3
  vector 65–6
vaccinia
  generalized 623, *624*
  progressive 623, *624*
vaccinia immunoglobulin (VIG) 571, 623
vaccinia virus 569, 622–3
  Modified Ankara strain (MVA) 66
  see also smallpox vaccines/vaccination
vagina
  barriers to infection 296, 299
  normal flora 47–8, 299, *300*
vaginal discharge 300

valaciclovir 151
valganciclovir 151, 349
vancomycin 134–5, **144**, 405
  mechanisms of resistance 127
vancomycin intermediate *Staphylococcus aureus* (VISA) 403, **404**
vancomycin resistant enterococci (VRE) 45, 134, 405
vancomycin resistant *Staphylococcus aureus* (VRSA) 403, **404**, 405
var genes, *Plasmodium falciparum* 466
varicella *see* chickenpox
varicella zoster immune globulin (VZIG or VZV IgG) 62, 346
varicella zoster virus (VZV) *198*, 423, *424*
  congenital infection 344–6
  diagnosis of infections 197–200, 426
  drug treatment 151, 152
  immunocompromised host 374
  meningitis 276
  primary infection in adults 341–2
  recurrent infection 424, **425**
  respiratory infections 254, 263, 341, 344
  skin rash 196–7
  transmissibility 195
  vaccine 344, **426**
  see also chickenpox; shingles
variola *see* smallpox
variola virus 621–2
vectorborne diseases 34–6
  travel related 523, 532–43
  viral hemorrhagic fevers 555, *556*, 562–3
  see also specific diseases
vectors, disease 34, 162
  control measures 472, 562–3, 588, 591–2
  see also mosquitoes; ticks
vector vaccines 65–6
vehicles 162
venereal disease *see* sexually transmitted diseases
ventilator associated pneumonia (VAP) 400
verotoxins 228
vertical transmission 11
vesicles 415
vesicular fluid, samples 87
vesicular rashes 196–201, 415
Vibrio 5, 528
Vibrio cholerae 527, 528–30
viral encephalitis 278–82
  as biological weapon **609**
  microbiology and pathogenesis 286–9
  mosquito-borne 287–8
  primary 279
  secondary 279, 281
  see also specific infections
viral entry inhibitors 154
viral hemorrhagic fevers (VHFs) 196, 553–66
  as biological weapons **609**
  clinical features 558–9
  diagnosis 555, *557*, *558*, *559*
  epidemiology 554
  infection control/containment 562–3
  management and treatment 560–2
  origins/routes of transmission 554–5, *556*

viral hemorrhagic fevers (VHFs) (*cont'd*)
    outcomes 563–4
    prevention 564
    virology 553
viral hepatitis 491–505
    clinical features 491–3
    interferon therapy **497**
    see also specific types
viral infections
    congenital 341–9
    diarrheas 222–4, 228–31, 236
    healthcare associated **403**
    host defences *59*
    immunocompromised host **365**, 374
    immunosuppressive effects 81, 373
    meningitis 276, 277, **278**, 286–7
    myocarditis 244–6
    neonatal/perinatal 356–9
    pericarditis **245**, 246–7
    pneumonia 253, 263
    respiratory tract 250–4
    skin 194–202
    traveler's diarrhea 531
    see also specific infections
viral transport medium (VTM) 86
viridans streptococci
    identification *94*, 243
    infections in neutropenia 373
    infective endocarditis 240, **242**, 243
virions 9–10
virulence 162
    molecular/genetic basis 76–8
virulence factors 66, 76, 78
viruses 9–11
    antiviral susceptibility tests 115–16
    classification 28, 29, **30**
    culture 100
    detection of products 101
    diagnostic identification 100, **375–6**
    electron microscopy 89, *91*, *92*
    host-specificity 10
    immune avoidance mechanisms 80–1
    immune escape mechanisms 81–2
    immune-mediated pathogenesis 79–80
    life cycle 26–9
    as parasites 30–1
    pathogenesis of disease 78–80
    structure and component function 25–31
    transmission 10–11
vitamins, of bacterial origin 46
voriconazole 146
vulvovaginitis 299–301
VZV *see* varicella zoster virus

warfare, biological *see* biological warfare agents
warts 201–2
    genital *201*, 303–4
water activities, recreational 543, **544**
waterborne infections 212–21
    healthcare settings 399
    travel related 523
    see also specific infections
Western blots 105–6, *107*
Western equine encephalitis 288
West Nile encephalitis 288, 585
West Nile virus (WNV) 583–8
    clinical features of infection 584–5, **586–7**
    diagnosis and virology 585–8
    introduction to USA **584**
white blood cells (WBCs), urinary 323
white powder scare **16**
WHO *see* World Health Organization
whooping cough *see* pertussis
winter-vomiting disease **215**, **222**, **223**, 224
World Health Organization (WHO)
    dengue guidance 590–1
    influenza pandemic alert system 517, **518**
    influenza surveillance 506, 514–15
    smallpox eradication 619
wound
    botulism **70**, 613
    exudates 87
    infections 400
Wuchereria bancrofti **13**, *118*, **149**

yeasts 11
yellow fever 523, 541–3
    epidemiology 541–2, 555, *556*
    outcome 563–4
yellow fever vaccine 543, 564
yellow fever vaccine-associated viscerotropic disease
    (YEL-AVD) 543
yellow fever virus 542, 554, *559*
Yersinia pestis **609**, 614–18
    microbiology 617
    see also plague

zalcitabine (DDC) 152
zanamivir 29, 154–5, 512–13
zidovudine 152
Ziehl–Neelsen staining **90**, 452
zoonoses 10, 507
    travel related 523, 543–7
zoster *see* shingles